# THE WASHINGTON MANUAL® OF PEDIATRICS

## Third Edition

*Editor*

**Andrew J. White, MD**
James P. Keating, MD, Professor of Pediatrics
St. Louis Children's Hospital
Washington University School of Medicine
St. Louis, Missouri

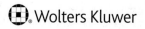

. Wolters Kluwer

Philadelphia • Baltimore • New York • London
Buenos Aires • Hong Kong • Sydney • Tokyo

*Acquisitions Editor:* James Sherman
*Development Editors:* Thomas Celona, Stacey Sebring
*Editorial Coordinator:* Chester Anthony Gonzalez
*Editorial Assistant:* Victoria Giansante
*Marketing Manager:* Kirsten Watrud
*Production Project Manager:* Catherine Ott
*Manager of Graphic Arts and Design:* Stephen Druding
*Manufacturing Coordinator:* Beth Welsh
*Prepress Vendor:* Straive

Third Edition

**Cataloging in Publication data available on request from publisher.**
**ISBN: 978-1-9751-9058-3**

MKO522

*This book is dedicated to pediatric trainees everywhere. Your time commitment, frontline effort, and investment in the health of our children is second to none. A special thanks to my mentors, including my father, A. James White, MD; my colleagues, Jonathan Gitlin, MD, and Alan Schwartz, PhD, MD; and of course, my mother, Linda J. White, RN—you have all been an inspiration to seek, acquire, and share knowledge.*

*—Andrew J. White, MD*

# Contributors

**Anne Marie Anderson, MD**
*Fellow, Pediatric Emergency Medicine*
*Department of Pediatrics*
*Washington University School of Medicine*
*St. Louis, Missouri*

**Carine Anka, MD**
*Pediatric Resident Physician*
*St. Louis Children's Hospital*
*Washington University School of Medicine*
*St. Louis, Missouri*

**Ana María Arbeláez, MD, MSCI**
*Division Chief of Pediatric Endocrinology*
*Co-Director TL1 Predoctoral Clinical*
*  Research Training Program*
*Washington University School of Medicine*
*St. Louis, Missouri*

**Adrienne D. Atzemis, MD, FAAP**
*Associate Professor of Pediatrics*
*Chief, Section of Child Abuse Pediatrics*
*Department of Pediatrics*
*Washington University School of Medicine*
*St. Louis, Missouri*

**Marie Batty, MD**
*General Pediatrician*
*Blue Fish Pediatrics*
*Washington University Clinical Associates*
*St. Louis, Missouri*

**Sima Bhatt, MD, MSCI, FAAP**
*Assistant Professor of Pediatrics*
*Assistant Medical Director for Cellular*
*  Therapies*
*Division of Hematology and Oncology*
*St. Louis Children's Hospital*
*Washington University School of Medicine*
*St. Louis, Missouri*

**Tarin M. Bigley, MD, PhD**
*Pediatric Rheumatology/Immunology Fellow*
*Department of Pediatrics*
*Washington University School of Medicine*
*St. Louis, Missouri*

**Kelleigh Briden, MD**
*Assistant Professor of Pediatrics*
*Department of Pediatrics*
*Washington University School of Medicine*
*St. Louis, Missouri*

**Katherine Burgener, MD**
*Pediatric Endocrinology Fellow*
*Division of Pediatric Endocrinology and*
*  Diabetes*
*Department of Pediatrics*
*St. Louis Children's Hospital*
*Washington University School of Medicine*
*St. Louis, Missouri*

**Lily Chen, MD**
*Resident Physician*
*Department of Dermatology*
*Washington University School of Medicine*
*St. Louis, Missouri*

**Tara Conway Copper, MD, MS**
*Associate Medical Director*
*Emergency Department*
*St. Louis Children's Hospital*
*Assistant Professor of Pediatrics*
*Department of Pediatrics*
*Washington University School of Medicine*
*St. Louis, Missouri*

**Samuel Cortez, MD, FAAP**
*Endocrinology and Diabetes*
*  Fellow*
*Department of Pediatrics*
*St. Louis Children's Hospital*
*Washington University School of Medicine*
*St. Louis, Missouri*

**Cameron Crockett, MD**
*Neuromuscular Medicine Fellow*
*Division of Pediatric Neurology*
*Department of Neurology*
*Washington University School of*
*  Medicine*
*St. Louis, Missouri*

**Vikas R. Dharnidharka, MD, MPH**
*Vice Chair for Clinical Investigation*
*Department of Pediatrics*
*Professor and Chief*
*Division of Pediatric Nephrology,*
  *Hypertension & Pheresis*
*St. Louis Children's Hospital*
*Washington University School of Medicine*
*St. Louis, Missouri*

**Sarah Dixon, MD**
*Clinical Assistant Professor*
*Department of Neurology*
*C.S. Mott Children's Hospital*
*University of Michigan*
*Ann Arbor, Michigan*

**Alexa Altman Doss, MD**
*Fellow, Allergy/Immunology*
*Department of Pediatrics*
*Washington University School of Medicine*
*St. Louis, Missouri*

**Amanda Reis Dube, MD**
*Instructor, Pediatric Hospital Medicine*
*Department of Pediatrics*
*Washington University School of Medicine*
*St. Louis, Missouri*

**Alexis Elward, MD, MPH**
*Professor, Pediatric Infectious Diseases*
*Washington University School of Medicine*
*St. Louis, Missouri*

**Melanie Fields, MD, MSCI**
*Assistant Professor*
*Departments of Pediatrics and Neurology*
*Washington University School of Medicine*
*St. Louis, Missouri*

**Ari Filip, MD**
*Fellow, Medical Toxicology*
*Department of Emergency Medicine*
*Washington University School of Medicine*
*St. Louis, Missouri*

**Cristina M. Gaudioso, MD**
*Neuroimmunology Fellow*
*Division of Pediatric and Developmental*
  *Neurology*
*Washington University School of Medicine*
*St. Louis, Missouri*

**Andrea Giedinghagen, MD**
*Assistant Professor*
*Division of Child and Adolescent*
  *Psychiatry*
*Department of Psychiatry*
*Washington University School of*
  *Medicine*
*St. Louis, Missouri*

**Catherine Gooch, MD**
*Assistant Professor of Pediatrics*
*Division of Genetics and Genomic*
  *Medicine*
*Washington University School of Medicine*
*St. Louis, Missouri*

**Jennifer L. Griffith, MD, PhD**
*Assistant Professor of Pediatric Neurology*
*Departments of Neurology and Pediatrics*
*Washington University School of Medicine*
*St. Louis, Missouri*

**Caroline C. Horner, MD, MSCI**
*Associate Professor of Pediatrics*
*Division of Allergy and Pulmonary*
  *Medicine*
*Department of Pediatrics*
*Washington University School of Medicine*
*St. Louis, Missouri*

**Jennifer Horst, MD**
*Assistant Professor of Pediatrics*
*Division of Pediatric Emergency Medicine*
*Washington University School of Medicine*
*St. Louis, Missouri*

**Chrissy Hrach, MD, SFHM, FAAP**
*Associate Professor of Pediatrics*
*Division of Hospitalist Medicine*
*Medical Director of Inpatient General*
  *Pediatric Medicine*
*Associate Pediatric Residency Program*
  *Director*
*St. Louis Children's Hospital*
*Washington University School of Medicine*
*St. Louis, Missouri*

**Andrew B. Janowski, MD, MSCI**
*Assistant Professor of Pediatrics*
*Department of Pediatrics*
*Washington University School of Medicine*
*St. Louis, Missouri*

**Will Johansen, MD**
*Assistant Professor of Pediatrics*
*Pediatric Advanced Care Team*
*Department of Newborn Medicine*
*St. Louis Children's Hospital*
*Washington University School of Medicine*
*St. Louis, Missouri*

**Carol M. Kao, MD**
*Assistant Professor*
*Department of Pediatrics*
*Washington University School of Medicine*
*St. Louis, Missouri*

**Robert M. Kennedy, MD**
*Professor Emeritus*
*Division of Emergency Medicine*
*Department of Pediatrics*
*Washington University School of Medicine*
*St. Louis, Missouri*

**Lila Kertz, DNP, APRN, CPNP-PC, AE-C**
*Clinical Director of the Severe Asthma Clinic for Kids*
*Division of Allergy and Pulmonary Medicine*
*Department of Pediatrics*
*Washington University School of Medicine*
*St. Louis, Missouri*

**Patti Kieffer, RN, BSN, CIC, FAPIC**
*Manager, Infection Prevention*
*Department of Quality, Safety and Practice Excellence*
*BJC Healthcare*
*St Louis Children's Hospital*
*Washington University School of Medicine*
*St. Louis, Missouri*

**Katherine Abell King, MD, FAAP, FACMG**
*Assistant Professor*
*Division of Genetics and Genomic Medicine*
*Department of Pediatrics*
*Washington University School of Medicine*
*St. Louis, Missouri*

**Abigail M. Kissel, MD, FAAP**
*Assistant Professor of Pediatrics*
*Division of Developmental Behavioral Pediatrics*
*University of Texas Southwestern Medical Center*
*Developmental Behavioral Pediatrician*
*Luke Waites Center for Dyslexia and Learning Disorders*
*Texas Scottish Rite Hospital for Children*
*Dallas, Texas*

**Maleewan Kitcharoensakkul, MD, MSCI**
*Assistant Professor of Pediatrics*
*Division of Rheumatology/Immunology*
*Division of Allergy and Pulmonary Medicine*
*Department of Pediatrics*
*Washington University School of Medicine*
*St. Louis, Missouri*

**Nikoleta Kolovos, MD**
*Associate Professor of Pediatrics*
*Division of Pediatric Critical Care Medicine*
*Washington University School of Medicine*
*St. Louis, Missouri*

**Jamie S. Kondis, MD, FAAP**
*Associate Professor of Pediatrics*
*Section on Child Abuse Pediatrics*
*Department of Pediatrics*
*Washington University School of Medicine*
*St. Louis, Missouri*

**Cadence Kuklinski, DO**
*Assistant Professor of Pediatrics*
*Division of Allergy and Pulmonary Medicine*
*Department of Pediatrics*
*Washington University School of Medicine*
*St. Louis, Missouri*

**Kathryn Leonard, MD**
*Assistant Professor of Pediatrics*
*Director of Educational Affairs*
*Division of Pediatric Emergency Medicine*
*Program Director*
*Pediatric Emergency Medicine Fellowship*
*Department of Pediatrics*
*Washington University School of Medicine*
*St. Louis, Missouri*

**Jennifer May, MD**
*Endocrinology and Diabetes Fellow*
*Pediatric Endocrinology*
*Washington University School of Medicine*
*St. Louis, Missouri*

**William McAlister, MD**
*Professor*
*Departments of Radiology and Pediatrics*
*Washington University School of Medicine*
*St. Louis, Missouri*

**Sarah Mermelstein, MD**
*Assistant Professor, Pediatrics*
*Division of Adolescent Medicine*
*Department of Pediatrics*
*Washington University School of Medicine*
*St. Louis, Missouri*

**Hoanh Nguyen, MD, FACMG**
*Clinical Geneticist and Clinical Biochemical Geneticist*
*Assistant Professor*
*Department of Pediatrics*
*Division of Medical Genetics & Genomics*
*Washington University School of Medicine*
*St. Louis, Missouri*

**Kevin O'Bryan, MD**
*Associate Chief Medical Informatics Officer, Assistant Professor*
*Department of Pediatrics*
*St. Louis Children's Hospital*
*Washington University School of Medicine*
*St. Louis, Missouri*

**Dean Odegard, MD, MS**
*Resident Physician*
*Department of Pediatrics*
*St. Louis Children's Hospital*
*Washington University School of Medicine*
*St. Louis, Missouri*

**William B. Orr, MD, FAAP, FACC**
*Assistant Professor of Pediatrics*
*Director, Pediatric Exercise Physiology Lab*
*Associate Director, Pediatric Cardiology Fellowship*
*Division of Cardiology*
*Washington University School of Medicine*
*St. Louis, Missouri*

**Katie Plax, MD**
*Ferring Family Professor of Pediatrics*
*Division Chief, Adolescent Medicine*
*Medical Director, The SPOT*
*Department of Pediatrics*
*Washington University School of Medicine*
*St. Louis, Missouri*

**Cassandra Pruitt, MD, FAAP**
*Medical Director, General Pediatrics and Complex Care Clinic*
*Professor of Pediatrics*
*Department of Pediatrics*
*Washington University School of Medicine*
*St. Louis, Missouri*

**Patrick J. Reich, MD, MSCI**
*Assistant Professor, Department of Pediatrics*
*Medical Director, Infection Prevention*
*Associate Program Director, Pediatric Residency Program*
*St. Louis Children's Hospital*
*Washington University School of Medicine*
*St. Louis, Missouri*

**Noor Riaz, MD, MPH**
*Assistant Professor of Pediatrics*
*Division of Hospitalist Medicine*
*Washington University School of Medicine*
*St. Louis, Missouri*

**Melissa M. Riley, MD**
*NICU Medical Director*
*St. Louis Children's Hospital*
*Associate Professor of Pediatrics*
*Division of Newborn Medicine*
*Washington University School of Medicine*
*St. Louis, Missouri*

**Katherine Rivera-Spoljaric, MD, MSCI**
*Associate Professor of Pediatrics*
*Medical Director, Home Ventilation Program and Severe Asthma Clinic for Kids*
*Co-Director, Office of Faculty Development*
*Division of Allergy and Pulmonary Medicine*
*Department of Pediatrics*
*Washington University School of Medicine*
*St. Louis, Missouri*

**Joan L. Rosenbaum, MD, FAAHPM**
*Professor of Pediatrics*
*Director, Pediatric Palliative Care*
*Department of Pediatrics*
*Washington University School of Medicine*
*St. Louis, Missouri*

**Robert J. Rothbaum, MD**
*Section Chief*
*Division of Pediatric Gastroenterology, Hepatology, and Nutrition*
*Department of Pediatrics*
*UCSF School of Medicine*
*Oakland, California*

**David A. Rudnick, MD, PhD**
*Associate Professor of Pediatrics*
*Associate Professor of Developmental Biology*
*Pediatric Gastroenterology, Hepatology and Nutrition*
*Department of Pediatrics*
*St. Louis Children's Hospital*
*Washington University School of Medicine*
*St. Louis, Missouri*

**Erica Schmitt, MD, PhD**
*Instructor*
*Division of Rheumatology/Immunology*
*Department of Pediatrics*
*Washington University School of Medicine*
*St. Louis, Missouri*

**Baddr Shakhsheer, MD, FACS**
*Assistant Professor of Surgery*
*Division of Pediatric Surgery*
*Department of Surgery*
*Washington University School of Medicine*
*St. Louis, Missouri*

**Leonid Shmuylovich, MD, PhD, FAAD, FA**
*Assistant Professor, Pediatric Dermatologist, Director of Vascular Anomalies Clinic*
*Division of Dermatology in the Department of Medicine*
*Departments of Radiology and Pediatrics*
*Washington University School of Medicine*
*St. Louis, Missouri*

**Jennifer N. Avari Silva, MD, FHRS, FAHA**
*Professor, Pediatrics and Biomedical Engineering*
*Director, Pediatric Electrophysiology*
*Faculty Fellow in Entrepreneurship*
*Department of Pediatrics & Biomedical Engineering*
*Washington University School of Medicine*
*St. Louis, Missouri*

**Paul S. Simons, MD**
*Associate Professor of Pediatrics*
*Developmental and Behavioral Pediatrics*
*Division of Academic Pediatrics*
*Washington University School of Medicine*
*St. Louis, Missouri*

**Jessica Sims, MD**
*Pediatric Chief Resident*
*St. Louis Children's Hospital*
*Washington University School of Medicine*
*St. Louis, Missouri*

**Kelsey Sisti, MD, FAAP**
*Assistant Professor of Pediatrics*
*Medical Director, Newborn Nursery*
*Missouri Baptist Hospital*
*Division of Pediatric Hospital Medicine*
*Department of Pediatrics*
*Washington University School of Medicine*
*St. Louis, Missouri*

**Mythili Srinivasan, MD, PhD**
*Professor of Pediatrics*
*Division of Hospitalist Medicine*
*St. Louis Children's Hospital*
*Washington University School of Medicine*
*St. Louis, Missouri*

**Ashley Steed, MD, PhD**
*Assistant Professor of Critical Care Medicine*
*Department of Pediatrics*
*Washington University School of Medicine*
*St. Louis, Missouri*

**Jeffrey Stokes, MD, FAAAAI, FACAAI**
*Professor in Pediatrics*
*Department of Pediatrics*
*Washington University School of Medicine*
*St. Louis, Missouri*

**Stephen Stone, MD, FAAP**
*Instructor in Pediatrics*
*Department of Pediatrics*
*Washington University School of Medicine*
*St. Louis, Missouri*

**Brian R. Stotter, MD, FAAP**
*Assistant Professor of Pediatrics*
*Division of Pediatric Nephrology,*
*  Hypertension & Pheresis*
*Department of Pediatrics*
*Washington University School of Medicine*
*St. Louis, Missouri*

**Ting Y. Tao, MD, PhD**
*Assistant Professor*
*Section Chief, Pediatric Radiology*
*Department of Radiology*
*Washington University School of Medicine*
*St. Louis, Missouri*

**Stefani Tica, MD, MPH**
*Fellow*
*Division of Pediatric Gastroenterology,*
*  Hepatology, and Nutrition*
*Department of Pediatrics*
*Washington University School of Medicine*
*St. Louis, Missouri*

**Ashley Turner, MD**
*Clinical Fellow*
*Division of Pediatric Critical Care*
*St. Louis Children's Hospital*
*Washington University School of Medicine*
*St. Louis, Missouri*

**Sarah Tycast, MD**
*General Pediatrician*
*The Children's Clinic*
*Tualatin, Oregon*

**Elizabeth C. Utterson, MD**
*Associate Professor of Pediatrics*
*Division of Pediatric Gastroenterology*
*Washington University School of Medicine*
*St. Louis, Missouri*

**Cynthia Wang, MD, MPHS**
*Dermatology Resident*
*Division of Dermatology*
*Washington University School of Medicine*
*St. Louis, Missouri*

**Brad W. Warner, MD**
*Jessie L. Temberg, MD, PhD*
*Distinguished Professor of Pediatric Surgery*
*Washington University School of Medicine*
*Surgeon-in-Chief*
*St. Louis Children's Hospital*
*St. Louis, Missouri*

# Preface

The first edition of *The Washington Manual® of Pediatrics* was created from *The Washington Manual® Pediatric Survival Guide* to provide concise and quickly accessible information to interns, residents, and medical students while they care for children in the hospital on the inpatient wards, in the intensive care units, in the emergency department, and in subspecialty outpatient clinics. In this third edition, we have expanded the content to be useful for all those caring for children, including hospitalists working in various community locations, those working at academic centers, as well as anyone staffing urgent care centers or working in primary care. The book provides established clear-cut approaches to the diagnosis and treatment of many of the most common pediatric problems and cuts out much of the fluff that bogs down similar works. In addition, it supplies evidence-based references when they are available, supporting the described management approaches.

The authors of this manual are interns, residents, nurse practitioners, chief residents, subspecialty fellows, and faculty at St. Louis Children's Hospital and Washington University School of Medicine, some of whom have moved beyond our walls. These talented, enthusiastic, and caring physicians have worked together to create a useful manual for all those in pursuit of knowledge about pediatric health and disease. In addition to the hard work of the many current authors, a special thanks goes out to Drs. Susan Dusenbery, Ana Maria Arbelaez, and Tami Garmany, whose efforts on the first edition and on the *Pediatric Survival Guide* set the stage for this current version.

Finally, this book would not exist without the unwavering support and encouragement of Dr. Gary Silverman, Chairman of Pediatrics at Washington University, and Dr. Hilary Babcock, Vice President and Chief Quality Officer of BJC Healthcare, who provided tireless enthusiasm, sage advice, and strategic guidance, and were both paramount in ultimately bringing this work to fruition.

*Andrew J. White, MD*

# Contents

# 1

# Primary Care and the Continuity Clinic

Marie Batty and Cassandra Pruitt

## INTRODUCTION

- Introduced by the American Academy of Pediatrics (AAP) in 1992, a "medical home" is an approach to providing comprehensive patient care that promotes partnerships between patients and families, clinicians, and medical staff. In a medical home, medical care should be accessible, comprehensive, family-centered, coordinated, and culturally appropriate.
- The first part of this chapter outlines important topics to discuss at every well child visit.
- The second part of this chapter will outline common childhood concerns often addressed by primary care pediatricians.

## TIMING OF WELL CHILD CARE VISITS

The AAP recommends pediatrician visits at 3-5 days of life, 1 month, 2, 4, 6, 9, 12, 15, 18, 24, and 30 months, 3 years, and then yearly through age 18-21.

## GROWTH AND NUTRITION

### Normal Growth Patterns for Age

- Pediatricians monitor weight, height, and head circumference over time. Deviation from norms can identify children with nutritional deficiencies, endocrinopathies, and other underlying conditions. (See Appendix C for CDC and WHO growth charts.)
- The Centers for Disease Control and Prevention (CDC) and AAP recommend using World Health Organization (WHO) growth charts from birth through 24 months of age, regardless of the patient's method of feeding.
- At age 2, pediatricians should transition to using the CDC growth charts to monitor the growth of patients compared to other children in the United States.

#### Weight
- It is normal for a newborn's weight to decrease up to 10% below birth weight in the first week of life due to limited intake and excretion of extravascular fluid. By 2 weeks of age, the weight is typically regained and may exceed birth weight.
- Term infants should grow by 30 g/day in the first 1-3 months of life, 20 g/day during 3-6 months of age, and 10 g/day between 6 and 12 months of age. Typically, birth weight doubles by 4 months and triples by 1 year.
- Children gain approximately 2 kg/year between age 2 and the onset of puberty. Children who gain <1 kg/year should be monitored closely for nutritional deficiencies.

*Height*
- Term infants should grow 25 cm in the 1st year, 10 cm during the 2nd year, and 7.5 cm during both their 3rd and 4th years. Height should increase by 50% in the 1st year and double by 4 years.
- Children grow approximately 5 cm/year between age 4 and the onset of puberty. Prepubertal growth is nonlinear with spurts of growth and times of slower growth.

*Head Circumference*
Term infants' head circumference should increase 2 cm/month in the first 3 months, then 1 cm/month between 3 and 6 months, and then 0.5 cm/month between 6 and 12 months. It typically increases by 2 cm from 1 to 2 years, and head growth is mostly complete by 4 years of age.

*Preterm Infants and Other Variants from Typical Growth Patterns*
- Preterm infant growth goals differ from term infants, and while further study is needed to understand the nutritional needs of preterm infants, the following growth goals can be used as a guide: weight should increase by 15 g/kg/day, length by 1 cm/week, and head circumference by 0.7 cm/week.
- Please see Chapter 18, Endocrinology, for detailed information on causes of short stature and deviations from typical growth patterns.

## Normal Diet

*Infants*
Breastfeeding
The AAP recommends breastfeeding for the first 12 months of life and exclusively for the first 6 months. Breastfeeding infants should receive 400 IU of supplemental vitamin D per day.

Formula Feeding
- Although breast milk should be the first choice for infant nourishment, there are many infant formulas that provide adequate nutrition (Table 1-1).
- Iron-fortified infant formula is the recommended substitute for infants who are not breastfed. The recommended intake amount is 100 kcal/kg/day. In newborns, this is 2-3 oz every 3-4 hours, which increases to 4 oz every 3-4 hours at 1 month of age. Infants who are formula fed should also receive 400 IU of supplemental vitamin D until they take approximately 30-32 oz of formula per day.
- While it is common practice to switch formulas in infants with difficulty gaining weight, frequent physiologic reflux, or other feeding difficulties, there are limited data for this practice.

Complementary Foods
- Complementary nutrient-dense foods (any foods and beverages other than human milk or formula) can be introduced starting between 4 and 6 months of age, when the infant is developmentally ready. Breast milk or formula should remain the primary source of nutrition for an infant in their first year of life.
- There is no specific recommended sequence for introducing foods, as long as essential nutrients that complement breast milk or formula are provided. In general, parents should start with single-ingredient foods and introduce them one at a time at 2- to 5-day intervals. Parents can gradually offer foods 2-3 times per day.
- After an infant tolerates initial introduction of complementary foods, it is recommended to introduce common food allergens (peanut butter, egg, etc.) between 4 and 6 months of age to decrease the risk of subsequent food allergy. For more

**TABLE 1-1** Common Infant Enteral Nutrition

| Formula | Carbohydrate | Protein | Fat | Clinical use |
|---|---|---|---|---|
| Breast milk | Lactose | Whey:casein = 80:20 | 100% LCT | Infant nutrition |
| Enfamil Neuro Pro, Similac Advanced | Lactose | Cow milk whey:casein = 60:40 | 100% LCT | Standard formula |
| Similac Isomil Soy | Glucose polymers, sucrose, lactose free | Soy protein isolate | 100% LCT | Cow's milk protein intolerance |
| Enfamil ProSobee | Glucose polymers, lactose free | Soy protein isolate | 100% LCT | Cow's milk protein intolerance, galactosemia |
| Enfamil Gentlease | Glucose polymers, reduced lactose | Whey:casein 60:40, partially hydrolyzed | 100% LCT | Fat/protein malabsorption, cholestasis |
| Nutramigen | Glucose polymers, lactose free | Casein hydrolysate | 100% LCT | Fat/protein malabsorption, cholestasis |
| Alimentum | Glucose polymers, sucrose, lactose free | Casein hydrolysate | 66% LCT, 33% MCT | Fat/protein malabsorption, cholestasis |
| Pregestimil | Glucose polymers, lactose free | Casein hydrolysate | 45% LCT, 55% MCT | Fat/protein malabsorption, cholestasis |
| EleCare, Neocate | Glucose polymers, lactose free | Amino acids | 67% LCT, 33% MCT | Severe cow's milk protein intolerance or multiple food allergies |

LCT, long-chain triglycerides; MCT, medium-chain triglycerides.
Adapted from Martinez JA, Ballew MP. Infant formulas. Pediatr Rev 2011 May;32(5):179–189.

information on introduction of high-allergen foods, please see Chapter 11, Allergic Diseases and Asthma.
- Before 12 months of age, cow's milk, honey, and hard, round foods that are a choking hazard should be avoided.

### Toddlers, Children and Adolescents
- At 12 months of age, children can be transitioned from breast milk or formula to whole milk containing calcium and vitamin D. Earlier transition to whole milk is associated with the development of iron deficiency anemia.
- Children should eat a variety of foods from all food groups including fruits, vegetables, whole grains, and lean meat. Nutritional needs should be met through nutrient-dense foods that provide vitamins and minerals but have little or no added sugars, saturated fat, and sodium.
- The United States Department of Agriculture (USDA) created a food guidance system called MyPlate. Key messages include portion control, making half of your plate fruits and vegetables, making half of your grains whole grains, switching to fat-free or 1% milk, choosing foods with lower sodium, and drinking water instead of sugary beverages.
- Feeding schedules include three meals plus 2-3 snacks per day. The amount of intake increases as a child's weight and energy needs increase. Children are able to self-regulate their energy intake by feeding themselves.
- Nutrient needs should be met primarily by consuming a variety of healthful foods, but in some cases, dietary supplements may be necessary to ensure adequate intake of one or more nutrients.
  - Females of childbearing age should take 400 μg of folate per day from fortified foods, a supplement, or both, in addition to a varied diet.
  - Recommendations for iron intake include the following:
    - Children ages 9-13 years: 8 mg/day
    - Females 14-18 years old: 15 mg/day
    - Males 14-18 years old: 11 mg/day
  - Recommendations for calcium intake include the following:
    - Children 4-8 years old: 1000 mg/day
    - Children and adolescents 9-18 years old: 1300 mg/day
    - Adolescents and adults 19 years and above: 1000 mg/day
- Limit carbonated soda and fruit drinks. Allow no more than 4-6 oz of 100% fruit juice daily due to its high calorie and sugar content.

## ELIMINATION PATTERNS

### Urinating
- Normal newborns have one wet diaper in the first day of life, and this increases by one each day until the infant makes at least 6-8 wet diapers per day.
- Less than three episodes of urine output per day is concerning for dehydration.
- At 2-4 years of age, children are developmentally ready to begin toilet training.

### Stooling
- The first stools after birth are meconium. The first stool should pass within 48 hours of birth.
- Infants have loose, yellow seedy stools that occur frequently.

- Stool frequency varies, and the normal range is wide, from 1 per week to 8 per day. Once children begin to eat solid food, their stools become firmer.
- Please refer to Chapter 17, Gastrointestinal Symptoms and Associated Diseases, for more information on stooling variants seen in children.

## SLEEP

- Sleep duration in a 24-hour period decreases as children age, with infants sleeping 16-20 hours per day and adolescents requiring 8-9 hours of sleep.
- The ability to sleep through the night usually develops between 3 and 6 months of age.
- There is a dramatic decrease in daytime sleep between 18 months and 5 years of age.
- Sleep hygiene is important to ensure quality of sleep. It is recommended to turn off all screens at least 60 minutes before bedtime and to not allow TVs, computers, or other screens in children's bedrooms.

## DEVELOPMENT

- Acquisition of developmental milestones occurs at specific times during childhood and in a particular sequence. Children are monitored for acquisition of milestones, and those who do not develop these skills as predicted require further evaluation.
- Table 1-2 lists gross motor, fine motor, cognitive, language, and social milestones and the typical age at which these skills are acquired for children 1 month through 8 years.
- Two commonly used screening tools to assess a child's development at well child visits are the Ages and Stages Questionnaire (ASQ) and Denver Developmental Screening Test. Please see Chapter 13, Developmental and Behavioral Pediatrics, for more information.

## VACCINATIONS

- Vaccinations are the most important preventive therapy that pediatricians provide to children. The up-to-date vaccine schedule and catch-up schedule for children and adolescents are available on the CDC website.
- Risks and benefits of vaccines should be discussed with patients and parents prior to administration. Contraindications and precautions to vaccine administration as well as information about preventing and managing adverse reactions are provided by the Advisory Committee on Immunization Practices (ACIP).
- Vaccine manufacturers and health care providers are required to report adverse events to the Vaccine Adverse Event Reporting System (VAERS).

## SCREENINGS

### Postpartum Depression

- The AAP recommends screening for postpartum depression in mothers at the 1-, 2-, 4-, and 6-month well child visits.
- The Edinburgh Postnatal Depression Scale (EDPS) is the most common screening tool for postpartum depression. A score of 10 or more indicates possible postpartum depression. The mother should be referred to her primary physician for further evaluation and treatment. Immediate action is necessary if the questionnaire indicates possible suicidality or the mother expresses concern for her or her infant's safety.

| TABLE 1-2 | Developmental Milestones by Age | | |
|---|---|---|---|
| Age | Gross motor skills | Fine motor skills | Cognitive, language, and social skills |
| 1 month | Head up while prone | Hands fisted | Fixes and follows to midline, startles to voice |
| 2 months | Chest up while prone | Hands fisted 50% of the time, grasps a rattle placed in hand | Follows past midline, regards speaker, social smile, coos |
| 4 months | Up on hands in prone, rolls front to back, no head lag | Keeps hands open, reaches for and retains objects in hand, brings hands to midline | Orients to voice, laughs, vocalizes when speaker stops talking |
| 6 months | Sits unsupported, rolls back to front | Raking grasp, transfers hand to hand | Discriminates strangers, consonant babbling |
| 9 months | Crawls, pulls to stand, cruises | Brings 2 toys together, finger feeds | Plays peek-a-boo, uncovers hidden objects, follows a pointed finger, says "dada" and "mama" indiscriminately, orients to name, understands "no" |
| 12 months | Cruises, walks alone | Mature pincer grasp | Says "dada" and "mama" appropriately, 1-2 additional words, immature jargoning, follows command with gesture |
| 15 months | Walks alone, stoops to pick up a toy, creeps up stairs | Builds tower of 2 cubes, imitates scribbling, uses a spoon and cup | 3-5-word vocabulary, follows simple commands, names one object, says "no" meaningfully, points to one or two body parts |
| 18 months | Throws ball while standing, walks up stairs with support, sits in a chair | Builds tower of 3-4 cubes, initiates scribbling | 10-25-word vocabulary, mature jargoning, points to three body parts and to self |

| Age | | | |
|---|---|---|---|
| 24 months | Jumps in place, kicks ball, throws overhand, walks up and down stairs with support | Builds tower of 6 cubes, imitates vertical stroke | 50+-word vocabulary, 2-word phrases, uses pronouns, 50% intelligible, follows two-step commands, refers to self by name, points to 6 body parts, parallel play |
| 3 years | Pedals a tricycle, alternates feet ascending stairs | Builds tower of 9 cubes, independent eating, copies a circle, draws 3-part person, unbuttons clothing | 200+-word vocabulary, uses plurals, 75% intelligible, gives full name, knows age and gender, counts to 3, recognizes colors, toilet trained |
| 4 years | Alternates feet descending stairs, hops on one foot | Builds tower of 10 cubes, able to cut and paste, copies a square, buttons clothing, catches a ball | 100% intelligible, uses "I" correctly, dresses and undresses with supervision, knows colors, tells tales, group play |
| 5 years | Skips, walks on tiptoes | Copies a triangle | 2000+-word vocabulary, identifies coins, names four to five colors, can tell age and birthday |
| 6 years | Tandem walk | Ties shoes, combs hair, copies a diamond | 10,000+-word vocabulary, reads 250 words, knows left vs. right, days of the week, and own telephone number |
| 7 years | Rides a bicycle | Bathes independently | Tells time to the half hour |
| 8 years | Reverse tandem walk | | Tells time within 5 min, knows months of the year |

## Hearing

- The AAP recommends objective hearing screens at birth and ages 4, 5, 6, 8, 10, 11-14, 15-17, and 18-21 years of age.
- For infants born in a hospital, it is recommended they undergo hearing screening prior to discharge. Otoacoustic emissions (OAEs) and auditory brainstem response (ABR) are the two most common hearing screens.
- Between the hearing screen at birth and the beginning of objective hearing screens at age 4, the pediatrician should assess the patient's hearing based on parental concerns, achievement of developmental milestones, auditory skills, and middle-ear examination.
- The most common objective hearing screen used in a pediatrician's office is pure-tone testing. During this screening test, a child is asked to raise her hand when a sound is heard. A child who fails this hearing screen should be referred for formal audiologic testing.

## Vision

- The AAP and American Academy of Ophthalmology (AAO) have outlined recommendations for vision screening based on a child's age. If any of these vision screens results in an abnormality, the pediatrician should consider referring the child for further evaluation by Ophthalmology.
- Newborns' eyes should be checked for a red reflex with an ophthalmoscope. Pediatricians should also assess for blink and pupillary response.
- Between 6 and 12 months of age, a pediatrician should check an infant for healthy eye alignment and movement.
- Between 12 and 36 months, a pediatrician can start using instrument-based vision screening. These devices are endorsed by the AAP and U.S. Preventative Services Task Force (USPSTF) as a valid method of vision screening for young children. These devices do not directly assess visual acuity but can identify ocular risk factors for early vision loss and detect ocular conditions known to cause amblyopia.
- Once a child is 6 years or older, they can participate in visual acuity testing using an optotype-based vision chart positioned at 10 or 20 feet away from the child. This screening should be repeated every 1-2 years.

## Lead

- Risk assessment screening for lead exposure should be performed at 6 months, 9 months, 1 year, and then annually through age 6.
- Lead levels should be obtained at 12 and 24 months.
- Evaluate for risk factors including the following:
  - Living in a home built before 1978
  - Living in a home with chipping paint or that has been recently renovated
  - History of pica (eating nonnutritive substances such as soil or paint chips)
  - Family member occupational exposures such as lead smelting, or hobbies such as pottery, fishing, or hunting
  - History of a sibling or close friend being treated for lead poisoning
  - History of owning imported pottery or eating imported canned food
  - Deficiency of iron, zinc, protein, calcium, or vitamin C, which can result in increased absorption of ingested lead

- Most commonly, patients are asymptomatic. However, even low lead levels (<5 µg/dL) can affect IQ and behavior. Poor school performance, aggression, hyperactivity, and inattention may be seen.
- When present, symptoms include headaches, abdominal colic, constipation, lethargy, growth failure, weight loss, vomiting, ataxia, and dental caries. As levels rise, symptoms progress to seizures, encephalopathy, and coma.
- Physical examination findings are nonspecific but may show developmental delay (particularly language delay), short stature, and mental status changes or seizures with severe toxicity.
- Venous samples are more accurate than fingerstick capillary values. Confirm elevated fingerstick results with a venous sample.
- A CBC with smear may show microcytic, hypochromic anemia with basophilic stippling.
  - Primary prevention is the preferred management, and chelation therapy does not reverse neurocognitive defects in children with lead neurotoxicity.
  - See Table 1-3 for recommended management.

## Iron Deficiency Anemia

- The AAP recommends universal screening for iron deficiency anemia with a hemoglobin level and assessment of risk factors at age 1. Selective screening can be performed at any time when risk factors are identified.
- CBC with smear shows low hemoglobin and hematocrit, elevated red cell distribution width (RDW), low mean corpuscular volume (MCV), and microcytic, hypochromic red blood cells.
- For more information regarding diagnosis and management of iron deficiency anemia, please refer to Chapter 19, Hematology and Oncology.

## Lipid Screening

- AAP guidelines recommend universal cholesterol screening with a nonfasting lipid panel between 9 and 11 years of age and again between 17 and 21 years of age.
- Selective screening is warranted for children between ages 2 and 10 with a family history of lipid and cholesterol disorder or premature heart disease, an unknown family history due to adoption, or personal characteristics associated with heart disease, such as high blood pressure, diabetes, or obesity.

## Depression and Anxiety

- The USPSTF recommends screening for depression in adolescents ages 12-18 years of age.
- The most common screening tool for depression is the PHQ-9, which consists of nine questions to diagnose major depressive disorder, determine severity of symptoms, and assess treatment response when used at follow-up visits.
- The Screen for Child Anxiety Related Emotional Disorders (SCARED) is most commonly used to screen patients ages 8-18 for childhood anxiety disorders, including generalized anxiety disorder, separation anxiety disorder, panic disorder, social phobia, and school phobia.
- For more information on diagnosis and management of depression and anxiety, please refer to Chapter 10, Adolescent Medicine, and Chapter 12, Child Psychiatry.

## Substance Use

- The Substance Abuse and Mental Health Services Administration (SAMHSA) recommends universal substance use screening, brief intervention, and/or referral to treatment (SBIRT) as part of routine adolescent health care.

| TABLE 1-3 | Assessment and Management of Confirmed Elevated BLL |
|---|---|
| **BLL (µg/dL)** | **Intervention** |
| <5 | Environmental history |
| | Assessment of nutritional and developmental milestones |
| | Follow up testing recommended based on child's age |
| 5-9 | Environmental history |
| | Risk reduction education—dietary and environmental |
| | Obtain confirmatory venous sample |
| | If elevated on confirmatory test, report BLL to local health department |
| | Based on venous sample, retest within 3 months |
| 10-19 | Follow actions for 5-9 µg/dL |
| | Repeat testing in 1 month for new cases, 1-3 months for known cases |
| 20-44 | Follow actions for 10-19 µg/dL |
| | Complete history and examination with neurodevelopmental assessment |
| | Hemoglobin, hematocrit, iron status |
| | Environmental investigation (lead inspection, abatement) |
| | Lead hazard reduction |
| | Abdominal plain radiographs (if lead particulate ingestion is suspected) with bowel decontamination if needed |
| | Repeat testing in 1 month for new cases, 1-3 months for known cases |
| 45-69 | Follow actions for 20-44 µg/dL |
| | Consider free erythrocyte or zinc protoporphyrin testing |
| | Oral chelation therapy may be considered in consultation with a medical toxicologist or pediatric environmental health specialty unit |
| | Consider hospitalization if lead-safe home cannot be assured |
| | Confirm BLL 24-48 hr before beginning chelation therapy |
| | Recheck BLL 1-3 weeks after chelation |
| ≥70 | Hospitalize and start chelation therapy in conjunction with medical toxicologist while confirming BLL emergently |
| | Follow actions for 20-44 µg/dL |
| | Consider free erythrocyte or zinc protoporphyrin testing |
| | Recheck BLL 1-3 weeks after chelation |

Adapted from Advisory Committee on Childhood Lead Poisoning Prevention (ACCLPP). Low level lead exposure harms children: a renewed call for primary prevention. Atlanta, GA: US Department of Health and Human Services, CDC, ACCLPP; 2012. Available at http://www.cdc.gov/nceh/lead/ACCLPP/Final_Document_010412.pdf

- Screening can be conducted as part of a detailed social history (HEEADSSS mnemonic—home, education and employment, eating, activities, drugs, sexuality, suicidality/depression, and safety) or with validated screening tools.
- CRAFFT (car, relax, alone, friends/family, forget, trouble) screening tool quickly assesses for problems related to substance use.
- Refer to Chapter 10, Adolescent Medicine, for more information on the diagnosis and management of substance use disorders.

## Sexually Transmitted Infections

- Pediatricians should screen for sexually transmitted infection (STI) risk by routinely and privately asking all adolescent and young adult patients about sexual activity, the type of sexual intercourse, and characteristics of sexual partners.
- The CDC and AAP have provided guidance for screening sexually active adolescents and young adults for STIs:
  - All sexually active adolescents ages 13 or older should be tested for HIV at least once. With a history of unprotected sex, HIV testing should occur at least once a year.
  - All sexually active women younger than 25 should be tested for gonorrhea and chlamydia yearly.
  - All sexually active gay or bisexual men should be tested at least once a year for syphilis, Chlamydia, and gonorrhea. This population may also require more frequent HIV testing.
- For more details on STI screening in the pediatric and adolescent population, please refer to Chapter 10, Adolescent Medicine, the CDC website or the Red Book.

## Tuberculosis

- Annually at each well child examination, pediatricians should screen for tuberculosis (TB) risk factors with recommended screening questions. The questions asked may vary based on geographic location and patient population.
- If a patient or parent answers yes to any screening questions, further clarification is needed to determine the extent of the risk. If any risk factor is present, test the child for TB or latent TB with a tuberculin skin test (TST).
- For more information about screening, diagnosis, and treatment of tuberculosis, refer to Chapter 21, Infectious Diseases.

## ANTICIPATORY GUIDANCE

### Health Promotion

*Exercise and Physical Activity*
- All children need physical activity starting in infancy. According to the AAP:
  - Infants need at least 30 minutes throughout the day of tummy time or interactive play while awake.
  - Children ages 3-5 need at least 3 hours of physical activity per day or approximately 15 minutes per hour while awake.
  - Children ages 6 and older need 60 minutes of moderate to vigorous physical activity most days of the week. For older children and adolescents, it is recommended they participate in muscle and bone strengthening activities 3 times a week.
- Children who engage in regular physical activity experience improved self-esteem, leadership and team building skills, decreased stress and anxiety, and improved physical and brain health.

*Reading to Your Child*
- Reading proficiency by the third grade is the most important predictor of high school graduation and career success; however, two-thirds of children in the United States each year do not develop reading proficiency by the end of third grade.
- The AAP recommends that pediatric providers promote early literacy development in children by encouraging parents to read aloud with their children and counseling families on developmentally appropriate shared-reading activities.

*Dental Care*
- Eruption of primary teeth begins at 5-7 months with mandibular central incisors and is complete by eruption of second molars at 20-30 months.
- Shedding of primary teeth occurs between 6 and 13 years, starting with mandibular central incisors.
- Secondary tooth eruption is complete by 17-22 years.
- Thumb and pacifier sucking habits usually cease spontaneously and are only a dental problem if they persist for a long time. If this behavior is ongoing at age 3 years, a mouth appliance may be recommended.
- Children should see a dentist when their first tooth appears, but no later than his/ her first birthday, and every 6 months thereafter. The American Academy of Pediatric Dentistry (AAPD) encourages families to establish a dental home for their children by age 1 year.
- Teeth should be cleaned at least twice daily with fluoridated toothpaste.
  - Age <2 years: Once teeth are present, use an infant toothbrush with a grain of rice-sized amount of fluoridated toothpaste.
  - Age 2-5 years: Brush teeth with a pea-sized amount of fluoridated toothpaste.
  - Ages 5+ years: Monitor child for effective brushing technique.
  - Ages 12 years and older: Use a 1-inch strip of fluoridated toothpaste.
- Fluoride supplementation is recommended to reduce tooth demineralization and promote remineralization. Important fluoride sources include toothpaste, community drinking water, infant formula, and prepared foods.
- Dental fluorosis occurs when a child is exposed to excess fluoride and results in changes to the tooth enamel including staining and pitting.

## Behavior
*Discipline*
- Discipline is a tool parents can use to modify and guide a child's behavior.
  - It should incorporate positive reinforcement (e.g., praise) for desired behavior and negative reinforcement (e.g., time-out) for undesired behavior.
  - Discipline is most effective when it is consistent, when the relationship between child and parent is positive and supportive, and when clear expectations are set.
  - Time-out is a preferred method of negative reinforcement because it removes the child from participation in desired activities. Time-out should be equal in minutes to the child's age in years.
  - The AAP recommends against corporal punishment, as it is of limited effectiveness and may have harmful consequences.

## Injury Prevention
*Safe Sleep*
- The AAP has recommendations to help parents make their infant's sleep environment as safe as possible:

- Infants should be placed on their backs to sleep for every sleep until age 1. If the baby falls asleep in a car seat, stroller, or swing, they should be moved to their crib and placed on their back as soon as possible.
- Infants should be placed on a firm sleep surface covered by a fitted sheet with no other bedding or soft objects in the sleep area.
- Infants should sleep in their parents' room, close to the parents' bed but on a separate surface (room sharing without bed sharing) for at least 6 months but preferably a year.
- Consider offering a pacifier at naptime and bedtime once breastfeeding has been firmly established. Studies have found a protective effect of pacifiers on the incidence of SIDS.
- Avoid second-hand smoke exposure.
- Dress the infant appropriately for sleep, with no greater than one layer more than an adult would wear for that environment.

### Childproofing the Home
Once an infant begins to be mobile, it is important to discuss childproofing the home with parents.

### Car Seats
- Because of the wide variety of car seats and car seat manufacturers, parents should refer to the manufacturer recommendations of their specific car seat for the height and weight limits.
- The AAP recommends that all infants and toddlers be restrained in a rear-facing car seat in the back seat of a car until at least 2 years of age.
- Children who have outgrown their rear-facing car seat should use a forward-facing car seat with a harness for as long as possible.
- Children who exceed the weight limit for their forward-facing car seat should be transitioned to a booster seat. They may discontinue use of a booster seat once the vehicle seat belt fits properly across their chest and lap, typically when they are 4 feet 9 inches tall (8-12 years of age).
- Children younger than 13 should ride in the back seat only.

### Firearm Safety
- The most effective way to prevent unintentional gun injuries, suicide, and homicides is to avoid having guns in the home and in the community.
- For families who decide to keep guns in their home, it is insufficient to just teach kids about gun safety. Safe storage of firearms is essential to keeping kids safe.
- All guns in the home should be stored unloaded in a locked box, with the ammunition stored and locked separately. Make sure children and teens in the home cannot access the keys or combinations to the locked boxes.

## COMMON CHILDHOOD CONCERNS

### Enuresis
- Enuresis in children older than 5 years of age is defined as two nighttime bed-wetting episodes (nocturnal enuresis) or daytime clothes-wetting episodes (diurnal enuresis) per week for 3 consecutive months.
- The prevalence varies with age and occurs in 7% of boys and 3% of girls at 5 years of age, 3% of boys and 2% of girls at 10 years, and 1% of men and <1% of women at 18 years.

- Clinical Presentation
  - The history should include questions about the frequency and amount of urination during the day and night, presence of dysuria, and history of constipation.
  - Parental history of enuresis is important to elicit, as children have a 44% incidence of enuresis when one parent was enuretic as a child and a 77% incidence when both parents were enuretic.
  - Evaluate for organic causes of enuresis in history and physical examination, including urinary tract infections, diabetes mellitus, neurologic abnormalities, medications, and chronic kidney disease.
- Laboratory Evaluation
  - Perform a urinalysis to look for signs of infection, glucosuria, or low specific gravity.
  - In children with diurnal enuresis, bladder ultrasound should be performed when the bladder is perceived to be full and when empty.
- Treatment
  - Though most enuresis resolves spontaneously, psychosocial consequences of bed-wetting may warrant therapy.
  - Begin with behavioral modification, including rewards for staying dry, urinating before bedtime, avoiding liquids at least 2 hours before bedtime, and waking the child 2-3 hours after falling asleep to void.
  - If enuresis persists, urine alarm treatment for 8-12 weeks has a 75-95% success rate.
  - Oral desmopressin (DDAVP) is a second-line treatment for nocturnal enuresis and works to reduce urine output overnight.
  - Both the alarm and DDAVP have a high relapse rate when discontinued.

## Physiologic Reflux

- During the first year of life, most infants experience regurgitation or "spitting up" of small amounts of food after eating.
- Clinical Presentation
  - Benign regurgitation occurs shortly after feeding, is nonforceful, and is not associated with weight loss or dehydration. Physical examination is within normal limits.
- Treatment
  - If no red flags such as weight loss, dehydration, projectile emesis, or bilious emesis are present, reassurance is indicated. If there are concerning findings on history or physical examination, consider other diagnoses such as pyloric stenosis, malrotation/volvulus, metabolic disorders, or increased intracranial pressure.
  - Physiologic reflux typically resolves spontaneously by 1 year of age as the lower esophageal sphincter function matures.
  - Measures to decrease regurgitation include frequent burping during feeds and propping the infant at a 30-degree angle following feeds.
  - See Chapter 17, Gastrointestinal Symptoms and Associated Diseases, for further information on regurgitation and vomiting.

## Colic

- Colic is defined as intermittent, unexplained, excessive crying that occurs >3 hours per day, >3 days per week, for >3 months.
- Clinical Presentation
  - Colic begins around 2 weeks of age, peaks at 6 weeks, and resolves by 3-4 months. Colic is usually worse in the late afternoon and evening.

- There are multiple unproven theories about the cause of colic, including gas, gastroesophageal reflux, food allergies, and cow's milk protein intolerance.
- Diagnostic Evaluation
  - Colic is a diagnosis of exclusion. A complete differential diagnosis should be considered when evaluating a child with excessive crying.
  - The physical examination is normal. Laboratory testing is not needed to make the diagnosis.
- Treatment
  - Parents should be reassured that they have a healthy infant. Studies have not shown significant improvement in colic with various therapies including simethicone drops and soy formula. There is some evidence that eliminating certain foods from the breastfeeding mother's diet may be effective in some infants, but this should be monitored closely and continued only if it is effective.

## Failure to Thrive

- Failure to thrive (FTT) is a physical sign of undernutrition. It is typically detected in the outpatient setting through serial monitoring of growth at routine well child visits.
- Causes of FTT can be grouped into one of four main categories:
  - Inadequate Intake
    ○ Insufficient food offered (e.g., food insecurity, neglect, lack of understanding of child's caloric needs, formula dilution)
    ○ Child's inability to take food (e.g., food aversion, oromotor dysfunction, developmental delay)
    ○ Emesis (e.g., due to functional or physical obstruction or elevated intracranial pressure)
  - Malabsorption
    ○ Underlying syndrome such as cystic fibrosis, Celiac disease, or food protein insensitivity or intolerance
  - Increased metabolic demands
    ○ Chronic disease such as congestive heart failure, chronic renal dysfunction
    ○ Hyperthyroidism
    ○ Various syndromes such as Turner syndrome, Down syndrome or Russell-Silver syndrome
    ○ Congenital infections (TORCH)
    ○ Insulin resistance as in patients with history of intrauterine growth restriction (IUGR)
    ○ Malignancy
  - Impaired Utilization
    ○ Inborn errors of metabolism
    ○ Chromosomal abnormalities
    ○ Endocrine disorders
    ○ Renal tubular acidosis
- Lack of expected weight gain is sometimes defined as <3rd to 5th percentile of weight for age or falling two percentiles over time. Height and weight measurements can be converted to z-scores, which are values that represent the number of standard deviations from the mean height and weight values for age. Z-scores are helpful when assessing a child whose height and weight falls well below or above standard percentile values. However, these mathematical definitions do not replace the pediatrician's clinical judgment.

- There may be long-term neurodevelopmental consequences of undernutrition.
- Clinical Presentation
  - History
    - History should include questions about diet, stooling, and growth patterns, pregnancy and birth complications, family history, patient and family meal-time behaviors, and social history with special attention to potential high-risk situations (e.g., poverty, multiple caregivers, teenage parents or parents with mental illness or intellectual disability).
    - A full review of systems should be performed to aid in the detection of underlying conditions that could cause FTT.
  - Physical Examination
    - Plot weight, height, and head circumference on growth charts to evaluate percentiles and compare to previously documented records.
    - Calculate the z-scores for height and weight to compare to the means for age.
    - Evaluate for dysmorphology that may suggest an underlying genetic cause of FTT.
    - Observe the child while eating, taking note of any oromotor dysfunction.
- Laboratory Evaluation
  - Studies have shown little added value of laboratory data in the evaluation of FTT; however, reasonable screening labs include a complete blood count (CBC) with differential, complete metabolic panel (CMP), sweat chloride test, anti-tissue transglutaminase (TTG) antibodies and total IgA, urinalysis (UA), and stool studies of fat content and reducing substances. Newborn screen results should be reviewed.
  - Second-line laboratory evaluation might include fat-soluble vitamin levels, urine organic acids, and serum amino acids. If length is also affected, consider thyroid stimulating hormone (TSH), free T4, and growth hormone measurement.
- Treatment
  - Focus of treatment should be nutritional repletion. Specific management should address the underlying cause.
  - Improvements in weight gain are best measured in weeks and months, so outpatient therapy is preferred. Hospitalization may be required in cases of severe malnutrition. During both outpatient and inpatient management, weight must be monitored frequently and caloric intake should be calculated to determine whether the child's caloric needs are being met.
  - Breastfeeding mothers can pump and provide expressed breast milk in a bottle to better quantify the volume of milk provided.
  - Access to a multidisciplinary team is key to successful treatment. This might include occupational, physical, and speech therapists, psychologists and psychiatrists, a dietician, and a social worker.
  - For children admitted to the hospital for FTT, discharge goals often include steady weight gain over several days and a stable feeding regimen to ensure ongoing weight gain at home.

## Picky Eating

- Toddlers may reduce their food intake as their rate of growth slows and assert independence by displaying their dislikes of certain foods. Over time, these patients tend to eat a well-balanced diet and have normal growth.
- Clinical Presentation
  - Examination is usually normal.

- Diagnostic Evaluation
  - Determine the extent of the diet by history, including the amount of cow's milk intake.
  - A CBC to evaluate for iron deficiency anemia may be indicated, particularly in patients with a large volume of milk intake.
  - If history and physical examination are concerning, further evaluation for food allergy, oral aversion, vitamin deficiency, or other underlying abnormalities may be warranted.
- Treatment
  - Provide a variety of foods at each meal in all of the basic food groups and allow the child to make choices. Do not pressure the child to eat any particular food as this may result in more significant feeding problems.
  - Children with highly restrictive diets or iron deficiency anemia may need vitamin and mineral supplementation.

## Overweight and Obesity

- Definition
  - Overweight is defined as BMI in the 85th to 94th percentile for age.
  - Obese is defined as body mass index (BMI) ≥95th percentile for age.
- Diagnostic Evaluation
  - Focus on the medical consequences of obesity such as hypertension, type 2 diabetes and insulin resistance, coronary artery disease, hypercholesterolemia, left ventricular hypertrophy, obstructive sleep apnea, mechanical stress on joints, pseudotumor cerebri, and hepatic steatosis.
- Laboratory Evaluation
  - Initial workup should include a fasting glucose (or hemoglobin A1c), fasting lipid panel, AST, and ALT. For patient convenience, the provider can elect to obtain nonfasting labs.
  - Other labs and studies to consider, depending on patient's age and degree of obesity, include vitamin D, GGT, uric acid, fasting serum insulin, urine microalbumin/creatinine ratio, C-peptide level, sleep study, or liver ultrasound.
- Treatment
  - Recognize overweight and obese patients and educate about the health consequences of obesity.
  - Schedule frequent visits with overweight and obese patients to encourage small but consistent diet and lifestyle modifications. These conversations should address the entire family to be most successful.
  - Medications for weight loss have limited data in pediatric patients.
  - Bariatric surgery is an extreme but effective treatment in adolescents with severe obesity.

## Dental Caries

- Dental caries are a preventable condition due to acid produced by bacterial fermentation of food debris on tooth surfaces. Acid demineralizes and destroys tooth enamel, dentin, and cementum, causing caries.
- Early Childhood Caries (formerly known as "baby bottle tooth decay" or "nursing bottle caries") is defined as the presence of one or more decayed, missing or filled tooth surfaces in any primary tooth between birth and age 6.
- Classified as early childhood caries (ECC) or severe-ECC based on age of onset and number of caries.

- Prevention is mainstay of management. In addition to adequate dental hygiene and screening, the AAPD recommends the following:
  - Avoid high frequency consumption of sugary liquids and solids in a bottle or no-spill training cup.
  - Do not put infants to sleep with a bottle containing milk or sugary beverages.
  - Wean from baby bottle between 12 and 18 months of age.

## Sleep Disorders

### Behavioral Insomnia of Childhood

- Clinical Presentation
  - There are two types of behavioral insomnia of childhood:
    - Sleep-onset association disorder is seen in infants and toddlers who learn to fall asleep only under certain conditions and do not develop the ability to self-soothe.
    - Limit-setting disorder involves delayed sleep onset due to the child stalling or refusing to fall asleep followed by frequent demands for attention once in bed.
- Treatment
  - Parents must establish a regular sleep schedule and bedtime routine.
  - Allowing the child to self-soothe at bedtime will allow them to fall back asleep more easily with night awakenings. Children should be put to bed drowsy but awake.
  - Parents should be prepared for worsening of the behavior before improvement.

### Night Terrors

- Clinical Presentation
  - Peak occurs between 4 and 12 years of age.
  - Arousal occurs from deep, slow-wave sleep usually in the first third of the night.
  - Presentation is consistent with intense fear including screaming or crying, tachycardia, tachypnea, skin flushing, diaphoresis, and increased tone.
  - The child has partial or complete amnesia of the event.
  - After the event, the physical examination is normal.
- Diagnostic Evaluation
  - Diagnosis is made based on the typical history.
  - History should also focus on an etiology for disrupted sleep including restless legs syndrome, obstructive sleep apnea, or seizures.
  - Polysomnography is not routinely indicated.
- Treatment
  - Parental reassurance, education, and good sleep hygiene are most important. These episodes are self-limited and cease with puberty as slow-wave sleep decreases.
  - Scheduled awakenings may be used for frequent episodes. The parent should awaken the child 15-30 minutes prior to the typical time of the episode for several weeks until the episodes stop.
  - Short-acting benzodiazepines can be used in rare, severe circumstances when the child is at risk of injury.

### Nightmares

- Clinical Presentation
  - Nightmares occur during REM sleep and, therefore, later in the night than night terrors.
  - Nightmares result in arousal, significant anxiety after awakening and potentially refusal to return to sleep.

- Children can recall the event.
- The physical examination is normal.
- Diagnostic Evaluation
  - The diagnosis is made by the classic history.
- Treatment
  - Good sleep hygiene is important. Nightlights and security blankets may be effective.
  - The child should avoid frightening television shows before bedtime.
  - In severe cases, assessment by a developmental pediatrician may be warranted.

### Sleepwalking

- Clinical Presentation
  - Peak age of presentation is 4-8 years old.
  - The child arouses during slow-wave sleep in the first third of the night and ambulates in a state of altered consciousness. Bizarre behaviors may occur during the episode.
- Diagnostic Evaluation
  - The diagnosis is made by the classic history.
  - Polysomnography is rarely indicated unless there is suspicion of obstructive sleep apnea or restless leg syndrome as precipitating factors.
- Treatment
  - Protect the child from harm. Make sure the bedroom is in a safe place, away from stairs.
  - Parents may place a bell or alarm on the child's door so that they know when the arousal occurs.
  - Rarely, in severe cases, benzodiazepines may be used.

## SUGGESTED READINGS

American Academy of Pediatrics. Literacy promotion: an essential component of primary care pediatric practice. Pediatrics 2014;134(2):404–409.

American Academy of Pediatrics. SIDS and other sleep-related infant deaths: updated 2016 recommendations for a safe infant sleeping environment. Pediatrics 2016;138(5):1–12.

American Academy of Pediatrics. The medical home: medical home initiatives for Children with Special Needs Project Advisory Committee. Pediatrics 2002;110:184–186.

American Academy of Pediatric Dentistry (AAPD). Policy on Early Childhood Caries (ECC): Classifications, Consequences, and Preventative Strategies. Chicago, IL: American Academy of Pediatric Dentistry (AAPD), 2016:79–81.

American Academy of Pediatrics Institute for Healthy Childhood Weight. Algorithm for the Assessment and Management of Childhood Obesity in Patients 2 Years and Older. 2015.

Barlow SE. Expert committee recommendations regarding the prevention, assessment and treatment of child and adolescent overweight and obesity: summary report. Pediatrics 2007;120(4):S164–S192.

Buz Harlor AD, Bower C. Hearing assessment in infants and children: recommendations beyond neonatal screening. Pediatrics 2009;124(4):1252–1263.

Committee on Practice and Ambulatory Medicine, Bright Futures Periodicity Schedule Workgroup. Periodicity schedule: policy statement 2021 recommendations for pediatric preventive health care. Pediatrics 2021;147(3):1–2.

Donahue SP, Baker CN. Procedures for evaluation of the visual system by pediatricians. Pediatrics 2016;137(1):1–9.

Earls MF, Yogman MW, Mattson G, Rafferty J. Incorporating recognition and management of perinatal depression into pediatric practice. Pediatrics 2019;143(1):1–9.

Hagan JF, Shaw JS, Duncan PM, eds. Bright Futures: Guidelines for Health Supervision of Infants, Children and Adolescents. 4th Ed. Elk Grove Village, IL: American Academy of Pediatrics, 2017.

Kliegman RM, St Geme JW, Blum NJ, et al., eds. Nelson Textbook of Pediatrics. 21st Ed. Philadelphia, PA: Elsevier, 2020.

Lobelo F, Muth ND, Hanson S, Nemeth BA. Physical activity assessment and counseling in pediatric clinical settings. Pediatrics 2020;145(3):1–21.

Siu AL US Preventive Services Task Force. Screening for depression in children and adolescents: US Preventive Services Task Force Recommendation Statement. Pediatrics 2016;137(3):1–8.

U.S. Department of Agriculture and U.S. Department of Health and Human Services. Dietary Guidelines for Americans, 2020-2025. 9th Ed. December 2020. Available at Dietary-Guidelines.gov

Workowski KA, Bolan GA. Sexually transmitted diseases treatment guidelines, 2015. MMWR Recomm Rep 2015;64(3):3–140.

# Newborn Nursery

Kelsey Sisti and Noor Riaz

## NEWBORN PHYSICAL EXAMINATION

- Vital signs: Temperature 36.5°C-37.9°C (hypothermia is just as important as hyperthermia), heart rate: 120-160 beats per minute, respiratory rate: 30-60 breaths per minute.
- Gestational age assessment for uncertain gestational age at birth.
  - Ballard examination is an estimation of gestational age by determining the infant's neuromuscular and physical maturity.
- Growth parameters: weight (percentile), length (percentile), OFC (percentile)
  - Appropriate for gestational age is ≥10% to ≤90% on Fenton growth curve.
  - Small for gestational age is <10% on Fenton growth curve.
  - Large for gestational age is >90% on Fenton growth curve.
- General appearance
  - Color: pink, pale, cyanotic, jaundiced
  - Activity: level of alertness, response to stimuli
- Head
  - Size, shape, and anterior fontanelle. Sutures: Separation may be palpable or they may be overriding.
  - Trauma: Caput succedaneum (hemorrhagic edema), which is superficial and crosses suture lines. Cephalohematoma is a circumscribed region of hemorrhage overlying the skull and beneath the periosteum, thus cannot cross sutures. Subgaleal hemorrhage is blood within the space above the periosteum and below the galea aponeurosis, a large potential space, and this can lead to severe hypovolemia and shock. Scalp lesions.
  - Eyes: Evaluate for reactivity to light and red reflexes, absence of which may indicate cataracts, corneal clouding, intraoccular pathology.
  - Ears: Note shape and position. Low set, posteriorly rotated, or other malformation may suggest congenital syndromes. Stiffness of cartilage is also an indication of gestational age.
  - Nose: Assess nares patency.
  - Mouth: Assess lip and palate both visually and by palpation to assess for clefts, tongue size. May see inclusion cysts on gums, Epstein's pearls on palate, or natal teeth.
- Neck: Assess for webbing, branchial cleft remnants, thyroglossal cysts, and goiter.
- Clavicles: Erythema, edema, or crepitus may indicate fracture.
- Chest: Symmetry, nipple location.
- Lungs: Clarity and symmetry of breath sounds. Accessory muscle use, retractions, and grunting are signs of respiratory distress.
- Heart: Activity of precordium, rhythm, murmurs on auscultation, as well as femoral pulses for both quality and symmetry.

- Abdomen: Assess shape (distended, scaphoid), quality (soft, firm), bowel sounds, presence of masses, spleen, and liver, which may be palpable 1-2 cm below right costal margin.
- Genitourinary
  - Male: Assess phallus and testes for hypospadias, chordee, torsion, hernia, hydrocele, undescended testes.
  - Female: Assess urethral meatus, introitus, clitoris for hypertrophy, labial masses. Vaginal discharge is common.
- Anus: Position and patency.
- Back: Spinal defects, dimples, pigmented lesions or tufts of hair, myelomeningocele, vascular malformations overlying the spine.
- Extremities: Symmetry and movement, Erb palsy, contractures, stability of hips with the Ortolani and Barlow maneuvers, foot creases for gestational age.
- Skin
  - Color: pink, pale, plethoric, jaundiced, meconium stained, acrocyanosis. Cracking or peeling suggests advanced gestational age
  - Petechiae or bruising
  - Pigmented lesions: café au lait spots, nevus, Mongolian spots
  - Rashes: erythema toxicum, pustular melanosis, milia
- Neurologic
  - General: alertness, jitteriness, response to handling
  - Cranial nerves: response to light, facial symmetry with cry, response to sound, gag, suck and swallow
  - Motor: resistance to passive movement, which increase with gestational age, resting posture, and tone
  - Primitive reflexes: Rooting: opens mouth and turn toward object stroking cheek. Moro: opening of hands, extension and abduction of arms, followed by anterior flexion and audible cry; disappears by 6 months

## ROUTINE CARE

- Hepatitis B vaccination: Recommended for all newborns within 24 hours of birth.
- Vitamin K: Recommended for all newborns within 6 hours of birth.
- Erythromycin eye ointment: Recommended for all newborns.
- Refusal of care: Discussion should be had with family about benefits of treatment and risks associated with refusal. Documentation of discussion and parents' acknowledgment of risks should be completed.

## FEEDING

- Breastfeeding: AAP recommends exclusive breastfeeding until 6 months and then with supplemental foods until 1 year of age. WHO recommends breastfeeding until the age of 2 years.
  - Human milk has the optimal nutrient composition for term and late preterm infants. Breast milk also has anti-infective properties that reduce the incidence of acute infections in newborns. It also provides passive immunity via secretory IgA from the mother, as well as oligosaccharides, nucleotides, and growth factors to enhance the infant's immune system.
  - Breastfeeding should be initiated within the first hour after delivery if possible. Infants should room in with their mother and breastfeed an average of 8-12 times

a day. If concerns for ineffective breastfeeding, encourage mother to begin pumping or expressing breast milk and offer any expressed breast milk to the infant. Frequent assessment of latch and quality of breastfeeding should be done to facilitate exclusive breastfeeding.

- Supplemental feedings are generally not necessary for healthy term infants and may impair breastfeeding relationship.
  - Late preterm infants, SGA infants, craniofacial anomalies, or those who cannot breastfeed well will benefit from supplemental feedings.
  - Recommend using paced bottle feeding and slow-flow nipples to help maintain a breastfeeding relationship.
  - We recommend assessing weight loss on the Newt (Newborn Weight Loss Tool) prior to supplemental feedings.
- Exclusively breastfed infants need vitamin D supplementation as breast milk contains <25 IU/L, which is insufficient to prevent vitamin D deficiency, and in extreme cases, rickets.
- Ankyloglossia is the persistence of midline sublingual tissue that restricts the infant's tongue and impairs the infant's ability to lift and/or extend the tongue. An infant's inability to effectively empty the breast or cause excessive trauma to the mother's nipple can cause poor weight gain and impair the breastfeeding relationship secondary to maternal trauma. Frenotomy is a simple procedure that improves the infant's tongue mobility, which often improves breastfeeding in cases of ankyloglossia.
- Formula is an adequate substitution for infants who are not breastfeeding due to various reasons including maternal preference, inborn errors of metabolism, maternal HIV infection, hepatitis C infection with cracked or bleeding nipples, and mothers who are receiving chemotherapy or other contraindications.
- Formula as a significantly different composition of whey/casein ratios than breast milk, as well as different protein, carbohydrate, and fat sources.
- Formula is unable to provide anti-infective and immune support that breast milk provides.

## LATE PRETERM

- Late preterm gestational age is defined as 34 0/7 weeks-36 6/7 weeks.
- NICU admission is recommended for those <35 0/7 weeks and/or <2 kg.
- Late preterm infants are at risk for respiratory distress, hypothermia (temperature <36.5°C), poor feeding, hypoglycemia, infection, and/or hyperbilirubinemia.
  - Respiratory distress: Please see Neonatology (Chapter 7) for the approach to the neonate with respiratory distress.
  - Hypothermia: Vital signs should be assessed every 4 hours. After 24 hours, neonate should be able to maintain temperature in appropriate clothing, single-wrapped blanket, and hat. If patient has 2 temperature drops, consider if patient needs higher level of care for thermoregulation support. Sepsis must also be considered with temperature instability.
  - Poor feeding: Late preterm infants may not be able to exclusively breastfeed till their due date. Consider supplementation with expressed breast milk and/or formula. If neonate is not feeding well by bottle, consider speech therapy/occupational therapy consult. Patient may need an NG tube if not meeting feeding goals.
  - Hypoglycemia: Blood sugars should be checked before feeding for 24 hours. Please see "hypoglycemia."

- Infection: Late preterm neonates are at higher risk for infection compared to full-term neonates. Please see "Sepsis" for more information.
- Hyperbilirubinemia: Bilirubin levels should be checked daily starting at 24 hours unless other indications to check sooner. Depending on neurotoxicity risk factors, late preterm infants would plot on medium or high risk curves on the treatment nomograms.
- Discharge criteria
  - Meets routine discharge criteria
  - Feeding well by breast that was assessed by experienced staff or taking 30 mL via bottle well prior to discharge
  - Pass a car seat test prior to discharge
  - Close follow-up with pediatrician in 24-48 hours

## BIRTH TRAUMA

- Cephalohematoma: should be monitored and documented on every examination
- Subgaleal hemorrhage
  - Neonates with subgaleal hemorrhage should have vital signs monitored and head circumference measured every 4 hours.
  - If subgaleal hemorrhage is increasing in size, obtain CBC to monitor hemolysis and bilirubin levels to monitor hyperbilirubinemia. Consider transfer to the NICU.
  - If subgaleal hemorrhage is increasing in size and infant demonstrates tachycardia, lethargy, respiratory distress, then transfer to higher level of care.
- Clavicle fracture
  - Can consider obtaining an plain radiographs.
  - Carefully examine the arm position, Moro reflex, and palmar grasp to rule out brachial plexus injury.
  - No treatment is necessary for an isolated clavicular fracture.
- Humerus fracture
  - Obtain plain radiographs of affected humerus.
  - Carefully examine the arm position, Moro reflex, and palmar grasp to rule out brachial plexus injury.
  - Immobilized the affected arm.
  - Recommend follow-up with Orthopedics 1 week after birth.
- Brachial plexus injury
  - Can occur after shoulder dystocia, breech delivery, or prolonged labor.
  - Examine the arm position looking for a waiter's tip, Moro reflex, and palmar grasp. Auscultate the lungs and monitor for respiratory distress.
  - Consult and refer to a brachial plexus center for further care.

## CONGENITAL ANOMALIES

- Cleft lip/palate
  - Monitor feedings closely. May require specialized bottle and feeding therapy.
  - Should have close follow-up with Cleft Palate Team.
- Club feet
  - No imaging or treatment is required in the Newborn Nursery.
  - Should have close follow-up with Orthopedics.

- Trisomy 21
  - Recommend consultation with Genetics.
  - Work-up includes FISH, karyotype, echocardiogram, CBC and may consider further work-up based on Genetics recommendations.
  - Monitor feedings closely. May require speech/occupational therapy.
  - Should have follow-up with Genetics or Down Syndrome Clinic.

## SEPSIS

- Most common causes of early-onset neonatal sepsis include group B streptococcus and *Escherichia coli*. Followed by other gram-positive organisms, viridans group streptococci and enterococci, and less commonly other gram-negative organisms, *Staphylococcus aureus* and *Listeria monocytogenes.*
- Physiologic abnormalities associated with sepsis: tachycardia with heart rate ≥160, tachypnea with respiratory rate ≥60, temperature instability with hyperthermia ≥38°C or <36.4°C.
- Screening indications
  - 35- to 37-week EGA with PROM > 18 hours, inadequate GBS prophylaxis, maternal intra-amniotic infection or if mother is treated for possible intra-amniotic infection
    - Maternal fever 39°C once or >38°C AND one of the following: maternal leukocytosis, purulent cervical discharge, fetal tachycardia
  - Any physiologic abnormality of the newborn
- Risk assessment guidelines: Our facility has transitioned to the Neonatal Early-Onset Sepsis Risk Calculator, using the CDC incidence of sepsis of 0.5/1000 live births.
  - Well appearing: no persistent physiologic abnormalities
  - Equivocal: persistent physiologic abnormality ≥4 hours after birth or ≥2 abnormalities for 2 hours
  - Clinically ill: persistent need for respiratory support, hemodynamic instability, neonatal encephalopathy, need for supplemental oxygen ≥2 hours after delivery
- Empirical treatment with ampicillin 100 mg/kg IV q8h and gentamicin 5 mg/kg/dose IV q24h is first line therapy for EOS pending speciation and sensitivities.

## MATERNAL INFECTIONS

- Gonorrhea
  - If mother was positive for gonorrhea during pregnancy and has a negative test of cure, no further treatment is indicated for baby except routine erythromycin eye ointment.
  - If mother has active infection at time of delivery or no test of cure available prior to discharge, per AAP Red Book recommends ceftriaxone 25-50 mg/kg, max 125 mg, one dose, route IV or IM.
- Chlamydia
  - If mother was positive for chlamydia during pregnancy and has a negative test of cure, only treatment indicated is routine erythromycin eye ointment.
  - If mother is positive at delivery or no test of cure is available, the pediatrician needs to be notified to monitor for possible sequelae, including pneumonia.
- Syphilis: Please see Infectious Diseases (Chapter 21).
- Hepatitis B: Please see Infectious Diseases (Chapter 21).
- Hepatitis C: Please see Infectious Diseases (Chapter 21).
- HIV: Please see Infectious Diseases (Chapter 21).

## HYPOGLYCEMIA

- Indications for screening
  - Late preterm infants, small for gestational age infants, large for gestational age infants, infant of a diabetic mother, infant of a mother who received β-blockers or was on steroids within 72 hours of delivery, or received poor prenatal care
- Symptoms
  - Mild: irritability, tremors, jitteriness, exaggerated Moro reflex, weak or high-pitched cry, tachypnea
  - Severe: seizures, hypotonia, apnea, lethargy, cyanosis, eye rolling, poor feeding
- Monitoring
  - Initial glucose at 2 hours of life, then preprandial glucose POC.
  - In the first 4 hours, if the glucose level is <40 mg/dL or <45 mg/dL at >4 hours, the infant requires intervention.
  - Duration
    ○ Infants that are LGA or mother's had IDM must be monitored for a minimum of 12 hours with preprandial glucose levels.
    ○ Infants that are SGA, LPT, maternal h/o steroids or β-blockers, poor prenatal care, or if they have become symptomatic at ANY time should be monitored for 24 hours with preprandial glucose levels.
  - All infant must have two consecutive screens >50 mg/dL in the first 48 hours, and if >48 hours of age, must have two >60 mg/dL to complete monitoring.
- Treatment
  - Feeding: If the infant has a low glucose, feed immediately if otherwise stable.
    ○ Encourage formula supplementation if repeated event or glucose <25 mg/dL.
  - Dextrose gel: When given in concurrence with feeding, it decreases incidence of mother and infant separation, as well as improves rates of breastfeeding.
  - If the point of care glucose is <25 or the infant has severe symptoms, immediately give a D10 bolus, send a stat serum glucose and may give dextrose gel while preparing the IV.

## HYPERBILIRUBINEMIA

- Physiologic hyperbilirubinemia is unconjugated elevated bilirubin that peaks in the first 3-5 days of life.
- Physiologic hyperbilirubinemia can lead to examination findings of jaundice, and rarely, kernicterus.
- Elevated bilirubin occurs due to high rate of bilirubin production, increased entero-hepatic circulation of bilirubin, and immature hepatic glucuronosyltransferase enzyme.
- Common risk factors for developing hyperbilirubinemia include hemolysis due to ABO, Rh, or minor antibody incompatibility, breastfeeding jaundice, late preterm birth, hemolysis due to birth trauma resulting in cephalohematoma, subgaleal hemorrhage, or excessive bruising.
- Less common risk factors for developing physiologic hyperbilirubinemia include genetic conditions such as G6PD deficiency, hereditary spherocytosis, Gilbert syndrome, Crigler-Najjar, sepsis, metabolic disorders, and certain medications.

## Evaluation

- Per AAP guidelines, all babies should have bilirubin testing performed by transcutaneous (TcB) or by serum (TsB) before discharge.
- If TcB plots in high-intermediate risk or >12 mg/dL, then send serum bilirubin. If sending serum bilirubin, total and direct levels should be evaluated.
- Jaundice should be assessed on every physical examination. Visual assessment is not a reliable measure of bilirubin level. If concerned for hyperbilirubinemia, obtain TcB or TsB.
  - Coombs positive babies should have bilirubin level assessed by TcB or TsB the first 6, 12, and 24 hours of life, and then daily. If concerned for rapidly rising bilirubin or meets threshold for phototherapy in the first 24 hours of life, also obtain CBC and retic.
  - Late preterm babies should have bilirubin level assessed every day starting at 24 hours of life.
- Bilirubin levels should be plotted on both nomograms for risk of developing severe hyperbilirubinemia and treatment threshold.
  - For those with levels below treatment threshold, use the risk nomogram to help determine follow up after discharge.
  - Treatment thresholds are based on gestational age and neurotoxicity risk factors of isoimmune hemolytic disease, G6PD deficiency, asphyxia, significant lethargy, temp instability, sepsis, acidosis, or albumin <3. Treatment thresholds are not changed based on hyperbilirubenima risk factors alone.

## Treatment

- Phototherapy is the treatment for hyperbilirubinemia that does not meet exchange transfusion threshold.
- Phototherapy should not be routinely initiated below treatment thresholds.
- Phototherapy surface area should be maximized with overhead lights and bili blanket. Infants should wear eye protection while receiving phototherapy.
- Phototherapy should be provided in mother's room when possible to maximize bonding opportunities and breastfeeding.
- Once phototherapy is started, bilirubin levels should only be assessed by serum bilirubin. TcBs will no longer be accurate.
- Bilirubin levels should be checked every 6-12 hours depending on bilirubin level, neurotoxicity risk factors, and degree of hemolysis.
- Discontinuation of phototherapy can occur when levels drop to 13-14 mg/dL or decreases 4-5 mg/dL but also is a clinical decision based on neurotoxicity risk factors, gestational age, and follow-up time frame.
- Rebound bilirubin can be considered based on based on neurotoxicity risk factors, gestational age, and follow-up time frame.
  - Level should be checked no earlier than 6 hours after discontinuation of phototherapy and ideally, 12-24 hours after discontinuation.
- Levels above phototherapy thresholds should be plotted on the exchange transfusion nomogram. For those demonstrating signs of acute bilirubin encephalopathy or meeting exchange transfusion thresholds, transfer to NICU should be initiated. Please see Neonatology chapter for further information.

## Conjugated Hyperbilirubinemia

- Conjugated hyperbilirubinemia is a direct bilirubin level >1 mg/dL when total bilirubin concentration is 5 mg/dL. For total bilirubin concentration >5 mg/dL, then conjugated hyperbilirubinemia is when the value of the direct bilirubin in >20% of the total concentration.

- Conjugated hyperbilirubinemia can be caused by biliary atresia, Dubin-Johnson syndrome, Rotor syndrome, sepsis, galactosemia, and thyroid abnormalities.
- Conjugated hyperbilirubinemia should not be treated with phototherapy and can cause bronzing of the skin.
- Consultation with Pediatric GI is strongly recommended for further workup.

## MURMUR

- Newborn with a murmur at >24 hours of life
- Pathologic signs: diastolic, continuous, late or pan systolic, >3/6, loudest in the back
  - Evaluate infant assessing respiratory rate, work of breathing, pulses. Obtain 4 quadrant blood pressures, preductal and postductal pulse oximetry, EKG.
    - If normal, obtain an ECHO. Disposition planning pending ECHO results and cardiology recommendations.
    - If abnormal, obtain ECHO, chest plain radiographs, ABG, consider septic workup. Consult Cardiology.
- Nonpathologic signs: systolic ejection murmur heard best in axilla consistent with physiologic peripheral pulmonary stenosis; high pitched systolic ejection murmur at left upper sternal border consistent with PDA, usually resolves in 2-3 days; low pitch soft systolic murmur at left lower sternal border, usually resolved by day 3-4
  - Follow-up with primary care physician within 2-3 days. If this cannot be arranged, consider ECHO prior to discharge.

## ANURIA AND DELAYED PASSAGE OF MECONIUM

- Anuria in a newborn for more than 24 hours should be evaluated. Most common cause of anuria in a newborn is an undocumented void in the delivery room or by parents. Review prenatal records to look for documentation of oligohydramnios or abnormal prenatal ultrasounds. Assess feeding adequacy. Physical examination to look for abdominal distention and infant genitalia should be done. If continued anuria, consider bladder and renal ultrasound, renal function panel, and possible catheterization.
- Meconium passage typically occurs in the first 24 hours and the majority by 48 hours of life in full-term infants. If the infant has not passed stool in the first 24 hours, they should be evaluated for feeding quality, presence of emesis. Physical examination should assess for abdominal distention, bowel sounds, and patent anus. If there is delayed passage of meconium beyond 48 hours or at any time the infant is symptomatic with poor feeding or bilious emesis, further evaluation should be done: abdominal plain radiograph and consider barium enema pending clinical presentation.

## JITTERY INFANT

- Examine the infant and complete a neurologic assessment.
- If concern for seizure, stabilize patient, and transfer to NICU.
- For suppressible movements, consider hypoglycemia, SSRI exposure, nicotine withdrawal, hypocalcemia, sleep myoclonus, and drug withdrawal including opioids.

## NEONATAL ABSTINENCE SYNDROME

- Withdrawal can be seen in infants from in utero exposure to prescribed medications and substances including opioids, benzodiazepines, barbiturates, methamphetamine, and cocaine.
  - Opioid withdrawal is most commonly seen.
  - Opioid withdrawal can occur from short- and long-acting opioids, including fentanyl, oxycodone, heroin, methadone, and suboxone.
- Testing: Recommend Urine Drug Screen and Meconium sent on babies with the following:
  - In utero exposure to opioids, benzodiazepines, barbiturates, or other illegal substances
  - Concern for substance use by mother's care team based on mother's clinical status
  - Infant with unexplained disturbed sleep, increased muscle tone, tremors, irritability, poor feeding, vomiting and diarrhea, sweating, tachypnea, and/or fevers
- Observation of babies exposed to opioids
  - Duration
    - ○ For mothers with a remote history of opioid use, $\geq 2$ weeks prior to delivery and negative UDS, we recommend monitoring for 48 hours
    - ○ For mothers with a recent history of opioid use, $< 2$ weeks prior to delivery, we recommend monitoring for 72 hours
    - ○ For mothers taking long acting opioids, such as methadone or suboxone, OR with illegal or illicit drug use at time of delivery, we recommend monitoring for 96 hours
  - Monitoring
    - ○ May use Finnegan tool, Modified-Finnegan tool, or ESC (Eat-Sleep-Console) tool
- Treatment
  - First-line treatment is nonpharmacologic care, including decreasing environmental stimuli, comfort measures including swaddling, skin to skin, rocking, and frequent small volume feedings.
  - Consider occupational, physical, and speech therapy early in course.
  - For those with increasing scores on Finnegan tool or not meeting goals on ESC, second-line treatment is pharmacologic with morphine.

## CIRCUMCISION

- Circumcision is the removal of the foreskin of an infant's penis and is the most common surgical procedure performed on pediatric patients.
- The AAP states that "the health benefits of newborn male circumcision outweigh the risks and the procedure's benefits justify access to this procedure for families who choose it" but do not currently make the recommendation that all infants should undergo circumcision.
- Benefits
  - Decreased risk of UTI from approximately 1 to approximately 0.1%. In infants with high-grade VUR, circumcision decreases their risk of UTI significantly more.
  - Decreased risk of squamous cell carcinoma of the penis
    - ○ This is relatively rare cancer, however, uncircumcision men were three times more likely to develop penile cancer. Data only showed correlation to men who had history of phimosis but did not correlate to uncircumcised men without phimosis

- Decreased risk of ulcerative STIs, most notably HSV
  - Does not decrease the risk of chlamydia, gonorrhea, or syphilis
- Decreased risk of HIV. Data show decreased transmission of HIV in circumcised men in areas of high HIV prevalence.
- Contraindications
  - Anatomic contraindications: chordee, hypospadias, penile torsion, webbed penis, buried penis, urethral hypoplasia, epispadias, and ambiguous genitalia including micropenis or bilateral cryptorchidism
  - Medical contraindications: acute illness, age <12-24 hours, familial history of bleeding disorder, or disorder of the skin or connective tissue that would impair healing, parental vitamin K refusal
- Complications are rare but include the following:
  - Increased risk of meatitis with subsequent meatal stenosis.
  - Bleeding: Apply pressure firmly for 10-20 minutes. If the bleeding continues, consider using a hemostatic agent. If continued bleeding, may consider applying silver nitrate, but avoid applying to glans or meatus. If persistent or arterial bleeding, consult Urology for evaluation for suturing.
  - Complete separation of circumcision line typically occurs after excessive skin removal. Unless excessive bleeding occurs, reassure families, most heal appropriately.
  - Infection is rare but can occur.
    - Granulation tissue often forms on the glans and is not a sign of infection.
  - Entrapped penis or Cicatrix is a later complication when the glans retracts proximal to the circumcision line, causing a secondary phimosis. This needs Urology follow-up.
  - Plastibell complications: When the Plastibell does not completely separate, which would require Urology to release it from the retained skin. The Plastibell can also slip proximally and become trapped on the glans causing distal edema, this requires emergent Urology consultation when seen.
  - Adhesions: Minor adhesions are common and resolve with time. Skin bridges can form and will require lysis on an elective basis if they are symptomatic.
  - Parental concerns: If the family is not satisfied with the cosmetic result, they can follow up with Urology.

## NEWBORN SCREENS

- Prior to discharge and recommended no earlier than 24 hours of life, the following screens should be obtained for all infants: hearing screen, CCHD (critical congenital heart disease screening), state Newborn Screen, and bilirubin level.
- Hearing screen: All infants should be screened prior to discharge via OAE (Oto-acoustic Emissions Testing) or ABR (Auditory Brain Stem Response).
  - OAE can be used as a screening examination for all infants.
  - ABR should be used for those who fail OAE, have an APGAR of 0-4 at 1 minute or 0-6 at 5 minutes, malformations of head or neck (cleft lip, cleft palate, ear malformations excluding ear pits and tags), family history of hearing impairment, Trisomy 21.
  - It is recommended that infants that qualify for an ABR, excluding failed OAE, have a repeat hearing screen at 12 months of life.
- Critical congenital heart disease screening
  - Pulse oximeter should be placed on right hand and either foot.

- Pass: Per AAP guidelines, pass is ≥95% in the right hand or foot and ≤3% differential between right hand and foot.
- Repeat screen: Oxygen saturation is <95% in the right hand and/or foot OR >3% absolute difference exists in oxygen saturation between the right hand and foot. Repeat screening is recommended 1 hour after the previous screen and for a total of three measures.
- Fail: <90% in hand or foot, oxygen saturation is <95% in the right hand and foot on three measures, each separated by 1 hour, or >3% absolute difference exists in oxygen saturation between the right hand and foot on three measures, each separated by 1 hour. Workup for hypoxia would be indicated at this time, including an echocardiogram.
- Newborn screen: Should be obtained at 24-48 hours of life.
- Bilirubin screen: Please obtain on day of discharge. Please see "Hyperbilirubinemia."

## DISCHARGE READINESS

- Well-established feeding plan and weight loss assessed with NEWT tool
- Voiding and stooling well
- Vital sign stability and sepsis risk assessed
- Anticipatory guidance given to families
- Completion of screenings
- Follow up with a pediatrician established

## SUGGESTED READINGS

American Academy of Pediatrics. In: Kimberlin DW, Brady MT, Jackson MA, et al., eds. Red Book: 2018 Report of the Committee on Infectious Diseases. 31st Ed. Elk Grove Village, IL: American Academy of Pediatrics, 2018.

American Academy of Pediatrics Task Force on Circumcision. Circumcision policy statement. Pediatrics 2012;130(3):585–586. doi: 10.1542/peds.2012-1989.

Ballard JL, Khoury JC, Wedig K, et al. New Ballard Score, expanded to include extremely premature infants. J Pediatr 1991;119(3):417–423. doi: 10.1016/s0022-3476(05)82056-6.

Benitz WE; Committee on Fetus and Newborn, American Academy of Pediatrics. Hospital stay for healthy term newborn infants. Pediatrics 2015;135(5):948–953. doi: 10.1542/peds.2015-0699.

Diller CL, Kelleman MS, Kupke KG, et al. A modified algorithm for critical congenital heart disease screening using pulse oximetry. Pediatrics 2018;141(5):e20174065. doi: 10.1542/peds.2017-4065.

Gartner LM, Greer FR; Section on Breastfeeding, Committee on Nutrition. Prevention of rickets and vitamin D deficiency: new guidelines for vitamin D intake. Pediatrics 2003;111(4):908–910. doi: 10.1542/peds.111.4.908.

Hall RT, Carroll RE. Infant feeding. Pediatr Rev 2000;21(6):191–200. doi: 10.1542/pir.21-6-191.

Knox I. Tongue tie and frenotomy in the breastfeeding newborn. NeoReviews 2010;11(9):e513–e519. doi: 10.1542/neo.11-9-e513.

Kocherlakota P. Neonatal abstinence syndrome. Pediatrics 2014;134(2):e547–e561. doi: 10.1542/peds.2013-3524.

Lauer BJ, Spector ND. Hyperbilirubinemia in the newborn. Pediatr Rev 2011;32(8):341–349. doi: 10.1542/pir.32-8-341.

Lewis CW, Jacob LS, Lehmann CU; Section on Oral Health. The primary care pediatrician and the care of children with cleft lip and/or cleft palate. Pediatrics 2017;139(5):e20170628. doi: 10.1542/peds.2017-0628. Erratum in: Pediatrics 2017;140(3):null.

Mackara N. (2021, January 11). PHM3 Do not initiate phototherapy in term or late PRETERM well-appearing infants WITH neonatal Hyperbilirubinemia if Their Bilirubin is below levels at which the AAP guidelines recommend treatment: Choosing Wisely. Available at https://www.choosingwisely.org/clinician-lists/phm3do-not-initiate-phototherapy-in-term-or-late-preterm-well-appearing-infants-with-neonatal-hyperbilirubinemia-if-their-bilirubin-is-below-levels-at-which-the-aap-guidelines-recommend-treatment/?highlight=phm. Last accessed on 4/30/21.

Newborn weight loss tool. (n.d.). Available at https://www.newbornweight.org/. Last accessed on 4/30/21.

Puopolo KM, Benitz WE, Zaoutis TE; Committee on Fetus and Newborn, Committee on Infectious Diseases. Management of neonates born at ≥35 0/7 weeks' gestation with suspected or proven early-onset bacterial sepsis. Pediatrics 2018;142(6):e20182894. doi: 10.1542/peds.2018-2894.

Tobian AAR, Gray RH, Quinn TC. Male circumcision for the prevention of acquisition and transmission of sexually transmitted infections: the case for neonatal circumcision. Arch Pediatr Adolesc Med 2010;164(1):78–84. doi: 10.1001/archpediatrics.2009.232.

Warren JB, Phillipi CA. Care of the well newborn. Pediatr Rev 2012;33(1):4–18. doi: 10.1542/pir.33-1-4.

Weston PJ, Harris DL, Battin M, et al. Oral dextrose gel for the treatment of hypoglycaemia in newborn infants. Cochrane Database Syst Rev 2016;(5):CD011027. doi: 10.1002/14651858.CD011027.pub2.

Wickremasinghe AC, Kuzniewicz MW, McCulloch CE, et al. Efficacy of subthreshold newborn phototherapy during the birth hospitalization in preventing readmission for phototherapy. JAMA Pediatr 2018;172(4):378–385. doi: 10.1001/jamapediatrics.2017.5630.

# Emergencies

Anne Marie Anderson and Tara Conway Copper

## INTRODUCTION

Patients presenting to the emergency unit (EU) often have undifferentiated illness with broad differential diagnoses. The severity of their presentations is variable and requires rapid assessment to determine the urgency of interventions and initial management.

### The Pediatric Assessment Triangle
- The Pediatric Assessment Triangle is a tool that allows for a rapid global assessment of patients using only visual and auditory clues even before any history is obtained.
- The three components of the Pediatric Assessment Triangle are appearance, work of breathing, and circulation to the skin (Fig. 3-1).
- If any of these categories are abnormal, the child is considered unstable, and more immediate intervention is needed. If all these areas are normal, the child is stable, and more time can be taken to assess for the etiology of the child's illness before intervention is required (Fig. 3-2).

#### Appearance
- Assess for age-appropriate tone, level of interaction, consolability, look or gaze (do they fix and follow, or do they have a blank stare?), speech (child), or cry (infant).
- An isolated abnormality of appearance may indicate altered mental status and may point to a central nervous system or metabolic abnormality.

#### Work of Breathing
- Assess for nasal flaring, retractions, abnormal airway sounds, or grunting.
- A child with increased work of breathing without abnormal appearance or circulation is in respiratory distress. Airway repositioning, suctioning, oxygen, or breathing treatments may be indicated depending on the cause of their respiratory distress.
- However, the combination of increased work of breathing and lethargy (abnormal appearance) may indicate respiratory failure. An advanced airway may be necessary.

#### Circulation to the Skin
- Assess for pallor, cyanosis, or mottling.
- Signs of poor circulation alone may be indicative of a shock state.
- The addition of altered appearance or alertness to poor circulation may indicate decompensated shock.

## CARDIOPULMONARY FAILURE

- Patients with the combination of abnormal appearance work of breathing, and circulation to the skin are suspected to be in cardiopulmonary failure and potentially on the verge of cardiac arrest.

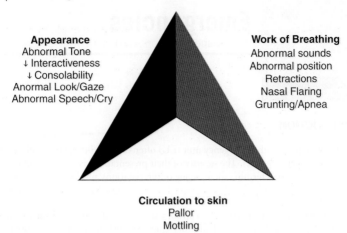

**Figure 3-1. Pediatric assessment triangle.** This tool allows for rapid assessment of children. (Adapted from Dieckmann RA, Brownstein D, Gausche-Hill M. The pediatric assessment triangle: a novel approach for the rapid evaluation of children. Pediatr Emerg Care 2010;26(4):312–315.)

• Cardiopulmonary failure and cardiac arrest can progress from initial states of isolated respiratory distress or failure, shock, or altered mental status. Most commonly in pediatrics, hypoxia from respiratory failure causes bradycardia, followed by cardiac arrest.
• In cases where you suspect cardiopulmonary failure and impending arrest, call for assistance and immediately begin resuscitation.

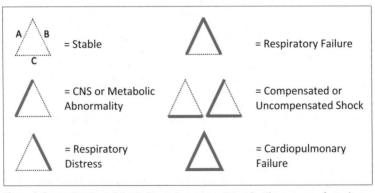

**Figure 3-2. Application of the Pediatric Assessment Triangle.** The presence of any abnormality (bolded line) in one or more sides of the Pediatric Assessment Triangle in Figure 3-1 suggests the underlying physiologic problem. A = Appearance, B = Work of Breathing, C = Circulation to the skin.

## Differential Diagnosis

- While providing resuscitation, a designated team member should obtain a rapid, focused history that can further guide resuscitation efforts.
- Based on history, the etiology of cardiopulmonary failure or cardiac arrest may be known, but consider the following differential for patients:
  - Trauma: motor vehicle crashes, burns, child abuse, firearms
  - Pulmonary: asthma, bronchiolitis, pneumonia, foreign body aspiration, smoke inhalation, drowning, acute respiratory distress syndrome (ARDS)
  - Infectious: sepsis, meningitis
  - Endocrine: diabetic ketoacidosis, adrenal failure
  - Central nervous system: head trauma, seizures, stroke, increased intracranial pressure, intracranial hemorrhage or mass
  - Cardiac: congenital heart disease, myocarditis
  - Others: sudden infant death syndrome (SIDS), poisoning, suicide, dehydration, congenital anomalies
- In your differential and work-up, consider the reversible causes of cardiac arrest, known as the Hs and Ts.
  - H: Hypovolemia, hypoxia, hypoglycemia, hypo/hyperkalemia, hydrogen ion (acidosis), hypothermia
  - T: Tension pneumothorax, tamponade, toxins, and thrombosis (pulmonary and coronary)

## Treatment

- Patients who receive delayed resuscitation or who present in asystole have a poor prognosis.
- All resuscitation begins with support of ventilation and circulation. Begin cardiopulmonary resuscitation (CPR) immediately in patients without a pulse or bradycardia with poor perfusion (Table 3-1).
- Identify and correct any reversible causes (Hs and Ts). Addressing Hs and Ts may help achieve return of spontaneous circulation (ROSC).
- Focus on providing high-quality CPR with minimal pauses. Target between 100 and 120 compressions per minute, at a depth of 1/3 to 1/2 the anterior-posterior diameter of the chest (approximately 1.5 inches in infants, 2 inches in children, and at least 2 inches in teenagers and adults). Make sure to allow full recoil of the chest. Assigning a CPR coach who gives feedback about depth and rate of compressions can help improve CPR efficacy.
- The goal of CPR is to optimize flow of oxygenated blood through the coronary arteries to the myocardium to achieve return of both electrical and mechanical cardiac function (ROSC). Effective cardiac compressions also deliver oxygenated blood to the brain and other essential organs.
- Minimize interruption of compressions. Each time compressions are stopped, blood flow through the coronary arteries stops, and upon resuming CPR, it takes several compressions to achieve return of optimal coronary perfusion.
- When an advanced airway is not in place, the ratio of compressions to ventilations is 30:2 for single rescuer and 15:2 for two-rescuer CPR. During CPR with an advanced airway, target a respiratory rate of 1 breath every 2-3 seconds (20-30 breaths per minute), accounting for age and clinical condition. Overventilation can compromise cardiac output.
- Refer to the American Heart Association's Pediatric Advanced Life Support (PALS) program for guidelines regarding the use of vasoactive medications and defibrillation during resuscitation.

| TABLE 3-1 | Basic Techniques of Pediatric Life Support |
|---|---|
| **Assess patient** <br> • Not breathing or only gasping <br> • No pulse palpated within 10 sec (carotid in adults, brachial or femoral in children) <br> • Call for help, AED | |
| **Compressions** | • Lower half of the sternum in child and adult <br> • One finger width below the mammary line in infants <br> • Two hands in adults, heel of one hand in child <br> • Two thumbs encircling the chest in infant with two rescuers <br> • Depth: at least 2 inches or 1/3 to 1/2 the AP diameter in adult, about 1.5 inches in child, or 1/3 to 1/2 the AP diameter in infant <br> • Rate: 100–120 compressions per minute <br> • Allow full chest recoil between compressions |
| **Airway** | • Position airway: head tilt-chin lift |
| **Breathing** (after first 30 compressions) | • 2 breaths at 1 sec per breath |
| **Compression/ventilation ratio** | No advanced airway: <br> • Single rescuer 30:2 <br> • Two rescuers: 15:2 up to puberty then 30:2 <br> After intubation: <br> • ~8–10 breaths/min, 1 breath every 6–8 sec, asynchronous with compressions |

Adapted from Topjian AA, Raymond TT, Atkins D, et al. Part 4: Pediatric basic and advanced life support: 2020 American Heart Association guidelines for cardiopulmonary resuscitation and emergency cardiovascular care. Circulation 2020;142 (16_suppl_2):S469-S523.

## ALTERED MENTAL STATUS

• Altered mental status is indicative of a CNS or metabolic process and has a broad differential.
• Take a focused history to help narrow the differential. Focus should include history of trauma, ingestion, seizures, neurologic deficits, prolonged fasting, and infectious symptoms.

### Differential Diagnosis

• CNS: Stroke, seizure, head trauma, increased intracranial pressure (ICP), CNS infection, ingestion (toxin or drug)
• Metabolic: Hypoglycemia, acidosis (sepsis, diabetic ketoacidosis, hypercarbia), uremia

## Physical Examination

- Note heart rate, blood pressure, respiratory pattern, and temperature. The combination of hypertension, bradycardia, and irregular respirations comprise Cushing triad, a late (near terminal) sign of increased ICP.
- Assess for pupillary size and response, focal neurologic signs, abnormal posturing, signs of trauma, and rash.
- Assign a Glasgow Coma Scale score (GCS). Note that this tool is only validated in the setting of trauma (Table 3-2).

## Work-Up

- Obtain a bedside glucose. Based on the clinical picture, consider CBC, electrolytes, transaminases, ammonia, lactate, venous blood gas, toxicology screen, and blood, urine and CSF cultures.
- If blood sugar is low without apparent etiology, quickly obtain critical hypoglycemia labs (see Chapter 18, Endocrinology for full list) and then correct hypoglycemia.
- In infants, also consider obtaining pyruvate, plasma amino acids and urine organic acids to assess for a possible inborn error of metabolism.
- Consider head CT or MRI depending on suspected cause of the neurologic insult.

| TABLE 3-2 | Glasgow Coma Scale | | | |
|-----------|--------------------|---|---|---|
| | **Infant** | | **Child/adult** | |
| **Eye** | | | | |
| | Spontaneous opening | 4 | Spontaneous opening | 4 |
| | Opens to speech | 3 | Opens to speech | 3 |
| | Opens to pain | 2 | Opens to pain | 2 |
| | None | 1 | None | 1 |
| **Verbal** | | | | |
| | Babbles | 5 | Spontaneous appropriate speech | 5 |
| | Irritable | 4 | Confused | 4 |
| | Cries to pain | 3 | Inappropriate words | 3 |
| | Grunts/moans to pain | 2 | Incomprehensible sound | 2 |
| | None | 1 | None | 1 |
| **Motor** | | | | |
| | Spontaneous movement | 6 | Obeys commands | 6 |
| | Localizes pain | 5 | Localizes pain | 5 |
| | Withdraws to pain | 4 | Withdraws to pain | 4 |
| | Decorticate flexion | 3 | Decorticate flexion | 3 |
| | Decerebrate extension | 2 | Decerebrate extension | 2 |
| | None | 1 | None | 1 |

## Treatment

- Support airway, breathing, and circulation (ABCs). Consider the use of an oral or nasopharyngeal airway for patients who are breathing spontaneously but have poor tone. If not protecting their airway or spontaneously breathing, most patients can be ventilated effectively using a bag and mask. Tracheal intubation may be necessary in the unresponsive patient to provide prolonged ventilation and decrease aspiration risk.
- If blood sugar is <40-60 mg/dL, administer dextrose intravenously (D10 at 2 mL/kg or D25 at 1 mL/kg). Repeat blood glucose in 15 minutes and repeat administration of dextrose as necessary.
- Consider naloxone for suspected opioid overdose. Flumazenil is appropriate for benzodiazepine overdose, but be aware that seizures may result. See Chapter 4, Poisonings for description of opioid and benzodiazepine toxidromes.
- If infection is suspected, start broad-spectrum antibiotics.

## TRAUMA

- Unintentional injury is the most common cause of death in children beyond the first year of life.
- In children ages 1-4, drowning is the most common cause of death.
- Otherwise, motor vehicle collisions (MVCs) are the leading cause of trauma-related deaths in children.
- When assessing a patient presenting with trauma, examination and initiation of interventions often precedes obtaining the history. When appropriate, the following elements of a focused history should be obtained. The mnemonic SAMPLE may be used: Symptoms, Allergies, Medications, Past medical history, Last oral intake, and Events leading up to the injury
  - Obtain information about the specific mechanism of injury, use of helmet, and loss of consciousness.
  - For MVCs, inquire about the speed of the vehicles involved, the side of impact relative to the patient, the degree of vehicle damage, whether or not the patient was restrained with an age-appropriate seat belt, if there was ejection from the vehicle, and the presence of injury or death in other passengers. These elements may help predict the severity of injury.

### Preparing for trauma patients

- For known critically ill trauma patients, prepare the trauma bay ahead of arrival. Set up monitors and airway equipment, and gather needed supplies based on the patient's known injuries.
- Gather a team of providers. In some institutions, a trauma page may alert a trauma team including trauma surgery. Identify a team leader and assign specific roles for the resuscitation. Ensure closed loop communication throughout evaluation of the patient.

### Primary Survey and Management of the Trauma Patient (ABCs)

The following algorithm is used in Advanced Trauma Life Support (ATLS) to assess trauma patients. It guides providers sequentially through assessment of a patient's Airway, Breathing, Circulation, Disability, and Exposure (ABCDE), with intervention provided at each step when needed. This is called the Primary Survey. ATLS is designed for resource-limited situations with fewer providers. In areas without resource limitation, the primary survey occurs simultaneously with resuscitation.

### Airway
- Assess airway patency. If the patient is able to speak, their airway is likely adequately protected. Inspect for blood, foreign objects, or loose teeth in the mouth.
- Intubate if necessary. Generally, advanced airways are placed in patients with GCS < 8, an absent gag reflex, oropharyngeal or airway trauma or edema, in those likely to receive prolonged ventilatory support, or when bag mask ventilation is difficult.
- Immobilize the cervical spine with an appropriately sized cervical collar or manual immobilization. In-line stabilization of the cervical spine is needed during placement of an advanced airway.

### Breathing
- Administer supplemental oxygen.
- Listen for symmetric breath sounds. Inspect the chest for symmetric chest rise, tracheal deviation, or open wounds. If pneumothorax is suspected, perform a needle decompression and consider chest tube placement.
- Consider orogastric tube placement to decompress the stomach.

### Circulation
- Heart rate and capillary refill are the best indicators of circulatory status in children. Hypotension occurs late. Cardiac output is maintained by tachycardia and increased systemic vascular resistance until compensatory mechanisms are overwhelmed.
- Apply direct pressure with sterile gauze to bleeding wounds. Consider the use of a tourniquet if bleeding is not controlled.
- Insert two large-bore intravenous (IV) catheters. Rate of fluid administration is directly proportional to the catheter's radius to the fourth power and inversely proportional to its length, so short, thick catheters are best suited for trauma resuscitations.
- Insert one or more intraosseous needles or a central venous line if peripheral IV access is delayed or the patient is unstable.
- Administer a rapid infusion of warmed isotonic fluid (normal saline or lactated Ringer's) of up to 20 mL/kg or 1 L maximum for adult-sized patients. Rapid infusion can be achieved with a pressure bag, push-pull system, or a rapid infusion device.
- If the patient remains unstable and blood loss is likely, give non–cross matched blood products and obtain emergent surgical consultation. Continue judicious blood product transfusion to maintain adequate perfusion, while also weighing that aggressive resuscitation before achieving control of bleeding is associated with increased mortality. Refer to your institution's policy regarding criteria for activation of a massive transfusion protocol, which promotes balanced resuscitation with 1:1:1 ratio of packed red blood cells to platelets and fresh frozen plasma.

### Disability
- Determine the following:
  - Level of consciousness. Assign a GCS.
  - Assess pupil size, equality, and responsiveness to light.
  - Assess muscle tone and strength.

### Exposure
- Expose the skin.
- Remove all clothing and keep the patient warm.

## Secondary Survey

- During your assessment, keep in mind potential sources of massive hemorrhage: external wounds and internal bleeding within the head, the chest, the abdomen, the retroperitoneum, the pelvis, and long bone fractures.
- Remove all clothing and perform a thorough head-to-toe evaluation looking for the following findings. This is called the Secondary Survey.
  - Neurologic: altered mental status, decreased GCS, abnormal muscle tone and sensation, decreased rectal tone sensation, rectal tone
  - Head-ear-eyes-nose-throat (HEENT): scalp, skull, or facial injury, signs of basilar skull fracture including bilateral periorbital ecchymosis (raccoon eyes) or mastoid ecchymosis (battle sign), hemotympanum (sign of temporal bone fracture), cerebrospinal fluid leak from the nose or ears, asymmetric pupil size or abnormal pupillary response, absent corneal reflex, hyphema, cervical spine tenderness or deformity, deviated trachea
  - Chest/abdomen/pelvis: clavicular deformity or tenderness, diminished breath sounds, distant or abnormal heart tones, rib tenderness or deformity, chest wall a symmetry, subcutaneous emphysema, abdominal tenderness or distension, bloody orogastric aspirates, splenic tenderness, pelvic instability
  - Genitourinary: blood in rectal vault or at the urethral meatus
  - Back: (patient log-rolled to their side with cervical spine stabilized) step-off along spinal column, tenderness along spine
  - Extremities: deformity or point tenderness, compartment syndrome (5 Ps: pain with passive movement of fingers/toes, paresthesia, pallor, pulselessness, poikilothermia)
  - Skin: delayed capillary refill, lacerations, abrasions, contusions, burns

## Laboratory Studies and Imaging

- Order the following laboratory tests:
  - CBC, CMP, type and cross, lipase, urinalysis, VBG, PT/PTT.
  - Consider a toxicology screen, ethanol level, and a urine pregnancy test.
- Obtain the following imaging:
  - Plain films: chest, pelvis, any extremity with pain or deformity, and cervical spine if not obtaining a cervical spine CT
  - Abdominal/pelvis CT with IV contrast
    - Consider obtaining in patients with blunt torso trauma, those who are complaining of pain, have tenderness on examination, have cutaneous abdominal or thoracic findings including seat belt sign, have diminished breath sounds, are vomiting, or have GCS < 13. Also obtain in injured patients with an AST or ALT > 200 units/L. Use an imaging threshold of AST or ALT > 80 units/L in patients with nonaccidental trauma.
  - Consider an emergent bedside echocardiogram if there is poor cardiac output despite volume administration, or distended neck veins as these findings may be indicative of cardiac tamponade.
  - Head CT: See imaging recommendations in section below, "Traumatic Brian Injury".
  - Additional imaging: Further CT imaging, including with angiography, may be needed.

## TRAUMATIC BRAIN INJURY

- When assessing for traumatic brain injury (TBI), carefully evaluate for external signs of trauma, altered mental status, and signs of focal neurologic symptoms. In the history, note the mechanism of injury and any history of loss of consciousness, vomiting, and severe headache. These elements guide decision-making about obtaining a head CT.

| TABLE 3-3 | PECARN Head CT Guidelines | |
|---|---|---|
| | **Younger than 2 years** | **2 years or older** |
| **Head CT recommended** | Altered mental status (or) | Altered mental status (or) |
| | GCS < 15 (or) | GCS < 15 (or) |
| | Palpable skull fracture | Signs of basilar skull fracture |
| **Observation vs. head CT** | LOC > 5 sec (or) | History of LOC (or) |
| | Nonfrontal scalp hematoma (or) | History of vomiting (or) |
| | Not acting normally (or) | Severe headache (or) |
| | Severe mechanism[a] | Severe mechanism[a] |
| **No head CT** | None of the above features present | None of the above features present |

[a]Severe mechanism: Head struck by high-impact object, pedestrian struck by motor vehicle, MVC if ejected, death of passenger, rollover, fall > 3 feet (<2 years) or >5 feet (≥2 years), bicyclist without helmet struck by motor vehicle (≥2 years only).
Adapted from Kuppermann N, Holmes JF, Dayan PS, et al. Identification of children at very low risk of clinically-important brain injuries after head trauma: a prospective cohort study. Lancet 2009;374(9696):1160–1170.

- The decision to obtain a head CT is guided by the Pediatric Emergency Care Applied Research Network (PECARN) Head Injury Algorithm. This stratifies the risk of intracranial injury to determine which children are at low risk for clinically important TBI and, therefore, do not require head CT.
- The algorithm guides providers to obtain a CT in children with a palpable skull fracture, signs of basilar skull fracture, altered mental status, or GCS < 15. (Table 3-3).

## Types of Injury
- TBI is often classified based on severity, taking into account GCS, duration of LOC, and imaging.
  - Severe TBI (GCS 3-8)
    - Patients have severely altered mental status requiring intubation and ventilation.
    - Head CT often shows a significant injury requiring neurosurgical intervention and ICP monitoring.
  - Moderate TBI (GCS 9-12)
    - Generally associated with prolonged loss of consciousness, focal neurologic deficits, and abnormal findings on head CT.
  - Mild TBI (GCS ≥ 13)
    - Patients typically have only temporary alterations in consciousness, normal neuroimaging, and no focal neurologic deficits.
    - This type of injury is often referred to as a concussion. Patients with concussions can have a variety of symptoms including headache, confusion, amnesia, double vision, nausea, vomiting, slurred speech, balance issues, personality changes, and sleep disturbances. These symptoms resolve over time with rest.

*Epidural Hematoma*
- Extra-axial collection of blood located between the dura and skull.
- Lens-shaped opacity on CT.
- An associated skull fracture is common, most often overlying the middle meningeal artery.
- Natural history includes a loss of consciousness followed by a lucid interval then decreasing responsiveness, usually within 2-3 hours. If not surgically drained urgently, it may result in rapid deterioration and herniation.
- Infants may take longer to show lethargy because open sutures separate to accommodate mass effect of an expanding hematoma.

*Subdural Hematoma*
- Extra-axial collection of blood located under the dura and over the brain, often associated with cerebral contusion, cerebral edema, or more significant brain injury than epidural hematoma.
- Crescent-shaped opacity on CT.
- Typically caused by injury to a bridging vein.
- Usually there is no lucid interval.
- Large lesions and those causing midline shift typically require neurosurgical evacuation.

*Subarachnoid Hemorrhage*
- Extra-axial collection of blood between the arachoid and pia mater.
- Traumatic subarachnoid hemorrhage is more commonly seen in the cerebral sulci than in the Sylvian fissure or basal cisterns on CT.

*Contusion*
- Often associated with skull fractures.
- Focal symptoms may be present at site of injury or at contrecoup site.

**Management**

*Moderate and Severe TBI*
- In all patients with TBI, ensure oxygenation, normalize ventilation, prevent hypotension, and maintain midline cervical spine positioning with head of bed elevated to 30 degrees to minimize secondary brain injury.
- Patients with a GCS of 8 or less (severe TBI) should be immediately intubated.
- Quickly identify lesions requiring neurosurgical intervention.
- Identify patients with signs of increased ICP including hypertension, bradycardia, and irregular breathing (Cushing triad), and pupillary changes, which may indicate impending herniation.
- While awaiting neurosurgical intervention, osmotic solutions including hypertonic saline and mannitol can be used to lower ICP. Hyperventilation can also be used as a temporizing measure, but be aware that this reduces cerebral blood flow.

*Mild TBI (Concussion)*
- Limiting aerobic and cognitive exertion is essential to optimizing recovery after concussion.
- Patients should be advised to follow a return to play protocol in which they return to activities in a stepwise manner based on resolution of symptoms.
  - For the first few days, patients should practice full cognitive and physical rest.
  - Patients and parents should monitor for resolution of the cognitive and physical symptoms and as they begin to feel better, gradually return to regular (nonstrenuous) activities.
  - Activity may then progress to light aerobic activity, then moderate then heavy sport-specific noncontact training, followed by full contact training, and finally competitive play.

- Each step should last a minimum of 24 hours, and athletes should only move to the next step if they do not have any new symptoms at the current step.
- This progression should be halted with return of symptoms, whereby patients should return to the last step in which they were symptom free.
- When discharging patients with concussions, be certain that the parents understand care instructions, warning signs, and anticipated symptoms. It is not necessary to instruct parents to wake children periodically during the night. Indicators for seeking medical attention include persistent headache, persistent vomiting, drowsiness, weakness, blurry or double vision, or ataxia. Irritability or change in behavior, neck pain, seizures, fever, and watery discharge from the nose or ears warrant return to the ED for repeat medical evaluation.

## NECK INJURIES

In any patient presenting with trauma, especially TBI, always evaluate for cervical spine fracture or dislocation.

### Diagnosis and Treatment

- Immobilize the cervical spine with a properly fitted cervical collar. A spine board is unnecessary.
- The cervical spine can be cleared without radiographs if the following criteria are met:
  - The patient is alert and responds to commands.
  - There is no midline neck pain on palpation.
  - The neurologic examination is normal.
  - There is no major distracting injury (e.g., long bone fracture).
- If imaging is obtained, the cervical collar should be left in place during imaging.
- Plain radiographs (anteroposterior, lateral, and open mouth views) can be used to clear C-spine precautions in the following patients:
  - Patients with normal mental status, who do not have focal neurologic complaints or findings on physical examination, and cervical spine tenderness is resolved.
  - Patients with limited range of motion or complaints of midline tenderness.
  - Also consider in patients with significant torso injury, high-risk MVC, diving injury, or predisposing conditions including Down syndrome.
- CT of the cervical spine should be considered in the following patients:
  - Patients with altered mental status.
  - Patients with persistent focal neurologic complaints.
  - Patients with abnormal plain radiographs.
- If there are symptoms of spinal cord injury, consult neurosurgery, and obtain a non-contrast MRI of the cervical spine to rule out spinal cord hematoma, edema, and stenosis.
- Patients can return to play when they have a full, pain-free range of motion, normal strength and sensation, normal lordosis of the cervical spine, and have been able to be cleared from their cervical collar.

## BURNS

- Classified by burn severity
  - Superficial (formerly 1st degree): involves the epidermis only; painful and erythematous.
  - Partial thickness (formerly 2nd degree): involves the epidermis and dermis, sparing dermal appendages. Superficial partial-thickness burns are red, blistered and painful. The erythema blanches with pressure. Healing occurs within

about 3 weeks with minimal scarring. Deep partial-thickness burns may be white and painless, do not blanch with pressure, and may require grafting. Healing occurs in 3-8 weeks, with scarring.
* Full thickness (formerly 3rd degree): involves full skin thickness and subcutaneous structures. Full-thickness burns are leathery and painless, often requiring grafting.
* Obtain history about the mechanism of the injury including how long they may have been entrapped in a closed space, and history of electrical or chemical burns.

## Diagnosis and Treatment

* Early initiation of fluid resuscitation, identification of associated injuries, and referral to pediatric burn center are key to optimizing outcome.
* Morbidity and mortality are largely determined by the body surface area involved (BSA), depth of burn, and presence or absence of airway injury.
* Use a burn chart to estimate BSA of burns. The Modified Lund-Browder Chart is preferred over the Rule of Nines for children (Fig. 3-3).
* As with all trauma patients, first manage their ABCs.
  * Airway
    ○ Evaluate for signs of potential inhalational injury including facial burns, singed nares, carbonaceous material in nares or mouth, cough, hoarseness, shortness of breath, or wheezing.
    ○ Administer humidified oxygen.
    ○ Airway edema and obstruction may be imminent if any of the above findings are present. Intubate early if airway is involved.
  * Breathing: Monitor closely for signs of distress.
    ○ May be compromised in the setting of altered consciousness, toxin exposure, or circumferential burns of the chest or abdomen.
    ○ Pulse oximeters overestimate arterial oxygenation if the carbon monoxide level is significant. Obtain $PaO_2$ from an arterial blood gas measurement.
  * Circulation
    ○ Give a 20 mL/kg bolus of isotonic fluid (normal saline or lactated Ringer's) if involved BSA is >10% in infants or >15% in children. Patients with burns >15% TBSA will require additional fluids, per modified Parkland formula. See Fluid Management section below.
    ○ If hypotensive, first manage according to trauma principles. Maintain at least 1 mL/kg/hr urine output.
* Obtain a CBC, and electrolytes, type and screen, and blood gas in patients with significant burns. Obtain a carboxyhemoglobin level and arterial blood gas in patients who sustained flame burns in an enclosed space to assess for carbon monoxide toxicity.

### Fluid Management

* For burns with 15% or greater TBSA, additional fluid resuscitation is needed.
  * Use modified Parkland formula (plus maintenance fluids) to calculate estimated fluid needs for the first 24 hours after the burn.
  * Modified Parkland fluid volume = 3 mL LR x weight (kg) x % TBSA partial- and full-thickness burns
  * Give half of the Parkland fluid volume over the first 8 hours since the time of the burn, subtracting any fluids given previously by emergency personnel or the trauma team.
  * Give the other half of the Parkland volume over the subsequent 16 hours.
  * Parkland fluid volume should be given in addition to maintenance IV fluids (D5LR).
  * Modified Parkland fluid calculations form an estimate of fluids needed. Titrate to age-appropriate urine output. The maintenance fluids should not be titrated.

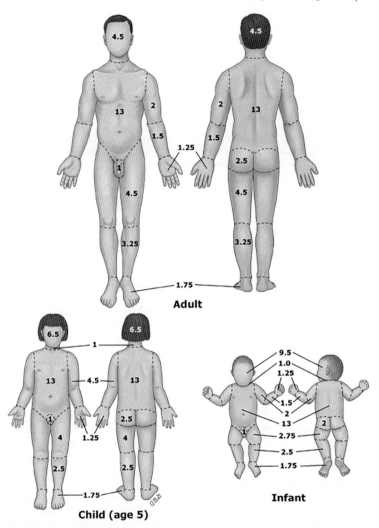

**Figure 3-3. Modified Lund Browder chart.** (Reprinted from Rice PL, Orgill DP. Assessment and classification of burn injury. In UpToDate, Post TW (Ed), UpToDate, Waltham, MA, 2021. Copyright © 2021 UpToDate, Inc. and its affiliates and/or licensors. All rights reserved.)

*Secondary Burn Management*
- Provide appropriate analgesia. Consider IV route for more severe burns.
- GI: Consider nasogastric tube placement and begin $H_2$ blocker for stress ulcer (Curling ulcer) prophylaxis.
- Consider inpatient burn management for the following patients. Keep in mind that the character of a burn may change over the first few days after the injury.
  - Burns >10% BSA in infants or >15% in children

- Electrical or chemical burns
- Burns that involve the face, hands, feet, perineum, or joints, or circumferential burns
- Inhalation injury
- Children with unsafe environment at home or uncertain follow-up

### Electrical and Chemical Burns

- Electrical burns often involve tissues in excess of the superficial skin damage. This may not be reflective of skin involvement.
  - Monitor for arrhythmias.
  - High voltage may cause rhabdomyolysis and development of compartment syndrome. This is more typical of industrial, not household, currents.
- Chemical burns require irrigation to wash away remaining chemicals on the patient. Remove all clothing as it may contain the chemical.

## CARBON MONOXIDE AND CYANIDE POISONING

- Inhalational injury is frequently encountered with fires in enclosed spaces.
- Carbon monoxide and cyanide are dangerous by-products produced during fires.

### Carbon Monoxide

- The need for CPR in burn patients is often indicative of high carbon monoxide levels or prolonged hypoxia.
- Carbon monoxide has a higher affinity for hemoglobin than oxygen, resulting in decreased oxyhemoglobin and decreased oxygen delivery to the tissues.
- Administer oxygen at 100% $FiO_2$ until a patient's carboxyhemoglobin level results, as carbon monoxide impairs the accuracy of $SpO_2$ monitors.
- Consult medical toxicology to discuss whether the patient is a candidate for hyperbaric oxygen therapy. Consider in those who are unconscious, have neurologic deficits, EKG with ischemic changes, severe acidosis, or carboxyhemoglobin >25%.

### Cyanide

- Cyanide is produced by combustion of many common household items including wool, silk, polyurethane found in insulation and upholstery, and plastics.
- Cyanide interferes with oxidative phosphorylation of the electron transport chain within cellular mitochondria resulting in inability to produce ATP and a shift to anaerobic metabolism. This leads to progressive metabolic acidosis.
- High levels of carboxyhemoglobin and cyanide impair utilization of oxyhemoglobin and may result in a bright red appearance of venous blood and a "cherry red" color of patients' skin. However, this finding is not reliable. Therefore, maintain a high clinical suspicion for carbon monoxide and cyanide toxicity following enclosed space fires.
- Cyanide toxicity can be treated with hydroxocobalamin (known as a Cyanokit). Know that hydroxocobalamin results in temporary red to purple discoloration of the urine, mucous membranes, and skin. The previous antidote of sodium thiosulfate and sodium nitrite are no longer routinely used due to risk of methemoglobinemia.

## DROWNING

- Drowning is defined as primary respiratory impairment from submersion or immersion in a liquid medium. The terms near-drowning, wet drowning, or dry drowning are no longer used. Rather, drowning is described as either fatal or nonfatal.

- Drowning is a leading cause of morbidity and mortality in children, with young children being most affected. Drowning can occur in large open bodies of water, pools, and also in small collections of water such as buckets and bathtubs when children are unsupervised.

## Pathophysiology

- In drowning victims, there is often initial panic and attempts to breath hold. Hypoxemia and hypercarbia result.
- Air hunger and hypercarbia trigger reflex breathing patterns resulting in aspiration of water and laryngospasm further contributing to hypoxemia.
- Hypothermia is often concomitant with drowning.
- Drowning has profound effects on many organ systems:
  - Pulmonary: Aspirated water disrupts surfactant, impairing pulmonary compliance and gas exchange. Pulmonary edema results from capillary and alveolar membrane damage.
  - CNS: Hypoxemia often leads to loss of consciousness. If persistently anoxic, permanent CNS damage can result within 4-6 minutes.
  - Cardiac: Progressive hypoxemia results in reduced myocardial oxygen delivery, peripheral vasoconstriction, and decline in cardiac output. Tissue hypothermia develops and causes further vasoconstriction, third spacing of fluids, and diuresis, which leads to intravascular hypovolemia and further worsening of cardiac output.
  - Tissue hypoxemia leads to metabolic acidosis, further impacting organ dysfunction.

## Management

- Management of all drowning victims should begin with assessment and management of ABCs.
  - Intubation is indicated in patients unable to protect their airway or in those unable to maintain oxygen saturations above 90% with noninvasive ventilation.
  - Oxygen should be administered at 100% $FiO_2$, even if the child has regained spontaneous ventilation, to mitigate tissue ischemia and acidosis.
  - Support hemodynamics with warmed crystalloid fluids and continue CPR if indicated.
- Neurologic status should be carefully assessed. Lack of pupillary response is associated with poor outcomes.
- Patients should be actively warmed to at least 32°C to optimize hemodynamic function. Subsequently, passive rewarming should be provided.
- A full trauma assessment should be performed. The cervical spine is rarely impacted unless there is history of diving into shallow water.
- Laboratory and imaging evaluation
  - Obtain a blood gas, electrolytes, and CBC.
  - Obtain a CXR.
  - Obtain cervical spine imaging only if history is concerning for neck trauma such as a dive into shallow water.
  - Head CT may be considered if signs of head trauma are present, or for altered mental status that is not otherwise explained by anoxic brain injury.
- Disposition
  - Patients without any respiratory distress, who have normal saturations on room air, normal CXR and pulmonary examination, and GCS of 15 should be observed for at least 6-12 hours and then may be discharged.

- Patients who do not meet the above criteria should be admitted to the floor or ICU depending on clinical status.
- Patient outcomes are often predicted by duration of submersion, amount of water aspirated, and the timeliness and effectiveness of initial resuscitation or CPR at the scene.

## HUMAN BITES

- Children may present for treatment of bites sustained from other children. Adult bites should raise suspicion for nonaccidental injury. If a bite mark needs to be investigated, photos of the bite with a proper measuring device should be obtained for further evaluation by a forensic analyst or dentist. Trace evidence collection for forensic laboratory DNA analysis may also be needed.
- The human mouth contains bacteria that can cause bites to become infected. The most common organisms involved are anaerobes, *Staphylococcus aureus*, and streptococci.
- Treatment
  - Use saline or a povidone-iodine solution to irrigate wounds. Approximately 150-200 mL of fluid per cm of laceration is needed, with 5-8 pounds per square inch (PSI) of pressure irrigation to adequately remove debris and reduce the risk of infection.
  - Leave the wound unsutured if it is not in a cosmetically important location.
  - If cosmetically significant, after irrigating the wound thoroughly, suture loosely, and inspect in 2-3 days for evidence of infection.
  - Do not use tissue adhesive due to high risk of infection.
  - Surgical exploration and washout is indicated for wounds with joint involvement.
  - Administer tetanus prophylaxis if necessary (Table 3-4).

| TABLE 3-4 | Tetanus Prophylaxis | |
|---|---|---|
| **Clinical scenario** | **Clean wound** | **Dirty, tetanus-prone wound** |
| Fully immunized and <5 years since last booster | None | None |
| Fully immunized and 5-10 years since last booster | None | Age appropriate tetanus containing vaccine[a] |
| Fully immunized and >10 years since last booster | Age appropriate tetanus containing vaccine[a] | Age appropriate tetanus containing vaccine[a] |
| Incompletely immunized or unknown | Age appropriate tetanus containing vaccine[b] | Age appropriate tetanus containing vaccine [a]and tetanus immunoglobulin |

[a]DTaP is recommended for children <7 years of age. Tdap is preferred to Td for persons aged 11 years or older who have not previously received Tdap.
[b]Persons aged 7 years or older who are not fully immunized against pertussis, tetanus, or diphtheria should receive one dose of Tdap (preferably the first) for wound management and as part of the catch-up series. If additional tetanus toxoid-containing doses are required, either Td or Tdap vaccine can be used.

- Consider antibiotic prophylaxis (amoxicillin-clavulanic acid or clindamycin and trimethoprim-sulfamethoxazole in those with penicillin allergy). Indications include for moderate or severe wounds, punctures, deep or closed facial bites, bites on hands, feet, or genitals, or in immunocompromised patients.

## ANIMAL BITES

- Determine circumstances of the injury, the state of health and vaccination status of the animal, and the current location of the animal.
  - Cat bitet: often a puncture wound and therefore more difficult to irrigate and at high risk for infection.
  - Dog bite: a crush-type injury resulting in infection-prone, devitalized tissue.
  - The mouths of dogs, cats, and other animals contain bacteria that can cause bites to become infected. The most common organisms involved are anaerobes, Staphylococcus aureus, group A streptococci, and Pasteurella multocida.
  - Bat bite: most commonly arises following discovery of a dead bat and uncertain circumstances of an actual "bite." Rabies prophylaxis is recommended if any possibility of a bat bite exists , or if a child is unable to reliably state whether they came into contact with the bat. Children sleep heavily and may not awaken from the presence of a small bat in their room, and a bat bite can be superficial and not easily noticed.
  - Contact the local health department to assess local risk of rabies.
  - Treatment: wound management is the same as for human bites.
  - Rabies prophylaxis should be considered when a domesticated animal cannot be monitored for at least 10 days following the bite. When monitoring is possible, defer postexposure prophylaxis. If the animal develops rabies symptoms during the observation period, it should be tested and postexposure prophylaxis should be initiated.
  - Rabies prophylaxis is also warranted following bites from certain high-risk animals including bats, skunks, raccoons, foxes, coyotes, bobcats, and woodchucks, if the animal cannot be tested. Other wildlife animals such as rabbits, squirrels, chipmunks, mice, and rats have low risk of harboring rabies and, therefore, postexposure prophylaxis is not indicated.
  - Rabies postexposure prophylaxis consists of rabies IVIG (injected into the wound) and rabies vaccine (given over days 0, 3, 7, and 14; injected at a site distant from the IVIG injection).

## LACERATIONS

- Most lacerations, including those on fingers and toes, can be anesthetized with topical gels, such as lidocaine (4%) plus epinephrine (1:1000) plus tetracaine (0.5%) (LET), to reduce patient anxiety.
- If additional local anesthesia is needed, lidocaine or lidocaine with epinephrine should be buffered 1:10 with standard 8.4% sodium bicarbonate and injected slowly using a 30-gauge needle to minimize injection pain.
- Many superficial hand and foot lacerations <2 cm in length that do not involve tendons or neurovascular structures heal well without need for suturing. Approximate wound edges with a bandage and keep dry and clean for 3-7 days.
- Choose suture type and size based on location of the injury. Most institutions have guidelines in place. When possible, use absorbable sutures to minimize the need for suture removal, which can cause further distress for children.

- Most lacerations can be repaired with simple interrupted sutures. Occasionally, deep sutures are needed to prevent large potential spaces.
- After repair, apply topical antibiotic ointment. Wounds can be gently washed and patted dry during healing. Give instructions to return for signs of infection. Once sutures are dissolved or removed, scarring can be mitigated by limiting sun exposure.

## INJURY PREVENTION

- Injury prevention strategies are essential in preventing traumatic injury in children. The following anticipatory guidance can help prevent significant morbidity and mortality.
- Children should always wear a helmet when riding a bicycle.
- Keep all medications, tools, and potentially dangerous equipment out of reach of children.

### Motor Vehicle Safety

- All infants and toddlers should be placed in a rear-facing car seat until they reach the weight or height specifications listed by the car seat manufacturer.
- Once children have outgrown rear-facing seats, children should be placed in a forward-facing car seat with a harness for as long as possible until they have reached the height or weight specifications listed by the car seat manufacturer. Most seats allow for children up to 65 lb or more.
- All children who have outgrown forward facing seats should be in a booster seat and seat belt with shoulder straps until they have reached a height of 4 feet 9 inches (57 inches) and are aged 8-12 years.
- Once children outgrow booster seats, they should be restrained in a shoulder and lap belt seat belt. All children younger than 13 years old should ride in the back seat.

### Drowning Prevention

- Children can drown even in a few inches of water.
- Children should be closely supervised in or near any pools, bodies of water, bathtubs, or standing water.
- Always empty buckets or kiddie pools after use.
- Remove pool toys after use to prevent tempting children from entering an unsupervised area.
- Encourage swimming lessons and water safety training.
- Encourage life vest use.
- All pools should have four-sided fencing or locking pool cover in place.

### Burn Prevention

- Ensure smoke alarms are functioning properly. Develop a home safety plan for fires.
- Keep working fire extinguishers in the home.
- Set hot water temperature to no more than 120°F.
- Never leave a heated stove unattended.

### Firearm Safety

- All firearms should be stored locked and unloaded with ammunition locked separately.

- Parents should be encouraged to inquire about the presence and storage of firearms prior to their child visiting the home of other family, friends, and neighbors.
- Children should be educated to not touch any firearm they see and inform an adult about its presence.

## PROCEDURAL SEDATION IN CHILDREN

- Indications and strategies for procedural sedation should be individualized in every patient. If procedural pain can be effectively managed with local anesthesia and/or oral analgesia, many children do not require sedation. For young children, allowing the parent to participate greatly reduces the child's anxiety and the need for sedation (e.g., suturing while a toddler sits in the parent's lap or provides distraction).
- For urgent and emergent procedures, the risks and benefits of sedation should be carefully considered, and the lightest effective sedation used. For children sedated in the ED, the risk of vomiting correlates poorly with the length of fasting. The risk of pulmonary aspiration is unknown but rare.
- Inhaled nitrous oxide or intranasal midazolam can respectively provide sedation and anxiolysis without the need for a frightening intravenous catheter. Nitrous oxide also has analgesic properties. When an IV is in place, ketamine can be used to achieve both sedation and analgesia.
- For additional information about sedation, see Chapter 31, Sedation.

## BEDSIDE ULTRASOUND

- Bedside point of care ultrasound (POCUS) is a tool with increasing utility and widespread application in Pediatric Emergency Medicine.
- Ultrasound is commonly used in the following clinical scenarios to guide diagnosis and management:
  - Skin and soft tissue infections: helpful to delineate the presence of a drainable fluid collection
  - E-FAST (Extended Focused Assessment with Sonography in Trauma) examination: can be useful in trauma to assess for free intraperitoneal or pericardial fluid and to evaluate for pneumothorax or pleural effusion (presumed to be hemothorax in trauma patients).
  - Bladder ultrasound: helpful to determine response to fluids, evidence of urinary retention, and likelihood of successful bladder catheterization
  - Cardiac examination
    - Bedside echocardiogram can be helpful for rapid assessment of myocardial contractility, the presence of effusion, and assessment of volume status.
    - Consider bedside ultrasound when cardiogenic shock is on your differential or if patients are not responding to fluid resuscitation as expected.
    - The compressibility of the IVC can help assess volume status.
- Ultrasound is also helpful for guidance in placing intravenous catheters and central lines.

## SUGGESTED READINGS

Chandy D, Weinhouse GL. Drowning (submersion injuries). In: Post TW, ed. UpToDate. Waltham, MA: UpToDate, 2021.

Dieckmann RA, Brownstein D, Gausche-Hill M. The pediatric assessment triangle. Pediatr Emerg Care 2010;26(4):312–315.

Fleisher GR, Ludwig S. Textbook of Pediatric Emergency Medicine. 8th Ed. Philadelphia, PA: Wolters Kluwer, 2020.

Halstead ME, Walter KD; The Council on Sports Medicine and Fitness. Sport-related concussion in children and adolescents. Pediatrics 2010;126:597–615.

Holmes JF, Lillis K, Monroe D, et al. Identifying children at very low risk of clinically important blunt abdominal injuries. Ann Emerg Med 2013;62(2):107–116.e2.

Jamshidi R, Sato T. Initial assessment and management of thermal burn injuries in children. Pediatr Rev 2013;34(9):395–404.

Kuppermann N, Holmes JF, Dayan PS, et al. Identification of children at very low risk of clinically-important brain injuries after head trauma: a prospective cohort study. Lancet 2009;374(9696):1160–1170.

Leonard JC, Kuppermann N, Olsen C, et al. Factors associated with cervical spine injury in children after blunt trauma. Ann Emerg Med 2011;58:145–155.

Mitaweh H, Bell MJ. Management of pediatric brain injury. Curr Treat Options Neurol 2015;17(5):348.

Quinn J, Cummings S, Callahan M, et al. Suturing versus conservative management of lacerations of the hand: randomized controlled trial. BMJ 2002;325:299–301.

Rice PL, Orgill DP. Assessment and classification of burn injury. In: Post TW, ed. UpToDate. Waltham, MA: UpToDate, 2021.

Rupprecht CE, Briggs D, Brown CM, et al. Use of a reduced (4-Dose) vaccine schedule for postexposure prophylaxis to prevent human rabies: recommendations of the advisory committee on immunization practices. MMWR Recomm Rep 2010;59(RR-2):1–9.

Shock and fluid resuscitation. In: Advanced Burn Life Support Course, Provider Manual. Chicago: American Burn Association, 2018:31–38.

Topijan AA, Raymond TT, Atkins D, et al. Part 4: pediatric basic life and advanced life support: 2020 American Heart Association guidelines for cardiopulmonary resuscitation and emergency cardiovascular care. Circulation 2020;142:S469–S523.

Trott A. Wounds and Lacerations: Emergency Care and Closure. 4th Ed. Philadelphia, PA: Saunders (Elsevier), 2012.

White NJ, Kim MK, Brousseau DC, et al. The anesthetic effectiveness of lidocaine-adrenaline-epinephrine gel on finger lacerations. Pediatr Emerg Care 2004;20(12):812–815.

# Poisonings

Jennifer Horst, Ari Filip, and Robert M. Kennedy

## INTRODUCTION

- When a patient has been a victim of poisoning, whether accidental or intentional, the etiology is often unclear. Victims of ingestions often present with altered mental status, leaving the clinician with a broad differential. **Remember to keep ingestion on the list**. This is a simpler task when faced with a patient who presents with a classic toxidrome (remember "mad as a hatter, dry as a bone"), but patients, particularly young children, often do not present with "classic symptoms."
- History and physical are critical, as many toxicants or medications are not part of a comprehensive drug screen.
- When drawing blood during the acute phase of illness, always secure extra samples when possible.
- **Poison control centers** can be an excellent source of information.
  - The National Capital Poison Center can be reached at **1-800-222-1222.**
  - This number will route to your state/region poison control center.

## CLASSIFICATION BY AGE

### Infants (<9 Months of Age)

- Accidental ingestions are rare in this age group due to limited developmental capabilities. Instead, consider the following:
  - Misuse of a medication (e.g., administering a medication prescribed for another household member to an infant)
  - Inappropriate dosing (concentration or measurement error) of a prescription or over-the-counter medication

### Toddlers (1-3 Years of Age)

- Toddlers have a potentially deadly developmental combination of independent mobility, evolving manual dexterity, and impulsivity.
- According to the 2019 Annual Report of the American Association of Poison Centers' National Poison Data, 31.3% of all exposures occurred in children younger than 3 years of age and children ≤5 years age comprised of 42.8% of human exposures.
- There is a male predominance for ingestions in children <12 years of age.
- In 2019, The 5 most common *exposures* in children are cosmetics/personal care products, cleaning substances, analgesics, foreign bodies/toys miscellaneous, and dietary supplements/herbals/homeopathic preparations. The five most common categories of substances involved in pediatric (≤5 years) *deaths* are fumes/gases vapors, unknown drug, analgesics, batteries, and anesthetics.

## School-Aged Children

Children in this age group with normal developmental achievement **do not** typically ingest toxic substances unless they are improperly stored (e.g., antifreeze stored in a soda container) or disguised as a treat (THC in gummies, etc.).

## Adolescents

- Intentional poisonings are more commonly recognized in this age group.
  - Suicide attempts
  - Recreational ingestion for amusement/altered perception/intoxication leading to unintentional overdose
  - More severe clinical effects of toxin due to higher volume ingestion
  - Higher associated morbidity and mortality with intentional poisonings (suicide attempts or deliberate poisonings) in all age ranges

## DIAGNOSIS

### History

- Often minimal or no history available due to altered mental status or impaired consciousness.
  - The number one chief complaint of poisoning victims is **altered mental status**.
- Ask detailed questions regarding the home environment, caretakers, timeline, access to substances, and attempted interventions before seeking medical care.
- Conduct a developmental assessment of the child, whether based on physical examination (sometimes complicated by altered mental status) or by history.
  - This can be key in validating the mechanism of access to the substances (e.g., a 3-month-old child could not pick up a pill and coordinate its transfer to his or her mouth, but an 11-month-old child could).
- Recent introduction of a new compound into the environment
  - Examples: Car's brake fluid was just changed and the container left accessible in the driveway
- New caretaker
  - Possible lower level of attentiveness to child's activity
  - New household members, such as elderly relatives, taking prescription medications that may be accidentally stored within arm's reach of a small child or accidently dropped on the ground
- Inquire about prescription and nonprescription medications as these are another common culprit.
  - They are available to all household members: **child-resistant caps are not child-proof**.
  - Illicit drugs are common causes of severe ingestion. Ask about drugs or THC-infused edibles.

### Clinical Presentation (Table 4-1)

- See Table 4-1.
- Physical exam findings to note:
  - Vital signs.
  - Pupillary exam: Make note of miosis versus mydriasis, or if nystagmus is present.
  - Mucous membranes: Dry versus profuse salivation.
  - Skin: Dry versus diaphoretic; *Always look for bruising.*

**TABLE 4-1** Toxidromes

| Category | Symptoms | Comments |
|---|---|---|
| Anticholinergic (antimuscarinic): antihistamines, tropane alkaloid plants, TCAs | Tachycardia, mydriasis, xerostomia/dry skin, flushing, urinary retention, ileus, delirium, hyperthermia | Delirium may manifest as "picking" behaviors: reaching or picking at objects. Hyperthermia is a morbid feature |
| Cholinergic | Salivation, lacrimation, urination, diarrhea, vomiting. Severe: bronchorrhea, bronchospasm, bradycardia, seizure, fasciculations, and muscle paralysis | "Killer B's": bronchorrhea, bronchospasm, and bradycardia are most concerning features. Mortality typically from respiratory cause (bronchorrhea, bronchospasm, diaphragmatic weakness/paralysis) |
| Neuroleptic malignant syndrome (NMS) | Confusion, rigidity (lead-pipe), hyperthermia, leukocytosis, CK elevation | May be confused with serotonin syndrome. Distinguished by more indolent time course (days-weeks), presence of lead pipe rigidity (vs. clonus) |
| Opioid | Miosis, constipation, respiratory depression, CNS depression | Pronounced respiratory depression, but other signs of autonomic dysfunction should not be present unless premorbid |
| Sedative-hypnotic | Sedation, hypothermia, CNS depression, respiratory depression, mild hypotension/bradycardia possible | Autonomic changes will typically be mild compared to level of sedation. Pupils will typically be unaffected compared to opioid or sympatholytic toxidrome |
| Sympatholytic toxicity: (e.g. clonidine or alpha-2 agonist) | Miosis, bradycardia, hypotension, respiratory depression and CNS depression | Similar features as opioid toxidrome (miosis, sedation, bradypnea), but bradycardia and hypotension may occur. Typically, respiratory depression is less pronounced |
| Sympathomimetic | Tachycardia, hypertension, mydriasis, diaphoresis, abnormal motor movements | Similar features to anticholinergic toxidromes, but patients will be sweating. Young patients may manifest with abnormal motor behaviors, vomiting, or may be agitated/inconsolable |
| Serotonin toxicity/serotonin syndrome | Tachycardia, mydriasis, diarrhea, hyperreflexia, clonus, agitation, hyperthermia | Toxicity exists on a spectrum, from mild serotonin toxicity to severe cases (serotonin syndrome). SSRIs, MAOIs, and TCAs are typical culprits, but other serotonergic drugs may contribute to this syndrome (e.g., tramadol, meperidine, bupropion, lithium, valproate, linezolid, amphetamines) |

- Breath sounds: Note respiratory rate and if wheezing is present.
- Listen for bowel sounds.
- Neuro exam
  - Mental status: Is patient arousable, agitated, picking at objects, responding to internal stimuli?
  - Check for clonus, reflexes, and rigidity.

## Laboratory Studies

- All patients presenting with suspected *intentional* poisoning should have the following studies obtained:
  - CBC, CMP, acetaminophen level, salicylate level, urine drug screen, and EKG.
  - Other studies, such as ethanol level or venous blood gas, may be indicated based on history and physical.
    - Salicylate and acetaminophen levels can be obtained at many hospitals and guide early care (NAC administration, etc) (Figs. 4-1 and 4-2).
- Point of care glucose: Obtain on all altered patients!
  - KULTS for anion gap metabolic acidosis: **K**etones, **U**remia, **L**actic Acid, **T**oxic alcohols, **S**alicylates
    - Ketones: DKA, starvation ketosis, alcohol ketoacidosis

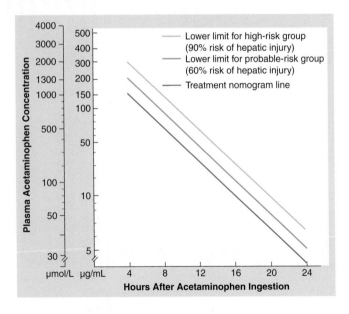

**CAUTIONS FOR USE OF THIS CHART:**
1. The time coordinates refer to time post ingestion.
2. Serum levels drawn before 4 hours may not represent peak levels.
3. The graph should be used only in relation to a single acute ingestion.
4. Given nuances to acetaminophen poisoning, consultation with poison center or toxicology service is generally recommended

**Figure 4-1. Nomogram showing plasma or serum acetaminophen concentration versus time post acetaminophen ingestion.**

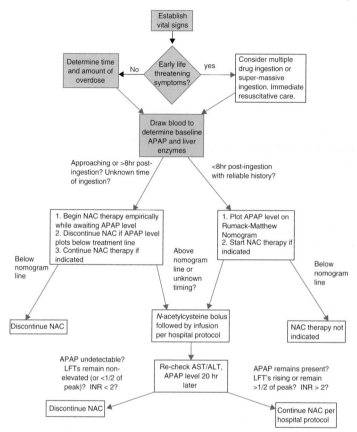

**Figure 4-2. Treatment algorithm for acetaminophen poisoning.**

- ○ Uremia: renal failure
- ○ Lactic acid: cyanide, carbon monoxide, metformin
- ○ Toxic alcohols: ethylene glycol, ethanol, methanol, propylene glycol
- ○ Salicylates: aspirin, methyl salicylate (oil of wintergreen)
- • Osmolar gap and co-oximetry can be helpful in the right context.
- • Drug screen
  - • Urine and serum "comprehensive" drug screens are not completely comprehensive.
    - ○ It is imperative to know your hospital's routine urine and serum drug screening panel.
  - • Drug screens at most institutions are immunoassay-based screening tests: antibodies recognize similar molecular structures among drug classes and their metabolites.
    - ○ Prone to false positives and false negatives.
    - ○ Drug classes without common metabolites may not be picked up (e.g., lorazepam, and clonazepam will often be missed on benzodiazepine screening).
      - – Some drug classes have similar effects but widely variable chemical structures (e.g., opiate screens will not pick up synthetic opioids like hydrocodone, oxycodone, fentanyl, and methadone).

| TABLE 4-2 | St. Louis Children's Urine Drug Screen |
|---|---|

| Compound | Cutoff concentration (ng/mL) |
|---|---|
| Benzoylecgonine (BEG) | 1 |
| Cocaine | 1 |
| EDDP (methadone metabolite) | 1 |
| Fentanyl | 1 |
| Ketamine | 1 |
| Lysergic acid diethylamide (LSD) | 1 |
| Methylenedioxyamphetamine (MDA) | 1 |
| Methylenedioxyethamphetamine (MDEA) | 1 |
| Methylenedioxymethamphetamine (MDMA) | 1 |
| Methylbenzodioxolylbutanamine (MBDB) | 1 |
| Methylphenidate | 1 |
| Phencyclidine (PCP) | 1 |
| Quetiapine | 1 |
| Bupropion | 1 |
| 6-Hydroxybupropion | 1 |
| Amphetamine | 5 |
| Methamphetamine | 5 |
| Methadone | 10 |
| Nordiazepam | 10 |
| Naloxone (Narcan) | 10 |
| Oxazepam | 10 |
| 7-Aminoclonazepam | 10 |
| Tramadol | 10 |
| Norbuprenorphine | 10 |
| Buprenorphine-3-glucuronide | 10 |
| Venlafaxine | 10 |
| 11-Nor-9-carboxy-Δ9-tetrahydrocannabinol-glucuronide | 20 |
| 6-Monoacetylmorphine | 25 |
| Alprazolam (Xanax) | 25 |
| Lorazepam | 25 |
| Codeine | 25 |
| Nalorphine | 25 |
| Oxycodone | 25 |
| Clonidine | 50 |
| Flunitrazepam (Rohypnol) | 50 |
| Hydromorphone | 50 |
| Oxymorphone | 50 |
| O-Desmethyltramadol | 50 |

| TABLE 4-2 | St. Louis Children's Urine Drug Screen (*Continued*) |
|---|---|

| Compound | Cutoff concentration (ng/mL) |
|---|---|
| Lorazepam-3-glucuronide | 100 |
| Hydrocodone | 100 |
| 11-Nor-9-carboxy-Δ9-tetrahydrocannabinol (THC) | 100 |
| Morphine | 100 |
| Morphine-3-glucuronide | 250 |
| Pentobarbital | 1000 |
| Phenobarbital | 1000 |
| Secobarbital | 1000 |
| Amobarbital | 1000 |
| γ-Hydroxybutyrate (GHB) | 10,000 |

Courtesy of St. Louis Children's Hospital.

- ○ Some drug classes may have metabolites that cause false positives (e.g., lamotrigine and PCP, trazodone and amphetamines). Positives should be confirmed by Gas chromatography-mass spectrometry (GC-MS).
- GC/MS is the gold standard for drug identification: can be used to confirm drug screen positives
  - ○ Not available at most institutions (i.e., must be sent out to external lab)
  - ○ Highly sensitive and specific for detection of the exact compound in question
  - ○ Exact library of compounds detected changes by institution:
  - ○ See Table 4-2
    - – Performed by mass spectrometry, with excellent specificity
- Specific quantitative drug assays
  - Antiepileptic medications (phenytoin/valproic acid/carbamazepine), analgesics (acetaminophen, salicylates), and metals (iron, lithium) are commonly encountered substances in pediatric ingestion cases, and levels are typically readily available.

## Other Useful Diagnostic Studies

- Electrocardiography
  - May refer to QT nomogram (Fig. 4-3) to identify high-risk QT prolongation
  - Tachyarrhythmias
    - ○ **Tricyclic antidepressants (TCAs)** may present with prolongation of the QRS intervals due sodium channel blockade, which could progress to fatal ventricular arrhythmias; QT may be prolonged as well.
    - ○ **Antipsychotic medication ingestion** may cause QT prolongation, making patient susceptible to *torsades de pointes*.
    - ○ **Sympathomimetics** (cocaine, amphetamines) can present with sinus tachycardia or other tachyarrhythmias.
  - Bradyarrhythmias
    - ○ β-**Blockers, calcium channel blockers, and clonidine** typically present with sinus bradycardia but can present with AV block.

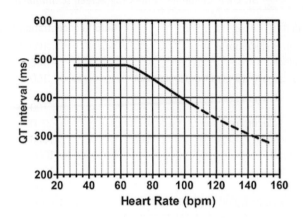

solid line indicates heart rates that are not tachycardic
dashed line is extrapolated to allow assessment of faster heart rates

The QT nomogram is a plot of the QT interval versus the heart rate. A QT–heart rate pair above the line is associated with an increased risk of torsades de pointes.

**Figure 4-3. QT nomogram.** (Reprinted from Isbister GK. Risk assessment of drug-induced QT prolongation. Aust Prescr 2015;38(1):20–24. Reproduced and adapted from WikiTox www.wikitox.org.)

- Radiography
  - Radiopaque foreign bodies that have been ingested or aspirated by the child may be visualized on chest or abdominal films.
  - Iron (ferrous sulfate), lead, or enteric-coated tablets may be seen in the gastrointestinal tract.
  - A negative radiograph does not exclude ingestion or aspiration.

## TREATMENT

### Elimination of Ingested Poisons

- Activated charcoal is often unhelpful; should be weighed against aspiration risk, clinical course, and severity of poison. Recommend discussing with poison center.
- May be considered if <1 hour after ingestion; the dose is 0.5-1 g/kg (30-50 g.
  - Agents absorbed by activated charcoal: barbiturates, colchicine, digitalis, amphetamines, phenytoin, salicylates, theophylline, and TCAs.
  - Most metals (iron, lead, lithium) are not absorbed by activated charcoal.
- Methods of secondary elimination
  - Whole bowel irrigation (polyethylene glycol); select cases, such as iron
  - Alkalinization: for barbiturates, salicylates
    - Administer $NaHCO_3$ and follow urine pH.
  - Hemodialysis, hemofiltration, or exchange transfusion (e.g., methanol, ethylene glycol, lithium, salicylates). Consult poison control or toxicologist

### Specific Antidotes/Therapy

See Tables 4-3 to 4-5.

**TABLE 4-3** Common Findings and Management Approach in Prescription Drug Ingestions

| Poison | Signs and symptoms | Antidote/treatment | Comments |
|---|---|---|---|
| Antimalarials (hydroxychloroquine, chloroquine, quinine) | Hypokalemia, QRS prolongation, QT prolongation, ventricular arrhythmia, hypotension | Electrolyte replacement, sodium bicarbonate bolus/hypertonic saline, vasopressors, high-dose diazepam (1 mg/kg) | Particularly dangerous medication in exploratory ingestions in young children |
| Antipsychotics | Akathisia, extrapyramidal reaction, anticholinergic effects, sedation, neuroleptic malignant syndrome (rare) | Diphenhydramine 1-2 mg/kg/dose (max 50 mg) if extrapyramidal symptoms, benzodiazepines in severe cases | Extrapyramidal symptoms predominate in 1st generation (e.g., haloperidol). Anticholinergic symptoms in second generation (e.g., olanzapine) |
| Barbiturates and anticonvulsants | Slurred speech, hypothermia, nystagmus, ataxia, CNS depression, seizures, arrhythmias | Charcoal, urine alkalinization, dialysis | Dialysis in select/severe cases: valproic acid, phenytoin, carbamazepine, phenobarbital |
| Beta-blockers | Bradycardia, heart block, hypotension, hypoglycemia | Glucagon (0.05-0.15 mg/kg boluses) + infusion, vasopressors, high-dose insulin, intravenous lipid emulsion, ECMO | Requires telemetry, heart block and bradycardia may be refractory to pacing |
| Benzodiazepines | Respiratory depression, CNS depression | Flumazenil 0.2 mg IV bolus, then 0.2 mg/min up to max 3 mg | Administration of flumazenil can precipitate seizures in habituated patients |
| Calcium channel blockers | Hypotension secondary to vasodilation/vasoplegia (dihydropyridines) vs. bradycardia and cardiogenic shock (nondihydropyridines). Selectivity is lost in overdose, and features of both may be present<br><br>Hyperglycemia from pancreatic islet cell blockade | Calcium chloride (target 13-15 mg/dL), vasopressors, high-dose insulin, methylene blue, intralipids, ECMO | Requires telemetry, heart block and bradycardia may be refractory to pacing |

(Continued)

**TABLE 4-3    Common Findings and Management Approach in Prescription Drug Ingestions (Continued)**

| Poison | Signs and symptoms | Antidote/treatment | Comments |
|---|---|---|---|
| Digitalis | Arrhythmia, hypotension, hyperkalemia | Fab fragments; 80 mg inactivates 1 mg of digoxin. 5–10 vials in unstable patient or unknown ingestion | Requires telemetry. Hyperkalemia in acute overdose portends high mortality risk |
| Imidazolines (clonidine and guanfacine) | Bradycardia, hypotension, bradypnea, miosis, CNS depression | Naloxone may be helpful, but at much higher doses than opioid overdose (10 mg independent of weight) | May need repeated re-assessment and stimulation. Intubation and vasopressors rarely needed |
| Insulin | Hypoglycemia, sweating, dizziness, pallor, syncope, seizure, coma | Continuous infusion of dextrose-containing fluids | Frequent blood glucose checks are warranted to reach appropriate glucose infusion rate. Encourage oral intake of complex carbohydrates, proteins, and fats as well |
| Iron | Nausea, bloody diarrhea, abdominal pain, leukocytosis, metabolic acidosis, shock, coma, hepatic failure, GI stricture (delayed) | Deferoxamine: 5 mg/kg/hr up to 15 mg/kg/hr as tolerated by BP, whole bowel irrigation, serial plain bowel radiograph | Toxic dose 20-60 mg/kg iron High toxic dose >60 mg/kg Lethal dose 200-300 mg/kg Deferoxamine for 4 hr iron level >500 µg/dL or systemic toxicity |
| Opioids | Hypoventilation, miosis, sedation, hypothermia, ileus | Naloxone 0.1 mg/kg IV | Half-life of opioid may exceed that of naloxone (half life 1 hr) and require redosing. Long-acting opioid (e.g., methadone) may require naloxone infusion |

| Agent | Symptoms | Treatment | Comments |
|---|---|---|---|
| Oral hypoglycemics such as sulfonylureas (e.g., glipizide, glyburide, etc.) | Severe hypoglycemia in pediatrics, resulting in lethargy, coma, seizures<br><br>Act by increasing pancreatic insulin release<br><br>Symptoms may occur 18-24 hr after the ingestion | Treatment of hypoglycemia includes octreotide 1 μg/kg SC q12h, which should be given for any symptomatic patient. IV dextrose bolus and/or infusion may be added, but at risk of stimulating more insulin production from pancreas<br><br>Glucagon 0.1 mg/kg (max 1 mg) may be considered as well<br><br>Unpleasant side effects: nausea, vomiting | Hypoglycemia may be resistant to IV dextrose; frequent monitoring of blood glucose is necessary<br><br>Sulfonylurea overdoses should be observed for 24 hr |
| Selective serotonin reuptake inhibitors (SSRIs) | Serotonin syndrome: tachycardia, mydriasis, diarrhea, hyperreflexia, clonus, agitation, hyperthermia | Cyproheptadine 0.25 mg/kg/day (mild-moderate cases only), benzodiazepines (moderate-severe), cooling/deep sedation (severe) | Usually precipitated by combination of serotonergic agents or massive single agent ingestion |
| Tricyclic antidepressants | Serotonin syndrome as above, sodium channel blockade (widened QRS), QT prolongation, tachycardia, hypotension, anticholinergic effects, seizures | Benzodiazepines, sodium bicarbonate or 3% hypertonic saline boluses (1-2 mEq/kg), vasopressors, physostigmine in rare cases, ECMO | Fatality common from widened QRS and ventricular arrhythmia |

**TABLE 4-4    Common Findings and Management Approach in Nonprescription Substance Ingestions or Exposures**

| Poison | Signs and symptoms | Antidote/treatment | Comments |
|---|---|---|---|
| Acetaminophen | Toxic dose >150 mg/kg. Nausea, vomiting, lethargy; at >24 hr: liver damage, jaundice, encephalopathy; at >7 days: renal failure | N-Acetylcysteine: IV infusion (Acetadote): 150 mg/kg bolus over 1 hr, then infusion: either 50 mg/kg over 4 hr, followed by 100 mg/kg over 16 hr (total 21-hr infusion) OR 12.5 mg/kg/hr × 20 hr | See toxicity nomogram and treatment algorithm (Figs. 4-1 and 4-2). Check level 4-hr postingestion. Effectiveness of NAC diminishes after 8 hr, NAC should be continued past 20 hr if signs of ongoing hepatotoxicity (LFT's rising or greater than half of peak level, INR rising or >2) |
| Alkaline corrosives | Dysphagia, oral and esophageal burns | Do not give emetic, charcoal, or gastric lavage. If eye or skin contact: rinse with water until pH 7.0, contact ophthalmology | Esophagoscopy within 24 hr of ingestion if indicated |
| Antihistamines/anticholinergics | Dry mouth, mydriasis, tachycardia, hyperthermia, TCA-like effects (1st gen. antihistamines) | Physostigmine 0.02 mg/kg IV, max 1 mg, benzodiazepines, sodium bicarbonate boluses (diphenhydramine) | Physostigmine has several contraindications: use should merit discussion with Poison Center or Toxicologist |
| Camphor | Delirium, seizures, methemoglobinemia, intravascular hemolysis | Methylene blue, blood transfusion, benzodiazepines for seizure, supportive care | |

| | | | |
|---|---|---|---|
| Carbamates/organophosphates | Cholinergic toxidromes: salivation, lacrimation, urination, diarrhea, vomiting. Severe: bronchorrhea, bradycardia, seizure, respiratory muscle paralysis | Airway protection; atropine aggressively titrated to drying of bronchial secretions; pralidoxime (organophosphates only); benzodiazepines for seizure | Decontamination of both patient and staff is imperative. Consider NG tube to remove residual toxin |
| Carbon monoxide | Headache, lethargy, seizure, coma, cardiovascular collapse | Delivery of supplemental oxygen, consider hyperbaric oxygen in consultation with toxicologist or poison control center (CoHb > 15%) | Pulse oximetry and arterial blood gas analysis may be normal. Diagnosis by co-oximetry |
| Cyanide | Altered mental status, hypotension and/or cardiovascular collapse, seizure, metabolic acidosis with high lactate | Hydroxocobalamin 70 mg/kg IV infusion over 15 min, max 5 g. May repeat ×1 if favorable response | Consider this in patients who have been in an enclosed fire. Should presumptively treat for metabolic acidosis with lactate of 10 or higher |
| Ethanol (also present in perfume, aftershave, mouthwash) | Slurred speech, delirium, nausea, vomiting, hypoglycemia, hypothermia, ataxia, respiratory depression, coma | Airway management<br>Dextrose-containing IV fluids<br>Supportive care (warming)<br>Give thiamine 500 mg TID IV/IM in chronic abuse cases to avoid neurologic injury if concern for Wernicke encephalopathy | Younger children with smaller glycogen stores are more likely to present with low blood sugar |

(Continued)

**TABLE 4-4** Common Findings and Management Approach in Nonprescription Substance Ingestions or Exposures (*Continued*)

| Poison | Signs and symptoms | Antidote/treatment | Comments |
|--------|--------------------|--------------------|----------|
| Hydrocarbons | Inhalation/aspiration can lead to respiratory distress and failure, sometimes delayed up to 12–24 hr after exposure | Supportive care Steroids controversial without evidence-based medicine support | Remember that symptoms of respiratory distress may be delayed. Radiographic findings may also lag clinical features |
| Methemoglobinemia (exposure to sulfonamide, local anesthetics, mothballs, nitrates and nitrites, dapsone) | Can have a normal $PaO_2$ and calculated oxygen saturation, although pulse oximetry may be low | Methemoglobinemia of >30% is treated with methylene blue 1–2 mg/kg IV administered over several minutes. Repeat dosing may be necessary | **Methylene blue is contraindicated in patients with glucose-6-phosphate deficiency since it can cause severe hemolysis** |
| Oil of wintergreen (up to 98% methyl salicylate) | Salicylate poisoning (see below). One tsp is equivalent to approximately 20 tablets of full-strength (325 mg) aspirin | Sodium bicarbonate for enhanced elimination, dialysis in severe cases | Particularly dangerous medication in exploratory ingestions in young children |
| Salicylate | GI upset, tinnitus, metabolic acidosis, hyperventilation/primary respiratory alkalosis, seizures, CNS depression, hypoglycorrhachia, ARDS | Activated charcoal if <1 hr or levels rising Urine alkalinization (keep urine pH: 7.5–8) with potassium supplementation Hemodialysis if renal failure, hypoxia, salicylate level >100 mg/dL, mental status changes, or severe poisoning | Obtain level at admission and at 4-hr postingestion. Absorption and kinetics may be erratic. Unit of measurement not standardized (mg/dL vs. mg/L) |

| Toxic alcohols such as ethylene glycol (antifreeze, brake fluid, motor oil) and methanol | Metabolic acidosis, compensatory respiratory alkalosis (tachypnea); renal failure with oxalate crystal deposition and acute tubular necrosis (ethylene glycol); blindness, CNS depression, and basal ganglia lesions (methanol) | Alcohol dehydrogenase blockade via fomepizole (15 mg/kg loading dose +10 mg/kg q12h). May substitute ethanol to maintenance level of >100 mg/dL if fomepizole unavailable. Dialysis may assist in removing the toxic alcohol and its metabolites if acidosis already present | Fluorescein and oxalate crystals in urine may be present, but these findings are neither sensitive nor specific |

**TABLE 4-5** Common Findings and Management Approach in Drugs of Abuse

| Poison | Signs and symptoms | Antidote/treatment | Comments |
|--------|--------------------|--------------------|----------|
| Cocaine | Tachycardia, hypertension, agitation, diaphoresis, mydriasis, vomiting, hyperthermia | Benzodiazepines (high doses may be required) | Relatively short lived. Drug screen looks for major metabolite: benzoylecgonine |
| Benzodiazepine | Miosis, respiratory depression | Flumazenil 0.2 mg IV bolus, then 0.2 mg/min up to max 3 mg | Administration of flumazenil can precipitate seizures in habituated patients |
| Methamphetamine/ amphetamine | Tachycardia, hypertension, agitation, diaphoresis, mydriasis, vomiting, hyperthermia, dystonia/rigidity | Benzodiazepines (high doses may be required), haloperidol helpful if abnormal motor findings | Amphetamine drug screen may be positive if on certain medications for ADHD |
| Barbiturates | Slurred speech, ataxia, CNS depression, respiratory depression | Charcoal, urine alkalinization (phenobarbital), dialysis (severe cases) | Long half-life may be present |
| Fentanyl | Miosis, lethargy, respiratory depression, coma | Naloxone (often single dose) | Observe at least 4 hours after naloxone dosing |
| Methadone | Miosis, lethargy, respiratory depression, coma | Naloxone (frequently requires infusion) | Long half-life (>24 hr), requires admission if patient needing naloxone reversal |
| Other opioids (heroin, prescription painkillers) | Miosis, lethargy, respiratory depression, coma | Naloxone | Variable half-lives, disposition depends on need for redosing naloxone, opiate screen may not detect synthetic opioids |

| | | | |
|---|---|---|---|
| THC | Lethargy, CNS depression, bradyarrhythmia in young children | Supportive care | Edible THC ingestions becoming more prevalent, may have very high concentration of THC |
| Synthetic cannabinoids | Variable psychoactive effects with either lethargy and CNS depression vs. tachycardia, agitation, psychosis, rhabdomyolysis, hyperthermia | Supportive care, benzodiazepines (if agitation present) | Pharmacologically diverse compounds, not detected on standard drug screens, variable psychoactive effects |
| Psychoactives/ dissociatives (psilocybin, LSD, PCP, MDMA) | Psychosis, agitation, rhabdomyolysis | Supportive care, benzodiazepines (if agitation present) | MDMA may also precipitate sympathomimetic toxidrome (underlying amphetamine structure). PCP may cause excited delirium as well |

## SUGGESTED READINGS

Hoffman RS, Burns MM, Gosselin S. Ingestion of caustic substances. N Engl J Med 2020;382(18):1739–1748. doi: 10.1056/NEJMra1810769.

Isbister GK, Page CB. Drug induced QT prolongation: the measurement and assessment of the QT interval in clinical practice. Br J Clin Pharmacol 2013;76(1):48–57. doi: 10.1111/bcp.12040.

Lowry JA, Fine JS, Calello DP, et al. Pediatric fatality review of the 2013 National Poison Database System (NPDS): focus on intent. Clin Toxicol (Phila) 2015;53(2):79–81.

Nelson L, ed. Goldfrank's Toxicologic Emergencies. 11th Ed. New York: McGraw-Hill Education, 2019.

Nelson L, Shih RD, Balick MJ, et al. Handbook of Poisonous and Injurious Plants. 2nd Ed. New York: New York Botanical Garden, 2007.

Rumack BH, Matthew H. Acetaminophen poisoning and toxicity. Pediatrics 1975;55(6):871–876.

Spyres M. The KULTS of Toxicology. EMCrit Blog. Published July 2, 2018. Available at https://emcrit.org/toxhound/kults-of-toxicology/. Last accessed on 4/30/21.

# Basic Orthopedics

Kathryn Leonard and Dean Odegard

## MUSCULOSKELETAL TRAUMA

### Fractures

In general, ligaments in children are functionally stronger than bones. Therefore, children are more likely to sustain fractures than sprains. The physis (growth plate) is a cartilaginous structure at the ends of long bones that is generally weaker than the surrounding bone and therefore predisposed to injury.

Physeal fractures are classified using the **Salter-Harris system** (Table 5-1). In general, the prognosis for normal healing worsens as the classification increases.

- **Type I:** Fracture through the physis that separates the metaphysis and epiphysis. These are often difficult to appreciate radiographically and are diagnosed clinically when point tenderness is found over the growth plate.
- **Type II:** Fracture extends through the physis and into the metaphysis.
- **Type III:** Fracture extends through the physis and epiphysis into the intra-articular space.
- **Type IV:** Fracture involves the epiphysis, physis, and metaphysis.
- **Type V:** A crush injury of the physis resulting from axial compression and is often difficult to diagnose radiographically.

### Evaluation

- The assessment of the pediatric patient with suspected fracture should include:
  - History: Patient's age, mechanism, and timing of injury are important details.
  - Physical exam
    - ○ Gross deformity
    - ○ Areas of point tenderness
    - ○ Range of motion of the affected extremity
    - ○ Neurovascular status distal to the injury—sensation, motor function, pulses
    - ○ Lacerations concerning for associated "open" fracture
- Radiographic evaluation should generally include the joint above and below the fracture and at least two views of the injured region (generally anteroposterior and lateral).

### General Management

- Keep patients NPO in case sedation or surgery is required.
- Cover open wounds with a sterile dressing. Open fractures require tetanus prophylaxis, antibiotics, and urgent débridement in the operating room (OR).
- Early pain management involves splinting and analgesia, for example, oral oxycodone 0.2 mg/kg.
- The need for closed reduction is multifactorial and related to patient age (potential for remodeling), bone(s) involved, and angle(s) of displacement.
- Closed reduction can be accomplished under sedation, followed by immobilization with a splint or bivalved cast (Fig. 5-1). Casts or splints should encompass the joint proximal and distal to the site of the injury.

**TABLE 5-1  Types of Salter-Harris Fractures**

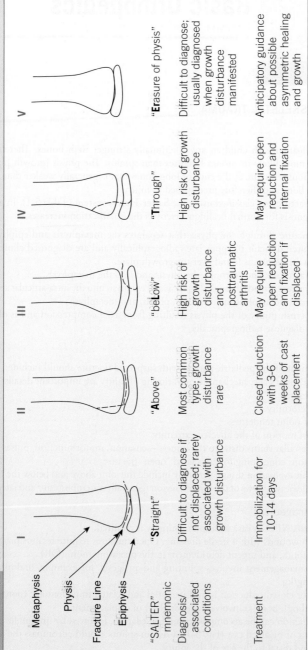

| | I | II | III | IV | V |
|---|---|---|---|---|---|
| "SALTER" mnemonic | "**S**traight" | "**A**bove" | "be**L**ow" | "**T**hrough" | "**E**rasure of physis" |
| Diagnosis/associated conditions | Difficult to diagnose if not displaced; rarely associated with growth disturbance | Most common type; growth disturbance rare | High risk of growth disturbance and posttraumatic arthritis | High risk of growth disturbance | Difficult to diagnose; usually diagnosed when growth disturbance manifested |
| Treatment | Immobilization for 10-14 days | Closed reduction with 3-6 weeks of cast placement | May require open reduction and fixation if displaced | May require open reduction and internal fixation | Anticipatory guidance about possible asymmetric healing and growth |

Metaphysis
Physis
Fracture Line
Epiphysis

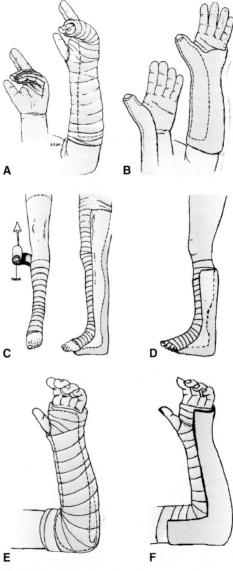

**Figure 5-1. Splints for various fractures. A.** Ulnar gutter; Boxer's fracture. **B.** Thumb spica; scaphoid or thumb fracture. **C.** Posterior long leg; knee injury and/or spiral fracture. **D.** Posterior ankle; ankle sprain or fracture of foot, ankle, or distal fibula. **E.** Sugar tong; distal radius and wrist fracture. **F.** Posterior long arm; elbow and wrist injury.

- Open reduction in the OR is indicated in failed closed reduction, displaced intra-articular fractures (Salter-Harris types III and IV), unstable fractures, open fractures, and fractures with significant neurovascular compromise.
- After placement of a cast or splint, it is important to monitor for signs and symptoms of **compartment syndrome**, described by the "Ps."
  - **P**ain out of proportion to the injury or pain with passive movement of fingers/toes (earliest sign)
  - **P**aresthesia distal to the cast
  - **P**allor or cyanosis distal to the cast
  - **P**ulse weak or thready distal to cast
  - Other signs include: marked swelling of tissues distal to the cast, increasing agitation, or increasing analgesic requirements

## Concerns Related to Nonaccidental Trauma

While no fracture is pathognomonic, certain types and patterns of fractures should raise the clinician's suspicion for nonaccidental injury, particularly if an implausible or inconsistent history of injury is provided. When considering a pediatric patient who is younger than 3 years of age or nonverbal, the following fractures should raise suspicion for child abuse.

### Multiple Fractures
- A patient who is younger than 3 years of age and presents without a plausible mechanism of injury needs a complete skeletal survey to evaluate for the presence of additional fractures.
- Multiple fractures that are unaccounted for in the history should generate a reasonable suspicion for nonaccidental trauma.
- Fractures in various stages of healing should be concerning for repeated injury.

### Complex Skull Fractures
- These skull fractures contain more than one line of fracture, sometimes described as a stellate pattern, and they may be accompanied by displacement or diastasis.
- Most accidental injuries are the results of falls onto a flat surface with resultant linear fractures over the convexity of the skull. A complex skull fracture suggests a greater level of force applied to the skull than would be expected from such a fall (e.g., off a bed or couch onto the floor).

### Rib Fractures
- Rib fractures may be present posteriorly, laterally, or anteriorly along the rib shaft.
- Posterior rib fractures are common from child abuse and are usually caused by anteroposterior thoracic compression.
- Lateral and anterior rib fractures may also result from anteroposterior compression but can also occur from direct blows to the chest.
- Closely examine the ribs above and below a known fracture because a direct blow often fractures several ribs simultaneously. The addition of oblique views increases the ability to detect rib fractures in cases of suspected abuse.

### Classic Metaphyseal Lesions ("Corner Fractures" or "Bucket-Handle Fractures")
- Think of these as avulsion fractures at the growth plate, in which either a crescent (bucket handle) or fragment (corner) of the bone is torn from the zone of provisional calcification and contained by the periosteum.
- These generally result from pulling or twisting forces.
- These injuries usually are not acute and represent previous injury to the physis.

*Humerus Fractures*

These are the most common long bone injuries associated with abuse, particularly in children <3 years of age.

*Femur Fractures*

These are the second most common fractures seen in child abuse and are extremely suspicious for abuse in a nonambulatory child without plausible mechanism.

## UPPER EXTREMITY MUSCULOSKELETAL INJURIES

### Clavicular Fracture

- This is the most common fracture in children. It may occur as a result of birth trauma, falling onto an outstretched arm, or a direct blow to the shoulder.
- Treatment
  - Clavicle fractures in neonates require care with lifting and swaddling but no further immobilization.
  - Most fractures (especially in children <12 years of age) are treated nonoperatively with immobilization via sling ± swathe, with bony union expected at 2-4 weeks. A bony callus may be prominent and will become less obvious over 6-12 months.
  - Surgery is reserved for open fractures, fractures with associated neurovascular injury or risk (e.g., posteriorly displaced fractures near the sternum), and fractures that compromise the skin.

### Shoulder Dislocation

- These are less common in the skeletally immature as most injuries tend to produce fractures.
- When shoulder dislocation does occur, 90% are anterior dislocations.
- These patients present with significant pain, arm held in adduction and internal rotation, and loss of normal contour of the shoulder (i.e., prominent acromion).
- Gentle closed reduction should be performed, followed by postreduction radiographs to ensure that there is no associated fracture (e.g., Hill-Sachs deformity, Bankart lesion). An axillary lateral plain radiograph should be done to confirm reduction.
- Patients should be immobilized in a sling and swathe for at least 3 weeks and referred for orthopedic follow-up.
- Recurrence is common, with an incidence of 50-95% and a greater rate of recurrence associated with younger age at first dislocation.

### Proximal Humerus Fracture

- The majority of these fractures will remodel and can be managed with a sling and swathe for 2-4 weeks (no splint or cast required) and referred for close orthopedic follow-up.
  - In children <12 years old with Salter-Harris type I or II fractures, up to 40 degrees of angulation and displacement of one-half the width of the shaft may be acceptable and treated as described above.
  - In adolescents, 20 degrees of angulation and displacement <30% the width of the shaft may be acceptable.

### Elbow Injuries

- Elbow injuries are common in children. Orthopedic consultation is necessary for most.

- A careful neurovascular examination to evaluate for distal pulses, capillary refill, and motor/sensory function of the radial, ulnar, and median nerves is essential, as neurologic or vascular compromise (usually transient) can be present with these injuries.
- On a lateral radiograph of the elbow, special attention must be made to the following:
  - **Anterior humeral line:** This line should intersect the middle third of the capitellum to rule out posterior displacement of the distal humerus.
  - **Radiocapitellar line:** A line drawn through the middle of the radial head should intersect the center of the capitellum. Failure of this line to intersect with the center of the capitellum indicates radial head dislocation.
  - **Posterior fat pad sign:** This lucency posterior to the distal humerus is generally visible on in the setting of moderate to large joint effusions. Fractures are present >70% of the time when a posterior fat pad is seen on plain radiograph.
  - **Anterior fat pad sign:** Elevation of the anterior fat pad is called the "sail sign" and indicates an effusion. This too suggests possible associated fracture.
- If no fracture is seen on the lateral plain radiograph, and the capitellum is not posteriorly displaced, but a posterior fat pad is present, apply a posterior long-arm splint (Fig. 5-1) and refer to orthopedic surgery for follow-up for presumed radio-occult fracture.
- Common elbow injuries include supracondylar humerus fractures, lateral condyle fractures, medial epicondyle fractures, and elbow dislocations.

### Supracondylar Humerus Fracture

- These account for the majority of elbow fractures in children. They generally occur after a fall onto an outstretched arm with hyperextension of the elbow or direct trauma. Transient median and radial nerve neurapraxia may occur.
- Treatment is dependent on the degree of displacement of the fracture.
  - **Type I:** Nondisplaced. Treated with immobilization in a long-arm cast or posterior splint with the elbow flexed at 60-90 degrees.
  - **Type II or III:** Displaced fractures require orthopedic consultation and may need to be treated with closed reduction and percutaneous pinning, or open reduction with internal fixation if unstable.

### Radial Head Subluxation ("Nursemaid's Elbow")

- The classic history is a child younger than 5 years of age who cries with pain and refuses to use the arm after being pulled or lifted by that arm (excessive axial traction). The child will hold the arm pronated and slightly flexed at the elbow and will refuse supination or pronation.
- Radiographs are unnecessary if reduction is successful. If plain radiographs are obtained, positioning of the arm for multiple views often results in reduction.
- Reduction is performed by either hyperpronating the wrist or supinating the wrist and fully flexing the elbow; a "pop" is felt over the radial head at the elbow.
- The patient will use that arm normally within 5-10 minutes. If there is no evidence of recovery, the diagnosis should be reconsidered.
- Note that radial head/neck fractures may mimic nursemaid's elbow. History and careful examination for areas of significant point tenderness and swelling are very important.

## Forearm Fractures

- Fractures of the radius and ulna are extremely common in children. The majority of these fractures involve the distal forearm.

- **Colles fracture:** fracture of the distal radius with displacement, resulting in classic "dinner fork" deformity of the wrist.
- Buckle fractures of the distal radius or ulna can be treated with a prefabricated wrist splint if pain on supination/pronation is minimal. If a parent is concerned the child will not leave the splint on, or if there is significant pain with movement of the wrist, a sugar-tong splint can be applied.
- Fractures of one or both cortices should be immobilized in a posterior long-arm or sugar-tong splint to immobilize the elbow and prevent pronation and supination (Fig. 5-1).
- Fractures with significant displacement or angulation are unstable and require reduction followed by immobilization as above.
- Fractures of the **radial and ulnar shafts** deserve special mention.
  - The potential for remodeling decreases in the diaphysis and in older children. Very little angulation is acceptable, and most of these injuries require orthopedic referral.
  - The thick periosteum of the radius and ulna contributes to greenstick or bowing fractures, which must be recognized and referred to an orthopedic specialist due to limited potential for remodeling with these injuries.
- When isolated fractures of the ulna or radius occur, careful review of images of the elbow and wrist is important to rule out associated dislocation patterns.
  - A **Monteggia fracture** is an ulnar fracture with associated radial head dislocation.
  - A **Galeazzi fracture** is a radial shaft fracture with disruption of the radioulnar joint distally.

## Hand Fractures

### Scaphoid Fracture

- This is the most common carpal bone fracture and typically occurs in adolescents. It generally occurs with direct trauma or falling onto an outstretched arm with hyperextension of the wrist.
- Characteristics include wrist pain and swelling, snuffbox tenderness, pain with supination against resistance, or pain with longitudinal compression of the thumb.
- Radiographs may be normal, even with dedicated scaphoid views. If physical findings suggest a scaphoid fracture (despite normal radiographs), treat with a thumb spica splint or cast (Fig. 5-1) and refer to orthopedics for follow-up.
- There is a risk of malunion or avascular necrosis with these fractures, although this is less common in the pediatric population, it can be devastating if missed.

### Boxer Fracture

- This is a fracture of the fifth metacarpal with apical dorsal angulation. It generally occurs after an object has been struck with a closed fist.
- Assess for malrotation by having the patient flex his or her fingers to make a fist and evaluate for overlapping of the fingers ("scissoring"). The malrotation should be reduced before placement of an ulnar gutter splint.
- Treatment
  - Attempts at closed reduction are usually ineffective since these fractures are unstable. Place an ulnar gutter splint (Fig. 5-1) with the metacarpals flexed at 70-90 degrees, and refer to a hand surgeon for consideration of operative pinning, especially those with angulation >30-40 degrees.

## LOWER EXTREMITY MUSCULOSKELETAL INJURIES AND ABNORMALITIES

Fractures near the pediatric hip should be considered an **emergency**, and orthopedic consultation should be sought immediately.

### Slipped Capital Femoral Epiphysis

• Slipped capital femoral epiphysis (SCFE) is displacement of the femoral head relative to the femoral neck at the physeal plate, akin to a Salter-Harris type I fracture (Table 5-1).
• SCFE is the most common hip disorder in adolescents. It typically presents between ages 8 and 15 years, with a mean age of 12 years in girls and 13.5 years in boys (related to timing of pubertal development).
• The male:female ratio is approximately 2:1. SCFE is more frequent in pubertal obese children and some specific ethnicities (African Americans, Latinos).
  • SCFE also occurs more frequently in children with endocrinopathies; thus, children presenting with SCFE who are outside the usual age range, <50th percentile for weight, or with suggestive signs/symptoms should be referred for an endocrine evaluation.
• Between 25% and 50% of cases are eventually bilateral.
• The classic presentation is dull, nonradiating, aching pain in the hip, groin, thigh, or knee that is worse with physical activity.
  • Acute onset of severe symptoms suggests acute or acute-on-chronic slippage. These patients present with significant pain and inability to bear weight.
• On examination, patients typically have limp and hold their leg at rest in neutral position, that is, flexion and external rotation. Flexion, internal rotation, and abduction of the affected hip are limited and painful. When the hip is passively flexed, the thigh abducts and externally rotates.
• Radiographic evaluation should include AP views of the pelvis and frog-leg views of the hips for side-to-side comparison.
  • A line parallel to the lateral aspect of the femoral neck (**Klein line**) should intersect a portion of the femoral epiphysis, but in cases of SCFE, the line will pass outside the epiphysis.
• Treatment includes immediate non–weight-bearing status and orthopedic consultation for surgical pinning.

### Legg-Calvé-Perthes Disease

• Legg-Calvé-Perthes disease (LCPD) is idiopathic avascular necrosis of the femoral head.
• LCPD occurs in children between the ages of 4 and 8 years and is five times more common in males. It is associated with delayed bone age, coagulopathy, and ADHD.
• Prognosis is better with younger bone age at onset of symptoms.
• Patients present with insidious onset of limp, referred knee pain, and limited hip internal rotation and abduction.
• For longer-standing cases, diagnosis is made by radiographs with AP and frog-leg views of the hips, which show fragmentation and then healing of the femoral head. Early in the avascular process, plain radiographs may be normal and magnetic resonance imaging (MRI) may be needed for diagnosis.
• All patients must be referred for orthopedic evaluation.

## Knee

### Fractures

- Fractures are more common in skeletally immature children.
- The distal femoral physis is the site most vulnerable to injury due to epiphyseal attachments of the medial and lateral collateral ligaments.
- Other injury sites include tibial spine avulsion at the insertion of the anterior cruciate ligament and fractures of the tibial tuberosity (most commonly sustained in adolescent males during sporting activities).
- Patella fractures can occur as a result of direct trauma to the knee or as an avulsion fracture during extension.

### Ligamentous Injuries

When ligamentous injuries occur, they are generally the result of direct trauma or sporting activities in skeletally mature patients (Table 5-2).

### Dislocations

- Knee (tibiofemoral) dislocation
  - Infrequent injury that is most commonly produced by high-velocity trauma but can occur during sporting activities.
  - Results from the rupture of two or more major ligaments of the knee.
  - The patient should be evaluated for associated neurovascular injury after reduction.
- Patellar dislocation
  - Lateral patellar dislocation is most common and typically occurs as a result of a pivoting motion with the foot planted or, less commonly, a direct blow to the medial knee.

| TABLE 5-2 | Injuries to Ligaments of the Knee | | |
|-----------|-----------|-----------|-----------|
| **Ligament** | **Injury** | **Physical examination** | **Management** |
| Medial collateral | Twisting or lateral blow to the knee | Pain and swelling at ligament; limitation of motion acutely; laxity with valgus stress | RICE, NSAIDs, no weight bearing, referral for orthopedic consult |
| Anterior cruciate | Pivoting with foot planted and knee flexed or direct blow during hyperextension | Displacement on Lachman or anterior drawer test; hemarthrosis, and avulsion fracture acutely | Crutches, +/− knee immobilizer, activity restrictions, referral for orthopedic consult |
| Posterior cruciate | Direct blow to tibia while knee is flexed | Displacement on posterior drawer test; posterior knee tenderness and small effusion | RICE, NSAIDs, no weight bearing, referral for orthopedic consult |

- The patella is often displaced laterally on examination, with associated swelling of the knee joint and limited range of motion.
- Radiographs should be obtained after reduction to assess for associated fractures.
- After reduction, patients should be treated with non–weight-bearing status; crutches; knee immobilizer or brace; rest, ice, compression and elevation (RICE); nonsteroidal anti-inflammatory medications (NSAIDs); and referral for orthopedic follow-up.

### Osgood-Schlatter Disease

- This painful, chronic microavulsion fracture of the tibial apophysis occurs due to repeated vigorous traction across the quadriceps in a growing child. It is most common in adolescents between the ages of 11 and 15 years, particularly those in sports with running and jumping.
- Physical examination reveals point tenderness at the tibial tubercle (i.e., insertion of patellar tendon). Additional maneuvers that elicit pain include active knee extension, squatting, and jumping.
- It is unnecessary to obtain plain radiographs if the presentation is classic. If obtained, elevation or fragmentation of the tibial tubercle is seen.
- Treatment and anticipatory guidance
  - Symptoms may persist with aggravating activities (e.g., jumping, climbing stairs) until tibial epiphyses close.
  - NSAIDs, ice, and rest for any pain.
  - Knee strap may help tolerance of painful activities; knee immobilizer and crutches if pain is severe.
  - Regular stretching of quadriceps and hamstrings.

## Lower Leg

### Tibial Shaft Fractures

- These common fractures are often the result of direct trauma.
- Most can be managed with closed reduction and casting.

### Toddler Fracture

- This is an oblique, nondisplaced spiral fracture of the distal tibia in an ambulating child under the age of 3. It generally occurs as a result of low-energy forces, and patients often present without history of injury.
- The child presents with antalgic gait and refusal to bear weight. There is often minimal tenderness to palpation, but pain is elicited with internal or external rotation of the ankle.
- Radiographs are not revealing >50% of the time; sensitivity is improved with an oblique view of the tibia. Ultrasound can sometimes detect a fracture hematoma.
- Treatment: immobilization with splint, cast, or walking boot for 3 weeks.

## Foot/Ankle

### Ankle Sprains

- These injuries occur due to inversion during plantar flexion, with talofibular ligament disruption being the most common injury.
- Patients present with pain anterior to the lateral malleolus, swelling, and ecchymosis.
- **Ottawa ankle and foot rules** indicate that radiographs should be obtained if:
  - Ankle pain is near the malleoli and *either:*
    - The patient is unable to bear weight (four steps) immediately after the injury **and** at the time of assessment *or*
    - Bone tenderness is present at the posterior edge or tip of either malleolus.

- Foot pain is present in the midfoot and *either:*
  - The patient is unable to bear weight as above *or*
  - Bone tenderness is present over the navicular base or the base of fifth metatarsal.
- Ankle sprains are classified as follows:
  - **Grade I:** mild stretching of the ligament
    - Presents with mild swelling and tenderness, no joint instability, and ability to bear weight and ambulate with minimal assistance
  - **Grade II:** incomplete tear of the ligament
    - Presents with moderate pain, swelling, tenderness, and ecchymosis; mild joint instability and limited range of motion; and painful weight bearing and ambulation
  - **Grade III:** complete tear of a ligament
    - Presents with severe pain, swelling, tenderness, and ecchymosis; significant joint instability; and inability to bear weight or ambulate
- Treatment
  - **Grade I:** elastic wrap or stirrup compression splint, ice, elevation, NSAIDs, and weight bearing as tolerated
  - **Grades II and III:** cast or posterior splint for 3 weeks
  - If there is suspicion of Salter-Harris I (point tender over physis): cast or splint, elevation, and orthopedic consult in 1 week
  - **RICE** (treatment mnemonic for sprains)
    - **R**est: Ambulation is allowed if it is not painful and does not result in swelling.
    - **I**ce: With the skin protected by cloth, ice area for 15-20 minutes every 2 hours while awake for the first 48 hours after injury.
    - **C**ompression: Use Ace wrap or air cast.
    - **E**levation: Keep the injury elevated as often as possible. The child may need a note for school.

*Sever Disease (Calcaneal Apophysitis)*
- This is an overuse injury of insidious onset, generally affecting children ages 10-12 years old (males more often than females) who play sports with running and jumping, especially those requiring cleats.
- Physical examination reveals point tenderness at the insertion of the Achilles tendon on the calcaneus.
- Treatment consists of RICE, regular gastrocnemius, and soleus stretching and return to play only when pain is resolved. Heel pads in shoes may provide some comfort.

## EVALUATION OF A CHILD WITH A LIMP

The differential diagnosis for a child presenting with a limp or refusal to bear weight is broad and varies by age (Table 5-3). A thorough history and physical examination are essential to differentiate benign from potentially life-threatening etiologies. The most common causes of limping are trauma (fracture, soft tissue injury, overuse injury), infection (septic arthritis, osteomyelitis), inflammation (transient synovitis, rheumatologic disorders), or other hip disorders (developmental dysplasia of the hip [DDH], SCFE, LCPD). The most important disorders to rule out are those that are potentially life- or limb-threatening; these include infectious etiologies (discussed below), tumors, DDH, and SCFE.

| TABLE 5-3 | Differential Diagnosis of Limp by Age | |
|---|---|---|
| **Toddler (0-5 years old)** | **School age (5-12 years old)** | **Adolescent (13-18 years old)** |
| Septic arthritis | Septic arthritis | Septic arthritis |
| Osteomyelitis | Osteomyelitis | Osteomyelitis |
| Transient synovitis | Transient synovitis | SCFE |
| DDH | Overuse syndromes | Overuse syndromes |
| Congenital limb anomaly | Growing pains | Fracture |
| LCPD | LCPD | Contusion |
| Toddler fracture | Fracture | Sprain/strain |
| Nonaccidental injury (child abuse) | Contusion | Patellofemoral pain syndrome |
| Contusion | Strain/sprain | Osteochondritis dissecans |
| Foreign body | Foreign body | |
| Neurologic disorders | Limb length discrepancy | Scoliosis |
| Rheumatic disease (JIA) | Neurologic disorders | Rheumatic disease (JIA, SLE, IBD) |
| Tumor | Rheumatic disease (JIA, ARF, HSP, dermatomyositis) | Tumor |
| | Tumor | |

DDH, developmental dysplasia of the hip; LCPD, Legg-Calvé-Perthes disease; SCFE, slipped capital femoral epiphysis; JIA, juvenile idiopathic arthritis; ARF, acute rheumatic fever; HSP, Henoch-Schönlein purpura; SLE, systemic lupus erythematous; IBD, inflammatory bowel disease.

## History

The history should focus on:

• Onset and duration of the limp
• Pain versus weakness
• Trauma
• Fever or other systemic symptoms

## Physical Examination

• Gait: The child should be undressed to an appropriate state and gait closely assessed.
• Limb: The entire limb should be palpated for evidence of point tenderness, joint effusion, or warmth. Full range of motion should be assessed in all joints. Limb lengths should be assessed.
• Neurologic: A thorough examination should look for any motor deficits or tone abnormalities. Assess deep tendon reflexes.
• Back, abdomen, and groin: Pain may be referred from these sites and may be the cause for limp.

## Evaluation

• Plain radiographs of the affected area are indicated to evaluate for evidence of fracture, effusion, lytic lesions, or other abnormalities.

- Routine laboratory workup is generally not indicated in afebrile children with a normal examination or obvious mechanism of traumatic injury. If the child is febrile or ill appearing, a complete blood count (CBC), erythrocyte sedimentation rate (ESR), C-reactive protein (CRP), and blood culture should be obtained.
- Additional workup should be guided by the initial evaluation.

## INFECTIOUS ETIOLOGIES

### Septic Joint

Bacteria can enter a joint via hematogenous spread, direct inoculation, or extension of infection. The organisms to consider are gram-positive organisms *Staphylococcus aureus* (most common) and streptococcal species, as well as gram-negative organisms *Kingella kingae* and *Neisseria gonorrhea* (primarily in adolescents). This diagnosis is an **orthopedic emergency**.

#### Clinical Presentation
- The majority of septic joints occur in the lower extremities, with the knee and hip being the most commonly affected joints. Multifocal infections are more common in neonates.
- Classic presentation is acute onset of fever, joint pain, and swelling, with limited range of motion of the affected joint and/or refusal to bear weight. Neonates may present with septic appearance, irritability, or pseudoparalysis of the affected limb.
- The joint may appear warm, red, swollen, and tender (although this is less common with involvement of the hip). With hip involvement, the hip tends to be held in abduction and external rotation (neutral position) to maximize comfort.

#### Evaluation
- Laboratory evaluation should include:
  - CBC with differential. White blood cell (WBC) count is elevated in about 50% of these patients.
  - Blood culture.
  - Synovial fluid analysis (cell count and differential, Gram stain, culture). Synovial fluid culture frequently does not grow even when clearly infected.
  - ESR and CRP, which are elevated in 90-95% of these patients. These markers are useful for trending during the illness and recovery. CRP will rise and fall earlier than ESR.
- Plain radiographs may show subtle signs of joint effusion, such as widening of the joint space, soft tissue swelling, obliteration of normal fat planes, or osteomyelitis. Ultrasound may show joint effusion.

#### Diagnosis
- The **Kocher criteria** can be used to aid diagnosis of septic arthritis in children with a painful joint.
  - The criteria include (1) nonweight bearing on the affected side, (2) ESR > 40 mm/hr, (3) history of fever >38.5°C, and (4) WBC > 12,000 μL.
  - A child with four of the criteria has a 99% likelihood of septic arthritis. With three criteria, the likelihood is 93%. With just two or one, the likelihood drops to 40% or 3%, respectively.
- The definitive diagnosis is made in microscopic examination of synovial fluid obtained through **arthrocentesis**. Hip aspirations are usually done under fluoroscopic guidance. If synovial fluid has >50,000 WBC, the hip may be opened and irrigated in the OR.

*Management*

Empiric parenteral antibiotic therapy targeted at *S. aureus* should be initiated *after aspiration of the hip joint* and the joint should be surgically drained and irrigated.

## Osteomyelitis

Osteomyelitis occurs most commonly in patients younger than 5 years of age. Infants and neonates are more likely to have multifocal osteomyelitis and concurrent septic arthritis. Hematogenous seeding is the most common pathway of infection, and the highly vascular metaphyses of long bones provide an ideal environment for spread of infection (although any bone may be affected). *S. aureus* is the most common pathogen (70-90%), with an increasing incidence of cases attributed to community-acquired methicillin-resistant *S. aureus* (MRSA). Group A β-hemolytic *Streptococcus* is the second most common pathogen. *K. kingae* is frequently isolated in toddlers and preschool-aged children and often has a more subtle clinical presentation with less inflammation.

*Clinical Presentation*
- The patient is usually febrile. Point tenderness over the bone is present; however, in contrast to the child with a septic joint, the child allows range-of-motion evaluation of the affected extremity. Redness and swelling may overlie the area of tenderness but are not consistently present.
- Neonates may present with irritability and pseudoparalysis of the affected extremity.

*Evaluation*
- Laboratory evaluation includes CRP, ESR, blood culture, and CBC. Elevated WBC count is often surprisingly absent.
- Standard plain films may not display destructive changes to bone in the first 10-14 days of illness. MRI or a bone scan can offer more information.
  - MRI is more sensitive and helps to detail subperiosteal abscesses in need of surgical drainage, but it often requires sedation in this age group.
  - Bone scan may be more helpful if considering multifocal disease.

*Management*
- Empiric parenteral antibiotic coverage should be aimed at the most common organisms and local sensitivity patterns. Blood cultures and bone aspirates should ideally be obtained before the initiation of antibiotics in the clinically stable child.
- Clindamycin or vancomycin are two commonly chosen initial agents. Oxacillin and gentamicin are empiric coverage for neonates. Patients with sickle cell disease are predisposed to *Salmonella* osteomyelitis, and use of a third-generation cephalosporin should be considered.
- Many patients will require antibiotics for 3-6 weeks, which may or may not need to be parenteral. Antibiotic duration and administration rely on clinical judgment, objective diagnostic data, and oral bioavailability of pertinent antibiotics.

## Transient Synovitis

This benign, self-limiting inflammatory condition is a diagnosis of exclusion. It is the most common cause of acute hip pain in children ages 3-10 and must be differentiated from a septic joint.

*Presentation*

These children typically have a nontoxic appearance with little or no fever, although they resist range-of-motion assessment and weight bearing.

*Evaluation*
- ESR, CRP, and WBC are generally normal. Synovial fluid, when obtained, is sterile, often with WBC < 50,000 cells/μL.
- Radiographs are recommended to exclude other possible diagnoses. Ultrasound is also frequently performed to confirm the presence of an effusion.

*Management*
These patients may be followed clinically and managed conservatively with NSAIDs. The prognosis is excellent, although a small percentage of cases recur.

## DEVELOPMENTAL MUSCULOSKELETAL DISORDERS

### Developmental Dysplasia of the Hip

DDH is a spectrum of abnormalities in which the femoral head and acetabulum are misaligned or have abnormal development. Etiologies include mechanical (abnormal in utero positioning), primary acetabular dysplasia, or ligamentous laxity.

*Epidemiology*
- Risk factors include breech presentation, female sex, oligohydramnios, first-born infant, postnatal positioning, white ethnicity, and family history. **However, most affected children do not have identifiable risk factors.**
- The left hip is more likely to be affected than is the right.
- Associated conditions include torticollis, clubfoot (metatarsus adductus), scoliosis, plagiocephaly, and low-set ears.

*Evaluation*
- The American Academy of Pediatrics (AAP) recommends that infants and toddlers be screened for DDH at every health supervision visit until the child is walking normally.
- Key physical examination findings include:
  - Asymmetry of gluteal and thigh folds.
  - Leg length discrepancy. A positive Galeazzi sign may be present on physical examination (Fig. 5-2).
  - Limited abduction (<45 degrees) in children >3 months of age.
  - Hip instability with Ortolani and Barlow maneuvers can be seen in infants up to 12 weeks of age (Fig. 5-2). Hip clicks without a sensation of instability are clinically insignificant.

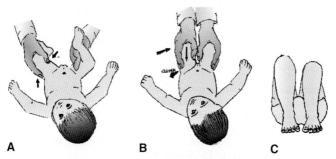

**A**   **B**   **C**

**Figure 5-2. A.** Ortolani maneuver (hip is dislocated). **B.** Barlow maneuver (hip is able to be dislocated). **C.** Allis or Galeazzi sign (leg length discrepancy).

- Diagnostic imaging
  - Ultrasound is the primary imaging modality for diagnosis until 4-6 months of age. After 4-6 months, radiographs are more helpful.
    - The AAP advises consideration of a screening hip ultrasound after 6 weeks of age for any infant positioned breech in the third trimester, with a family history of DDH, with a hip examination abnormality that subsequently normalized, or a history of improper swaddling.
    - Proper swaddling allows free movement at the hip and does not force hip adduction and extension.

*Management*
- The natural history of DDH depends on the severity and the age of the patient. Most hip instability in newborns is physiologic, and up to 90% of cases stabilize by 8-12 weeks of age. Patients with untreated DDH may develop altered gait or hip pain as they get older.
- Any child with limited hip abduction or asymmetric hip abduction after 4 weeks of age should be referred to an orthopedic specialist.
- Treatment method by age
  - 0-6 months
    - Pavlik harness for abduction bracing; wear 23 hours a day for at least 6 weeks.
    - Triple diapering as a treatment is not recommended.
  - 6-18 months, or Pavlik failure
    - Closed reduction and spica casting for 3 months
    - Open reduction followed by spica casting if closed reduction is unsuccessful
  - Older than 18 months
    - Open reduction and spica casting or osteotomy

## Scoliosis

Scoliosis is defined by lateral curvature of the spine >10 degrees, with associated coronal or rotational deformities. Classification depends on magnitude, location, direction, and etiology. About 80% of cases are idiopathic and occur during adolescent growth spurts. Congenital or neuromuscular etiologies are also possible. Pulmonary function is typically preserved unless thoracic curvature exceeds 70 degrees. The incidence of back pain, except in patients with thoracolumbar curvature, is no greater than in the general population.

*Epidemiology*
- Approximately 2-3% of the population has scoliosis. Females are affected more often and with greater incidence of curve progression. There is often a positive family history.
- Curve progression is more likely in skeletally immature patients and those with curves >30-40 degrees at skeletal maturity.

*Evaluation*
- Screening at routine health supervision visits should begin at 8 years of age.
- Physical examination should evaluate body asymmetry (hips, shoulders, scapulae, spine) when looking from behind.
  - Adams forward bend test (Fig. 5-3): with hands together, posterior ribs prominent on convex side; a scoliometer reading (angle of trunk rotation) of 5-7 degrees correlates with a Cobb angle of 15-20 degrees.
  - Leg length differences are most apparent when palpating the iliac crest.

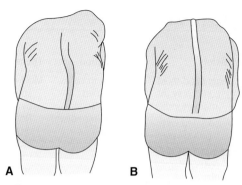

**Figure 5-3. Scoliosis. A.** Deformity. **B.** Normal spine.

- Diagnosis is made with *standing* full-length PA and lateral views of the spine. The **Cobb angle** measures the degree of angulation and is the gold standard for diagnosis.

*Management*
- Refer patients with:
  - Cobb angle >30 degrees in any patient
  - Cobb angle >20-29 degrees in a premenarchal girl, or boy aged 12-14 years
  - Angle of trunk rotation >7 degrees
  - Progression of curvature >5 degrees in any patient
- The choice of therapy depends on the degree of curvature and the potential for further growth.
  - Cobb angle 11-20 degrees: observation with serial examinations and radiographs as indicated
  - Cobb angle 21-40 degrees: bracing indicated for skeletally immature patients with growth potential
  - Cobb angle >40 degrees: surgery indicated for skeletally immature patients with curves ≥50 degrees and some skeletally immature patients with curves between 40 and 50 degrees

## In-toeing

- In general, feet pointing toward midline during gait is a common developmental variation that resolves spontaneously as the child grows.
- On examination, determine the foot progression angle, range of internal and external hip rotation, thigh-foot angle, and degree of metatarsus varus.
- In-toeing is characteristic of femoral anteversion, internal tibial torsion, and metatarsus adductus. Long-term functional problems are unusual, and severe or persistent cases should be referred to an orthopedist (Table 5-4).

## Out-toeing

Feet pointing away from midline during walking usually spontaneously resolves over time. Indications for referral include unilateral/asymmetric out-toeing or persistence of symptoms >8 years of age causing limitation of activity.

| TABLE 5-4 | Types of In-toeing | | |
|-----------|--------------------|---|---|

| Condition (incidence) | History | Physical examination | Therapy |
|-----------------------|---------|----------------------|---------|
| Metatarsus adductus (5-10%) | Diagnosed most commonly in infants/toddlers<br><br>Associated with hip dysplasia<br><br>Common to have positive family history | Forefoot in varus, C shaped (metatarsals point in midline) | Most cases resolve spontaneously by age 2 years. Referral to orthopedics is indicated if rigid (may require serial casting) or persistent. |
| Internal tibial torsion (5-10%) | Diagnosed at 1-4 years old, after ambulatory<br><br>More frequent when sitting or sleeping on feet with feet turned in | Abnormal (internal) thigh-foot angle (normal: 0-20 degrees at birth; 20 degrees by age 2-3; 0-40 degrees adults) | Growth corrects the majority of cases by 5 years of age.<br><br>Refer to specialist if no improvement over first year of walking.<br><br>Surgery may be indicated in severe cases in children >8-10 years old. |
| Femoral anteversion (80-90%) | Diagnosed between 3 and 8 years of age | Patella face medially when standing and point toward midline when walking<br><br>Increased internal rotation and decreased external rotation of both hips | Usually resolves by 8-12 years old<br><br>Surgery is indicated if internal rotation ≥80 degrees, or severe gait disturbance persists >11 years of age. |

## Bowlegs (Genu Varum)

Physiologic genu varum is common in children younger than 2 years. It is typically bilateral, improves slowly starting around 18 months of age, and disappears by 3-4 years of age.

- Differential diagnosis
  - Physiologic varus is most common.
  - Rickets.
  - Familial bowlegs.
  - Posttraumatic growth disturbance.
  - Skeletal dysplasia.
  - **Blount disease**, a pathologic growth disturbance of the medial epiphysis of the tibia that often results in progressive bowing. Risk factors include a family history, obesity, African American ethnicity, and early walking. There are two types.

○ Early-onset Blount disease is diagnosed before 10 years of age (usually before 3 years of age). It is often bilateral, typically worsens after walking has begun, and may be treated with braces or epiphysiodesis.

○ Late-onset Blount disease is diagnosed after 10 years of age and is rarely bilateral. It is strongly associated with obesity. Osteotomy is commonly required.

• Bowlegged children who merit orthopedic referral include those with severe or progressive bowing, persistent bowing after 3 years of age, unilateral/asymmetric bowing, short stature, or history of metabolic disease, trauma, infection, or tumor.

## Knock Knees (Genu Valgum)

Physiologic genu valgum is often first noticed around 2-3 years of age, progresses for 1-2 years, and spontaneously corrects at 3-4 years of age. It should not worsen after 7 years of age.

• Differential diagnosis
  • Physiologic valgus is most common.
  • Rickets.
  • Skeletal dysplasias.
  • Posttraumatic growth disturbance.
• Features suggestive of pathology that merit orthopedic referral include severe or progressive deformity after age 4-5 years, persistent knock knees after 7 years, unilateral or asymmetric deformity, and history of metabolic disorder, trauma, infection, or tumor.

## SUGGESTED READINGS

Beaty JH, Kasser JR, eds. Rockwood and Wilkins' Fractures in Children. 7th Ed. Philadelphia, PA: Lippincott Williams & Wilkins, 2009.

Connolly LP, Connolly SA. Skeletal scintigraphy in the multimodality assessment of young children with acute skeletal symptoms. Clin Nucl Med 2003;28(9):746–754.

Craig C, Goldberg M. Foot and leg problems. Pediatr Rev 1993;14:395.

Egol K, Koval KJ, Zuckerman JD. Handbook of Fractures. Philadelphia, PA: Wolters Kluwer, 2015.

Fleisher GR, Ludwig S, eds. Textbook of Pediatric Emergency Medicine. 6th Ed. Philadelphia, PA: Wolters Kluwer/Lippincott Williams & Wilkins, 2010:324–336, 345–358, 372–377, 1336–1375, 1568–1586.

Kleinman PK. Diagnostic Imaging of Child Abuse. 3rd Ed. Cambridge, UK: Cambridge University Press, 2015.

Marsh J. Screening for scoliosis. Pediatr Rev 1993;14:297.

Plint AC, Bulloch B, Osmond MH, et al. Validation of the Ottawa ankle rules in children with ankle injuries. Acad Emerg Med 1999;6:1005.

Shaw BA, Segal LS; Section on Orthopaedics. Evaluation and referral for developmental dysplasia of the hip in infants. Pediatrics 2016;138(6):e20163107.

US Preventive Services Task Force. Screening for developmental dysplasia of the hip: recommendation statement. Pediatrics 2006;117:898–902.

# 6

# Child Maltreatment

Adrienne D. Atzemis and Jamie S. Kondis

## INTRODUCTION

Child maltreatment is a common cause of childhood morbidity and mortality, leading to more than 1800 child deaths per year in the United States. Failure to recognize signs and symptoms of child maltreatment and to appropriately respond can result in death. The types of child maltreatment are as follows:

- Neglect: A child is not provided with adequate basic needs, such as safety, nutrition, housing, education, and medical and dental care.
- Physical abuse: A child is physically harmed by another's nonaccidental actions.
- Sexual abuse: A child is subjected to developmentally inappropriate sexual material or activities by someone in a caretaking role or is subjected to sexual activity without his or her consent.
- Caregiver-fabricated illness: A child is subjected to unnecessary medical care because of a caregiver's fabrication, exaggeration, or inducing of symptoms.
- Emotional abuse: A child is emotionally harmed by a caretaker's actions or verbal statements.

It is estimated that over one million children are victimized by some type of child maltreatment each year. Maltreatment spans all social, economic, educational, racial, and cultural spectrums, although there are risk factors for an increased incidence, including the following:

- Child factors: young age, unplanned or unwanted pregnancy, prematurity, developmental delay, cognitive impairment, and having a "difficult" temperament
- Caregiver factors: social isolation, mental illness, substance abuse, personal history of victimization, poverty, lack of parenting skills, and unrealistic expectations of child
- Community factors: violence, poverty, lack of resources, and failure to address community needs

## MANDATORY REPORTING OF CHILD MALTREATMENT

- Laws for reporting child maltreatment vary from state to state, but in every US state, medical providers are mandated to report child maltreatment.
- Health care providers should be aware of their legal obligations as mandated by their country or state, as well as their institutional policies addressing abuse concerns.
- Failure to report abuse can result in fines and/or imprisonment and/or loss of medical license.

## RECOGNIZING AND RESPONDING TO NEGLECT CONCERNS

- Types of neglect include physical, supervisional/abandonment, endangering/safety, emotional, educational, and medical/dental.

- Neglect may manifest as inadequate hygiene (child is obviously smelly or filthy), or poor hygiene may contribute to medical problems, such as a wound infection.
- The child may be wearing clothes that are too small or are inappropriate for the environment.
- A child's injuries may be the result of inadequate supervision, or the family may delay in seeking care for the injuries.

## RECOGNIZING AND RESPONDING TO PHYSICAL ABUSE CONCERNS

- A provider's ability to correctly recognize child physical abuse is first dependent on his or her willingness to accept maltreatment as a potential cause of a physical finding.
- It is then dependent on the provider to recognize concerning elements of the history and recognize suspicious physical findings.
  - Concerning history
    - No history to account for an injury.
    - Delay in seeking medical care.
    - Past history of abuse.
    - Substantial variation in the history, either by the same caregiver over time or by two different caregivers.
    - The history provided is implausible.
    - The history lacks contextual details.
    - The historian gives a vague timeline.
  - Concerning injury
    - The injury is discordant with the developmental stage of the patient.
    - There is a proposed minor mechanism leading to a major injury.
    - The injury is patterned or geometric.
    - The injury has sharply demarcated borders or transition zones.
    - The injury sites are unusual for an accidental injury.
    - There are multiple sites, types, or stages of healing injury.
    - The injuries are bilateral or involve multiple planes of the body.
- Many communities have identified local experts who are experienced providing medical care to victimized children within the context of local legal regulations and expectations. Inexperienced providers are encouraged to utilize the assistance of local experts before a final diagnosis is provided.
- Presume that the medical record will be reviewed by local investigatory agencies and may be used in legal proceedings. Therefore, ensure that the record is complete and legible and provides enough information for nonmedical professionals to reasonably understand the findings.

### Bruises

- Bruises are common in active healthy children and are also the most common presenting injury in an abused child.
- See Table 6-1 for common characteristics of abusive versus accidental bruises.
- See Figures 6-1–6-3, for examples of slap mark, loop-shaped mark, human bite.

### Fractures

- Fractures are the second most common injury caused by child abuse.
- Abusive fractures are frequently occult and do not have overlying bruise.

| TABLE 6-1 | Common Characteristics of Abusive versus Accidental Bruises | |
|---|---|---|
| | **Accidental** | **Abusive** |
| Location | Anterior | Posterior |
| | Bony prominences | Softer areas |
| | Forehead | Cheeks |
| | Elbow | Ears |
| | Knees | Abdomen |
| | Shins | Thighs |
| | | Buttocks |
| Shape | Circular | Linear |
| | Oval | Looped |
| | | Patterned |
| | | Human bite |
| Number | Solitary | Clustered |
| | Few | Many |
| Developmental status | Cruising active child | Nonmobile infant |
| Color | All bruises undergo a progression of color changes with time; the color of a bruise cannot be used to distinguish abuse or accidental cause. Bruises cannot be accurately dated as older or newer than another bruise. | |

- Any fracture type may be inflicted, but there are fractures that are considered highly specific for an inflicted mechanism including the following:
  - Classic metaphyseal lesion (CML)/classic metaphyseal fracture (CMF), also known as Corner fracture or Bucket-Handle fracture, these fractures are highly specific for abuse in infants <1 year old and most common in <6 months old.
  - Rib fractures: Abusive rib fractures can result from compression of the chest or a direct impact. Posterior rib fractures are typically caused by an anterior-posterior squeezing of the chest.
  - Scapular fracture.
  - Spinous process fracture.
  - Sternal fracture.
- Fractures that are considered moderately specific for inflicted mechanism are as follows:
  - Multiple fractures, especially bilateral
  - Fractures of different ages
  - Epiphyseal separations
  - Vertebral body fractures and subluxations
  - Digital fractures
  - Complex skull fractures
- Fractures that have low specificity for abuse and are commonly accidental in nature include the following:

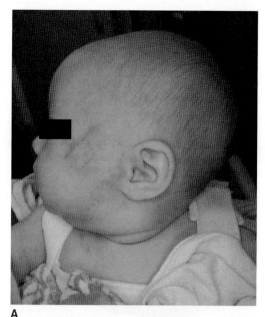

A

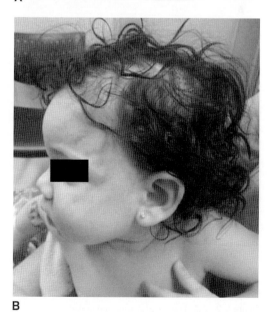

B

Figure 6-1. A,B. Hand slap marks.

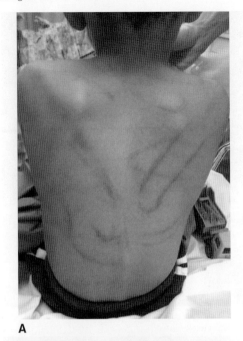

A

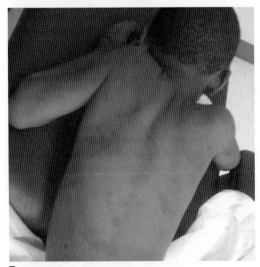

B

**Figure 6-2. A,B.** Loop marks, acute and healed.

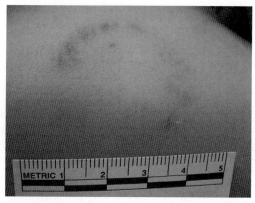

**Figure 6-3.** Human bite mark.

- Clavicular fractures
- Long bone shaft fractures
- Supracondylar fracture
- Linear skull fractures
- Both accidental and abusive fractures can be transverse, oblique, or spiral and depend on the direction of forces during the trauma mechanism. A spiral fracture can result from any rotational movement of a limb, which can occur in both accidental and abusive events.
- A medical evaluation into possible medical disease leading to brittle bones or other bone disease that can be misinterpreted as fracture should be performed if there is medical indication that such a condition exists.

## Burns

- Abusive burns may be thermal, chemical, or electrical.
- Scald burns from tap water are the most common forms of abusive burns.
- The mean age for abusive burns is 2-4 years.
- Abusive burns to the hands and feet from immersion in a hot liquid may have a "stocking" or "glove" pattern with a sharp demarcation between burns and normal skin. There may be sparing to the soles of the feet or palms of the hands or the buttocks because the spared area is pressed to a cooler surface. There may be sparing of the flexor or extensor surfaces if the extremities were held in protective positions.
- Burns with a solid object can lead to burns with a pattern in the configuration of that object. They are typically deeper than are accidental contact burns with an object. Commonly seen objects include curling irons, clothes irons, or heaters.
  - Cigarette burns from inflicted trauma are deeper and more rounded than are accidental burns from a cigarette, which have a flame-/brush-shaped pattern. Cigarette burns can be confused with impetigo, varicella, insect bites, or alternative healing practices.

## Abusive Head Trauma (AHT)

- This is the most fatal form of child abuse.
- Injuries are related to impact forces or angular acceleration/deceleration or inertial forces or a combination of those.

- The acceleration-/deceleration-related injury was previously known as "shaken baby syndrome." The term "abusive head trauma" is preferable since shaking is only one mechanism of trauma that can lead to these injuries.
- The average age of victims of AHT is 3-6 months, which coincides with a period of time in which infants often have an unrelenting cry and caregivers become frustrated.
  - The infant's behavior is often viewed as "demanding."
  - Only the infant and the caretaker are present in 99% of cases.
  - There is often a delay in seeking medical care.
  - A nonbiologic male caretaker is the most common perpetrator of AHT.
- Intracranial injuries that can be seen in AHT include subdural hemorrhage and/or subarachnoid hemorrhage, retinal hemorrhages, hypoxic encephalopathy, cerebral infarction, parenchymal contusion, cerebral edema, and herniation. Ultimately, these can lead to death in the most severe cases.
- Injuries to other body regions are seen approximately 50% of the time. These include rib fractures, CMFs, long bone fractures, or intra-abdominal injuries. Often, there are no signs of external trauma.
- Retinal hemorrhages are an important marker for a traumatic rotational injury. They occur in approximately 85% of infants diagnosed with AHT.
  - While retinal hemorrhages can occur in other situations (such as birth, or accidental traumas), in those situations, they are typically few and confined to the posterior pole. Retinal hemorrhages that are extensive, throughout the retina and vitreous, reach to the periphery, and involve multiple layers are associated with abusive mechanisms.

## Abdominal Trauma

- This is the second most fatal form of child abuse.
- Severe and fatal cases peak at the toddler age. In all cases of fatal child physical abuse, approximately 14% have abdominal injuries.
- Abusive abdominal trauma is often occult because caregivers present with a false or misleading history, and symptoms can initially be confused for other conditions, such as a gastrointestinal virus or a more minor illness.
- Inflicted abdominal injuries include duodenal hematoma, bowel contusion/rupture, liver laceration, pancreatic fracture (and subsequent pseudocyst formation), adrenal hematoma, renal injury, mesenteric avulsion, and vessel injuries.
- Abdominal injuries are rarely isolated; more than 60% have other injuries including cutaneous injuries, fractures, or head trauma.
- The liver is the most common organ injured by abuse (nearly two-thirds of cases), and the most common site of contusion and laceration is the left lobe.

## Medical Workup for Physical Abuse

- History: The medical provider should not be hesitant to obtain a complete history from available caretakers. An open, honest, and nonjudgmental approach is advised and generally well accepted by caretakers. Older, verbal children should be given an opportunity to provide a history in private. A complete history should include the following:
  - Trauma history of each known injury, including the mechanism of the injury and a time line of when the child was last injury-free
  - Birth and newborn history, including the maternal health history, information about the pregnancy, labor and delivery, vitamin K status, and if there was any excessive bleeding during circumcision or to the umbilical cord stump

- Growth and nutrition, including reviewing all growth charts and inquiring about any alternative nutrition practices and whether the infant is exclusively breastfed or formula fed
- Prior health problems, any history of "easy bruising," any prior injuries, emergency room visits, or urgent care visits
- Developmental history including if the child is able to roll, crawl, scoot, pull to stand, cruise, walk, run, climb, or use language
- Social history including asking about any caregivers, the parents' occupations, what type of housing, and if there are any animals in the home
- Family history of any bleeding, bone, or other heritable disorders, such as hemophilia or osteogenesis imperfecta
- Physical examination: Every child being evaluated for possible physical abuse should receive a comprehensive physical examination with special attention to the following:
  - Skin examination
    - Be sure to visualize all skin surfaces, including areas frequently missed such as behind the ears, genitals, and buttocks.
    - Document skin findings such as bruises, abrasions, and burns via a written description, using body diagrams (drawings) and with photographs.
    - Describe congenital findings such as congenital melanosis or birthmarks to distinguish them from possible injuries.
  - HEENT examination
    - Carefully evaluate the scalp, moving hair as necessary, to detect possible head injury.
    - Visualize the oral cavity to detect intraoral injuries (palate, frenulum) and dental decay/injuries.
  - Eye examination
    - A dilated retinal examination performed by a skilled examiner should be performed in cases concerning for AHT with intracranial injuries.
  - Torso examination
    - Palpate the chest for evidence of rib abnormality or crepitus.
    - Abdominal examination should be thorough to detect possible abdominal injury.
  - Extremity examination
    - Carefully palpate the extremities for evidence of acute or healing fracture.
  - Genital examination
    - Maltreated children often are subjected to multiple abuse types. Sexual abuse should be considered.
  - Developmental evaluation
    - Document the developmental milestones observed during examination, as it may reveal inconsistency with the history provided or may reveal developmental delay associated with chronic neglect.
  - Any signs of a medical disease that may be an alternative explanation for abuse concern.
- Laboratory evaluation
  - Verbal children with evidence of acute inflicted injury and all nonverbal children undergoing an evaluation for possible recent physical abuse should receive basic laboratory evaluation to screen for occult trauma. This data may also reveal a concern for an alternative medical diagnosis.
    - Complete blood count
    - Comprehensive metabolic panel (including AST and ALT)

- Lipase
- A noncatheterized urinalysis
- Additional laboratory data if specific concern exists
  - Stool for blood (in select cases with concern for abdominal trauma)
  - Serum myoglobin or creatinine kinase (if concern for muscle injury)
  - Troponin (if concern for cardiac injury)
  - Urine drug screen and/or specific drug testing (if concern for drug exposure)
- Children with bruising/bleeding (including internal bleeding like subdural hematoma) or historical/clinical concern for bleeding disorder should be screened for bleeding disorder:
  - PT/PTT.
  - Factor VIII level.
  - Factor IX level.
  - Von Willebrand activity.
  - Further evaluation may require obtaining a hematology consult.
- Any historical or physical indication of possible medical disease that may be responsible for abuse concern should be appropriately evaluated by laboratory means, if necessary.
- Imaging
  - Plain radiographs of bone
    - Regardless of age, any symptom or clinically apparent physical sign of possible fracture should be imaged.
    - Skeletal survey: All children <3 years of age with concern for abuse, children age 3-5 years on a case by case basis (chronically debilitated or have other serious abusive injuries present), and rarely children >5 years should receive a complete skeletal survey.
      - A complete skeletal survey should always include skull (AP and lateral) four views if suspected skull fracture, AP radii/ulnae, C spine (AP and lateral), PA hands, lumbar spine (lateral), AP femurs, thorax (AP, lateral, right and left oblique) including thorax and upper lumbar spine, AP tibias/fibulae, pelvis, abdomen (AP) to include mid lumbar–sacral spine, AP or PA feet, and AP humeri.
      - Accepting less than the recommended views will result in an unacceptable error rate. The "babygram," which is an AP view on 1-2 radiographs, should never be accepted as complete.
      - A follow-up skeletal survey should be performed 2-3 weeks after the initial skeletal survey. The follow-up skeletal survey can detect callous formation denoting an underlying fracture that was not apparent on the initial skeletal survey and can clarify questionable fractures. To decrease radiation exposure, a modified skeletal survey, which eliminates the skull and possibly the abdomen and pelvis, is acceptable for the follow-up testing since there is a low yield for finding new fractures in those areas.
  - Abdominal imaging
    - Indications include peritoneal signs, AST or ALT elevation >80, pancreatic enzyme elevation, hematuria, abdominal or lower thoracic wall bruises, encephalopathy, or hemodynamic instability of unknown etiology.
    - Abdominal CT is considered the gold standard imaging technique and should include IV contrast for solid organs, bladder and visceral injury, and PO contrast to detect hollow viscus injury.

○ Abdominal ultrasound is not routinely recommended and is considered less reliable to detect specific injuries, but ultrasound may occasionally indicate concerning signs of intra-abdominal injury, such as free fluid, which should then be thoroughly evaluated.
• Neuroimaging
  ○ Regardless of age, any historical or clinical evidence of acute intracranial injury should be evaluated with neuroimaging.
  ○ Clinical evidence of chronic intracranial injury is best evaluated by brain MRI.
  ○ Young infants being evaluated for physical abuse (<6 months of age, multiple fractures, witnessed abuse, sibling with evidence of AHT) should have neuroimaging to screen for occult head injury. If there is any concern for an acute injury requiring treatment, a CT of the head should be obtained. Brain MRI may be more appropriate in cases not requiring emergent neuroimaging.
  ○ Any patient with a brain injury finding on CT or a patient who still has neurologic sign of possible brain injury after a normal CT should also receive a brain MRI.
  ○ Spine imaging (CT or MRI as clinically indicated) should be performed if there is any historical or clinical indication of spine injury. There should be a low threshold for obtaining spine imaging in infants with suspected AHT.

## RECOGNIZING AND RESPONDING TO SEXUAL ABUSE CONCERN

• Sexual abuse occurs when a child is engaged in sexual activities that she or he cannot comprehend, for which she or he is developmentally unprepared and cannot give consent and/or violate law or social taboos.
• Perpetrators of child sexual abuse:
  • Are in a position of responsibility, trust, or power
  • Are typically a known and trusted caregiver or family member
  • Rarely use violence, but manipulation of the child's trust
  • Seek sexual gratification from the child, regardless of their usual sexual partner preferences
• Sexual assault is any sexual act where consent is not obtained or freely given.
• Perpetrators of sexual assault:
  • Are known or unknown to the victim
    ○ 90% of perpetrators are someone who the child knows and trusts.
  • May use threats, violence, alcohol or drugs, or manipulation to overcome the protective efforts of their victim
• By age 18 years, 1 in 4 females and 1 in 13 males have experienced a sexual abuse/assault event.

### Medical Evaluation of Sexual Abuse

• Children may present to medical providers in a variety of ways, but most commonly, a child has made a verbal disclosure of abuse. Children who disclose sexual abuse typically disclose only a portion of the abuse events after a significant time has passed. This process of disclosure should not be interpreted as evidence of a false history.
• Less commonly, a child will present for a sexual abuse evaluation because of a concerning symptom or sign.
• Concerning symptoms/signs of sexual abuse include the following:
  • Inappropriate sexual behaviors

- Diagnosis of a sexually transmitted infection
- Genital pain or injury
- Behavioral indicators
- Sexual promiscuity or prostitution
- Pregnancy
- Every child with a credible concern of sexual abuse/assault should be offered a timely medical evaluation by a provider who is skilled in performing such evaluations.
- History: The medical provider should not be hesitant to obtain a complete history from available caretakers. An open, honest, and nonjudgmental approach is advised and generally well accepted by caretakers. Caregivers should be provided a quiet and private area to discuss sexual abuse concerns, away from the child, who may become upset by seeing an upset loved one.
  - A general past medical history and review of systems from an available caregiver.
  - A collection of available incident history from available caretakers and/or investigators who may have knowledge about the events leading to a sexual abuse concern.
  - Older, verbal children should be given an opportunity to provide a history in private.
    - Many institutions employ experienced staff members who have received training in the best practices of obtaining a history of abuse from a child.
    - All questions asked of the child should be open ended and nonleading. Suggestions "What happened?" "What happened next?" "How is your body feeling right now?"
    - Any question asked and the response of the child should be documented verbatim.
- Physical examination: If done without sensitivity to the emotional aspects of sexual abuse/assault, a physical examination can be interpreted as traumatic by victims. Patients, including young children, should not be forced or intimidated to consent to a physical examination or any aspect of medical care for sexual abuse/assault. Care should be taken to offer the patient as much control over the medical process as possible. Every child being evaluated for possible sexual abuse should be offered a comprehensive physical examination with special attention to the following areas:
- Any signs of a medical disease that may be an alternative explanation for abuse concern
- Skin examination
  - The examiner should visualize all skin surfaces.
  - Attention to skin injuries such as abrasions, bruises, and bite marks, which may be present in areas targeted to restrain (such as the neck and wrists) as well as targets of sexual activity (such as the neck, breast, inner thighs, genitals).
- Abdominal examination
  - Sexual assault victims may have intra-abdominal injury from blunt force or from a penetrating injury through the genital-urinary or GI tract.
- Genital/anal examination
  - Familiarity with normal genital anatomy and common variants is required, as many normal variations are misinterpreted as evidence of acute or healed injury.
  - See Figure 6-4 for anatomical image.
  - Most sexual abuse victims have normal genital examinations, without evidence of injury. This is attributed to multiple factors, including the following:
    - The sexual contact was such that injury would be unexpected.
    - The sexual contact included penetration of tissue that is resilient and elastic.
    - The sexual contact resulted in injury that has healed, leaving no evidence.

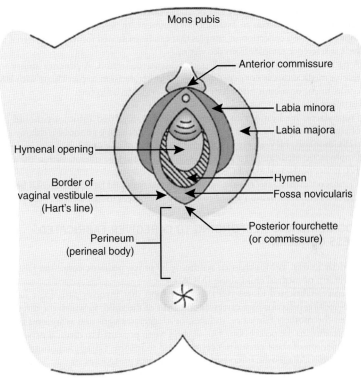

**Figure 6-4. Diagram of the genital anatomy of a prepubertal girl.** This drawing shows a crescent hymen. (From Pokorny SF. Pediatric and Adolescent Gynecology. New York: Chapman and Hall, 1996.)

- ○ Injuries that may be found include bruising, abrasion, and lacerations of any genital structure.
- ○ Child sexual abuse victims are at risk for sexually transmitted infections. Clinical indication of an infection should be addressed.
- Any abnormality should be documented in multiple forms, such as a written description, a drawing, and/or photograph. Photo or video documentation is considered a standard practice for sexual abuse evaluations.
- Laboratory testing
  - If there is historical or clinical indication of genital contact, then appropriate sexually transmitted infection testing should be performed according to CDC recommendations.
  - STI testing should be performed at the time of the acute assault, and then follow-up testing should be performed.
- Forensic evidence collection
  - Most jurisdictions suggest that evidence collection be performed within the first 72-120 hours postassault.
  - Most law enforcement agencies have specific procedures and kits to use during trace evidence collection. Be familiar with your local expectations.

- Trace evidence of the assault can be transmitted from assailant/environment to victim and from victim to assailant/environment; therefore, evidence collection should include a collection of samples that can be evaluated for foreign material as well as reference samples from the victim.
- A patient has the right to refuse trace evidence collection. A patient's ability to receive medical care is not dependent on his or her decision to participate with law enforcement or submit himself or herself for evidence collection.
- Treatment
  - Prophylactic medications to prevent sexually transmitted infections should be offered within the first 72 hours postsexual assault including gonorrhea, chlamydia, trichomoniasis, HIV, or Hep B, depending on risk of transmission.
  - Prophylactic medication to prevent pregnancy should be offered within the first 120 hours postsexual assault.
  - Victims of sexual abuse/assault and their caretakers should be offered mental health resources and information about community resources for assistance.

## RECOGNIZING AND RESPONDING TO CAREGIVER-FABRICATED ILLNESS CONCERN

- (Formerly known as Munchausen syndrome by proxy, pediatric condition falsification [PCF], or medical child abuse [MCA])
  - Caregiver-fabricated illness (CFI) is a situation that involves pathologic health care–seeking behavior by a caregiver on behalf of the child, in which the caretaker (often the mother) fabricates, induces, or exaggerates signs and symptoms of illness leading to the perception of an ill child when presented to medical personnel.
  - The creation of these circumstances may lead to incorrect diagnoses, unnecessary medications, diagnostic interventions, and surgical procedures.
  - Evaluation and treatment in such cases require the involvement of a multidisciplinary team familiar with the dynamics of CFI.
  - Open confrontation with the suspected caretaker should be avoided until agreed on by the institutional multidisciplinary team.
  - In the interest of the child's safety, do not hesitate to keep the child under close inpatient supervision (1:1 nursing, 1:1 sitter) should intentional administration of a harmful substance be suspected (i.e., covert administration of subcutaneous insulin, the willful contamination of a wound or catheter with feces, or any other type of harmful act with the result of inducing ill health).
  - The intentional killing of a child by poison is not necessarily synonymous with CFI. Typically, it lacks the repetitive health care–seeking and health care–shopping behaviors characteristic of CFI, although it is no less puzzling.

## SUGGESTED READINGS

Adams JA, et al. Updated guidelines for the medical assessment and care of children who may have been sexually abused. J Pediatr Adolesc Gynecol 2016;29(2):81–87.

Adams JA, Farst KJ, Kellogg ND. Interpretation of medical findings in suspected child sexual abuse: an update for 2018. J Pediatr Adolesc Gynecol 2018;31(3):225–231.

Anderst JD, Carpenter SL, Thomas C, et al.; the Section on Hematology/Oncology and Committee on Child Abuse and Neglect Clinical Report. Evaluation for bleeding disorders in suspected child abuse. Pediatrics 2013;131(4):e1314–e1322.

Bass C, Glaser D. Early recognition and management of fabricated or induced illness in children. Lancet 2014;383(9926):1412–1421.

Choudhary AK, Servaes S, Slovis TL, et al. Consensus statement on abusive head trauma in infants and young children. Pediatr Radiol 2018;48(8):1048–1065.

Christian CW; Committee on Child Abuse and Neglect. The evaluation of suspected child physical abuse. Pediatrics 2015;135(5):e1337–e1354. Pediatrics 2015;136(3):583.

Deutsch SA. Understanding abusive head trauma: a primer for the general pediatrician. Pediatr Ann 2020;49(8):e347–e353.

Escobar MA Jr, Wallenstein KG, Christison-Lagay ER, et al. Child abuse and the pediatric surgeon: a position statement from the Trauma Committee, the Board of Governors and the Membership of the American Pediatric Surgical Association. J Pediatr Surg 2019;54(7):1277–1285.

Flaherty EG, et al. Evaluating children with fractures for child physical abuse. Pediatrics 2014;133(2):e477–e489.

Henry MK, Bennett CE, Wood JN, et al. Evaluation of the abdomen in the setting of suspected child abuse. Pediatr Radiol 2021;51(6):1044–1050. https://doi.org/10.1007/s00247-020-04944-2

Jenny C. Child Abuse and Neglect: Diagnosis, Treatment, and Evidence. St. Louis, MO: Elsevier Saunders, 2011.

Johnson SB, Riley AW, Granger DA, et al. The science of early life toxic stress for pediatric practice and advocacy. Pediatrics 2013;131(2):319–327.

Knox BL, Alexander RC, Luyet FM, et al. Medical neglect in childhood. J Child Adolesc Trauma 2020;13(3):257–258.

Narang SK, Fingarson A, Lukefahr J; Council on Child Abuse and Neglect. Abusive head trauma in infants and children. Pediatrics 2020;145(4):e20200203.

Palusci VJ; Council on Child Abuse and Neglect, Kay AJ, et al. Identifying child abuse fatalities during infancy. Pediatrics 2019;144(3):e20192076.

Pawlik MC, Kemp A, Maguire S, et al.; ExSTRA investigators. Children with burns referred for child abuse evaluation: burn characteristics and co-existent injuries. Child Abuse Negl 2016;55:52–61.

Pierce MC, Kaczor K, Lorenz DJ, et al. Validation of a clinical decision rule to predict abuse in young children based on bruising characteristics. JAMA Netw Open 2021;4(4):e215832.

Ravanfar P, Dinulos JG. Cultural practices affecting the skin of children. Curr Opin Pediatr 2010;22(4):423–431.

U.S. Department of Health & Human Services, Administration for Children and Families, Administration on Children, Youth and Families, Children's Bureau. Child Maltreatment 2019. 2021. Available at https://www.acf.hhs.gov/cb/research-data-technology/statistics-research/child-maltreatment

# 7 Neonatology

Kelleigh Briden and Melissa M. Riley

## APPROACH TO THE NEONATE IN RESPIRATORY DISTRESS

- You are looking at a newborn infant in respiratory distress.
  - Assessment and appropriate treatment of this neonate should be the immediate goal.
  - Determination of the underlying causes should be the secondary goal.
- The algorithm in Figure 7-1 summarizes the approach to the infant in respiratory distress.

### History

- Is the neonate term, late preterm, or preterm?
- Are there any risk factors for sepsis in maternal history?
- Was meconium noted at delivery?

### Physical Examination

- Assess vital signs, important in assessing the severity of the respiratory distress, and also indicate the urgency for intervention.
- Note color, capillary refill, pulse strength.

### Etiology

- Signs of respiratory distress such as flaring of alae nasi, chest wall retractions, and grunting point to a respiratory (alveolar) etiology.
- An inspiratory stridor indicates upper airway obstruction.
- An inspiratory stridor with poor cry suggests vocal cord paralysis.
- Tachypnea (respiratory rate >60 breaths per minute) without chest wall retractions is a good clue to an underlying cardiac etiology or retained interstitial fluid. For more information about cardiac causes, see Figure 7-2.
- Hyperpnea (deep sighing respirations) suggests metabolic acidosis (sepsis, shock, inborn error of metabolism).

### Laboratory Studies and Imaging

- A chest radiograph to differentiate parenchymal (hyaline membrane disease, pneumonia, meconium aspiration, fluid in the minor fissure) from pleural (effusion, pneumothorax) or chest cavity causes (diaphragmatic hernia) of respiratory distress
- Blood gas interpretation
  - pH
    - Normal 7.35-7.45.
    - Acidosis ≤7.35.

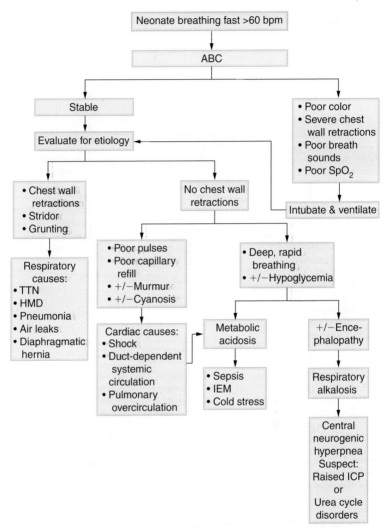

**Figure 7-1. Approach to respiratory distress in a neonate.** ABC, airway, breathing, circulation; TTN, transient tachypnea of the newborn; HMD, hyaline membrane disease; IEM, inborn error of metabolism; ICP, intracranial pressure.

- ○ Alkalosis ≥7.45.
- ○ Derangements may be respiratory, metabolic, or mixed in origin.
- PaCO$_2$
  - ○ Normal 35-45
  - ○ Respiratory alkalosis ≤35
  - ○ Respiratory acidosis ≥45

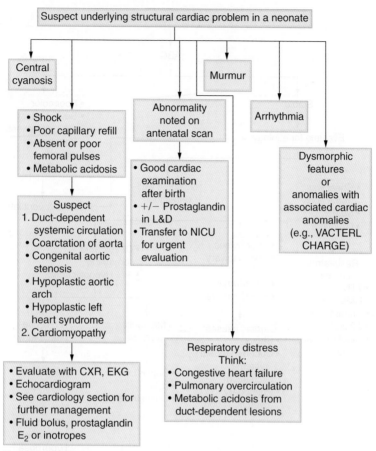

**Figure 7-2. Algorithm to use when cardiac disorder should be suspected in a neonate.** Look at relevant sections and algorithms for further information about the symptoms and signs mentioned here.

- $PaO_2$
  - To interpret, can utilize the following:
  - Oxygenation index $(OI) = \dfrac{MAP \times FiO_2}{PaO_2} \times 100$
  - Alveolar arterial (A-a) gradient $= PAO_2 - PaO_2$
    - $PAO_2 \approx FiO_2 \left( P_{ATM} - pH_2O \right) - \dfrac{PaCO_2}{R}$
      - $P_{ATM} = 760$ mm Hg at sea level
      - $pH_2O = 47$ mm Hg
      - $R = 0.8$

| TABLE 7-1 | Endotracheal Tube Size in Neonates | |
|---|---|---|
| Tube size (internal diameter in mm) | Weight (kg) | Gestational age (weeks) |
| 2.5 | <1 | <28 |
| 3 | 1–2 | 28–34 |
| 3.5 | 2–3 | 34–38 |
| 3.5–4 | >3 | >38 |

- $HCO_3$
  - Important base for buffering
  - $HCO_3^- + H^+ \leftrightarrow H_2CO_3 \leftrightarrow CO_2 + H_2O$
- Base excess
  - Takes into account other buffers in addition to $HCO_3^-$
- A blood culture is the gold standard for diagnosing or ruling out sepsis, although it can be false negative in 30% of cases for a variety of reasons (common causes: inadequate blood sample and pretreatment with antibiotics).

## Treatment

- Guidelines for intubation/surfactant therapy
  - Some indications for endotracheal intubation and mechanical ventilation of an infant include apnea, poor oxygen saturation despite supplemental oxygen by noninvasive respiratory support, and respiratory acidosis.
  - Surfactant administration is indicated for persistent oxygen requirement with indication of parenchymal lung disease.
  - See Tables 7-1 and 7-2 for further information about endotracheal intubation in neonates.

## Special Considerations: Persistent Pulmonary Hypertension of the Newborn (PPHN)

- Increased pulmonary vascular resistance resulting in right to left shunting across PDA or PFO, which results in severe V/Q mismatch, hypoxemia, and cyanosis.
- An early indicator of PPHN is poor tolerance of care with desaturation. Preductal and postductal saturation differential of >10% (differential cyanosis, pink hands, blue feet) indicates right-to-left shunting across the patent ductus arteriosus (PDA).

| TABLE 7-2 | Endotracheal Tubes and Depth of Insertion in Neonates[a] |
|---|---|
| Weight (kg) | Approximate depth of insertion (cm from upper lip) |
| 1 | 7 |
| 2 | 8 |
| 3 | 9 |
| 4 | 10 |

[a]Rule of thumb: Weight + 6 = depth of insertion.

Absence of this sign does not preclude the right-to-left shunting, which may be across the foramen ovale.
- It is advisable to maintain oxygen saturation of >95% in term infants until their disease process is identified and pulmonary hypertension is ruled out.

## APPROACH TO THE NEONATE WITH APNEA AND BRADYCARDIA

- History
  - What is the gestational age of the infant?
  - Are these events new or different from prior events?
  - Were there any precipitating factors?
- Physical examination
  - Assess vital signs. Have they returned to baseline?
  - Is the infant well or ill appearing?
  - Note upper airway sounds, breathing pattern, perfusion, and abdominal examination.
- Think about the etiology and additional appropriate evaluation/intervention after initial stabilization.

### Differential Diagnosis

- Events are recent in onset, and the neonate is ill appearing.
  - Sepsis: Evaluation may include a CBC, blood culture, chest radiograph (pneumonia) or 2-view abdominal radiograph (necrotizing enterocolitis), lumbar puncture, and commencement of antibiotics.
  - Respiratory distress: Intervene while awaiting for evaluation results; treatment may include noninvasive or invasive ventilation. Evaluation should include a chest radiograph and blood gas.
- Events are recent in onset, and the neonate is well appearing.
  - Sepsis: Indications for septic workup include a history of temperature instability, feeding intolerance, abdominal distension, and lethargy. See previous discussion for management.
  - PDA: Evaluate pulse volume, pulse pressure, and precordial pulsations. PDA can occur with or without a murmur. Timing of echocardiography should be discussed.
  - Anemia: Severe anemia in premature infants can present as new onset of apnea and bradycardia. Check Hgb, and if the infant is anemic, discuss transfusing pRBCs. Remember anemia can coexist with sepsis.
  - Blocked ectopic atrial beat: This is a common cause of heart rate drop in preterm infants and is self-limiting. It does not necessarily cause hemodynamic compromise but does warrant an ECG.
  - Obstructive apnea from uncoordinated suck and swallow, if associated with recently introduced oral feeds or noticed while the infant is feeding from a bottle.
  - Incorrect position of a feeding tube. Check with radiograph.
  - Eye examination for retinopathy of prematurity (ROP). This is a common cause of heart rate drop as a result of the vagal stimulation from eyeball compression during the examination (these infants could also have tachycardia from anticholinergic effects of cyclopentolate drops for the eye examination).
  - Vagus nerve induced: In a ventilated infant where the airway is patent (endotracheal tube), it is unlikely to be obstructive in origin and more likely to be central. Consider vagus nerve–induced bradycardia from increased intracranial pressure or more commonly a low-lying endotracheal tube irritating the carina.

- Intraventricular hemorrhage (IVH): Consider if it is the first 24 hours of life in an extremely premature infant (<26 weeks of gestation), especially if there is a rapid hemoglobin drop. An ultrasound of the head is diagnostic. IVH is most likely to occur in the 1st week of life.
- Hydrocephalus: Consider if an infant with known IVH has an increasing occipitofrontal circumference, bulging fontanelle, and increasing frequency of heart rate drops. Weekly ultrasounds should be considered.
- Events are not new in onset, and the neonate has a history of heart rate drops.
  - Benign: Consider whether the infant may have had heart rate drops in the past and may need only weight-appropriate dose adjustments of caffeine. Term infants can have lower resting heart rate (80-100) when sleeping and is often not pathologic. Can evaluate with EKG to rule out conduction abnormality.
  - Seizures: These should be considered in all neonates with no good explanation for apnea. Heart rate increases with subtle seizures. Think of seizures if apnea is associated with abnormal eye or limb movements. Look for seizures with an EEG, if the baby has meningitis or a recent onset/progression of IVH.
- Apnea of prematurity: This is a diagnosis of exclusion and hence mentioned at the end. It is due to immaturity of the respiratory center. It could be central or obstructive but usually is mixed in etiology and can be treated with caffeine and/or respiratory support.

## APPROACH TO THE NEONATE WITH AN UNACCEPTABLE BLOOD GAS ANALYSIS RESULT

- Promptly examine the infant as an impending emergency may be progressing. Vital signs, color, inspection of the respiratory support devices, and pulmonary examination will guide decision-making.
- Chest radiographs can aid in making a diagnosis.
  - A malpositioned ETT, atelectasis versus pneumonia, and air leaks may be identifiable on chest radiograph.
  - Radiographs will not identify diagnoses such as patient-ventilator asynchrony and PDA.

### Etiology and Treatment
- Problem: DOPE
  - DOPE mnemonic from PALS is useful.
  - D: **D**isplacement of endotracheal tube. If the chest wall is not expanding well with ventilator breaths, auscultate the chest for presence of breath sounds. Use a $CO_2$ detector (if the $CO_2$ detector turns yellow, the tube is in the trachea; if the indicator remains purple, the tube is likely not in the trachea). Direct laryngoscopy can verify tube positioning.
  - O: **O**bstruction. Can you pass a suction catheter through the endotracheal tube?
  - P: **P**neumothorax. Are breath sounds unequal (atelectasis or pneumothorax)? Transillumination with fiberoptic light and observing for the "halo" around the light source may diagnose pneumothorax in a premature neonate (false-negative and false-positive results possible).
  - E: **E**quipment malfunction. Disconnecting the infant from the ventilator and mechanical bagging with a flow-regulated breathing bag can help determine the

adequate pressure required to move the chest wall (if higher than the current peak inspiratory pressure, then the lung compliance has worsened). If the chest wall moves with the current inspiratory pressure, then there is an equipment malfunction.
  • Treatment involves fixing the identified problem.
• Problem: possible asynchrony
  • Does the neonate exhale when the ventilator delivers its breath? Does it appear that there is a seesaw movement of the chest and abdomen? This indicates patient ventilator asynchrony. This is uncommon with synchronized intermittent mandatory ventilation available on modern ventilators.
  • Treatment (in pressure ventilation)
    ○ Increasing the ventilator rate or providing pressure support for breaths initiated by the neonate can improve the ventilation without switching the mode of ventilation (if the ventilator allows this mode).
    ○ Switching to assist mode of ventilation so that each breath is ventilator supported can also be tried (this is a poor mode for weaning support).
    ○ Sedating the infant so that he or she does not "fight" the ventilator. Use the smallest dose of opioids to start and titrate to effect. It is very important to prevent this phenomenon in large-term infants to prevent pneumothorax.
• Problem: changing (worsening) lung compliance
  • Discuss with the respiratory therapist whether the tidal volume delivered by the ventilator is decreasing over a period of time; this indicates worsening lung compliance.
    ○ Check the position of endotracheal tube (is it at the same level where it was originally taped? Has it slipped in or out?).
    ○ Do you hear a murmur or feel bounding peripheral pulses (is the ductus arteriosus patent and causing decreased compliance)?
    ○ Is there temperature instability? Has the character of endotracheal secretions changed (such as an increased amount of secretions or a change in secretion color to yellow)? If these secretion changes are seen, this indicates that the patient may have pneumonia, which would worsen lung compliance.
    ○ Is the infant on the ventilator for a long time and developing chronic lung disease?
  • In volume control mode of ventilation, suspect all the above possibilities if you note increasing pressure generated by the ventilator to deliver the same volume.
• *Sometimes, it is good to think outside the box.*
  • Is the blood gas result unacceptable because of an extrapulmonary cause?
    ○ Is the abdomen distended and tense (necrotizing enterocolitis, spontaneous intestinal perforation, or intestinal obstruction)? Is the abdominal distension compromising the tidal volume of the lung? This is seen in infants with ascites (hydrops) or unrepaired abdominal wall defects who are being treated with a silastic pouch (silo), and the contents of the silo are progressively reduced into the abdominal cavity.
  • Does the infant have sufficient ventilatory drive?
    ○ Is he or she too sedated?
    ○ Does the ventilator rate need to be increased? (In nurses' parlance: the infant is "riding the vent.")
  • Is the endotracheal tube very old? Think of changing it even if there are protests; a blocked endotracheal tube can cause respiratory acidosis.

## APPROACH TO THE NEONATE WITH CONCERN FOR ABDOMINAL PATHOLOGY

- History
  - What was their gestational age and what is their corrected gestational age?
  - What is their stooling pattern? Hematochezia?
  - Any emesis? Hematemesis? Bilious emesis?
  - Any prior abdominal surgery or antenatal concern for abdominal pathology?
- Physical examination
  - Appearance of abdomen (color or change from previous), feel of abdomen and bowel sounds.
  - Additionally infants with significant abdominal pathology may demonstrate clinical signs of shock or compensated shock (take note of heart rate, blood pressure, pulses, and perfusion).

### Diagnosis and Treatment

*Necrotizing Enterocolitis (NEC)*

- Clinical features may include ill-appearing infant (although sometimes well appearing); abdominal distension; abdominal discoloration (erythematous, gray, blue); absence of bowel sounds.
- Stop enteral feeds, decompress the stomach with continuous nasogastric (Replogle) suction (to prevent emesis and aspiration as well as respiratory compromise), evaluate for sepsis (CBC, blood, urine, and possibly cerebrospinal fluid culture), and evaluate for pneumatosis intestinalis on radiograph.
- Start antibiotics. Metronidazole is typically reserved for intestinal perforation.
- Consult surgery if evidence of free air or if worsening in clinical status.
- The neonate should be monitored closely with frequent clinical examinations, CBCs, electrolytes, blood gases, and abdominal radiographs (anteroposterior and lateral decubitus films) for these parameters.
- Depending on the degree of illness severity, infants may need increase in respiratory support and/or hemodynamic support.

*Intestinal Obstruction*

- Bilious emesis in a neonate is concerning for bowel obstruction/volvulus and should be treated as an emergency.
- Clinical features may include an ill-appearing infant; abdominal distension; hyperactive/hypoactive bowel sounds; incarcerated hernia. Often, these infants will be well appearing with a normal examination, but bilious emesis is alarming on its own to prompt further evaluation.
- Mainstays of treatment: Stop enteral feeds, nasogastric (Replogle tube) decompression of stomach, and administer parenteral fluid or nutrition.
- Radiologic investigations, such as plain abdominal radiograph and contrast studies, can confirm the diagnosis and help delineate the cause. Surgical consultation may be indicated.

## APPROACH TO THE NICU PATIENT WITH HYPOGLYCEMIA

For a similar discussion of hypoglycemia in the well baby nursery, please see Chapter 2.

### History

- What was the gestational age? Chronologic age?
- How is their nutrition received: parenteral/enteral/combination? Any recent changes?

- What medications have they been exposed to? Have there been any recent medication changes?
- How was the blood sugar obtained?

## Physical Examination
- Well appearing or ill appearing? Jittery? Concern for seizure?
- On vital signs, make note of infant temperature.

## Diagnosis and Treatment
- Diagnosis of symptomatic hypoglycemia should not delay treatment but often the two can be done simultaneously.
- Serum glucose should be obtained after hypoglycemia detected with glucometer.
- Obtain the following laboratory tests in conjunction with serum glucose: insulin; TSH, thyroxine; growth hormone, cortisol, lactate, pyruvate, and urine ketones.
- Follow institution-specific guidelines for hypoglycemia management in regard to asymptomatic levels at which to treat.
- Treatment for symptomatic hypoglycemia is 2 mL/kg/dose of 10% dextrose.

### Diminished Glucose Supply
- Inadequate glycogen stores
  - Prematurity: Glycogen is deposited in the 3rd trimester.
  - Intrauterine growth restriction (IUGR): May have reduced glycogen stores.
- Impaired glucose production
  - Inborn errors of metabolism
  - Endocrine disorders: pituitary hormone deficiencies or adrenocortical insufficiency resulting in low cortisol or growth hormone
  - Liver failure: impaired gluconeogenesis; glycogenolysis
- Iatrogenic
  - Rapid wean in glucose infusion rate including when infant loses IV access unexpectedly
  - Missed feedings or change in feedings (volume/fortification)

### Increased Glucose Utilization
- Hyperinsulinism
  - Infant of a diabetic mother
  - IUGR
  - Beckwith-Wiedemann Syndrome: present in half of neonates with this diagnosis
  - Perinatal stress
  - Persistent hyperinsulinism secondary to gene mutations

## APPROACH TO THE NEWBORN WITH JAUNDICE (FIG. 7-3)

- Examine the infant and review the history.
- Remember that neonatal jaundice can be unconjugated (lipid soluble, risk for kernicterus, responds to phototherapy) or conjugated (water soluble, no risk for kernicterus, and not treated with phototherapy).

## Epidemiology
- Identify the risk factors for jaundice as outlined in the AAP guidelines on jaundice. Note that these guidelines are for infants at a gestational age of ≥35

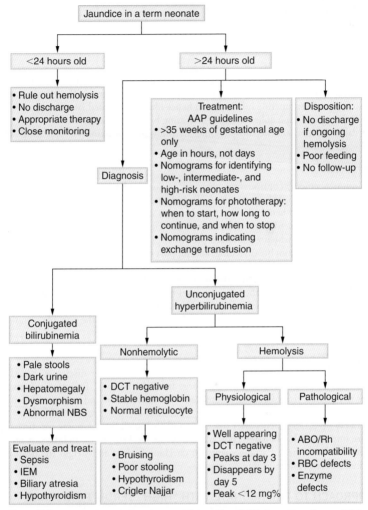

**Figure 7-3. Approach to a term neonate with jaundice.** DCT, direct Coombs test; IEM, inborn error of metabolism.

weeks. Management recommendations for preterm infants at a gestational age of <35 weeks are consensus based and should be used to guide therapies in this population.

• Emphasis should be on identifying risk factors for hemolysis and ruling out hemolysis in all infants with jaundice. Rapidly rising bilirubin, a high reticulocyte count, and falling hemoglobin (in the absence of extravascular bleeding) are good indicators of hemolysis. Risk factors for kernicterus should be identified.

## History and Physical Examination

- Note adequacy of feeding, passing stools, and voiding (risk factors for increased enterohepatic circulation of bilirubin).
- Examine for the following:
  - Well-being (no sepsis)
  - Growth parameters (Small for gestational age infants are likely to be plethoric, resulting in higher bilirubin and requiring earlier phototherapy. This may be symptomatic of intrauterine infection and hence likely conjugated jaundice.)
  - Bruising and cephalohematomas (increasing bilirubin production)
  - Pallor, edema, and hepatosplenomegaly (indicators of hemolysis and congestive heart failure)

## Treatment

- Commencement, continuation, discontinuation, and monitoring effectiveness of phototherapy should be as per the AAP guidelines. These guidelines are based on the age in hours, and hence, the exact age in hours should be remembered when deciding on the treatment (e.g., 17 hours, not day 1).
- Breastfed babies who are jaundiced present a special challenge. Mothers should not be discouraged from breastfeeding, and support from a lactation consultant (if available) should be sought.
- Double volume exchange transfusion is reserved for scenarios when intensive phototherapy fails to bring the bilirubin level below the neurotoxic range or for when the patient has signs of acute bilirubin encephalopathy (see Appendix E). Exchange transfusions should be performed in the NICU setting given the possible complications from exchange transfusion.

## Follow-Up

- Monitoring clinically with/without follow-up bilirubin after discharge should be arranged within 48 hours after discharge from the hospital. Breastfed infants are at the highest risk of getting readmitted with dehydration and increased bilirubin levels.
- Follow-up arrangements after discharge and the possible time frame for discharge are important. If discharge takes place over the weekend or on holidays, it means difficult home health arrangements for checking feeding and weight trends, home phototherapy, and bilirubin estimation.

## APPROACH TO THE NEONATE WITH "HIGH" SERUM POTASSIUM

Was the sample hemolyzed? If so, repeat a venous sample.

## Treatment

- Identify hemodynamic instability requiring urgent treatment.
  - Look at the bedside cardiac monitor for tall T waves or wide QRS complexes.
  - Look for poor capillary refill and hypotension.
- If you see any of the above, then irrespective of the level of potassium, the neonate is symptomatic and hence needs emergency treatment.
- Evaluate for causes of hyperkalemia after emergency treatment. Some of the common causes are excess potassium in total parenteral nutrition (TPN) or IV fluids, poor urine output, bruising, hemolysis, or metabolic acidosis.

*Emergency Treatment*
- IV fluids with potassium should be stopped immediately while awaiting calcium gluconate administration.
- IV 10% calcium gluconate is best because it has a directly protective effect on the myocardium. Potassium stops the heart in diastole, and calcium counteracts this with its positive inotropic effect. It is long lasting and very effective.
- Sodium bicarbonate is also useful because it causes metabolic alkalosis and shifts potassium intracellularly, reducing serum potassium. A 2 mL/kg/dose of 4.5% sodium bicarbonate should be used.

*Nonemergency Treatment*
- Emergency measures may not be required even if serum K levels are 5.5-6.5 mEq/L in preterm infants if:
  - There is no cardiac arrhythmia.
  - Urine output is adequate (>1 mL/kg/hr).
  - Potassium supplementation in the parenteral fluid is not excessive (2-3 mEq/kg/day).
  - Blood pH is not acidotic.
- It may be prudent to watch clinically and monitor serial potassium levels and urine output.
- Reducing potassium in the parenteral fluid is also an option.
- If serum potassium is >7.5 mEq/L, even without cardiac arrhythmia, removing potassium from parenteral fluid, increasing glucose infusion rate (to increase endogenous insulin, which will then shift potassium intracellularly) with or without insulin drip, or adding calcium to the parenteral fluid either all at once or sequentially is a reasonable option.
- It is necessary to continue monitoring for hemodynamic compromise.
- Continuous nebulizations with albuterol ($\beta_2$-receptor agonist) cause transcellular shift of potassium and reduce potassium.
- Lack of IV access is usually not an issue because hyperkalemia is seen in "micropreemies" (nonhemolytic hyperkalemia caused by bruising, poor urine output because of high antidiuretic hormone level, poor renal cortical blood flow, and low glomerular filtration rate) in the first few days of life when most neonates have umbilical lines.

## APPROACH TO THE NEONATE WITH HIGH BLOOD PRESSURE

- Hypertension is defined as blood pressure in the >95th percentile on Zubrow nomograms based on postconceptual age.
- Ideal conditions to measure blood pressure in an infant are:
  - 90 minutes after a feed
  - Sleeping or quiet for 15 minutes
  - In prone position
- Before ordering a battery of tests, check for the conditions under which blood pressure was measured as above.
- A correct-sized cuff should be used; the cuff should cover two-thirds the length of the arm and 75% of the limb circumference. Blood pressure should be measured in the arms rather than the legs (where it is normally higher).
- A single measurement is not diagnostic, and three successive readings at 2-minute intervals should be made before deciding on "hypertension."
- Rule of thumb: Systolic blood pressure >100 mm Hg in a term infant a few weeks old should be treated.

## Etiology

- Agitation and inadequate pain control are two common explanations for high blood pressure recorded.
- Caffeine, theophylline, and corticosteroids are common medications implicated.
- Excessive parenteral fluid and sodium administration over the past few days are two important causes that can be missed unless TPN prescriptions are scrutinized closely.

## History

- History of umbilical arterial lines is a common predisposing factor for renovascular hypertension.
- Stigmata of renal disease (as outlined previously) should increase suspicions of intrinsic renal disease (vesicoureteric reflux, multicystic dysplastic kidney, horseshoe kidney).
- An infant with chronic lung disease often has hypertension from multiple etiologies.
- Endocrine disorders are not seen commonly in neonates (except Cushing syndrome with steroid therapy, and neonatal hyperthyroidism, which is rare).

## Physical Examination

- Check for unequal pulses and blood pressure in arms and legs (coarctation of aorta).
- Palpate for ballottable renal mass and auscultate for renal bruit on either side of the umbilicus (renovascular causes are the most common causes of hypertension). Infants of diabetic mothers can present with gross hematuria. These infants should be evaluated for hypertension and palpable renal masses, which are indicative of renal vein thrombosis.

## Laboratory Studies and Imaging

- Laboratory evaluation involves the following:
  - Urine examination (macroscopy, microscopy, and culture; infection is still the most common cause of renovascular hypertension.)
  - Renal measures such as blood urea nitrogen, serum creatinine, and electrolytes
  - Renal ultrasound for anatomical anomalies
  - Doppler studies for vascular anomalies
  - Echocardiogram for coarctation of aorta
  - Ratio of serum renin to aldosterone levels
- The ratio of renin to aldosterone is recommended to distinguish primary from secondary hyperaldosteronism, but turnaround time for results is too long and interpreting the results in small "preemies" may not be very helpful clinically. If no cause is found in the initial screening tests, then it is hoped that the subspecialties would have become involved a while ago. Urinary levels of vanillylmandelic acid to diagnose pheochromocytoma are not required routinely.

## Treatment

- Treatment depends on the cause, but symptomatic drug therapy is beyond the scope of this discussion.
- ACE inhibitors such as enalapril are avoided in infants <44 weeks of gestational age. This medication can inhibit nephron growth, which continues up to 44 weeks.

## NUTRITIONAL REQUIREMENTS OF NEONATES

Human milk is the preferred source of nutrition whenever possible. Donor human milk is pasteurized and may be used as a substitute for mother's own milk.

### Calories

- Parenterally fed premature neonates require 90-100 kcal/kg/day to promote sustained growth.
- Enterally fed neonates require 120 kcal/kg/day.
- Factors that may increase caloric demand include thermal stress, increased metabolic rate (e.g., hyperthyroid state, postoperative recovery), and increased fecal losses (malabsorption).
- Maintenance fluid requirements for both term and preterm infants by the end of the 1st week are about 150 mL/kg/day.
- Human breast milk and formulas for mature, term infants provide 20 kcal/oz, whereas formulas for premature infants provide either 20 or 24 kcal/oz.

### Proteins

Adequate protein intake is estimated to be approximately 2.5 g/kg/day in term and 3.5-4.0 g/kg/day in preterm infants (approximately 0-15% of caloric intake). Parenterally, TrophAmine is used as a source of amino acids.

### Fats

- Approximately 40-45% of caloric intake should come from fat.
- Premature infants are unable to digest long-chain fatty acid in formula (lack of bile salts).
- Premature formulas use medium-chain fatty acids as a predominant source of fat. Parenterally, Intralipid 20% is used to provide fat calories. Infusion is initiated at 0.5 g/kg/day and gradually increased to 3 g/kg/day.

### Carbohydrates

- Approximately 40-45% of caloric intake comes from carbohydrates. Parenterally, dextrose is used as a carbohydrate source. Usual starting glucose infusion rates are 6-8 mg/kg/min. This is gradually advanced to deliver more calories, to a maximum of 10-12 mg/kg/min.
- Lactose is the predominant carbohydrate in human milk and formula, and it is well absorbed in premature infants.

### Strategies for Providing Nutrition

- In premature infants who are unstable after admission to the nursery, start an infusion of "starter total parenteral nutrition," or "starter TPN." This TrophAmine solution provides 2.5 g/kg/day of protein when infused at 50 mL/kg/day.
- To make up maintenance fluid requirements, $D_{10}W$ is "piggybacked" to the TPN at 30 mL/kg/day. Regular TPN with adjustment of fluid intake is commenced on day of life 1 with 2.5 g/kg/day of protein, 0.5 g/kg/day of Intralipid, and $D_{12.5}W$ ± electrolytes depending on weight loss, electrolytes, and urine output.
- For administration, a central catheter is preferred (central umbilical venous catheter, peripherally inserted central catheter). In peripherally placed lines, to avoid injury to

vessels, the maximum allowed concentration of dextrose is 12.5%. Central catheters require the addition of heparin to the TPN.
- Trophic feeds (up to 20 mL/kg/day) are usually started by gavage feeds on day of life 2-4, depending on the infant's clinical condition and the availability of human milk. The volume of initiating and the rate of advancement of feeds depend on the infant's birth weight and tolerance of feeds. The goal is to achieve full enteral nutrition by 10-14 days of life. Human milk is preferred and is fortified with human milk fortifier once intake reaches 75-100 mL/kg/day. Liquid fortifiers are typically used as they are sterile products.

## Nutrition Monitoring
- Parameters used to track growth are daily weights, weekly lengths, and occipitofrontal circumference.
  - Iron supplements are started at 2-3 weeks of life when at full feeds at 2-4 mg/kg/day.
  - Premature infants need higher amounts of calories, protein, calcium, phosphate, iron, and sodium intake compared with their term counterparts.
- Infants at high risk for metabolic bone disease (<30 weeks of gestation, prolonged TPN, diuretics, steroids) should have ionized calcium, phosphorus, and alkaline phosphatase levels monitored at 4 weeks of age and every 2 weeks thereafter.
- Infants on prolonged TPN should have the following laboratory tests every 2 weeks: serum electrolytes including calcium, magnesium, albumin, alkaline phosphatase, and phosphate.

### Expected Weight Gain
- Term infants: 20-30 g/day for the first 3 months, 15-20 g/day for the next 3 months, and 10-15 g/day for the next 6 months. These infants will double their birth weight in 5 months, triple it in 1 year, and quadruple it in 2 years.
- Preterm infants: 15 g/kg/day.

### Expected Increase in Head Circumference
- Term infants: 2 cm/month for first 3 months, 1 cm/month for the next 3 months, and 0.5 cm/month for the next 6 months
- Preterm infants: 0.5 cm/week

## RETINOPATHY OF PREMATURITY

- ROP is a disorder of the developing retinal vasculature that occurs with interruption of the forming retinal vessels. Constriction and obliteration of the advancing capillary bed are followed by neovascularization of the retina, which can extend into the vitreous (Fig. 7-4).
- The incidence varies inversely with gestational age.
- The most serious and feared complication of ROP is retinal detachment and associated loss of vision that may occur in 6-8% of infants.
- Disease occurs when vessels posterior to the ridge become dilated and tortuous.

### Classification (Table 7-3)
### Screening
- Who should be screened?
  - Infants with a birth weight of <1500 g or ≤ 30 weeks of gestational age **and** selected infants between 1500 and 2000 g or >30 weeks of gestation with an

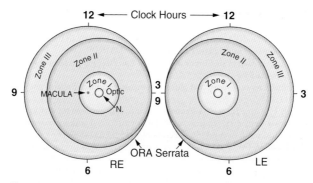

**Figure 7-4.** Schema of the right and left eye showing the zones and clock hours used in the description of retinopathy of prematurity.

unstable neonatal course (as defined by the neonatologist). Pupils are dilated using cyclopentolate and phenylephrine eye drops.
• Pacifiers and oral sucrose are recommended for comfort during the examination.
• When should screening take place?
  • ROP is not detected before 31 weeks corrected gestational age.
  • Infants born at 22-27 weeks of gestational age should be screened when at 31 weeks of age.
  • Infants born at 28-30 weeks of gestational age should be screened at 4 weeks of age.

## Treatment

• Laser photocoagulation is aimed at the avascular part to reduce the production of the growth factors responsible for exuberant vascular growth. There are well-defined criteria to identify infants needing laser therapy.
• Vascular endothelial growth factor inhibitors can be injected into the eye to avoid or delay laser therapy.
• Other therapeutic options include cryotherapy and scleral banding/vitrectomy for later stages.

| TABLE 7-3 | International Classification of Retinopathy of Prematurity |
|---|---|
| **Stage** | **Description** |
| 1 | A line of demarcation develops from the vascularized region of the retina and the avascular zone. |
| 2 | The line becomes a ridge that protrudes into the vitreous; there is histologic evidence of an atrioventricular shunt. |
| 3 | Extraretinal vascular proliferation occurs with the ridge; neovascular tufts can be found posterior to the ridge. |
| 4 | Scarring and fibrosis can occur when the neovascularization extends into the vitreous; this can cause traction on the retina, leading to retinal detachment. |
| 5 | Total retinal detachment |

## SUGGESTED READINGS

AAP. Clinical practice guideline: management of hyperbilirubinemia in the newborn infant 35 or more weeks of gestation. Pediatrics 2004;114(1):297–316.

Abrams S. Calcium and vitamin D requirements of enterally fed preterm infants. Pediatrics 2013;131:e1676–e1683.

Adamkin D. Clinical report—postnatal glucose homeostasis in late-preterm and term infants. Pediatrics 2011;127:575–579.

Butler TJ, Szekely LJ, Grow JL, et al. A standardized nutrition approach for very low birth weight neonates improves outcomes, reduces cost and is not associated with increased rates of necrotizing enterocolitis, sepsis or mortality. J Perinatol 2013;33:851–857.

Cornblath M, Hawdon JM, Williams A, et al. Controversies regarding definition of neonatal hypoglycemia: suggested operational thresholds. Pediatrics 2000;105:1141–1145.

Dionne JM, Flynn JT. Hypertension in the neonate. Neoreviews 2012;13:e401.

Ewer AK, Yu VY. Effect of fortifying breast milk on gastric emptying. Arch Dis Child Fetal Neonatal Ed 1996;74(1):F60–F62.

Fierson WM, et al. Policy Statement: American Academy of Pediatrics. Screening examination of premature infants for retinopathy of prematurity. Pediatrics 2013;131:189–195.

Maisels MJ, Watchko JF, Bhutani VK, et al. An approach to the management of hyperbilirubinemia in the preterm infant less than 35 weeks of gestation. J Perinatol 2012:32:660–664.

Nwanko MU, Lorenz JM, Gardiner JC. A standard protocol for blood pressure measurement in the newborn. Pediatrics 1997;99:e10.

Perlman JM, Wyllie J, Kattwinkel J, et al. Neonatal resuscitation: 2010 International Consensus on cardiopulmonary resuscitation and emergency cardiovascular care science with treatment recommendations. Pediatrics 2010;126(5):e1319–e1344.

SUPPORT Study Group of the Eunice Kennedy Shriver NICHD Neonatal Research Network; Finer NN, Carlo WA, Walsh MC, et al. Early CPAP versus surfactant in extremely preterm infants. N Engl J Med 2010;362(21):1970–1979.

Zubrow AB, Hulman S, Kushner H, et al. Determinants of blood pressure in infants admitted to neonatal intensive care units: a prospective multicenter study. J Perinatol 1995;15:470–479.

# Critical Care

Ashley Turner, Ashley Steed, and Nikoleta Kolovos

## RESPIRATORY FAILURE

Respiratory failure is defined as the inability of the respiratory system to provide adequate oxygen to meet the body's demands, excrete carbon dioxide, or both. This failure is characterized by hypoxemia (decreased oxygen content in the blood), which may lead to hypoxia (tissue oxygen deprivation) as well as hypercapnia (increased carbon dioxide [$CO_2$] content in the blood).

### Causes of Hypoxemia and Hypercapnia

*Alveolar Hypoventilation*: defined as inadequate minute ventilation

- Multiple etiologies including impaired respiratory drive from altered sensorium (i.e., sedation, coma, status epilepticus), upper airway obstruction, peripheral nervous system dysfunction (i.e., Guillain-Barré syndrome, botulism), or respiratory muscle weakness (i.e., muscular dystrophy, fatigue).
- Physical examination: encephalopathy/apnea/hypopnea often seen in those with impaired respiratory drive; stridor/suprasternal retractions with upper airway obstruction; neuropathy/myopathy with underlying neuromuscular disorders.
- Treatment: Supplemental oxygen may offset hypoxemia in mild cases, but non-invasive or invasive mechanical ventilation may become necessary. Proper patient position or placement of an oral or nasal airway device may alleviate upper airway obstruction. Helium and oxygen (heliox) gaseous mixtures may reduce turbulent flow and overcome increased resistance caused by upper airway obstruction.

*Ventilation/Perfusion (V/Q) Mismatch*: Ideally, ventilated lung units receive blood flow for gas exchange to occur. However, when ventilation and perfusion are not optimized, hypoxemia and hypercapnia can result. Ventilated alveoli not adequately perfused are termed dead space (V/Q > 1). In contrast, when alveoli receive blood but inappropriately ventilated, this blood is deemed "shunted" (V/Q < 1), and again no gas exchange occurs.

- Various causes of V/Q mismatch exist. An extreme example of V/Q > 1 is pulmonary embolism. Pneumonia, atelectasis, and asthma can lead to V/Q < 1.
- Physical examination: nonspecific signs of respiratory distress and increased work of breathing such as tachypnea, nasal flaring, and retractions. Specific etiologies may manifest with certain signs such as crackles in patients with pneumonia or wheezing and prolonged expiration in patients with reactive airway disease. A massive pulmonary embolism may result in cardiovascular collapse.
- Treatment: Aimed at treating the underlying cause (i.e., steroids for asthma or antibiotics for pneumonia). As with alveolar hypoventilation, supplemental oxygen may offset hypoxemia, but moderate-to-severe cases require escalation of respiratory support.

*Diffusion Impairment*: Oxygen diffusion from the alveolar space into the blood depends on the surface area available for exchange, the thickness of the alveolar wall, the partial pressure difference across the space, and the rate of blood flow. Less surface area available for gas exchange, increased thickness of the alveolar wall, decreased difference in the partial pressure of oxygen, or an increased rate of blood flow limit oxygen diffusion. $CO_2$ more readily diffuses across the alveolar surface, and thus its elimination is less affected by these alterations.

- Examples of diffusion impairment include pulmonary fibrosis and emphysematous changes.
- Physical examination: nonspecific signs of respiratory distress. Crackles or coarse breath sounds may be appreciated in patients with pulmonary fibrosis.
- Treatment: aimed at optimizing oxygen diffusion by increasing the surface area available for gas exchange. These include application of continuous positive airway pressure (CPAP), limiting any underlying disease process resulting in a thickened alveolar wall, and increasing the alveolar oxygen partial pressure with supplemental oxygen administration.

### Additional Causes of Hypoxemia

*Shunt*: Venous blood bypasses ventilated alveoli and mixes with oxygenated blood.

- Etiologies include anatomical shunts (i.e., intracardiac mixing, arteriovenous malformations). Extreme cases occur when no ventilation reaches some airspaces and local V/Q = 0. Hypoxic pulmonary vasoconstriction limits the latter by decreasing perfusion to lung areas with low ventilation via constriction of local pulmonary arterioles, thereby redirecting blood flow to ventilated alveoli.
- Physical examination: Findings vary from cyanosis without distress to shock due to the extreme decrease in overall oxygen content in blood.
- Treatment: aimed at the underlying process. For example, optimize the balance between pulmonary and systemic blood flow in patients with cardiac mixing defects until surgical correction is possible.

*Low Inspired Partial Pressure of Oxygen*: High altitudes have lower partial pressures of oxygen in the atmosphere, which directly diminishes the partial pressure difference driving oxygen transport across the alveoli wall. Supplemental oxygen can be used to increase the partial pressure of oxygen delivered to the alveoli.

## RESPIRATORY SUPPORT

### Noninvasive Support

Respiratory insufficiency can be supported with noninvasive strategies ranging from supplemental oxygen by nasal cannula to mechanical ventilation with a tight-fitting face or nasal mask depending on severity. This is distinguished from invasive support, which is supplied via an artificial airway (i.e., an endotracheal or tracheostomy tube).

*High-Flow Nasal Cannula (HFNC)*: HFNC provides heated, humidified gas (with varying amounts of supplemental oxygen) at increased flow rates (depending on the manufacturer but up to 60 L/min) compared to a simple nasal cannula that typically supports flows of 4 L/min.

- The benefits of HFNC are multifactorial, including the following:
  - Increased flow rates provide some low-level positive pressure.
  - Movement of oxygen-rich gas past the nasopharyngeal dead space results in $CO_2$ washout and improved alveolar ventilation.

- Heated, humidified gas at high-flow rates reduces inspiratory resistance through the nasal passages, improves mucociliary clearance, and reduces metabolic work.
- Indications: Nearly any cause of respiratory failure, including viral bronchiolitis and pneumonia, may improve with a trial of HFNC.
- Titration: Starting flow rate of 0.5-1.0 L/kg/min. The flow may be increased to 1.5 to 2 L/kg/min. Flows >2 L/kg/min may not provide additional clinical benefit.
- Advantages: well tolerated with a soft, flexible cannula adhered to the face. Humidification aids in secretion clearance. Patients typically tolerate enteral nutrition while receiving HFNC although this is dependent on alleviation of increased work of breathing. Continuous albuterol can be delivered through HFNC if indicated.
- Disadvantages: In the absence of biphasic positive pressure, respiratory support may be inadequate and necessitate escalation.

***Noninvasive Positive-Pressure Ventilation***: Noninvasive mechanical support can be delivered by targeting positive pressure during the respiratory cycle. Biphasic positive airway pressure (BiPAP) delivers a higher pressure during the inspiratory cycle (IPAP setting) and a lower pressure during the expiratory cycle (EPAP setting). The increased pressure delivery is triggered via the ventilator's sensing of the patient's inspiratory effort. CPAP can be applied without change in pressure throughout the respiratory cycle.

- Indications: multiple, including viral bronchiolitis, pneumonia, and severe asthma exacerbation. Chronic BIPAP may be indicated for static or slowly progressing neuromuscular disease, central hypoventilation, chronic respiratory insufficiency, and sleep apnea.
- Titration: Typical initial settings are IPAP 8-10 cm $H_2O$ and EPAP 5-6 cm $H_2O$ and are adjusted based on the patient's work of breathing, oxygen delivery, and ventilation. A backup rate may be set and is useful for patients with hypopnea or underlying neuromuscular weakness.
- Advantages: Avoidance of an artificial airway and therefore decreased sedation need as compared to that required for patient tolerance of an endotracheal tube (ETT). Consequently, patient interactivity is improved and mobility level less diminished.
- Disadvantages: Requires some patient cooperation and therefore may require some sedation to tolerate an appropriately fitted mask, particularly in younger children. These devices cannot deliver full ventilatory support, and assessment of pulmonary mechanics is less readily gauged than during invasive mechanical ventilation. Gaseous gastric distention may occur, limiting ability to provide enteral nutrition. Long-term use may result in pressure injuries to the skin.

## Invasive Support

Indications for invasive respiratory support include the following: respiratory failure, shock (with the goal of decreasing systemic oxygen consumption via decreasing the oxygen demand necessary for work of breathing), need for controlled ventilation as therapy (as for treatment of intracranial hypertension), to facilitate safety during procedures, to relieve upper airway obstruction, or inability to protect the airway in the setting of altered sensorium.

## Intubation

*Preparation*
- Have ready access to the following: oxygen, suction equipment, appropriately sized mask, ventilation bag, lighted laryngoscope (video laryngoscope if available) with appropriately sized blade, ETT of the expected size as well as one 0.5 mm larger and 0.5 mm smaller, stylet, $CO_2$ detector, pulse oximetry, secure intravenous (IV)

access, and ventilator. Consider having an appropriately sized laryngeal mask airway (LMA) in case of difficulty with intubation and oral airway in case of difficulty with bag mask ventilation.

- Position the patient in such a manner that the oral, pharyngeal, and tracheal axes are aligned to achieve optimal view of the airway.
- Pharmacologic agents (see Table 8-1). Sedatives and neuromuscular blocking agents are used for patient comfort and to facilitate visualization of the glottis.
- Review prior intubation history and records if available.

*Signs of a Difficult Airway*
Consider the presence of an anesthesiologist or otolaryngologist with advanced airway skills if the patient has signs of a difficult airway such as micrognathia, facial clefts, midface hypoplasia, maxillary protrusion, facial asymmetry, small mouth opening, short neck, limited cervical spine mobility (including need for c-spine precautions), foreign body, oral or upper airway bleeding, suspected pulmonary hemorrhage, or known history of difficult airway.

## AIRWAY MANAGEMENT

### Rapid Sequence Induction and Emergent Intubation

Rapid sequence induction is rarely used in pediatric critical care prior to intubation given many patients' inability to tolerate even brief lack of ventilation. However, patients at high risk for pulmonary aspiration (known recent oral intake or trauma) may require rapid sequence induction.

- This is accomplished by preoxygenation and denitrogenation of the lungs utilizing 100% oxygen and a tight-fitting face mask.
- A defasciculating dose of neuromuscular blockade may be considered in patients with intracranial hypertension or ocular injury.
- Patients may benefit from isotonic fluid administration, provided their cardiovascular status can withstand additional preload.
- Cricoid pressure should be administered to prevent aspiration of gastric contents.

### Bag-Mask Ventilation

Most patients should undergo bag-mask ventilation to facilitate gas exchange during induction and initial neuromuscular blockade.

- Depending on the patient's last enteral intake, minimization of time undergoing bag-mask ventilation is warranted to reduce aspiration risk.
- A well-fitting mask that covers the nose and mouth is essential. An oral or nasal airway may also be necessary if upper airway obstruction occurs due to poor airway tone after administration of sedation and neuromuscular blockade.
- Two people may be needed: one to ensure an optimal seal via patient positioning and one to operate the bag.
- If a patient cannot be ventilated via a bag and mask, consider placement of oral airway to aid in mouth opening and tongue displacement. Do not give neuromuscular blockade unless able to ventilate. If inability to ventilate persists, emergently consult anesthesiology or otolaryngology personnel while placing rescue airway devices, such as a LMA and supplying oxygen.

**TABLE 8-1** Medications for Intubation

| Class | Dose | Time of onset | Advantages | Disadvantages |
|---|---|---|---|---|
| **Sedatives** | | | | |
| Ketamine | 1 mg/kg dose may be repeated. | 30-45 sec | Nonnarcotic analgesic and anesthetic, increases systemic blood pressure, bronchodilator | May induce severe laryngospasm, increases cerebral blood flow (CBF), increases salivation, emergence can be complicated by delirium |
| Propofol | 1 mg/kg dose may be repeated. | 30-45 sec | Hypnotic, amnestic agent | Vasodilation, diminished CBF, pain at site of injection. Provides no analgesia |
| Fentanyl | 1 μg/kg dose may be repeated. | 1-2 min | Narcotic analgesic | Bradycardia and chest wall rigidity if given rapidly in large doses |
| **Neuromuscular blocking agents** | | | | |
| Rocuronium | 1-1.5 mg/kg. | 30 sec to 1.5 min | No hemodynamic effects, metabolized in the liver, lasts 15-30 min | Less ideal in patients with full stomach due to time of onset; however, higher doses (1.5 mg/kg) lead to faster onset |
| Succinylcholine | 1 mg/kg. | 30-60 sec | Rapid onset of action ideal for emergent intubation of patients with full stomachs, depolarizing agent, lasts 5-10 min | May increase ICP, may potentiate hyperkalemia in patients with crush injuries, spinal cord injuries, or neuromuscular disease, may trigger malignant hyperthermia |

*Ventilating Bags*
- Self-inflating bags (i.e., Ambu bag): do not require adequate seal or gas source to fill (can pull gas from environment) but will not provide any gas flow unless actively ventilating (cannot provide CPAP)
- Flow-inflating bags (i.e., anesthesia bags): fill only when connected to a gas source and have an adequate seal, require regulation of pressure delivery via a control valve, and allow operator to gauge lung compliance (change in lung expansion for a delivered pressure)

*Selection of Laryngoscopy Blade and Endotracheal Tubes*
- Blade types
  - Miller: straight blade with a slightly curved tip, positioned posterior to the epiglottis allowing visualization of glottis by lifting the epiglottis upward. Particularly helpful for those with a relatively large and floppy epiglottis as in an infant.
  - Macintosh: curved blade, positioned in the vallecula, anterior to the epiglottis, such that the epiglottis is lifted upward indirectly to expose the glottis.
- Endotracheal tubes (ETTs)
  - Selecting the proper ETT size is important for achieving effective mechanical ventilation and preventing tracheal injury.
  - Cuffed versus uncuffed ETTs: Cuffed ETTs allow better occlusion of the airway, potentially place less pressure on the tracheal mucosa, provide more reliable end-tidal $CO_2$ monitoring, and minimize aspiration risk. In general, cuffed ETTs are preferred.
  - The Cole formula estimates uncuffed ETT size based on age:
    - Uncuffed tube size (mm internal diameter) = [age in years/4] + 4.
    - Cuffed tubes should typically be 0.5 mm smaller than the Cole formula indicates.
    - The Cole formula is less reliable for infants and patients with discrepant age to size.
    - Infants are typically intubated with a 3.0- to 4.0-mm ETT.

*During and After Intubation*
- When the airway is visualized, the ETT should be observed to pass through the vocal cords into the glottis. Stop advancement after the cuff has passed through the glottis or at a predetermined placement as noted by marking on the tube or by the following approximation:

$$3 \times ETT \text{ size (in mm)} = \text{appropriate endotracheal tube depth (cm)}$$

- Position should be confirmed with $CO_2$ detection, symmetrical chest wall rise, equal auscultation over the chest wall, and favorable gas exchange.
- Chest radiography is useful to evaluate depth of ETT placement.

## Mechanical Ventilation
- Use of positive pressure to move gas into the lungs in order to achieve oxygenation and ventilation. Specifically, a ventilator delivers a regulated gas flow, which generates a pressure that is transmitted to the lungs (airway pressure) to move a volume (tidal volume) of gas.
- Major determinants of oxygenation are alveolar lung volume and fraction of inspired oxygen ($FiO_2$). Alveolar lung volume is affected primarily by measures that determine mean airway pressure (MAP), such as positive end expiratory pressure (PEEP), inspiratory time, and peak airway pressure. The major determinants of $CO_2$ clearance is

minute ventilation, defined as the amount of gas moved into and out of the lungs per minute. Minute ventilation is calculated as follows:

$$\text{Minute ventilation} = \text{tidal volume} \times \text{respiratory rate}$$

- The goals of mechanical ventilation are to maintain oxygenation and ventilation, while being comfortable to the patient, and minimizing ventilator-induced lung injury and complications such as pneumothorax, cardiovascular compromise, and respiratory muscle atrophy.

*Modes of Conventional Mechanical Ventilation*
- Ventilators provide multiple strategies of ventilation as determined by the mode selected. Modes differ by the parameters set by the clinician, such as the timing and pattern of breathing (mandatory, synchronized, or supported) as well as how that support is delivered (regulated by flow or pressure).
- Basic modes of mandatory and assisted ventilation are those in which the clinician sets a respiratory rate and either a tidal volume (volume control) or peak airway pressure (pressure control).
  - Volume control ventilation provides a constant inspiratory flow pattern compared to pressure control ventilation, which provides a decelerating inspiratory flow pattern. This subtle variation may affect patient comfort.
  - In volume control ventilation, the tidal volume is a set parameter; therefore, careful attention must be paid to the pressure required to achieve that target tidal volume. In pressure control ventilation, the driving pressure is a set parameter; therefore, careful attention must be paid to the tidal volume (and resultant minute ventilation) achieved with the set driving pressure. Variation in a patient's respiratory effort and respiratory system compliance affects each dependent factor.
- **Mandatory Ventilation**
  - In controlled mandatory ventilation, the ventilator delivers a set number of breaths per minute with a set tidal volume (volume control) or pressure (pressure control) with a fixed inspiratory time regardless of patient effort; no gas flow is provided between delivered breaths. The addition of a continuous gas flow allows for spontaneous breathing, and this mode of ventilation is called intermittent mandatory ventilation.
- **Synchronized Intermittent Mandatory Ventilation** (SIMV)
  - Synchronized intermittent mandatory ventilation (SIMV) is the most commonly used mode of conventional mechanical ventilation in the PICU. Unlike mandatory ventilation, SIMV uses a patient trigger to match the patient's desire for a breath to a delivered breath. This synchronization improves patient comfort.
  - Like mandatory ventilation, the ventilator delivers a set number of breaths per minute with a set tidal volume (volume control, SIMV-VC) or pressure (pressure control, SIMV-PC) with a fixed inspiratory time.
  - Pressure-regulated volume control (PRVC) combines features of both volume and pressure control ventilation. In PRVC, the ventilator adjusts the positive pressure provided as respiratory system compliance changes to achieve a target tidal volume. PRVC offers a fixed minute ventilation, unlike pressure control, and the decelerating inspiratory flow pattern is better tolerated by the patient than the constant flow pattern of volume control. In PRVC, a high-pressure limit terminates the breath to avoid high positive inspiratory pressures to protect the patient from ventilator-induced lung injury. In PRVC, the patient's positive inspiratory pressure must be monitored as an indication of changing lung compliance.

- In SIMV, the patient can take additional pressure-supported breaths beyond the ventilator's set rate. The pressure-supported breaths are patient triggered and supported with a driving pressure set separately from the volume control or pressure control breaths. If no patient effort is detected, the ventilator will deliver control breaths at the set ventilator rate.
- A common strategy for weaning from SIMV is to decrease the number of mandatory breaths and rely more on pressure-supported, spontaneous breaths.
- **Assist-Control Ventilation**
  - Like SIMV, assist control uses a patient trigger to match the patient's desire for a breath to a delivered breath. As with mandatory ventilation and SIMV, the ventilator delivers a set number of breaths per minute with a set tidal volume (volume control) or pressure (pressure control).
  - Unlike SIMV, with assist control, the ventilator delivers a full (volume or pressure control) breath with every patient initiation. As a result, if the respiratory rate is set at 20 and the patient is breathing 30 breaths per minute, decreasing the rate to 15 will not impact the amount of support provided.
  - While the assist-control mode of ventilation has been used for years, it has been largely replaced with SIMV.
- **Supported Ventilation**
  - Supported ventilation is defined as a breath that is triggered by the patient and assisted by the ventilator (volume or pressure). Therefore, supported ventilation is only used in patients with an intact ventilatory drive.
  - Pressure support (PS) ventilation is a mode in which the patient triggers the ventilator to deliver a flow of gas sufficient to provide a preset pressure. The tidal volume achieved is determined by the patient's inspiratory effort, the preset pressure support level, and respiratory system compliance. PS is a commonly used mode of ventilation when weaning toward extubation.
  - Daily extubation readiness tests (ERT) should be considered in all intubated patients. During an ERT, patients are placed in PS ventilation at a setting defined by their ETT size. Once in ERT settings, a patient's respiratory rate and tidal volume are monitored to determine readiness for extubation.
  - Volume support (VS) ventilation is a mode in which the patient triggers the ventilator to deliver a flow of gas sufficient to provide a preset volume. In patients with relatively constant respiratory rates, VS can more easily guarantee appropriate minute ventilation although the pressures needed to deliver a set tidal volume must be monitored as respiratory compliance changes.
- **Strategies for Conventional Ventilation**
  - SIMV-PC and SIMV-PRVC are the initial conventional ventilator modes trialed for most pediatric patients. SIMV-PRVC is often chosen due to the guaranteed minute ventilation and use of high-pressure limits to prevent ventilator-induced lung injury. SIMV-PC is useful for patients with a moderate leak around the ETT since the effect on ventilation due to the leak can be mitigated with increased pressure settings. (See Table 8-2 for a comparison of common ventilator strategies.)
  - With SIMV-PC, the following settings are defined: pressure control, PEEP, respiratory rate (RR), pressure support (PS), and $FiO_2$. With SIMV-PRVC, the following settings are defined: tidal volume, PEEP, RR, PS, and $FiO_2$. For both modes, an inspiratory time is set to determine the duration of a mandatory breath.
  - Tidal volume: The average resting tidal volume for a spontaneously breathing, non-intubated child is 5-7 mL/kg with larger "sigh" breaths periodically interspersed;

| TABLE 8-2 | Comparison of Common Conventional Ventilator Strategies | | |
| --- | --- | --- | --- |
| **Mode** | **Volume control (VC)** | **Pressure control (PC)** | **Pressure-regulated volume control (PRVC)** |
| Clinician-set parameter | Tidal volume. | Peak inspiratory pressure. | Tidal volume. |
| Dependent parameter | Peak inspiratory pressure. | Tidal volume. | Peak inspiratory pressure. |
| Mean airway pressure | Lower for given tidal volume, inspiratory time, and peak airway pressure. | Higher for given tidal volume, inspiratory time, and peak airway pressure. | Higher for given tidal volume, inspiratory time, and peak airway pressure. |
| Other set parameters | Rate, PEEP, inspiratory time, $FiO_2$. | Rate, PEEP, inspiratory time, $FiO_2$. | Rate, PEEP, inspiratory time, $FiO_2$. |
| Flow pattern | Constant inspiratory flow. | Decelerating inspiratory flow. | Decelerating inspiratory flow. |
| Advantages | Guaranteed tidal volume and minute ventilation, changes in respiratory system compliance detected by changes in peak inspiratory pressure. | Peak airway pressure is limited. Decelerating flow pattern may allow inflation of airspaces with longer time-constants and may be more comfortable to the patient. | Guaranteed tidal volume and minute ventilation with a decelerating flow pattern with similar advantages listed for pressure control. |
| Disadvantages | Peak airway and alveolar pressures may vary excessively. Continuous flow may cause patient discomfort, asynchrony, and increased work of breathing. | Tidal volume varies with compliance and therefore adequate minute ventilation may not be achieved if alterations in lung compliance are not noted. | If lung compliance worsens, the breath delivery may terminate due to high positive inspiratory pressures based on preset limits that may lead to inadequate minute ventilation. |

average adult tidal volumes are 350-600 mL depending on lung size. An appropriate tidal volume should generate adequate chest rise.
- Pressure control: For a patient in SIMV-PC, a pressure control is set to achieve a tidal volume of 6-8 mL/kg as discussed above.
- Rate: A physiologic norm for age is selected and then adjusted with particular attention paid to the patient's ability to fully exhale and $CO_2$ clearance as assessed by end-tidal $CO_2$ monitoring and blood gas analysis.
- Inspiratory time: A physiologic, age-specific time is selected, resulting in an average inspiratory:expiratory ratio of 1:2. Reasonable starting inspiratory times are 0.4-0.5 seconds for infants, 0.6-0.8 seconds for younger children, and 0.8-1.2 seconds for adolescents and adults. Particular attention must be paid to the patient's respiratory rate and inspiratory time such that full exhalation is achieved between breaths. In patients with obstructive pulmonary disease, this physiology is particularly important and may necessitate lower than normative set RRs on the ventilator.
- PEEP: Depending on the patient's lung compliance and the need for intubation, PEEP should be adjusted to maintain lung recruitment at functional residual capacity, which is the starting lung volume at which lung compliance is optimal. A starting PEEP value of 5 cm $H_2O$ is often sufficient for most patients with reasonable lung compliance; increases are typically made in 1-2 cm $H_2O$ increments. The hemodynamic effects of excessive PEEP require close attention. High levels of PEEP will decrease systemic venous return (leading to a decrease in right heart preload) and consequently impair cardiac output. In addition, under- or overdistension of the lung by suboptimal PEEP will impair gas exchange. Assessment of lung distention is aided by chest radiography.
- $FiO_2$: The need for supplemental oxygen is based on the pathophysiology necessitating intubation, and its use will be determined by clinical circumstances and titrated to maintain appropriate oxygen delivery to the body. Attempts should be made to limit its use to nontoxic levels, typically <60%, by also targeting optimal ventilator strategies and airway clearance.
- (See Acute Respiratory Distress Syndrome Network, Khemani, Malhotra, West, suggested readings.)

*High-Frequency Oscillatory Ventilation*
- High-frequency oscillatory ventilation (HFOV) is most often used in the pediatric setting as a rescue ventilation strategy for those patients with severe hypoxia or hypercapnia despite optimal conventional ventilator management. The mode of ventilation uses high MAPs to facilitate alveolar recruitment and maintenance with superimposed sinusoidal oscillations that achieve small changes in lung volumes at supraphysiologic frequencies (3-15 Hz corresponding to 180-900 cycles per minute). This form of ventilation may also induce less ventilator-associated lung injury by minimizing lung stretch.
- HFOV parameters
  - Mean airway pressure (MAP): This is the main determinant of oxygenation. This pressure is typically set 5 cm $H_2O$ above the MAP pressure used during conventional mechanical ventilation and increased until adequate oxygenation is achieved. When weaning pressure in HFOV, the MAP is typically decreased in increments of 1-2 cm $H_2O$. Transition to conventional ventilation is considered when MAP needed to achieve optimal gas exchange is feasible on a conventional ventilator (typically <20 cm $H_2O$).

- ΔP: The amplitude (i.e., size of the oscillations) is a key determinant of ventilation and is adjusted to achieve adequate gas exchange and vibration ("jiggle") of the patient, typically targeted to the level of the groin. Incremental adjustments to the amplitude are typically made by 2-3 cm $H_2O$.
- Frequency (hertz): The frequency also influences patient ventilation via inverse effects on tidal volume (i.e., the lower the hertz, the larger the tidal volume). Initial frequency settings are based on the patient's size with higher frequencies used in infants (12-15 Hz) titrating down to lower frequencies in adolescents (3-8 Hz). Adjustment to the frequency is typically made by 0.5-1 Hz to optimize ventilation. Higher frequency is considered to be more lung protective.
- Endotracheal cuff inflation: The amount of cuff inflation deserves particular attention in the patient on HFOV. By deflating the cuff partially or completely in order to achieve a leak around the ETT, passive elimination of carbon dioxide occurs, augmenting ventilation. However, the ability to achieve a high MAP may be compromised by a large leak. Therefore, the clinical circumstance and gas exchange will guide the adjustment of cuff inflation.
- Tips for initiation: Given end-tidal $CO_2$ cannot be followed while a patient is on HFOV, a transcutaneous $CO_2$ monitor should be placed for continuous $CO_2$ monitoring. Obtain blood gases frequently at the time of HFOV initiation and titration. Frequent chest plain radiographs are helpful to assess lung expansion.
- (See Arnold suggested reading.)

*High-Frequency Percussive Ventilation*
- High-frequency percussive ventilation is provided by the volume diffuse respirator (VDR). This mode of ventilation effectively mobilizes pulmonary secretions due to the unique gas flow and humification, which facilitates gas exchange. This ventilator was initially created for burn patients with inhalation injury, but its use has become more widespread recently in the pediatric population.
- The VDR is now predominantly used for patients with the following indications: airway secretion clearance, lung recruitment, and hypercapnia from reversible/recruitable increased physiologic dead space. Contraindications to the use of the VDR are unresolved high-resistance respiratory failure (such as status asthmaticus), which may worsen air trapping, and untreated pneumothorax.
- Setting VDR parameters
  - Settings affecting ventilation
    ○ Average inspiratory pressure (AIP)—equivalent to positive inspiratory pressure (PIP) in conventional mechanical ventilation. Usually set at 25-30 cm $H_2O$. Increasing the AIP will typically increase $CO_2$ clearance.
    ○ Inspiratory time/expiratory time—Traditionally, keep the inspiratory to expiratory ratio at 1:1 with 1-2 seconds for each (shorter times for younger patients). To increase $CO_2$ clearance, decrease the inspiratory time.
    ○ Pulse frequency—500-700 "breaths" per minute (higher for younger patients). Like the frequency of HFOV, lower frequencies correspond to larger changes in lung volumes and thereby increased ventilation. Higher frequencies are considered to be more lung protective.
  - Settings affecting oxygenation
    ○ Average expiratory pressure (AEP)—equivalent to PEEP. AEP is the sum of the demand (0-2 cm $H_2O$) and oscillatory (8-12 cm $H_2O$) PEEP. To improve oxygenation, increase the AEP, which increases the MAP.
    ○ $FiO_2$.

- Tips for initiation: As with patients on HFOV, a transcutaneous $CO_2$ monitor should be placed for $CO_2$ monitoring. Obtain blood gases frequently at the time of VDR initiation. Obtain a chest plain radiograph after initiation to assess lung expansion.
- Transition back to a conventional ventilator when VDR support is weaned with stable gas exchange and secretion burden is improved.

*Assessment of Mechanical Ventilation*
- In an intubated patient, frequent clinical assessment of aeration, chest wall movement, work of breathing, and evaluation of gas exchange are essential. If a patient appears distressed, ensure that he or she is receiving appropriate ventilator support and that the level of sedation is sufficient in order to prevent patient-ventilator dyssynchrony.
- Blood gas analysis is key to assessing adequacy of mechanical ventilation.
  - Arterial blood gas (ABG) provides the most information about gas exchange.
  - In patients without arterial access, a capillary blood gas will provide a good estimate of the pH and $PaCO_2$ but does not reflect oxygenation. A venous blood gas obtained from a central line can also be useful, but peripheral venous gases, particularly those obtained with a tourniquet, are less reliable.
  - The $PCO_2$ of a venous blood gas is typically 5 mm Hg higher than the arterial $PCO_2$ with an accordant slight decrease in the venous pH.
- Exhaled $CO_2$ monitoring: measured at the end of the ETT. Depending on the degree of dead space ventilation and/or obstructive pulmonary disease, this value at the end of exhalation can serve as a proxy for $P_ACO_2$, which should also correlate well with $PaCO_2$. When exhaled $CO_2$ is measured continuously in an intubated patient, the displayed waveform can also provide information about the degree of obstructive pulmonary disease.

*Respiratory Failure Refractory to Mechanical Ventilation*
In severe pulmonary disease with hypoxia or hypercapnia refractory to the above means of mechanical support and threatening oxygen delivery to the body, extracorporeal membrane oxygenation (ECMO) may be necessary. This support is achieved by continuously circulating the patient's blood through a gas exchanger outside the body. In venous-venous ECMO (VV-ECMO), the patient's venous blood undergoes gas exchange outside the body and then is returned to the patient's venous system where it enters the lungs having already undergone gas exchange.

## SHOCK

- Shock is a clinical syndrome characterized by inadequate tissue perfusion and subsequent poor oxygen delivery, which ultimately leads to deranged homeostatic mechanisms and irreversible cellular damage. It is a clinical diagnosis and is not solely based on measurement of blood pressure.
- Given that tissue perfusion depends on blood volume, vascular tone, and cardiac function, all shock states result from abnormalities in one or more of these entities.

## Classification

- Shock can be classified in many ways, and any classification system must allow for overlap. Some schemes have classified shock based on etiology (Table 8-3) and others based

| TABLE 8-3 | Classification of Shock | | | |
| --- | --- | --- | --- | --- |
| Types of shock | Hypovolemic | Distributive | Cardiogenic | Septic |
| Etiology | Dehydration<br>Gastroenteritis<br>Heat stroke<br>Burns<br>Hemorrhage<br>Major abdominal surgery/third spacing | Anaphylaxis<br>Neurogenic<br>Drug toxicity | Congenital<br>Ischemic<br>Traumatic<br>Cardiomyopathy<br>Drug toxicity<br>Tamponade | Bacterial<br>Fungal<br>Viral<br>Parasitic |
| Pathophysiology | Decreased intravascular volume → decreased venous return → decreased myocardial preload | Vasomotor tone abnormalities → maldistribution of circulatory volume → peripheral pooling and vascular shunting → vasodilation and decreased myocardial preload | Pump failure → inadequate cardiac output | Infection and inflammatory response → tissue damage and impaired endothelial function → capillary leak → decreased myocardial preload and vasodilation, potentially cardiogenic also |

*(Continued)*

**TABLE 8-3** Classification of Shock *(Continued)*

| Types of shock | Hypovolemic | Distributive | Cardiogenic | Septic |
|---|---|---|---|---|
| Diagnosis | Early presentation (compensated): poor skin turgor, sunken eyes, cool extremities, tachycardia, normotensive, increased systemic vascular resistance (SVR), decreased urine output, normal or near normal cardiac filling pressure<br><br>Late (uncompensated): hypotension, altered sensorium, cardiopulmonary failure, and anuria | Profound hypotension<br><br>Anaphylaxis → other manifestations such as angioedema, emesis<br><br>Spinal shock → bradycardia | Similar presentation to hypovolemic shock except normal skin turgor and lack of sunken eyes<br><br>May have crackles suggestive of pulmonary edema, hepatomegaly, enlarged cardiac silhouette on chest plain radiograph | "Cold" shock presents similarly to hypovolemic and cardiogenic shock except with evidence of infection. "Cold" shock is notable for increased SVR and thus, delayed capillary refill. "Warm" shock will present with hyperdynamic circulation, decreased SVR, and flash capillary refill.<br><br>Often abnormal thermal regulation (fever or hypothermia) |
| Initial treatment | Volume repletion (blood products if etiology is hemorrhage) | Volume repletion<br>Vasopressors | Inotropes, lusitropy<br>Afterload reduction<br>May require diuretics | Volume repletion<br>Vasopressors and inotropes (cold shock—consider epinephrine first; warm shock—consider norepinephrine first)<br>Antimicrobials |

on patient examination characteristics (such as "warm" or "cold" shock). Regardless of the classification, a thorough understanding of the etiologies is required in order to direct therapeutic efforts at optimizing tissue perfusion and oxygen delivery.

- A patient in shock, regardless of initial etiology, may exhibit pathophysiologic characteristics of different types of shock at different times during illness. Therefore, frequent assessment, including both physical examination and laboratory evaluation, is paramount to titrate therapy appropriately in a time-sensitive manner.

## Monitoring

- A high index of suspicion and knowledge of conditions predisposing to shock are essential for early recognition and intervention. A thorough but targeted history will often uncover the etiology and guide corrective measures.
- Signs of decreased tissue perfusion, as manifest by changes in body temperature, heart rate, respiratory rate, capillary refill, urine output, pulse characteristics, and alteration in mental status, should be assessed.
- Laboratory investigations should include serum electrolytes (including ionized calcium), renal and hepatic panels, and complete blood count with differential. An early type and screen is useful if the patient may ultimately require blood products; however, for the patient in acute hemorrhagic shock, transfusion with universal donor products may be necessary prior to laboratory cross-matching. Blood gas analyses (optimally arterial), central venous oxygen saturation, and lactate can provide additional information about the adequacy of tissue perfusion and oxygen delivery as well as guide therapy.
  - Central venous oxygen saturation (mixed venous oxygen saturation, $SvO_2$) is the oxygen saturation of venous blood returing to the heart and is used to understand the relationship between oxygen delivery and oxygen consumption. With decreased oxygen delivery or increased oxygen consumption, $SvO_2$ is decreased. Physiologic $SvO_2$ is 70-80%. This marker is often decreased prior to an elevation of lactate and thus serves as an early indicator of inadequate oxygen delivery.
  - Lactate is an end product of anaerobic metabolism; thus, an elevation in lactate may indicate inadequate oxygen delivery.
- Continuous cardiopulmonary monitoring, pulse oximetry, temperature, and blood pressure measurements are essential.
  - Central line placement may be necessary for volume resuscitation, provision of vasoactive infusions, central venous pressure (CVP) and $SvO_2$ monitoring, and frequent blood laboratory assessments.
  - Arterial catheters can be used for frequent blood gas analysis and continuous blood pressure monitoring.
  - Thermodilution techniques or pulmonary arterial pressure monitoring may be considered for determination of cardiac output, volume status, and systemic vascular resistance (SVR) to guide optimal management.
- Placement of a urinary catheter allows for assessment of renal perfusion as manifest by urine output (<1 mL/kg/hr suggests renal hypoperfusion).

## Treatment

- Management of shock is aimed at optimizing perfusion of critical vascular beds in order to optimize oxygen delivery while minimizing unnecessary oxygen demand. Eventually, if shock remains uncorrected, an irreversible state of multiorgan failure develops.

- Treatment of the underlying cause is mandatory (e.g., cessation of hemorrhage in a profusely bleeding patient or antibiotic therapy in a patient with bacterial sepsis).
- Unless cardiogenic shock is suspected, initial resuscitation often begins with administration of intravenous fluids. This measure to increase preload will benefit patients with hypovolemia and/or decreased SVR. Infuse 20 mL/kg of isotonic crystalloids (normal saline, lactated Ringer's solution) with continued assessment before repeating fluid boluses. Physical examination assessment is aimed at whether the fluid administration improved perfusion (mental status, capillary refill, improved heart rate, and urine output) or worsened examination findings (hepatomegaly, crackles on lung auscultation, or worsened tachycardia). Cautious intravenous fluid administration is warranted if cardiogenic shock is suspected, and small boluses (5-10 mL/kg) are recommended initially as evaluation ensues.
- Patients with septic shock may need repeat fluid boluses every 5-10 minutes and as much as 80-100 mL/kg to optimize perfusion. Multiple peripheral intravenous access points or a central venous line is necessary.
- Severe metabolic acidosis may be treated with 1-2 mEq/kg sodium bicarbonate intravenously. However, sodium bicarbonate should be given cautiously to patients with impaired ventilation as increased intracellular acidosis may occur.
- Use of medications with vasopressor effects, such as epinephrine, norepinephrine, and vasopressin, may be required to improve perfusion (Table 8-4). An understanding of the patient's pathophysiology is important to choose the optimal agent.
- Lusitropy and afterload reduction with milrinone to improve myocardial performance may be indicated for patients with severe cardiac dysfunction.
- End-organ dysfunction, including renal, gastrointestinal, hematologic (coagulation), and central nervous system (CNS), must be identified and treated. Supportive care of these organ systems is necessary while the underlying etiology of shock is addressed.
- Corticosteroids should be considered in patients who fail to respond to vasopressor therapy. Earlier treatment may be warranted for those at risk for adrenal insufficiency (history of CNS abnormality, chronic steroid use, purpura fulminans, hyperpigmentation suggesting chronic adrenal insufficiency, or intubation with etomidate). Hydrocortisone doses of 50 mg per body surface area per day divided every 6-8 hours have been recommended. Also, consider drawing a random cortisol level before administration of steroids. This information may aid in discontinuing steroids later once the patient is improved.
- If the patient's hemodynamic status remains ambiguous despite ongoing clinical assessment, consider either thermodilution techniques or pulmonary arterial pressure monitoring (via a Swan-Ganz catheter) for assessment of cardiac output, volume status, and SVR.
- In cases of catecholamine refractory shock, consider broad etiologies such as cardiac tamponade, new pneumothorax, ongoing blood loss, and intra-abdominal catastrophe (such as infected or necrotic tissue).
- In cases of severe cardiopulmonary failure refractory to the above therapeutic measures, venous-arterial ECMO (VA-ECMO) may be necessary. For patients in shock, this support is achieved by draining blood from a venous cannula, circulating the blood through a gas exchanger and then pumping it back into the patient's central arterial circulation. VA-ECMO does not address the underlying etiology of shock but instead offers support while ongoing diagnostics ensue and therapeutic measures take effect. Importantly, coagulopathic patients need careful consider-

| TABLE 8-4 | Vasoactive Medications Used in Shock | | | | |
|---|---|---|---|---|---|
| **Medication** | **Epinephrine** | **Norepinephrine** | **Vasopressin** | **Angiotensin II** | **Milrinone** |
| Indication | "Cold" septic shock, cardiogenic shock | "Warm" septic shock, distributive shock | "Warm" septic shock, distributive shock | Septic or distributive shock. Risk venous thromboembolism. Risk of rejection in patients who have undergone heart transplant | Cardiac dysfunction in patients with adequate blood pressure (caution in renal dysfunction) |
| Mechanism of action | Chronotropy, inotropy, and increases SVR | Increases SVR | Increases SVR, does not increase PVR | Vasoconstriction via the renin-angiotensin-aldosterone system | Inotropy, lusitropy, and decreases SVR |
| Typical dosage | 0.01-1 µg/kg/min | 0.01-1 µg/kg/min | 0.1-2 mU/kg/min | 2.5-80 ng/kg/min | 0.125-1 µg/kg/min |

Systemic vascular resistance (SVR), Pulmonary vascular resistance (PVR)

ation for ECMO candidacy as the ECMO circuit requires systemic anticoagulation. Timely consultation with a pediatric surgeon is necessary for any patient in whom ECMO support may be required.
- (See Weiss suggested reading.)

## INCREASED INTRACRANIAL PRESSURE

- Increased intracranial pressure (ICP) is a common sequela of a variety of CNS insults, including trauma, infection, ischemic injury, and metabolic disease.
- Therapy directed at decreasing ICP has been shown to improve outcomes in traumatic brain injury but may benefit other carefully selected patients.
- Increased ICP is exerted by entities that occupy the fixed intracranial space including brain parenchyma, blood, cerebral spinal fluid (CSF), and any intracranial pathology such as tumors, hematomas, abscesses, or other mass lesions.
- If the volume of one component in the intracranial space increases, the volume of the other components, usually blood or CSF, must be reduced to maintain ICP within normal limits.
  - Once the capacity for this mechanism fails, ICP increases.
  - If the pressure becomes sufficiently high, movement of the brain or brainstem across the tentorium or through the skull base will occur (herniation), which can lead to irreversible damage of the brain or brainstem and death.

### Cerebral Perfusion Pressure and Cerebral Autoregulation

- The brain depends on a constant blood supply to provide oxygen and metabolic substrates. This blood supply exerts a pressure, known as the cerebral perfusion pressure (CPP), which must be maintained to provide energy to the metabolically active brain tissue. CPP is used as a measure of cerebral blood flow (CBF) and can be calculated if the mean arterial pressure (MAP) and ICP are known (CPP = MAP − ICP). Note that if the CVP is higher than the ICP, then CPP is calculated as follows: CPP = MAP − CVP. While the optimal CPP in children is not known, striving to keep the CPP above age-specific thresholds (for children <6 years old 40-55 mm Hg and those >6 years old 50-60 mm Hg) is reasonable based on current evidence. ICP goals are <20 mm Hg.
- Autoregulation refers to the brain's ability to maintain CBF despite wide fluctuations in MAP. CBF is well maintained for MAPs ranging from 60 to 150 mm Hg in adults. However, outside this range, CBF directly varies with blood pressure. At low blood pressures, CBF may be inadequate and result in ischemia. At high blood pressures, CBF becomes excessive and may contribute to increased ICP.
- In the injured brain, autoregulation may be compromised or completely lost leading to the above pathology even when MAPs are within physiologic ranges.
- A major factor in autoregulation is the brain's response to changes in arterial $O_2$ and $CO_2$ levels. Hypoxia is a potent cerebral vasodilator, and hypocapnia is a vasoconstrictor. Although other aspects of autoregulation may be lost, these responses are usually preserved in the injured brain and can be therapeutically useful.

### ICP Monitoring

- In order to maintain CPP within a desirable target, ICP monitoring may be necessary. This monitoring is typically achieved with a fiberoptic pressure monitor placed in the brain parenchyma, subdural, or epidural space or with an intraventricular

catheter (external ventricular drain, EVD). The latter also offers the advantage of therapeutic CSF removal.
- Monitor-associated complications are rare but include infection, hemorrhage, seizures, and inaccurate readings.
- Indications for consideration of ICP monitoring include the following:
  - Glasgow Coma Score ≤8 after traumatic brain injury
  - Abnormal head computed tomography (mass lesion, contusions, cerebral edema, or compression of the basal cisterns) in the setting of an abnormal neurologic examination
  - Neurologic examination obscured by sedation or neuromuscular blockade in the above pathologic settings
- The presence of an open fontanelle and/or sutures does not negate the utility of monitoring as increased ICP, worsening brain injury, and herniation may still occur.

## Airway Management

- A secure airway is critical in patients with elevated ICP to prevent secondary damage from hypoxia and to control or therapeutically lower $pCO_2$ given its effects on CBF.
- The principal goals of a neuroprotective intubation are deep sedation without significant hemodynamic effects and avoidance of hypoxia. Preoxygenation is essential to mitigate any hypoxia during the intubation process. Careful selection of sedatives and nondepolarizing muscle relaxants is essential.
- Stimulation of the oropharynx and larynx produces a vagally mediated reflex increase in ICP. Consider administration of lidocaine (1 mg/kg IV), which directly inhibits this response in at-risk patients.

## Treatment

- While the primary injury may or may not be possible to mitigate (resectable brain tumor vs. traumatic brain injury), avoidance of secondary brain injury is paramount in patients with elevated ICP. This goal is achieved by maintaining adequate supply of oxygen and nutrients to the injured brain and avoiding further insults such as ischemia or excessive metabolic demands (i.e., seizures and hyperthermia). Therefore, hypotension and hypoxia must be meticulously avoided.
- Therapy is directed at maintaining CPP by ensuring that blood pressure is adequate and ICP low. If necessary, fluid or blood product administration and vasoactive medications may be needed.
- Surgical evacuation of mass lesions may be necessary. Timely consultation with a neurosurgeon is paramount. However, surgical management is often not sufficient due to significant residual brain edema that contributes to elevated ICP.
- Medical management is directed at minimizing cerebral metabolism (which increases cerebral blood volume) and controlling excessive CBF while maintaining CPP to ensure adequate delivery of oxygen and metabolic substrates to the brain.
  - Ensure normothermia. Increased metabolic demand from fever can increase cerebral blood volume and ICP. Cooling blankets and acetaminophen can be used. Excessive energy demand from shivering should be controlled with paralytic agents.
  - Elevate the head of the bed to 30 degrees, and ensure that the patient's head is midline. This position facilitates venous drainage thereby decreasing cerebral blood volume. Accordingly, ensure that bandages and cervical collars do not impede venous drainage.
  - Consider continuous EEG monitoring for seizure activity and implement antiseizure medications if necessary. Seizures greatly increase cerebral metabolism and blood flow

and therefore must be aggressively treated. If a patient requires muscle relaxation, continuous EEG monitoring will be necessary for seizure monitoring. For acute seizure control, the following antiseizure medications may be considered: lorazepam, levetiracetam, fosphenytoin, or phenobarbital. If further seizure activity occurs, pentobarbital infusion could be considered. Consultation with a neurologist is important for seizure management. Seizure prophylaxis, most commonly with levetiracetam, should be considered for patients at high risk for early posttraumatic seizures (penetrating brain injury, intracranial hematomas, and depressed skull fractures).

- Attention to fluid management is important with avoidance of overhydration (total fluid intake should not exceed 1500 mL/m$^2$ and goal CVP 5-10 mm Hg). Isotonic fluids such as lactated Ringer's or normal saline should be used, and hyponatremia must be avoided (Na > 140 mmol/L). Normoglycemia is important (generally 100-200 mg/dL) with particular attention paid to the avoidance of hypoglycemia.

- Decreasing brain metabolism and agitation with sedatives may help in controlling elevated ICP. Careful consideration to the use of paralysis with a nondepolarizing neuromuscular blocking agent may be considered in the patient with ventilator dyssynchrony or frequent coughing, both of which are associated with increased ICP. However, obfuscation of the neurologic examination except for pupillary examination must be acknowledged and considered.

- In patients with an intraventricular catheter, frequent CSF removal is often beneficial for ICP control. However, this therapy offers little benefit for patients with severe tissue edema and small ventricles without excess CSF to drain.

- Osmotic agents (mannitol, hypertonic saline) are effective at controlling elevated ICP in many patients.
  - Mannitol, dosed at 0.5-1 g/kg, may be given intermittently every 4-6 hours to lower ICP. This osmotic agent will also induce brisk diuresis and should not be given to patients who are hypotensive or have decreased vascular preload. Close monitoring of intravascular volume is important.
    - Critical hyperosmolality from mannitol administration is associated with renal toxicity; therefore, serum osmolality is measured in order to determine the safety of repetitive doses. The measured osmolality is compared with the calculated serum osmolality using the following equation: calculated serum osmolality = (2 × Na) + (BUN/2.8) + (Glucose/18) + 10. If the osmolar gap (measured osmolality − calculated osmolality) is <20 mOsm/L, repeat dosing of mannitol is considered safe.
  - Hypertonic saline (3% sodium chloride) given in boluses of 5 mL/kg may be effective at controlling elevated ICP. For every 1 mL/kg of 3% hypertonic saline, serum sodium is expected to increase by approximately 1 mmol/L. In patients with symptomatic cerebral edema or elevated ICP, titrate to a serum sodium of 155-165 mmol/L (corresponding to a serum osmolality of <360 mOsm/L). A 3% infusion of 1-3 mL/kg/hr may facilitate this goal. Given risk of renal injury at severe hypernatremia, titrate hypertonic infusion down by 0.25 mL/kg/hr if Na > 165 mmol/L and ICP allows.

- Hyperventilation leads to hypocapnia and resultant cerebral vasoconstriction, which decreases cerebral blood volume and consequently ICP.
  - PaCO$_2$ levels should be maintained between 35 and 40 mm Hg to prevent excessive cerebral blood volume.
  - Further hyperventilation (PaCO$_2$ < 35 mm Hg) should be avoided given concern for brain ischemia at markedly low CBF; however, transient aggressive hyperventilation may be considered in cases of refractory intracranial hypertension with impending herniation refractory to other immediate measures.

- Implementation of a barbiturate coma with pentobarbital will decrease CBF by decreasing cerebral metabolism and may be considered for patients with ICP refractory to maximal medical and surgical therapy.
  - Continuous EEG monitoring is important to titrate dosing to a burst-suppression pattern.
  - High-dose barbiturate therapy depresses cardiac output and produces hypotension; vasopressor therapy is often necessary to promote MAP and consequently improve CPP.
  - Should the patient demonstrate progression to brain death (see section below), the first brain death examination must be delayed until the barbiturate effect has cleared as these medications can confound this examination. This process may take days and serum barbiturate levels may be useful to monitor clearance.
- Steroid therapy is indicated for vasogenic edema caused by tumors, and consultation with a neurosurgeon is useful in determining benefit in relation to potential surgical intervention.
- In patients with refractory elevated ICP unresponsive to the above therapies, consultation with a neurosurgeon regarding a decompressive craniotomy may be warranted.
- (See Downard, Kochanek, Stopa suggested readings.)

## DEATH ON THE BASIS OF NEUROLOGIC CRITERIA (BRAIN DEATH)

### Definition

- Brain death is a clinical diagnosis based on neurologic assessment of irreversible damage to the brain, including the brainstem, resulting from a known etiology leading to coma. Ongoing cardiopulmonary support facilitates organ donation in patients with prior consent (or families who provide consent).
- The diagnosis of brain death cannot be made in the presence of conditions that could be responsible for the absence of detectable brainstem functions. Such conditions include the following:
  - Shock or persistently low blood pressure
  - Severe electrolyte, pH, or metabolic abnormalities
  - Temperature <35°C
  - Drug intoxication (barbiturate coma), poisoning, or neuromuscular blockade
- These conditions must be corrected before evaluation for brain death. Individual hospitals have policies regarding the diagnosis of brain death, and these documents should be consulted before any final determination.

### Brain Death Examination

- In most instances, physical examination criteria are sufficient to make the diagnosis of brain death. However, ancillary tests may be necessary when components of the physical examination cannot be performed safely, if uncertainty persists after the physical examination, if a medication effect may obfuscate examination findings, or to reduce the timing between brain death examinations.
- Two examinations must be performed by two attending physicians who are caring for the patient. These examinations should be separated in time by >24 hours for a neonate and >12 hours for infants older than 30 days and children. The first examination confirms the patient has met criteria for brain death determination, and the second examination confirms its irreversibility.

- The neurologic examination consists of the following components:
  - Coma with loss of consciousness and lack of responsiveness (rudimentary spinal cord reflexes such as triple flexion of the legs with painful stimuli may be present and require expertise to differentiate from retained motor responses).
  - Absence of brainstem reflexes with midpoint or dilated pupils that do not respond to light, lack of movement facilitated by the bulbar musculature, and absent gag, cough, corneal, and oculovestibular reflexes.
  - An apnea test demonstrating no respiratory effort in the presence of elevated $PaCO_2$. A baseline blood gas measurement is obtained to document normocapnia and then the patient is preoxygenated with 100% oxygen for 5 minutes before removing mandatory ventilation (such as disconnection from the ventilator while oxygen is provided by an anesthesia bag connected to the ETT). The patient is monitored for any respiratory effort over the observation time while serial blood gas measurement monitors elevation in $PaCO_2$. A rise of 20 mm Hg above baseline and $\geq 60$ mm Hg without respiratory effort in this setting indicates lack of neurologically mediated respiratory control.
  - If an apnea test cannot be safely performed given a medical contraindication or cardiopulmonary instability, an ancillary test should be undertaken. Cerebral angiography is considered an optimal test for determination of CBF although its availability is limited and may be technically difficult in small patients. Nucleotide cerebral perfusion scan is a commonly utilized ancillary test and can be performed at the patient's bedside. Demonstration of EEG silence may also be performed as an ancillary test. These studies require expertise in administration and interpretation.
- (See Greer, Martin suggested readings.)

## POSTOPERATIVE CARE OF PATIENTS AFTER CONGENITAL CARDIAC SURGERY

- Successful postoperative management of congenital cardiac patients requires the following:
  - Knowledge of preoperative anatomic diagnosis and pathophysiologic effects
  - Understanding of anesthetic and operative details as well as potential resultant complications
  - Knowledge of postoperative anatomy and physiologic consequences
  - Careful postoperative intensive care unit management

### Preoperative Details

- Prior to the surgical procedure, the ICU team should be familiar with the following important historical information:
  - Prenatal course and gestational age
  - Age and weight
  - Anatomic details of the congenital cardiac lesion
  - Pathophysiologic effects before surgery
  - General health of the patient
  - Noncardiac medical and surgical history
  - Results of any diagnostic procedures and radiographic studies (echocardiogram, CTA, MRI, and cardiac catheterization)

## Operative Details

- Details of the operation, including anesthetics used and the duration of cardiopulmonary bypass, aortic cross-clamp, and circulatory arrest should be noted.
  - During cardiopulmonary bypass, catheters are placed in both venae cavae to drain blood from the patient, which is then oxygenated and rewarmed before being returned to the patient via a catheter in the ascending aorta. This blood flow pattern leaves the patient's heart relatively devoid of blood, enabling proper visualization for operative procedures. However, cardiopulmonary bypass results in a nonphysiologic, nonpulsatile blood flow, which can trigger the inflammatory cascade and coagulopathy.
  - Aortic cross-clamp time is the time during which the coronary artery blood flow is interrupted via a clamp placed across the aorta. It reflects the ischemic time for the heart.
  - Circulatory arrest is the time that the patient is not perfused (including the brain) as all the blood is drained into the bypass system but not returned. This state is necessary for procedures on the proximal aorta. Hypothermia is employed in order to decrease cellular metabolism and oxygen demand during this time.
  - Longer ischemic or artificial perfusion times may lead to a greater systemic inflammatory response and end organ dysfunction.
- Details about the surgical approach, difficulty in disconnecting the patient from bypass, and intraoperative complications, such as arrhythmias, bleeding, or air embolism, are important to note. The presence of intracardiac lines, chest tubes, and temporary cardiac pacing leads should be conveyed during transfer of care in the intensive care unit.
- An echocardiogram is often obtained in the operating room to evaluate for residual defects.

## ICU Management: The First Several Hours

- After effective communication with the anesthesia and surgical team regarding the patient and procedure, the ICU team turns attention toward assessment and any further postoperative resuscitation needed while keeping in mind potential complications.
  - During transport from the operative room, tubes, wires, and lines may become inadvertently dislodged. Therefore, it is important to verify placement of the ETT and vascular assessment as well as chest tube placement. An immediate chest plain radiograph will aid in this assessment. Interrogation of temporary pacing leads is also important.
  - Assess the patient's hemodynamic status (skin color, central and peripheral pulses, capillary refill, core and extremity temperatures, heart rate, and blood pressure).
  - Obtain baseline postoperative laboratory evaluation (ABG, lactate, central venous oxygen saturation, serum electrolytes, ionized calcium, hemoglobin, platelet count, coagulation studies, and renal function).
  - Assess rhythm and interrogate pacemaker wires if applicable.
  - Evaluate tracing and pressures from all transduced lines (which may include the following: radial/femoral artery, superior vena cava, right atrium, pulmonary artery, and left atrium) in the setting of patient's postoperative anatomy.
- Provide respiratory support as necessary. Positive pressure ventilation hinders venous return to the heart but reduces left ventricular afterload. Knowledge of the patient's underlying physiology and appreciation of complex cardiopulmonary interactions

are vital to develop an optimal strategy to provide respiratory support. Certain anatomical defects or conditions require tailored ventilatory strategies to optimize cardiac output.

- If the patient has high pulmonary vascular resistance (PVR) or is prone to pulmonary hypertensive crises, sedation and neuromuscular blockade for 24-72 hours may be needed to ensure optimal pulmonary blood flow. Hyperventilation (by lowering $pCO_2$ and reversing acidosis), high inspired oxygen fraction, and, in some instances, nitric oxide may be used to facilitate pulmonary blood flow.
- If excessive pulmonary blood flow is problematic, such as in a patient with residual intracardiac shunt, hypoventilation and low inspired oxygen may be necessary to avoid pulmonary vasodilation.
- After the Glenn and Fontan operations, early extubation is often the goal, as positive pressure ventilation will diminish pulmonary blood flow in these passive pulmonary blood flow systems.

## ICU Management: Overnight

- Careful attention must be paid to bleeding (such as blood evacuated from the patient's chest tubes) postoperatively.
  - Excessive output (>4 mL/kg/hr for 2 hours or >10 mL/kg at any one instance) may indicate the presence of bleeding that can be surgically corrected. Immediate communication with the cardiothoracic surgeon is necessary since bleeding from large thoracic vessels requires chest reexploration and surgical ligation. Alternatively, excess bleeding may represent a medical coagulopathy that will require transfusion of any or all of the following: packed red blood cells, plasma, platelets, cryoprecipitate, protamine (if heparin from the bypass pump circuit has not been fully reversed), or recombinant factor VII. In the event of life threatening hemorrhage, activation of the hospital's massive transfusion protocol may be of benefit in providing the patient with an optimized ratio of blood products during the resuscitation.
  - Less output than expected may also be cause for concern. This situation could arise from a clot in the patient's thorax or in the chest tube itself, which can lead to nonevacuated and underappreciated bleeding. Excessive clot in the patient's thorax may lead to cardiac tamponade. Signs to watch for tamponade include tachycardia, hypotension, and elevation in CVP. This concern should also be brought to the immediate attention of the surgeon as the patient may require exploration of the chest cavity.
- Arrhythmias
  - Junctional ectopic tachycardia (JET) is a supraventricular arrhythmia that is most frequently seen in patients undergoing surgery that involves instrumentation of the ventricular septum (repair of atrioventricular canal defects, ventricular septal defects, and tetralogy of Fallot). The arrhythmia may be seen early postoperatively.
    - JET originates outside the sinoatrial (SA) node and often starts relatively slowly and then progressively speeds up; once the rate exceeds the SA node, it becomes the dominant pacemaker. The QRS may look normal, although retrograde p-waves may be apparent.
    - This rhythm may cause atrial-ventricular dyssynchrony, and therefore cardiac output may become compromised with a fall in systolic blood pressure. The rhythm is identified by the presence of cannon A waves (indicative of the right atrium contracting against a closed tricuspid valve) on the CVP tracing.

- ○ Treatment is aimed at slowing the rate in order to decrease myocardial energy demand and oxygen consumption while restoring full cardiac output. As JET can be potentiated by fever and elevated catecholamines, treatment efforts are aimed at minimizing their presence and effect. Cooling the patient's core and avoidance of heat lamps may be necessary. Reduction in catecholamine infusions should be strongly considered if physiologically tolerated. However, calcium infusions may be continued to promote inotropy. Increased sedation, especially dexmedetomidine as it is an α-2 agonist, may be necessary if the patient is agitated leading to increased circulating endogenous catecholamines. Antiarrhythmics, such as amiodarone, may be necessary; an amiodarone bolus (5 mg/kg) infused slowly over 30 minutes followed by a continuous infusion of 15 mg/kg/day is a typical treatment option. However, care must be maintained as intravenous amiodarone can cause hypotension and hypocalcemia, and thus patients require vigilant monitoring during its administration.
  - ○ If the patient has a pacemaker (or temporary wires left postoperatively), the patient can be atrially paced at a rate slightly exceeding the JET rate to achieve atrial-ventricular synchrony and improved cardiac output. However, atrial pacing at high rates (>180 beats per minute) also results in impaired cardiac output (given decreased ventricular filing and thus reduced stroke volume). Therefore, efforts to slow the JET rate are necessary prior to overdrive pacing.
  - ○ The arrhythmia often resolves in 12-24 hours and does not require long-term pacing or medications.
- • Complete heart block is the failure of atrioventricular (AV) node conduction, and consequently contraction of the atria and ventricles are not coordinated to maximize cardiac output. This arrhythmia is also seen in patients undergoing surgery involving the septum given the anatomy of the electrical conduction system.
  - ○ The underlying escape rate is junctional (originating from the AV node) or ventricular and often insufficient to maintain optimal cardiac output, especially in the setting of suboptimal stroke volume.
  - ○ Treatment typically involves pacing the ventricle every time an atrial beat is sensed, thereby restoring AV concordance.
  - ○ The condition often resolves in the first several days after surgery. If it persists longer than 2 weeks, a permanent pacemaker will be necessary.
- • AV nodal reentry tachycardia is another form of supraventricular tachycardia that can occur postoperatively and may be confused with JET. The distinction is important as the arrhythmias respond to different management.
  - ○ This arrhythmia often occurs with a rapid increase in heart rate compared to the relatively insidious rate increase that occurs in JET.
  - ○ If the patient is hemodynamically stable, vagal maneuvers may be attempted (such as ice to the face), or intravenous adenosine may be given.
  - ○ If the patient fails to convert to sinus rhythm with adenosine, other supraventricular arrhythmias, such as atrial flutter or ectopic atrial tachycardia, should be considered. These conditions require rapid overdrive pacing or cardioversion.
  - ○ If the patient is hemodynamically unstable, synchronized cardioversion should be attempted immediately. Alternatively, the patient may be overdrive paced at a rapid atrial rhythm (>300 beats per minute) for several seconds.
- • Postcardiopulmonary bypass, many patients exhibit physiology consistent with low cardiac output. This syndrome has been coined "low cardiac output syndrome" and typically reaches its nadir 6-12 hours postoperatively (see Parr, Wernovsky, suggested

readings). While the etiology is incompletely defined and likely multifactorial for each patient, supportive care is the mainstay of treatment.

- The intensive care physician must consider any additional factors that may contribute to or potentiate low cardiac output physiology such as the following: residual or unrecognized structural defects, continuation of perioperative ventricular dysfunction, reperfusion injury, effects of cardiopulmonary bypass, expected physiologic postoperative cardiopulmonary interactions, complications of surgery (such as compromised coronary arteries during repair of transposition of the great vessels), arrhythmias, pulmonary hypertension, and infection.
- Low cardiac output syndrome will be manifest by symptoms and signs of cardiogenic shock such as depressed mental status, core hyperthermia (with peripheral cooling), mottled extremities, tachycardia, narrowed pulse pressure or frank hypotension, poor urine output, decreased central venous hemoglobin oxygen saturations, and increased lactate production. Pulmonary edema on chest radiograph may be present.
- Treatment is supportive. Evaluation of central venous, right atrial, and left atrial pressures, as well as physical examination, can guide therapy.
  - Low filling pressures (uniformly low CVP, right atrial, or left atrial pressures) indicate hypovolemia and should be treated with sequential 5 mg/kg boluses of colloids or crystalloids with attention to fluid response.
  - Normal or elevated filling pressures (high CVP, right atrial, or left atrial pressures) indicate depressed myocardial function and should be treated with inotropic support, including calcium infusions.
  - Cool, poorly perfused extremities with normotension indicate borderline myocardial function; afterload reduction (milrinone 0.5-1 µg/kg/min) should be considered (see Roeleveld, suggested readings).
  - If the patient continues to exhibit poor cardiac output despite optimal medical therapy, ECMO support is indicated. Frequent communication with the cardiothoracic surgeon is critical.
    - Elective cannulation for ECMO may be considered in the patient exhibiting progressively worsening cardiac output, as evidenced by frequent physical examination and biochemical markers of organ perfusion (see Trittenwein, suggested readings).
    - ECMO should be considered in any patient with refractory hypotension, worsening metabolic acidosis, and/or inotropic requirement of >0.2 µg/kg/min of epinephrine in the postoperative period.
    - ECMO support may be required to bridge through low cardiac output syndrome, or if the patient is unable to separate from ECMO support to ventricular assist device placement and listing for transplantation.

## ICU Management: The Next Several Days

- Most postoperative cardiac surgery patients benefit from diuretic therapy by the 1st postoperative day.
- Nutrition is very important for postoperative cardiac patients. Glucose containing intravenous infusions are typically started in the immediate postoperative period and then transitioned to enteral or parenteral nutrition within 24-72 hours. Enteral nutrition is preferred except in cases in which there is concern for poor gut perfusion secondary to low cardiac output or vasopressor therapy or if the patient develops a postoperative ileus. In cases in which the patient requires prolonged mechanical

ventilation but otherwise can tolerate feeding, enteral nutrition is provided via the nasogastric or nasojejunal route.

• Chest tube output should be monitored continually, and output should diminish while also becoming more serous. The cardiothoracic surgeons will typically remove the chest tubes once drainage has met these criteria. Cloudy output may be a sign of chylous drainage, suggesting damage to the thoracic duct. Ongoing chylous drainage may impair the patient's ability to separate from mechanical ventilation.

  • Occasionally, the recurrent laryngeal nerves or phrenic nerves may be damaged intraoperatively. This injury may be permanent secondary to direct trauma or temporary as a result of thermal damage from therapeutic hypothermia intraoperatively or from stretch injury.

    ○ Given the role of the recurrent laryngeal nerves in vocal cord opening, damage is manifested by upper airway obstruction with stridor and respiratory distress becomes apparent after extubation. Diagnosis of vocal cord paralysis may be made in an extubated spontaneously breathing patient via a flexible bedside scope. In the setting of complete vocal cord paralysis, the patient will require reintubation and await return of nerve function or proceed with tracheostomy placement.

    ○ Phrenic nerve damage may be suspected from chest radiology demonstrating a persistently elevated diaphragm, particularly when unilateral in nature. Signs are consistent with respiratory distress, and patients demonstrate paradoxical abdominal wall retractions. Young infants are more prone to respiratory failure from diaphragmatic paralysis and may require surgical plication.

## MANAGEMENT OF CHILDREN WITH SINGLE VENTRICLE LESIONS

• Complete mixing of the blood supply from the systemic and pulmonary venous return is a common resultant physiology of a variety of congenital cardiac lesions. Examples of such mixing lesions include the single ventricle heart defects, and atresia of the atrioventricular valves is a common pathologic finding.

• The single ventricular output is divided into two parallel circulations, the systemic and pulmonary circuits, in order to provide blood flow to both the lungs and the rest of the body. The relative proportion of blood flow to these vascular beds is determined by the relative resistances to flow in each circuit (i.e., the PVR and the SVR).

• Therefore, the physiology of single ventricle defects can be considered in three broad categories that determine the preoperative management and the surgical treatment. These categories are patients with balanced circulations, those with excessive pulmonary blood flow, and those with insufficient pulmonary blood flow.

### Balanced Circulation

• In this situation, as in normal cardiac physiology, the pulmonary blood flow ($Q_p$) is equal to the systemic blood flow ($Q_s$). However, given pulmonary and systemic venous return mixing, the arterial oxygen saturation is approximately 75-85%. Immediate surgery or medical management may not be needed.

• A balanced circulation in a neonate with single ventricle physiology suggests that the PVR has not yet dropped to the normal physiologic range (lower than the SVR).

### Excessive Pulmonary Flow

• Excessive pulmonary blood flow implies that the $Q_p$ is greater than $Q_s$ and is expected physiology as PVR falls in the days after birth. Given more pulmonary blood flow, the arterial hemoglobin oxygen saturation is higher than that in a balanced circulation. However, this situation is not advantageous because, if untreated, it can lead to congestive heart failure as the single ventricle has to work harder to maintain adequate systemic blood flow in the face of mounting pulmonary vascular steal.

- Management is aimed at promoting more blood flow into the systemic circulation. One mechanism to achieve more systemic blood flow is by decreasing SVR. Left ventricular afterload reduction, such as with nitroprusside, milrinone, or angiotensin-converting inhibitors, may be used. Accordingly, medications that increase SVR are avoided. Alternatively, PVR may be increased by controlled hypoventilation with neuromuscular blockade (acidosis and increased $pCO_2$ increase PVR) and/or with decreased inspired oxygen. Increased hematocrit may contribute to increased PVR by increasing blood viscosity and thus decreasing pulmonary shunting.

- Medical treatment for excessive blood flow is insufficient long-term (given progression to heart failure), and therefore surgery is typically necessary after PVR decreases. Early consultation with a cardiothoracic surgeon is paramount to determine the optimal timing of surgical intervention. Pulmonary banding may be considered as an initial approach in order to restrict blood flow to the pulmonary vascular bed. This intervention involves placing a band around the main pulmonary artery. This band is tightened intraoperatively until aortic oxygen saturation is 75-85% or the gradient across the band is 40-60 mm Hg.

## Insufficient Pulmonary Blood Flow

- Insufficient pulmonary blood flow implies that the $Q_p$ is less than $Q_s$, and hypoxemia is resultantly present with arterial oxygen saturation that is typically 70% or lower. The goal of management is to increase pulmonary blood flow to aid in arterial hemoglobin oxygenation.

- One option to divert blood flow into the pulmonary circulation is by increasing the resistance to flow in systemic circulation by increasing SVR. Sometimes systemic vasoconstrictive agents, such as phenylephrine or vasopressin, may be necessary. Care should be used with inotropes such as epinephrine, however, as these medications increase the workload on the already comprised single ventricle.

- Another avenue to increase pulmonary blood flow is to decrease PVR. Increasing the fractional percent of oxygen and/or decreasing $pCO_2$ via hyperventilation and relative alkalosis will lower PVR and facilitate pulmonary blood flow. Also consider whether direct pulmonary vasodilators, such as nitric oxide and prostacyclin, may be helpful. Hypovolemia should be avoided, and euvolemia targeted.

- However, medical therapies may also become inadequate, and again, early consultation with a cardiothoracic surgeon is paramount. Depending on future planned surgical interventions, pulmonary valve dilation or atrial septostomy (to increase blood mixing at the atrial level) may be required.

  - The primary surgical intervention before complete palliation is establishment of a systemic-to-pulmonary shunt. A common approach is a modified Blalock-Taussig (BT) shunt, wherein a conduit is anastomosed in an end-to-side fashion to the subclavian artery (innominate artery in hypoplastic left heart syndrome) and the pulmonary artery. After successful surgery, arterial oxygen saturation is approximately 75-85%, indicative of a balanced circulation with more optimal oxygen delivery to end-organ tissues.

## Surgery

- Most patients with single ventricles ultimately undergo similar staged surgical operations aimed at ultimately unloading the single ventricle from providing both the pulmonary and systemic output by establishing stable extracardiac systemic to pulmonary connections.
- These procedures converge in the establishment of passive pulmonary blood flow, and thus successful outcome is dependent on low pulmonary resistance and low single ventricle end diastolic pressure. Therefore, cardiac catheterization is performed before these procedures to evaluate PVR and single ventricle end diastolic pressure.
- Without unloading via staged surgical procedures, the single ventricle is at high risk for failure over time.
- Alternately, the patient may be considered for heart transplantation at an appropriate center if the cardiac anatomy is not amendable for staged surgery.

### Norwood

- The traditional first operation for patients with hypoplastic left heart syndrome is known as the Norwood. This operation establishes systemic blood flow from the single ventricle and therein must establish alternative pulmonary blood flow via a shunt. Patients typically undergo this procedure once their intrinsically elevated PVR drops in the week after birth and pulmonary overcirculation thereby ensues.
  - The branch pulmonary arteries are excised from the main pulmonary artery, and the resultant pulmonary trunk is anastomosed to the hypoplastic aorta, creating a neoaorta. Aortic arch coarctation requires reconstruction, and atrial septostomy is performed as well.
  - Pulmonary blood flow is then established with either a modified Blalock-Taussig (BT) shunt or a Sano shunt.
    - The modified BT shunt allows for physiologic runoff of blood flow to the pulmonary vascular bed during diastole, the time when the coronary arteries are perfused. Therefore, the modified BT shunt may be complicated by coronary artery hypoperfusion, a significant risk in the already volume-overloaded heart.
    - The Sano shunt is a plastic conduit surgically placed to connect the right ventricle and the pulmonary arteries. The Sano shunt provides pulsatile pulmonary blood flow only during systole and avoids diastolic runoff and coronary steal.

### Hybrid

- The hybrid procedure is an alternate staged approach for patients with single ventricles. This procedure, as its name implies, utilizes both interventional cardiology techniques and surgery. Bands around the pulmonary arteries are surgically placed and tightened to achieve sufficient but not excess pulmonary blood flow. The interventional cardiologist creates an atrial septostomy and stents the ductus arteriosus. This portion of the procedure establishes stable intracardiac mixing and systemic blood flow. Reconstruction of the aortic arch in patients with hypoplastic left heart syndrome is delayed until the next stage.
- Use of this technique allows for avoidance of cardiopulmonary bypass and cardioplegia necessary for the Norwood operation in the young infant.

### Glenn Shunt

- The next surgery, the Glenn operation, is typically performed at approximately 4-6 months of age when PVR generally has dropped further, and pulmonary blood flow via the shunt no longer requires as much pressure from the ventricle. This time also coincides with when the patient outgrows the Sano or BT shunt (the amount of pulmonary blood flow is suboptimal due to limitations in the size of the conduit). The patient will exhibit decreased arterial oxygen saturations.

- During the Glenn operation, the previously placed modified BT shunt or Sano shunt is removed, and a cavopulmonary shunt is created by anastomosing the superior vena cava to the pulmonary artery. Blood flow is typically routed to the right and left lung, and the operation is termed a bidirectional Glenn. This procedure results in all blood flow from the superior vena cava now entering the pulmonary circulation without transversing the heart. Given that the resultant pulmonary blood flow is passive, the presence of low PVR is essential.
- If the patient previously underwent a hybrid procedure, this surgery becomes more involved as the operation includes removing the pulmonary artery bands, reconstructing the aortic arch and possibly pulmonary artery reconstruction, and lastly, creating the cavopulmonary shunt (superior vena cava to pulmonary artery).
- The patient will still exhibit cyanosis because blood return via the inferior vena cava empties into the single ventricle and mixes with oxygenated blood prior to systemic ventricular ejection.

*Fontan Shunt*
- The last operation to separate the pulmonary circulation from the systemic circulation is known as the Fontan procedure. This procedure, typically performed at approximately 2-3 years of age, involves anastomosing the inferior vena cava to the pulmonary artery.
  - Postoperatively, these patients will now have almost normal arterial oxygen saturations. A slight reduction occurs since the coronary veins, which contain little oxygenated blood, still empty into the ventricle.
- In many patients undergoing Fontan procedures, a small fenestration or hole is made between the Fontan circuit and the heart. This connection allows a right-to-left shunt or "pop-off" for blood flow to the heart in order to maintain cardiac output in the event that PVR is elevated and passive pulmonary blood flow is diminished.
  - When blood shunts through the fenestration, the patient will have systemic arterial desaturation and possibly cyanosis depending on the amount of shunted deoxygenated blood. However, without the shunt, a rise in PVR may lead to a decrease in cardiac output, leading to a dangerous combination of hypotension and arterial desaturation.
  - (See Kaplinski, Reemstem, Roeleveld suggested readings.)

## CONVALESCENCE AND RECOVERY

Most children recover from critical illness with survival rates over 97%. Prolonged intensive care unit stays may result in or worsen delirium and require management of sedative and narcotic habituation. Physical deconditioning may prolong ventilator needs and ICU length of stay. Children surviving critical illness and their families may experience psychosocial effects long past discharge from the pediatric intensive care unit.

### Delirium
- Delirium is now recognized as a frequent complication of ICU admissions and affects over 25% of critically ill children. Children <2 years of age and those with

existing medical conditions are at higher risk. The development of pediatric delirium is multifactorial but is associated strongly with the use of benzodiazepines. Pediatric delirium is associated with longer duration of mechanical ventilation, higher mortality, and cognitive impairment.

- Three types of pediatric delirium are recognized: hyperactive, hypoactive, and mixed. Children most commonly exhibit hypoactive or mixed delirium.
- Validated, pediatric-specific delirium screening tools exist; the Cornell Assessment of Pediatric Delirium (CAP-D) is applicable to children aged 0-18 years. Other validated tools exist; all allow for reliable and efficient screening.
- Treatment is multifactorial and includes environmental modification, promotion of sleep hygiene, and the use of atypical antipsychotics. Atypical antipsychotics are generally well-tolerated; screening and weekly electrocardiograms are useful to detect QTc prolongation.

## Narcotic and Sedative Tolerance

- The medications required to facilitate interaction with mechanical ventilation may result in tolerance and potentiate delirium. Rapid discontinuation of these medications may result in significant withdrawal symptoms. Patients should receive screening for withdrawal symptoms as medication doses decrease.
  - Patients receiving continuous infusions of narcotics or sedatives for <1 week generally do not require a medication taper.
  - Symptoms and signs of withdrawal include irritability, yawning, feeding intolerance, and tachycardia.
  - Utilizing the lowest effective dose of analgesic and sedative medications may reduce the risk of withdrawal syndromes.

## Early Mobility

- Early mobility in critically ill patients may reduce the negative effects of prolonged intensive care unit stays. Improvement in motor function and reduction in length of hospital stay are additional benefits. Early mobility programs require multidisciplinary collaboration including family involvement.
  - Assessment of pain, spontaneous breathing trials, management of delirium, and exercise are key elements in recovery.
  - Sleep hygiene and environmental modifications are important for overall health and recovery.
  - Family engagement and partnering is a key component of success. Services such as music and pet therapy can provide additional benefit.

## Postintensive Care Syndrome

- After recovery from critical illness, children may experience new or worsening physical and emotional impairments. For the family, prolonged intensive care unit stays are life-altering; many caregivers experience significant psychologic impact as a result of their loved one's illness. Postintensive care syndrome is an emerging area of study.
  - New or worsening global dysfunction is common following discharge from the pediatric intensive care unit. Residual effects persist in many at 6 months following discharge, but many children demonstrate improvement over time.
  - Physical, cognitive, emotional, and social health are important components of a child's recovery. New or worsening function in these areas may have long-lasting impacts on development and quality of life.

- Identification, screening, and follow-up of at-risk children are needed to optimize long-term outcomes for survivors of critical illness.
- (See Siegel, Amigoni, Watson, Society of Critical Care Medicine suggested readings.)

## SUGGESTED READINGS

Acute Respiratory Distress Syndrome Network. Ventilation with lower tidal volume as compared with traditional tidal volume for acute lung injury and the acute respiratory distress syndrome. N Engl J Med 2000;342:1301–1308.

Amigoni A, Mondardini MC, Vittadello I, et al. Withdrawal assessment tool-1 monitoring in PICU: a multicenter study on iatrogenic withdrawal syndrome. Pediatr Crit Care Med 2017;18(2):e86–e91.

Arnold HJ. High-frequency ventilation in the pediatric intensive care unit. Pediatr Crit Care Med 2000;(1):93–99.

Downard C, Hulka F, Mullins RJ, et al. Relationship of cerebral perfusion and survival in pediatric brain injured patients. J Trauma 2000;(49):654–659.

Duff JP, Topjian AA, Berg MD, et al. 2019 American Heart Association focused update on pediatric advanced life support: an update to the American Heart Association Guidelines for cardiopulmonary resuscitation and emergency cardiovascular care. Pediatrics 2020;145(1):e20191361.

Fuhrman BP, Zimmerman JJ. Pediatric Critical Care. 6th Ed. Philadelphia, PA: Mosby, 2022.

Greer DM, Shemie SD, Lewis A, et al. Determination of brain death/death by neurologic criteria: the World Brain Death Project. JAMA 2020;324(11):1078–1097.

Kaplinski M, Ittenbach RF, Hunt ML, et al. Decreasing interstage mortality after the Norwood procedure: a 30-year experience. J Am Heart Assoc 2020;9(19):e016889.

Khemani RG, Parvathaneni K, Yehya N, et al. Positive end-expiratory pressure lower than the ARDS network protocol is associated with higher pediatric acute respiratory distress syndrome mortality. Am J Respir Crit Care 2018;198:77–89.

Khemani RG, Smith LS, Zimmerman JJ, et al. Pediatric acute respiratory distress syndrome: definition, incidence and epidemiology: proceedings from the Pediatric Acute Lung Injury Consensus Conference. Pediatr Crit Care Med 2015;16(Suppl 5):S23–S40.

Kochanek PM, Tasker RC, Carney N, et al. Guidelines for the management of pediatric severe traumatic brain injury, third edition: update of the brain trauma foundation guidelines. Pediatr Crit Care Med 2019;20(Suppl 3):S1–S82.

Malhotra A. Low tidal-volume ventilation in the acute respiratory distress syndrome. N Engl J Med 2007;357:1113–1120.

Martin SD, Porter MB. Performing the brain death and the declaration of pediatric brain death. J Pediatr Intensive Care 2017;6:229–233.

Nichols DG, Shaffner DH, et al. Roger's Textbook of Pediatric Intensive Care. 5th Ed. Philadelphia, PA: Lippincott Williams & Wilkins, 2016.

Parr GVS, Blackstone EH, Kirklin JW. Cardiac performance and mortality early after intracardiac surgery in infants and young children. Circulation 1975;51:867–874.

Reemstem BL, Pike NA, Starnes VA. Stage I palliation for hypoplastic left heart syndrome: Norwood versus Sano modification. Curr Opin Cardiol 2007;22:60–65.

Roeleveld PP, Axelrod DM, Klugman D, et al. Hypoplastic left heart syndrome: from fetus to Fontan. Cardiol Young 2018;28(11):1275–1288.

Roeleveld PP, de Klerk JCA. The perspective of the intensivist on inotropes and postoperative care following pediatric heart surgery: an international survey and systematic review of the literature. World J Pediatr Congenit Heart Surg 2018;9(1):10–21.

Siegel E, Traube C. Pediatric delirium: epidemiology and outcomes. Curr Opin Pediatr 2020;32(6):743–749.

Society of Critical Care Medicine Clinical Resources: ICU Liberation Bundle. Available at https://www.sccm.org/Clinical-Resources/ICULiberation-Home/ABCDEF-Bundles. Last accessed on 5/5/2021.

Stopa BM, Dolmans RGF, Broekman MLD, et al. Hyperosmolar therapy in pediatric severe traumatic brain injury—a systematic review. Crit Care Med 2019;47(12):e1022–e1031.

Trittenwein G, Pansi H, Graf B, et al. Proposed entry criteria for postoperative cardiac extracorporeal membrane oxygenation after pediatric open heart surgery. Artif Org 1999;23: 1010–1014.

Ungerleider RM, Meliones J, McMillan KH, et al. Critical Heart Disease in Infants and Children. 3rd Ed. Philadelphia, PA: Elsevier, 2019.

Watson RS, Choong K, Colville G et al. Life after critical illness in children—toward an understanding of pediatric post-intensive care syndrome. J Pediatr 2018;198(7):16–24.

Weiss SL, Peters MJ, Alhazzani W, et al. Surviving sepsis campaign international guidelines for the management of septic shock and sepsis-associated organ dysfunction in children. Pediatr Crit Care Med 2020;21(2):e52–e106.

Wernovsky G, Wypij D, Jonas RA, et al. Postoperative course and hemodynamic profile after the arterial switch operation in neonates and infants: a comparison of low-flow cardiopulmonary bypass and circulatory arrest. Circulation 1995;92:2226–2235.

West JB. Respiratory Physiology: The Essentials. 11th Ed. Philadelphia, PA: Lippincott Williams & Wilkins, 2015.

# Surgery
Baddr Shakhsheer and Brad W. Warner

Pediatric surgical disease constitutes a wide breadth of pathology. Of the myriad of congenital and acquired problems that require the expertise of a pediatric surgeon, the most common are discussed in this chapter, with a focus on diagnosis and surgical management.

## CONGENITAL DISORDERS

### ABDOMINAL WALL DEFECTS

#### Definition and Anatomy
- Abdominal wall defects allow herniation of abdominal contents through the abdominal wall.
  - In **omphalocele**, the defect is at the umbilical ring. The defect has a thin membranous sac covering over the herniated abdominal contents. Rupture of the sac can occur, thus exposing the intra-abdominal organs. Omphalocele is associated with other midline defects.
  - In **gastroschisis**, the defect is to the right of the umbilicus/umbilical cord. The herniated contents are not covered by a sac.

#### Epidemiology
- The incidence of **omphalocele** is 1 in 4000 births.
- The incidence of **gastroschisis** is 1 in 6000-10,000 births.
- There is no gender predominance.
- Anomalies associated with the two defects differ.
  - **Omphalocele** is associated with Beckwith-Wiedemann syndrome; pentalogy of Cantrell; cloacal exstrophy; trisomies 13, 18, and 21; Turner syndrome; and Klinefelter syndrome.
  - **Gastroschisis** is typically not associated with any chromosomal anomalies, but intestinal atresia, short bowel syndrome, and poor intestinal motility may be present.

#### Etiology
- **Omphalocele** is thought to occur because of a failure of the intestines to return to the abdomen during gestation.
- **Gastroschisis** is thought to be a defect at the site of involution of the right umbilical vein.

#### History and Physical Examination
- Abdominal wall defects are associated with elevated maternal α-fetoprotein levels and can be diagnosed by prenatal ultrasound.

- In **omphalocele**, the small and large bowel, the stomach, and sometimes the liver may be visible through the membranous sac.
- In **gastroschisis**, the exposed bowel is thickened and may be covered in a fibrin peel. The entire midgut is generally herniated, but other organs, including the stomach or pelvic organs, may also herniate. There may be an associated intestinal atresia.

## Imaging

- **Prenatal:** Imaging involves thorough ultrasonographic examination to look for other anomalies. This initial imaging may further dictate the need for fetal echocardiography and amniocentesis for karyotyping. Cesarean section is only warranted if the liver is within the omphalocele sac. All other defects can be delivered vaginally unless dictated by other obstetric reasons.
- **Postnatal:** In combination with a detailed physical examination, imaging is directed at identifying other congenital anomalies. Commonly, abdominal ultrasound, cardiac echocardiogram, and other radiographic techniques are used.

## Treatment

*Postnatal*
- Nasogastric decompression at birth is mandatory.
- Any trauma to the omphalocele membrane should be avoided. Herniated bowel in gastroschisis should be treated similarly. Typically, to protect the abdomen immediately after delivery, the lower half of the neonate's body can be gently placed in a clear plastic bowel bag to maintain moisture and heat during transportation to a neonatal intensive care unit (NICU). Avoid placing saline-soaked gauze over the bowel as it can lead to significantly decreasing the neonate's body temperature. Wrapping the bowel with gauze should also be avoided since it prevents the ability to assess bowel perfusion and may create a tourniquet effect.
- A heat lamp may be necessary to maintain normothermia.
- Fluid losses can be significant and fluid status should be monitored closely and IV fluids at 1.5-2× maintenance.
- Antibiotics are indicated in gastroschisis, and in the case of omphalocele membrane rupture.
- The umbilical cord stump in cases of gastroschisis should be preserved in order to potentially utilize it for "sutureless closure."

*Surgery*
- Primary closure can be performed in infants with small defects when the volume of herniated contents is small. Sutureless closure may be appropriate in select patients where the umbilical cord remnant is utilized as a vascularized pedicle for coverage.
- Staged closure, using a silo that is placed at the bedside, is used for gastroschisis defects when the abdominal cavity at birth is too small to accommodate the herniated contents.
- Postoperative care in the NICU may include mechanical ventilation and monitoring for abdominal compartment syndrome. Intestinal ileus is expected after closure, especially for gastroschisis, and total parenteral nutrition (TPN) may be necessary.

*Results and Complications*
- Outcome is largely dependent on gestational age at birth and the presence of other congenital and genetic anomalies.

- Long-term complications include gastroesophageal reflux and adhesion-related bowel obstruction. Poor intestinal motility may also be a problem.
- Short bowel syndrome and need for long-term parenteral nutrition may be a significant problem in children with gastroschisis.

## CONGENITAL DIAPHRAGMATIC HERNIA

### Definition and Anatomy
- A congenital diaphragmatic hernia (CDH) is a defect in the diaphragm allowing herniation of abdominal contents into the thorax.
- Most cases (80%) are left sided. Rare cases are bilateral.

### Epidemiology
- Incidence is approximately 1 in 2000-5000 births.
- The condition is associated with pulmonary hypoplasia and pulmonary hypertension.

### Etiology
- The cause is a defect in diaphragmatic development.
- A genetic cause is not currently known. There is emerging evidence that vitamin A (retinol) may play an important role in diaphragm development.

### History
- Maternal history of polyhydramnios exists in 80% of cases.
- CDH can be diagnosed on prenatal ultrasound. Prenatal chromosomal analysis may be indicated.

### Physical Examination
- Tachypnea, grunting, cyanosis, and decreased breath sounds occur on the affected side.
- A scaphoid abdomen with an asymmetric and distended chest may be seen.
- Hypotension may be present as a result of mediastinal compression and obstruction of venous return to the heart.

### Laboratory Studies and Imaging
- Tests include blood gas analysis as well as preductal and postductal oximetry.
- A chest radiograph showing bowel in the chest and a paucity of bowel gas in the abdomen confirms the diagnosis.
- Cardiac anomalies can occur in up to 25% of infants with CDH; a cardiac echocardiogram is warranted. Major cardiac anomalies are associated with significantly lower survival rates.

### Differential Diagnosis
- Congenital diaphragmatic eventration
- Congenital cystic pulmonary airway malformations

### Treatment
Medical treatment may be indicated for pulmonary hypertension.

*Extracorporeal Membrane Oxygenation*
- Extracorporeal membrane oxygenation (ECMO) may be useful when there is inadequate oxygen delivery in the face of adequate volume resuscitation, circulating hemoglobin, pharmacologic support, and ventilation.
- Infants should generally be >34 weeks of gestation, weigh >2000 g, have no major intracranial hemorrhage, have been on a mechanical ventilator for <14 days, and have no lethal congenital anomalies.

*Surgery*
- Surgical repair is not an emergency; rather, it should be performed when the infant is physiologically stable and the pulmonary vascular tone has been maximally optimized.
- Preoperative treatment includes the following:
  - Nasogastric tube, intravenous fluid, intubation, and mechanical ventilation.
  - Ventilation by mask or "bagging" is contraindicated to avoid distension of the bowel.
  - Blood gas analysis, as well as preductal and postductal oximetry, should be monitored serially.

*Results and Complications*
- Mortality rates 20-52% (infants with CDH who require ECMO).
- Gastroesophageal reflux occurs in 45-85% of patients.

## ESOPHAGEAL ATRESIA AND TRACHEOESOPHAGEAL FISTULA

### Definition and Anatomy
- Esophageal atresia (EA) is a discontinuity in the esophagus. There may be an associated fistulous connection between the esophagus and the trachea, which is known as a tracheoesophageal fistula (TEF).
- Classification is based on the location of the TEF, if present. Eighty-five percent of patients have the type where there is a blind-ending upper pouch with a fistula between the trachea and distal esophagus.
  - Other types include a fistulous connection between the proximal portion of the esophagus with or without an atresia.

### Epidemiology and Etiology
- Incidence is approximately 1 in 4000 live births with a slight male predominance.
- About 50% have an associated congenital anomaly (e.g., VACTERL, Trisomy 18 and 21, CHARGE syndrome).
- Abnormal separation of the esophagus and trachea occurs during the 4th week of gestation.

### History
- Maternal polyhydramnios is characteristic.
- Diagnosis can be made by prenatal ultrasound.

### Physical Examination
- A newborn with EA has excessive drooling and episodes of cyanosis or respiratory distress. It is impossible to pass a feeding tube into the infant's stomach.

- A newborn with an isolated TEF swallows normally and does not drool but may choke and cough while eating.
- A newborn with a distal fistula or an isolated fistula may have a distended abdomen due to the inspired air communicating through the fistula.

## Laboratory Studies and Imaging

- Tests include complete blood count (CBC), electrolyte panel, and type and screen.
- Chest and abdominal radiographs after placement of a catheter into the infant's mouth show catheter location in the esophagus.
  - Coiling of the catheter tip in the proximal esophagus suggests an atresia, while air in the stomach suggests a distal or isolated fistula.
  - Patients with a proximal fistula or no fistula at all have a "gasless abdomen" without air in the loops of bowel.
- Echocardiogram determines the location of the aortic arch, which is important in operative planning, and evaluates for concomitant cardiac anomalies.
- Given the frequent association with other VACTERL (Vertebral, Anorectal, Cardiac, Tracheo-Esophageal, Renal, Limb) anomalies, a careful physical examination, along with chest radiography, sonography of the spine and kidneys, and an echocardiogram are also required.

## Treatment

*Surgery*
- Preoperative treatment includes the following:
  - The neonate is placed in an upright position and a nasoesophageal or oroesophageal tube is inserted to suction saliva and prevent aspiration. The infant should not be fed orally.
  - Mechanical ventilation is needed if the infant is in respiratory distress or has pneumonia. Bag-mask ventilation is contraindicated if a distal fistula is present because it causes worsening and clinically significant abdominal distension.
- The goal of surgery is to separate the esophagus from the trachea and restore esophageal continuity.

*Complications*
- Dysphagia is a common postoperative symptom.
- Gastroesophageal reflux (40%) and recurrent respiratory tract infections from silent aspiration may require fundoplication.
- Late complications include anastomotic stricture, anastomotic leak, tracheomalacia, food impaction, and sequelae of reflux.

## MALROTATION

### Definition and Anatomy

- Abnormal rotation of the midgut results in a narrow mesenteric base, conferring a risk of life-threatening midgut volvulus, bowel obstruction, and mesenteric vessel occlusion, which is a surgical emergency.
- Instead of the usual left-of-spine position, the ligament of Treitz lies to the right of the midline; there is a narrow mesenteric base and Ladd bands overlie the duodenum.

## Epidemiology and Etiology

- Seventy-five percent of infants present when <1 month of age and 90% are symptomatic within the 1st year.
- Malrotation can also present in childhood and adulthood.
- The incidence at autopsy is 0.5-1%.
- Associated anomalies occur in about 50% of patients and include CDH, abdominal wall defects, tracheoesophageal anomalies, intestinal webs and atresias, anorectal malformations, orthopedic and cardiac anomalies, situs inversus, and asplenia and polysplenia.
- Abnormal rotation and fixation of the small bowel occur during gestation.

## History

- The most common symptoms are bilious vomiting, colicky abdominal pain, and distension.
- Bilious emesis in a newborn infant is volvulus until proven otherwise. An emergent upper GI series is indicated.
- If midgut volvulus is present, this is an emergent situation. These patients may be lethargic, irritable, and in shock.
- Children who are not diagnosed in infancy may present with chronic abdominal pain, vomiting, diarrhea, and failure to thrive.
- Occasionally, malrotation is an incidental finding on a radiographic workup for another problem.

## Physical Examination

- Abdominal distension, dehydration, and possibly signs of shock are found.
- Abdominal tenderness and blood on rectal examination are suggestive of bowel ischemia.

## Laboratory Studies and Imaging

- Tests include CBC, electrolyte panel, and type and screen.
- Upper gastrointestinal (GI) contrast study is diagnostic. A malpositioned duodeno-jejunal junction is pathognomonic for malrotation.
- Reversed orientation of superior mesenteric artery and vein can be seen on ultrasonography.
- If the upper GI study shows normal duodenal anatomy, a small bowel follow-through can be done to document the position of the cecum. Nonfixation of the cecum can be seen.

## Treatment

### Surgery

- Preoperative treatment includes nasogastric tube decompression, fluid resuscitation, and correction of electrolyte and acid-base abnormalities. Antibiotic therapy is indicated in patients with midgut volvulus, peritonitis, or sepsis.
- The Ladd procedure involves division of Ladd bands over the duodenum and widening of the mesenteric base between the small and large bowel. The small bowel remains on the patient's right abdomen, and the large bowel remains on the patient's left abdomen. Lastly, an appendectomy is performed to avoid future diagnostic difficulty given the abnormal location of the appendix.

- Emergency surgery is required in cases of malrotation with midgut volvulus. Parents of children with asymptomatic malrotation awaiting surgery should be taught to recognize the signs and symptoms of this emergency.
- In cases when malrotation is diagnosed without midgut volvulus, the Ladd procedure is performed due to the associated risk for volvulus.

*Complications*

Long-term adhesion-related complications, including bowel obstruction, can occur in about 25% of surgical patients.

## INGUINAL HERNIA

### Definition

This hernia involves protrusion of intra-abdominal contents (e.g., omentum, bowel, and gonad) through a defect in the abdominal wall into the inguinal canal.

### Epidemiology and Etiology

- Most hernias in infants and children are indirect, originating lateral to the epigastric vessels.
- Inguinal hernia repair is the most common surgery performed on children.
- Its incidence in full-term neonates is 3-5% and as high as 30% in infants weighing <1 kg. The peak incidence is in the first 3 months of life.
- Etiology is a patent processus vaginalis, not due to muscle weakening (as in adults with direct hernias).

### History

Parents often give a history of intermittent bulging in the groin associated with crying or straining.

### Physical Examination

- A mass may be present in the groin, and in male infants, it may extend into the scrotum.
- Scrotal transillumination can help distinguish between a hernia and a hydrocele.
- A hernia that cannot be reduced is termed incarcerated. If the blood supply is compromised because of incarceration, the hernia is strangulated. All strangulated hernias are incarcerated, but not all incarcerated hernias are strangulated.

### Imaging

Ultrasound may be used if diagnosis is equivocal on physical examination.

### Differential Diagnosis

Hydrocele, testicular torsion, testicular tumor, and inguinal lymphadenopathy are possibilities.

### Treatment

*Surgery*

- Timing of inguinal hernia repair historically was guided by the postconceptual age (gestational plus postnatal age) of the infant and the known risk of incarceration. The risk of postoperative apnea from general anesthesia has been shown to be significantly increased with postconceptual age <60 weeks. Prospective studies are ongoing to compare early (prior to NICU discharge) versus late inguinal hernia repair in premature infants.

- The risk of incarceration after difficult manual reduction is significant; if reduction is challenging, the child should be admitted to the hospital and undergo hernia repair during the same hospitalization after 24-48 hours to allow for tissue edema to subside.
- A strangulated hernia mandates emergent surgical exploration and repair.
- Parents of children with an inguinal hernia awaiting surgery should be counseled to recognize the signs and symptoms of incarceration, and they should seek emergent medical care to reduce the hernia.
- Primary herniorrhaphy is appropriate. Contralateral exploration is made more feasible with the advent of laparoscopy. A laparoscope can be introduced via the hernia sac of the affected side to visualize the contralateral internal ring. This is generally done in children <1-2 years of age. A left-sided hernia may also be a relative indication as hernias are typically more common on the right.

*Complications*
- Preoperative complications include incarceration, strangulation, and bowel ischemia necessitating bowel resection.
- Complications associated with elective hernia repair are rare (2%) and include hematoma, wound infection, and gonadal ischemia.
- The surgical complication rate significantly rises in the setting of incarceration.
- In neonates, repair is associated with up to 8% recurrence. In older infants, the expected recurrence rate is 1%.

# ACQUIRED DISORDERS

## NECROTIZING ENTEROCOLITIS

### Definition and Anatomy
- Necrotizing enterocolitis (NEC) is an acute inflammatory process of the intestines that may progress to necrosis and perforation of intestinal tissue.
- NEC most commonly affects the terminal ileum and right colon but may involve any or all segments of the GI tract.

### Epidemiology and Etiology
- NEC occurs in 1-3 per 1000 live births.
- The incidence in the NICU is 2-4%.
- Etiology is multifactorial. Predisposing factors include prematurity and enteral feeds.
- Breast milk reduces but does not eliminate the risk for NEC.

### History
- Classic presentation includes the triad of abdominal distension, bloody stools, and pneumatosis intestinalis.
- The typical premature infant is 2-3 weeks of age and has recently initiated formula feeding.

## Physical Examination

- Abdominal examination may be notable for distension, abdominal wall erythema or discoloration, or a palpable mass (fixed dilated loop of bowel).
- A septic infant may also have tachycardia, hypotension, hypothermia, and signs of poor perfusion.

## Laboratory Studies and Imaging

- Trends of diminished leukocyte and platelet counts, as well as hemoglobin concentration, are useful. Electrolytes and blood gases are also followed.
- Blood cultures may aid in tailoring antibiotic coverage.
- Serial abdominal radiographs (anteroposterior, left lateral decubitus, or cross table lateral) looking for pneumatosis intestinalis, portal venous gas, and pneumoperitoneum are useful. Distended loops of small bowel are commonly seen but can be a nonspecific finding.
- Ultrasonography may be useful for detecting pneumatosis intestinalis and portal venous gas.

## Monitoring

Continuous hemodynamic monitoring and clinical examination are necessary.

## Treatment

*Nonoperative*

- Medical management is the treatment of choice for patients with NEC who do not show signs of persistent shock or pneumoperitoneum.
- Nonoperative management consists of antibiotics, fluid resuscitation, nasogastric or orogastric decompression, serial laboratory tests, and examinations. Enteral feeds are discontinued for at least 7 days in cases when pneumatosis intestinalis is present. Vasopressor support may be appropriate. Parenteral nutrition is also initiated.

*Surgery*

- Exploratory laparotomy, resection of necrotic or perforated bowel, and ostomy creation are the mainstay of surgical intervention. More recently, primary peritoneal drainage has been shown to be an alternative treatment with equivalent outcome in extremely low birth infants who present with pneumoperitoneum.
- Preoperative interventions include fluid resuscitation, and correction of electrolytes, anemia, and coagulopathy. Cross-matched blood products must be available for surgery.
- In infants who are gaining weight and are no longer critically ill, reversal of enterostomy is timed around 8 weeks after the initial operation.
- Survival in infants receiving surgical treatment is 70-80%.

*Complications*

- Recurrent NEC occurs in 4-6% of infants.
- Intestinal stricture is the most common complication.
- Short bowel syndrome and intestinal malabsorption can result depending on the amount of bowel needing to be resected.

## Differential Diagnosis

Sepsis-related ileus may present in a similar fashion for which medical management is indicated.

# INFANTILE HYPERTROPHIC PYLORIC STENOSIS

## Definition

Infantile hypertrophic pyloric stenosis (IHPS) is narrowing of the pyloric canal caused by circular muscular hypertrophy.

## Epidemiology and Etiology

- Incidence is 2-3 per 1000 live births.
- The male:female ratio is 4:1.
- Siblings of patients with IHPS are 15 times more likely to develop IHPS than are those with no family history.
- The cause is unknown but likely genetic and may be related to defects in nitric oxide synthase within the pyloric muscle.

## History and Physical Examination

- The classic presentation includes nonbilious vomiting that occurs most commonly in weeks of life 2 through 8. Initially, the infant may regurgitate feeds, but this generally progresses to a characteristic projectile nonbilious emesis.
- An olive-sized pyloric mass may be palpable. The abdomen is soft and nontender.
- Poor skin turgor and a sunken fontanelle accompany dehydration.

## Laboratory Studies and Imaging

- An electrolyte panel often reveals a hypochloremic, hypokalemic, metabolic alkalosis from excessive vomiting.
- Blood urea nitrogen and creatinine can indicate severity of dehydration.
- Abdominal ultrasonography is diagnostic if the pyloric muscle thickness is >3 mm and length >1.5 cm. If equivocal, an upper GI contrast study can also be obtained.

## Treatment

- IHPS is not a surgical emergency; fluid resuscitation, normalization of electrolytes, and correction of acid-base imbalances must be accomplished before operation.
- Correction of the metabolic alkalosis preoperatively minimizes the risk of postoperative apnea.
- Administration of potassium in the intravenous fluids should not be done until urine output has been established.
- Open and laparoscopic pyloromyotomy are acceptable.

### Results and Complications

- Feeding is initiated soon after surgery, and infants are usually discharged home on postoperative day 1 or 2.
- Perforation, wound infection, wound dehiscence, or incomplete myotomy may complicate pyloromyotomy.

# INTUSSUSCEPTION

## Definition and Classification

- Intussusception involves a segment of the bowel telescoping into a more distal segment.

- Peristalsis causes propulsion of the intussusception into the intussuscipiens, resulting in lymphatic and venous obstruction. Progression of this process leads to bowel wall edema, mucosal bleeding, arterial insufficiency, worsening mechanical intestinal obstruction, and eventually bowel necrosis.
- Classification is according to anatomy—most common is ileocolic.

## Epidemiology and Etiology

- Overall incidence is 1-4%. Typically, the patient is 3 months to 3 years of age.
- Approximately 95% of cases occur in children <2 years of age; intussusception is the most common cause of intestinal obstruction in this age group.
- Pathologic lead points should be suspected with increasing age. Medical conditions that can create a lead point within the bowel include, but are not limited to, Meckel diverticulum, intestinal duplication cyst, small bowel lymphoma, polyps, cystic fibrosis, and Henoch-Schönlein purpura.

## History

- The infant or child classically has a history of crying and drawing up his or her legs during intermittent episodes of abdominal pain. The child may be otherwise asymptomatic between episodes. Most children with intussusception are healthy and well nourished.
- Vomiting (80%) may initially be nonbilious but can become bilious as obstruction progresses. Children with intussusception are often lethargic and may pass bloody stools, known classically as "currant jelly stools," due to sloughing of the intestinal mucosa. This may be a late finding.
- A history of recent gastroenteritis or upper respiratory infection is sometimes elicited.

## Physical Examination

- Abdominal examination reveals an empty right lower quadrant and a tender "sausage-shaped" mass in the right upper quadrant in 85% of patients. As the process progresses, patients can develop abdominal distension and peritoneal signs.
- Mucosal bleeding can cause stool to be guaiac positive even in the absence of a history of bloody stool.

## Laboratory Studies and Imaging

- A CBC and electrolyte panel are necessary.
- Two-view plain abdominal radiographs have a much lower sensitivity than has ultrasound in detecting intussusception (62.3% vs. 98.4%). If obtained late in the process, the radiograph may show an obstructive bowel gas pattern or pneumoperitoneum from perforation.
- Ultrasonography has a sensitivity of 98.5% and 100% specificity.
- An air contrast enema is both diagnostic and therapeutic.

## Treatment

*Nonoperative*

- Hydrostatic reduction of the intussusception with saline or by air enema is performed by radiologists after notification of a pediatric surgeon. The success rate is 96% for contrast enema reduction and 92% for air contrast enema reduction. This procedure is contraindicated in patients who have peritonitis or signs of shock.

- Nonoperative reduction may be complicated by perforation, which is a surgical emergency.
- Successful reduction is followed by a period of observation dependent on patient status. This may be in the emergency department or inpatient setting.

*Surgery*
- Operative treatment is indicated in patients with peritonitis or shock.
- Patients with incomplete or unsuccessful reduction, multiple recurrences, or a pathologic lead point also require surgical reduction and/or resection.
- Preparation for surgery includes fluid resuscitation, and correction of electrolyte and acid-base abnormalities. Antibiotic therapy and NG decompression are indicated in patients who are septic or have peritoneal signs.

*Recurrence*
- The recurrence risk is up to 3.9% in the first 24 hours and up to 6.6% in the first 48 hours after nonoperative reduction.
- After operative reduction, recurrence is infrequent.

## APPENDICITIS

### Definition
Inflammation of the appendix may progress to necrosis and perforation.

### Epidemiology and Etiology
- Appendicitis is the most common surgical emergency in childhood.
- Peak incidence occurs at 10-12 years of age. The higher rate of perforation in children (30%) compared with adults is attributed to the fact that symptoms are often mistaken for gastroenteritis and to the child's inability to communicate pain.
- Blockage of the appendiceal orifice causes venous congestion that leads to arterial insufficiency.

### History
- Typically, vague periumbilical pain localizes to the right lower quadrant and can be accompanied by nausea, vomiting, anorexia, and/or fever.
- Diarrhea and dysuria may also be present from irritation by the adjacent inflamed appendix.

### Physical Examination
- Palpation of the abdomen in the right lower quadrant elicits pain. There may be rebound tenderness or guarding.
- Palpation of the left lower quadrant may result in reproduction of right lower quadrant pain (Rovsing sign).
- Rectal examination results in focal tenderness on the right if the appendix lies in the pelvis.
- If the child is otherwise stable and the diagnosis of appendicitis is uncertain, serial abdominal examinations should be performed to monitor the child's clinical trajectory.

### Laboratory Studies
- Patients with appendicitis usually have a low-grade leukocytosis with a neutrophilia.

• If presentation is not classic, liver enzymes, amylase, and lipase levels may be helpful to rule out other causes of abdominal pain.

## Imaging and Surgical Diagnostic Procedures

• Abdominal ultrasound is a fairly sensitive and specific test for appendicitis but may be difficult in patients who are obese or uncooperative. This should be the diagnostic modality of choice in experienced centers.
• Computed tomography (CT) may be required but should be done selectively due to radiation exposure risks. Magnetic resonance imaging (MRI) has also been described.
• Diagnostic laparoscopy is especially helpful in teenage girls in whom diagnosis of appendicitis is equivocal.

## Differential Diagnosis

Conditions to rule out are gastroenteritis, constipation, mesenteric adenitis, Crohn disease, urinary tract infection, pyelonephritis, and gynecologic pathology.

## Treatment

• Perforated appendicitis with intra-abdominal abscess formation in a hemodynamically stable patient may be managed with a percutaneous drain inserted by an interventional radiologist and antibiotic therapy. A pilot study randomizing pediatric patients to early appendectomy versus initial nonoperative management with IV antibiotics with or without a percutaneous drain did not show a significant difference in total hospitalization, recurrent abscess formation, or overall charges.
• Postoperative antibiotics and duration remain controversial.

*Surgery*
• Laparoscopic and open appendectomy are both standard. Recent studies suggest that laparoscopic appendectomy may be associated with a lower wound infection rate and a shorter hospital stay.
• Preoperatively, the patient should be kept nil per os and be given intravenous fluid maintenance. Broad-spectrum antibiotics to cover Gram negative and anaerobic organisms should be given once diagnosis of appendicitis is made.

*Complications*
• Early complications include intra-abdominal abscess and wound infection.
• Late complications include those that are adhesion related, including bowel obstruction.
• Infertility may be a risk in female patients with perforated appendicitis due to significant scar formation.

## ABDOMINAL TRAUMA

### Definition and Anatomy

• Solid organs commonly injured include the liver, spleen, kidneys, and pancreas.
• Hollow viscus injuries or perforation can occur anywhere along the GI tract.
• Vascular structures may also be injured.
• External landmarks for the boundaries of the abdomen are the nipples superiorly and the pelvis inferiorly.

## Epidemiology and Etiology

- The leading cause of mortality and morbidity in children is trauma.
- Motor vehicle accidents followed by firearm injury rank number one and two as mechanisms of death.
- Abdominal injuries are most often caused by blunt trauma.
- Despite careful primary and secondary surveys, injuries are still missed in 2-50% of children.

## History

- Pertinent history includes the mechanism of injury.
  - Was the mechanism penetrating or blunt?
  - Was the patient restrained?
  - Was the patient thrown on impact?
  - Does the injury pattern fit the history? If not, suspicion should be raised for non-accidental trauma.

## Physical Examination

- Primary survey for any trauma patient includes evaluating airway, breathing, and circulation (ABCs).
- A focused secondary survey follows and includes (but is not limited to) the neurologic, chest, abdominal, back, and extremity examinations.
  - Identify wounds that suggest a penetrating injury, looking for entrance and exit wounds.
- A tertiary survey consisting of a repeat heat to toe examination is performed within 24 hours of hospital admission to avoid missed injuries.

## Laboratory Studies and Imaging

- Trauma panel (CBC, electrolytes, liver enzymes, amylase, lipase, coagulation panel, type and cross-match, urinalysis) is often performed to guide further management or imaging.
- Chest and pelvis radiographs as well as abdominal and pelvic CT with intravenous contrast are useful and may reveal solid organ injury or free intraperitoneal fluid that may be concerning for hollow viscus perforation.
- Cervical spine series may be indicated in patients with significant mechanism of injury.

## Treatment

*Nonoperative*

- Patients with a significant mechanism of injury who have no identifiable injury on initial evaluation should undergo serial clinical evaluation with abdominal examination for 24 hours.
- Tetanus immunization, if not up to date, is imperative in penetrating trauma and burns.

*Surgery*

- Surgery is indicated if the patient has peritonitis, uncontrolled abdominal bleeding, or pneumoperitoneum. Surgery may be indicated if there was penetration of the abdominal wall through the fascia as there is concern for intra-abdominal bowel injury that may not be revealed by imaging.
- Preoperatively, placement of two large-bore intravenous lines, nasogastric decompression, and supplemental oxygen is necessary.

## SOFT TISSUE ABSCESS

### Definition
Purulent fluid collects in the skin and subcutaneous tissue.

### Epidemiology and Etiology
- Methicillin-resistant *Staphylococcus aureus* (MRSA) strains are becoming increasingly prevalent in children with community-acquired staphylococcal infections. The majority of these children have no identifiable risk factors.
- The cause is violation of the epidermis, with bacterial invasion of the skin and soft tissue.

### History
- There is often a history of progressive swelling, pain, erythema, and warmth in a localized region of skin.
  - There may be spontaneous drainage from the site of the infection.
  - Fever and leukocytosis may be present.
- It is important to ask about trauma to the skin.
- Other key elements of the history include previous abscesses, recurrent abscess, and family members with abscesses or with MRSA exposure.

### Physical Examination, Laboratory Studies, and Imaging
- Identify the abscess location, size, amount of induration, presence of fluctuance, quality and quantity of drainage, and area of erythema.
- CBC with differential is often obtained in febrile patients. If the lesion is incised and drained, a wound/fluid culture is obtained.
- Ultrasonography is helpful in some instances such as a suspected breast abscess.

### Surgical Diagnostic Procedures
If it is unclear whether there is a fluid collection to drain, needle aspiration under local anesthesia can be helpful.

### Treatment
*Medications*
- If MRSA is suspected, clindamycin or trimethoprim/sulfamethoxazole is recommended.
- Oral antibiotic therapy after adequate incision and drainage is still not well defined but typically continued for a few days.
- Systemic signs of infection (fever, leukocytosis) warrant intravenous antibiotics.

*Surgery*
- Incision and drainage procedures in children often involve use of sedation.
- Simple abscess may not require daily packing. More complex abscesses may benefit from a temporary drain placement to allow for easier cleansings of the area and dressing changes in the pediatric patient.
- Inadequate drainage could result in progressive spread of the infection.

### Referrals
A patient with recurrent abscesses should be referred to a specialist in immunology and infectious disease.

## Patient Education

Personal hygiene practices should be reviewed with the parent and child.

## SUGGESTED READINGS

Bergmeijer JHLJ, Tibboel D, Hazebroek FWJ. Nissen fundoplication in the management of gastroesophageal reflux occurring after repair of esophageal atresia. J Pediatr Surg 2000;35:573–576.

Fujimoto T. Hypertrophic pyloric stenosis. In: Puri P, Hollwarth M, eds. Pediatric Surgery. Heidelberg, Germany: Springer-Verlag, 2000:171–180.

Gahukamble DB, Khamage AS. Early versus delayed repair of reduced incarcerated inguinal hernias in the pediatric population. J Pediatr Surg 1996;31:1218–1220.

Gray MP, Li SH, Hoffmann RG, et al. Recurrence rates after intussusception enema reduction: a meta-analysis. Pediatrics 2014;134(1):110–119.

Henderson AA, Anupindi SA, Servaes S, et al. Comparison of 2-view abdominal radiographs with ultrasound in children with suspected intussusception. Pediatr Emerg Care 2013;29(2): 145–150.

Henry MCW, Gollin G, Islam S, et al. Matched analysis of non-operative management vs immediate appendectomy for perforated appendicitis. J Pediatr Surg 2007;42:19–24.

Lee SL, Gleason JM, Sydorak RM. A critical review of premature infants with inguinal hernia: optimal timing of repair, incarceration risk and postoperative apnea. J Pediatr Surg 2011;46(1):217–220.

Logan JW, Rice HE, Goldberg RN, et al. Congenital diaphragmatic hernia: a systematic review and summary of best-evidence practice strategies. J Perinatol 2007;27(9):535–549.

Malviya S, Swart J, Lerman J. Are all preterm infants younger than 60 week postconceptional age a risk for post-anesthetic apnea? Anesthesiology 1993;78:1076–1081.

Menon SC, Tani LY, Weng HY, et al. Clinical characteristics and outcomes of patients with cardiac defects and congenital diaphragmatic hernia. J Pediatr 2013;162(1):114–119.

Moss RL, Dimmitt RA, Barnhart DC, et al. Laparotomy versus peritoneal drainage for necrotizing enterocolitis and perforation. N Engl J Med 2006;354:2225–2234.

Murphy FL, Sparnon AL. Long-term complications following intestinal malrotation and the Ladd's procedure: a 15 year review. Pediatr Surg Int 2006;22:326–329.

Orzech N, Navarro OM, Langer JC. Is ultrasonography a good screening test for intestinal malrotation? J Pediatr Surg 2006;41:1005–1009.

Owen A, Marven S, Jackson L, et al. Experience of bedside preformed silo staged reduction and closure for gastroschisis. J Pediatr Surg 2006;41:1830–1835.

Somme S, To T, Langer JC. Factors determining the need for operative reduction in children with intussusception: a population based study. J Pediatr Surg 2006;41:1014–1019.

St Peter SD, Aguayo P, Fraser JD, et al. Initial laparoscopic appendectomy versus initial nonoperative management and interval appendectomy for perforated appendicitis with abscess: a prospective, randomized trial. J Pediatr Surg 2010;45(1):236–240.

Tirabassi MV, Wadie G, Moriarty KP, et al. Geographic information system localization of community-acquired MRSA soft tissue abscesses. J Pediatr Surg 2005;40:962–966.

Waag K. Intussusception. In: Puri P, Hollwarth M, eds. Pediatric Surgery. Heidelberg, Germany: Springer-Verlag, 2006:313–320.

Yagmurlu A, Vernon A, Barnhart DC, et al. Laparoscopic appendectomy for perforated appendicitis: a comparison with open appendectomy. Surg Endosc 2006;20:1051–1054.

# 10 Adolescent Medicine

Jessica Sims, Sarah Mermelstein, Sarah Tycast, and Katie Plax

## INTRODUCTION

- Adolescence is the time of transition from childhood to adulthood. Typically, it begins at 10-14 years of age and is characterized by rapid physical, cognitive, emotional growth, and sexual development (puberty).
- Adolescents also develop independence and separation from their parents. They may become less willing to participate in family activities and many concentrate on peer relationships and challenge parental authority.
- Adolescents often are increasingly concerned about their developing body, peer opinion, independence, and sexual exploration.
- Tips for the adolescent clinical interview
  - Interview the adolescent and the accompanying adult(s) together and then the adolescent alone.
  - Early in the interview and in front of the accompanying adult(s), discuss patient confidentiality. Be sure to say that you will keep your findings and all discussions confidential unless the patient is at risk of hurting himself or herself or others, or someone has hurt the patient.
  - Encourage the adolescent to discuss problems with his or her parents/caregivers, and encourage parents/caregivers to create a time in the day to be with their child.
  - The adolescent psychosocial history often includes a **HEADSS** assessment:
    - **H**ome dynamics and members
    - **E**ducation: school performance, school supports
    - **A**ctivities, **A**spirations
    - **D**rugs, **D**epression
    - **S**ex, **S**uicide, **S**afety, **S**trengths
  - Offer anticipatory guidance on diet, maturation, sexuality, injury prevention, and good health habits.
  - Other advice includes the following:
    - Before the physical examination, give the adolescent the option of being examined alone or accompanied by the parent/caregiver. Respect the patient's modesty.
    - When formulating a plan, it is important to reinforce the strengths and achievements of the adolescent both to the patient and to the parent/caregiver.
    - Use a shared decision-making strategy and youth-directed priorities if behavior change is needed.

## CONSENT AND CONFIDENTIALITY

- These issues are very important when caring for adolescents.
- Be familiar with your local laws, as they vary state-to-state.

## Definitions

- Consent is an agreement to medical care (examination, testing, treatment, surgical procedures).
  - Patients have the right to know about their health and treatment options, and the physician should respect their autonomy, rights, preferences (religious, social, cultural, philosophic), and decisions.
  - When obtaining consent, it is important to:
    - Provide information (studies, treatments, risks/benefits, alternative options)
    - Assess the patient's understanding
    - Assess the patient's capacity for decision-making
    - Ensure the patient's freedom to choose
  - In most situations, a parent or guardian's consent is required for the medical care of a minor; however, there are certain exceptions where adolescents may consent for their own medical care. Depending on the specific state laws, this may include the following:
    - An adult 18 years or older (for himself or herself).
    - A minor who is married, is active duty military, or is declared emancipated by the court.
    - A minor parent may consent for themselves as well as for a child in their legal custody.
    - A minor who present requesting treatment for pregnancy, contraception. STD testing and/or treatment, including HIV. However, most states require parental involvement or notification for a minor who chooses to have an abortion (https://www.guttmacher.org/state-policy/explore/parental-involvement-minors-abortions).
    - Minors may be able to consent for outpatient mental health and drug or substance abuse counseling, but this varies from state-to-state.
- Confidentiality is the agreement between the patient and the health care provider that information will not be shared without explicit permission of the patient.
  - The goals of confidentiality are to protect patient privacy, ensure access to health care, and encourage open and honest communication.
  - The Health Insurance Portability and Accountability Act (HIPAA) designates parents or guardians of unemancipated minors as "personal representatives" with access to their children's personal health information. This does **not** apply to evaluation and treatment of STDs, pregnancy, contraception, or outpatient substance abuse under most state laws. Depending on the state, if a minor seeks evaluation for pregnancy, STD, or drug or substance abuse and the results are negative, then a health care provider may be obligated to not release any of that information to parents.
  - The 21st Century Cures Act was signed into law on December 13, 2016, with recent expansion of the "Final Rule" on April 5, 2021. The Final Rule aims to promote transparency, increase patients' access to their own health information, and prohibit "information blocking" of medical records from patients and legal guardians. This rule mandates access to health information via the electronic health record (EHR) for adolescents and their proxies, typically parents or guardians. For now, the data that must be shared include clinical notes, immunizations, lab results, medications, objective data such as vitals and growth curves, and problem lists. This will expand include all health information in 2022. There are exceptions allowed under the Cures Act, most notably for adolescent care the Privacy Exception and the Preventing Harm exception. The law does not include any language that distinguishes between the handling of access to health information for adults from that of minors. As a result, providers should be aware of potential risks to patient confidentiality when documenting and should apply existing state and federal laws when appropriate.

○ It is important to know your state's specific statutes.
○ Further information about adolescent consent and confidentiality issues can be found at the Web site for the Center for Adolescent Health and the Law (www.cahl.org).
• Confidentiality cannot be maintained when the adolescent poses risk of harm to himself or herself or to others or someone has hurt him or her.

## SEXUALLY TRANSMITTED INFECTIONS

### Definition and Etiology
Sexually transmitted infections (STIs) can present as urethritis, vulvovaginitis, cervicitis, genital ulcers or growths, pelvic inflammatory disease (PID), epididymitis, abdominal pain, enteritis or proctitis, hepatitis, arthritis, pharyngitis, rash, or conjunctivitis.

### Screening and Prevention
• Condoms, when properly used, can greatly decrease the spread of STIs and should be encouraged.
• CDC screening recommendations (2015)
  • Annual screening for gonorrhea and chlamydia in sexually active females.
  • Consider screening cisgender men who have sex with cisgender women for chlamydia in high prevalence clinical settings or in populations with high burden of infection.
  • Routine screening for human immunodeficiency virus (HIV) between the ages of 13-64 and at least annual screening for people considered high risk (injection-drug users and their sex partners, persons who exchange sex for money or drugs, sex partners of HIV-infected persons, and MSM or heterosexual persons who themselves or whose sex partners have had more than one sex partner since their most recent HIV test).
  • Annual screening for syphilis, gonorrhea, chlamydia, and HIV in sexually active men who have sex with men (MSM). Screening in this population should include extragenital sites of contact (rectum, pharynx). Consider more frequent screening (every 3-6 months) in MSM who have multiple partners.
  • Hepatitis C screening (1) at least once in a lifetime for all adults aged ≥18 years, except in settings where the prevalence of HCV infection is <0.1%; (2) for all pregnant women during each pregnancy, except in settings where the prevalence of HCV infection is <0.1%; and (3) to all people with HIV, hepatitis C–infected partners, and who use intravenous (IV) drugs or have partners that do.
• Human papillomavirus (HPV) causes genital warts and cervical cancer. HPV vaccine is recommended by the Advisory Committee on Immunization Practices (ACIP) between 11 and 12 years of age; however, they recommend the vaccine for everyone between 9 and 26. If the vaccine is started before age 15, a two-dose series is given with the second dose given 6-12 months after the first dose.
  • Papanicolaou (Pap) smear screening recommendations still apply because the vaccine does not protect against all types of HPV.
  • Initiation of Pap smears should occur when the patient is 25 years old, regardless of age of onset of sexual activity. A pelvic examination and Pap smear is not required for initiation of birth control.

### Diagnosis and Treatment
• Table 10-1 summarizes the characteristics and treatment of the various STIs.
• Adolescents can consent for evaluation and treatment of STIs without parental consent and notification in most states.

| TABLE 10-1 | Characteristics and Therapy for Sexually Transmitted Diseases |
|---|---|

| Disease | Characteristics | Therapy |
|---|---|---|
| **Gonorrhea** | • Caused by *N. gonorrhoeae*<br>• Patients are often coinfected with *Chlamydia*, so *treat for both regardless of chlamydia result*<br>• Sexual partners should be treated<br>• May cause mucopurulent cervicitis<br>• Widespread resistance to quinolones | • **Uncomplicated urogenital, rectal, or pharyngeal:**<br>**Ceftriaxone** 500 mg IM single dose (or 1 g if patient weighs ≥150 kg)<br>**OR if cephalosporin allergic:**<br>**Gentamicin** 240 mg IM single dose **AND azithromycin** 2 g in a single oral dose PLUS test-of-cure |
| **Chlamydia** | • Caused by *C. trachomatis*<br>• Asymptomatic infection is very common among men and women<br>• Sexual partners should be treated<br>• May cause mucopurulent cervicitis<br>• Sexual abuse must be considered in preadolescent children with chlamydia | • **Uncomplicated urogenital:**<br>**Doxycycline** 100 mg PO bid for 7 days or **azithromycin** 1 g PO single dose<br>• **Pregnancy:** azithromycin 1 g PO single dose or amoxicillin 500 mg PO tid for 7 days with retesting 3 months after treatment |
| **Syphilis** | • Caused by *Treponema pallidum*<br>• Primary: painless ulcer or chancre<br>• Secondary: rash, mucocutaneous lesions, and adenopathy<br>• Early latent syphilis: *within a year of prior negative evaluation,* patient has seroconversion or unequivocal symptoms of primary or secondary syphilis, or sex partner with primary, secondary, or early latent syphilis<br>• All others should be considered to have late latent syphilis | • **Primary and secondary or early latent:**<br>**Benzathine penicillin G** 2.4 million units IM in a single dose (pregnant or not)<br>• **Penicillin allergy:**<br>**Doxycycline** 100 mg PO bid for 14 days **OR**<br>**Tetracycline** 500 mg PO qid for 14 days<br>• **Late latent:**<br>**Benzathine penicillin G** 2.4 million units IM every week for 3 weeks<br>• **Penicillin allergy:**<br>**Doxycycline** 100 mg PO bid for 28 days **OR**<br>**Tetracycline** 500 mg PO qid for 28 days |

*(Continued)*

| TABLE 10-1 | Characteristics and Therapy for Sexually Transmitted Diseases *(Continued)* |
|---|---|

| Disease | Characteristics | Therapy |
|---|---|---|
| | • Tertiary: CNS, cardiac, or ophthalmic lesions, auditory disturbances, gummas<br>• Diagnosis: VDRL or RPR (positive = fourfold change in titers)<br>  • Cannot compare one to the other—may turn negative after treatment<br>  • Treponemal serologic test to confirm infection (FTA-ABS)—stays positive for a lifetime<br>• Sexual partners should be treated | • **Tertiary syphilis:**<br>**Benzathine penicillin G** 2.4 million units IM every week for 3 weeks<br>• **Neurosyphilis:**<br>**Aqueous crystalline penicillin G** 4 million units IV q4h for 10-14 days followed by<br>**Benzathine penicillin G** 2.4 million units IM every week for 3 weeks at the completion of IV therapy |
| Trichomoniasis | • Caused by *Trichomonas vaginalis*<br>• Malodorous yellow-green discharge and irritation but may be asymptomatic<br>• Diagnosis: wet prep and rapid antigen testing<br>• Sexual partners should be treated<br>• Retest within 3 months of treatment | **Metronidazole** 500 mg PO bid for 7 days for people with a vagina and 2 g PO single dose for people with a penis **OR tinidazole** 500 mg PO bid for 7 days<br>**If unable to tolerate multiple doses:**<br>**Metronidazole** 2 g PO single dose<br>**OR tinidazole** 2 g PO single dose |
| Epididymitis | • Usually caused by chlamydia or gonorrhea<br>• Epididymal swelling, tenderness, discharge, fever, dysuria | **Ceftriaxone** 500 mg IM single dose<br>(or 1 g if patient weighs ≥150 kg)<br>**PLUS**<br>**Doxycycline** 100 mg PO bid for 10 days<br>For acute epididymitis most likely caused by enteric organisms, add levofloxacin 500 mg orally once daily for 10 days OR ofloxacin 300 mg orally twice a day for 10 days<br>Follow up in 72 hr to ensure response to therapy |

**TABLE 10-1** Characteristics and Therapy for Sexually Transmitted Diseases *(Continued)*

| Disease | Characteristics | Therapy |
|---------|-----------------|---------|
| Herpes | • Recurrent, lifelong viral infection<br>• May manifest as painful genital or oral ulcers, cervicitis, or proctitis or be asymptomatic<br>• Pregnant women who acquire infection near time of delivery have a higher risk of perinatal infection (30-50%) | **First episode:**<br>**Acyclovir** 400 mg PO tid for 7-10 days **OR**<br>**Famciclovir** 250 mg PO tid for 7-10 days **OR**<br>**Valacyclovir** 1 g PO bid for 7-10 days |
| Herpes | • Condoms reduce, but do not eliminate, risk of transmission<br>• Asymptomatic shedding can occur<br>• Treatment may shorten duration of lesions but does not eradicate the virus | **Recurrent episodes:**<br>**Acyclovir** 400 mg PO tid for 5 days **OR**<br>**Acyclovir** 800 mg PO tid for 2 days **OR**<br>**Famciclovir** 125 mg PO bid for 5 days **OR**<br>**Valacyclovir** 500 mg PO bid for 3 days<br><br>**Daily suppressive therapy if six recurrences or more per year** (↓ frequency of recurrences by 75%):<br>**Acyclovir** 400 mg PO bid **OR**<br>**Valacyclovir** 500-1000 mg PO once daily |
| Chancroid | • Caused by *Haemophilus ducreyi* and very rare in the U.S.<br>• One or more painful ulcers and tender suppurative regional lymphadenopathy<br>• All patients should be tested for HIV at time of diagnosis and 3 months after (it is a cofactor for HIV)<br>• Partners must be treated | **Azithromycin** 1 g PO single dose **OR**<br>**Ceftriaxone** 250 mg IM once **OR**<br>**Ciprofloxacin** 500 mg PO bid for 3 days **OR**<br>**Erythromycin** 500 mg PO tid for 7 days<br>• If treatment is successful, ulcers improve symptomatically in 3 days; complete healing may require >2 weeks |

*(Continued)*

**TABLE 10-1** Characteristics and Therapy for Sexually Transmitted Diseases *(Continued)*

| Disease | Characteristics | Therapy |
|---------|-----------------|---------|
| **Genital warts or condyloma acuminatum** | • Caused by human papillomavirus<br>• May manifest as visible genital warts or uterine, cervix, anal, vaginal, urethral, or laryngeal warts (types 6, 11)<br>• Associated with cervical dysplasia (types 16, 18, 31, 33, 35)<br>• Condoms reduce but do not eliminate risk of transmission<br>• Patient might remain infectious even though warts are gone<br>• Cervical and anal mucosa warts management should be by expert<br>• Treatment may induce wart-free periods but does not eradicate virus<br>• HPV vaccine now recommended for all children at 11-12 years of age | • **External warts:**<br>*Patient administered:*<br>**Podofilox 0.5% topical solution** bid for 3 days and then 4 days off; may repeat 4 times this cycle, **OR**<br>**Imiquimod 5% cream** apply at bedtime 3× per week then wash off in AM for up to 16 weeks<br>*Provider applied:*<br>**Cryotherapy OR**<br>**Podophyllin resin 10-25% OR**<br>**Trichloroacetic acid OR surgical or laser removal** |
| **Pediculosis pubis** | • Lice or nits on pubic hair<br>• Patients consult because of pruritus or visual nits | **Permethrin 1% cream:** apply for 10 min and rinse<br>**Pyrethrins with piperonyl butoxide:** apply for 10 min and rinse |
| **Scabies** | • Caused by *Sarcoptes scabiei*<br>• In adults may be sexually transmitted but not in children<br>• Pruritus and rash<br>• Treat partners and household contacts, plus household decontamination | **Permethrin 5% cream:** apply to body from neck down, and wash off after 8-14 hr **OR**<br>**Ivermectin** 200 μg/kg PO × 1 and then can repeat after 2 weeks<br>**Lindane 1% lotion**[a] |

| **TABLE 10-1** | Characteristics and Therapy for Sexually Transmitted Diseases *(Continued)* |
|---|---|

| Disease | Characteristics | Therapy |
|---|---|---|
| **Vaginitis** | | |
| **Bacterial vaginosis** | • Caused by *G. vaginalis*<br>• Most prevalent cause of pathologic vaginal discharge<br>• Symptoms may include vaginal discharge and odor, vulvar itching, and irritation, although up to 50% are asymptomatic<br>• Partners do not need treatment | **Metronidazole** 500 mg PO bid for 7 days **OR**<br>**Metronidazole gel 0.75%:** 5 g applicator intravaginally for 5 nights **OR**<br>**Clindamycin cream 2%:** 5 g applicator intravaginally for 7 nights[b] |
| **Candidiasis** | • Symptoms include pruritus, erythema, and white discharge<br>• Partners do not need treatment | **Fluconazole** 150 mg PO once<br>**Clotrimazole** 100-mg tablet: 2 intravaginal daily for 3 days or 1 daily for 7 days<br>**Clotrimazole** 1% cream 5 g intravaginally for 7 nights<br>**Miconazole** 200 mg vaginal suppository for 3 days |

[a]Do not use in patients <2 years of age due to neurotoxicity. Only use in cases of treatment failure or if patients cannot tolerate first-line treatments.
[b]Clindamycin cream is oil based and might weaken latex condoms and diaphragms for 5 days after use.

- Evaluation should include complete history and physical examination. In symptomatic people with a vagina, a pregnancy test, wet prep, assay for *Neisseria gonorrhoeae* and *Chlamydia trachomatis*, *Trichomonas*, and HIV testing should be performed if there is concern for STI. Consider rapid plasma reagin (RPR), depending on syphilis prevalence in your community. In people with a penis, a urine specimen should be taken for diagnosis of infection with *N. gonorrhoeae* and *C. trachomatis*, and HIV and RPR testing should also be completed. In MSM, oral and rectal testing for *N. gonorrhoeae* and *C. trachomatis* are also recommended if they are having oral and anal sex.
- If an STI is suspected and follow-up is uncertain, treat presumptively for at least gonorrhea and chlamydia.
  - All sexual partners should be evaluated and treated for STIs. Expedited partner treatment options facilitate partner treatment.
  - Encourage safer sex.

## Complications

Long-term sequelae of STIs include PID, chronic pelvic pain, ectopic pregnancy, cervical dysplasia, infertility, and cancer.

## PELVIC INFLAMMATORY DISEASE

### Definition and Etiology

* PID is a spectrum of inflammatory disorders of the upper female genital tract, including endometritis, salpingitis, and oophoritis. Complications may include tuboovarian abscess (TOA), perihepatitis, pelvic peritonitis, formation of scar tissue, increased risk for ectopic pregnancy, and infertility.
* The most common causal organisms are *N. gonorrhoeae* and *C. trachomatis*. Other organisms isolated are *Gardnerella vaginalis*, *Haemophilus influenzae*, enteric gram-negative rods, *Streptococcus agalactiae*, *Bacteroides fragilis*, and *Mycoplasma genitalium*.

### Diagnosis

Lower abdominal pain in a sexually active female with no other identifiable cause and:

* Minimum criteria
  * Adnexal/uterine tenderness OR
  * Cervical motion tenderness
* Hospitalization criteria
  * All pregnant women with suspected PID
  * If surgical emergency such as appendicitis cannot be excluded
  * Inability of patient to follow up or tolerate outpatient therapy
  * If the patient did not respond clinically to oral antimicrobial therapy
  * If the patient has severe illness, nausea and vomiting, or high fever
  * Patient with TOA

### Treatment

* Outpatient treatment
  * Ceftriaxone 250 mg IM PLUS doxycycline 100 mg PO bid for 14 days
  **OR**
  * Cefoxitin 2 g IM and probenecid 1 g PO PLUS doxycycline 500 mg PO bid for 14 days
* Metronidazole 500 mg PO bid for 14 days is often added for broader anaerobic coverage; will also treat BV that is often associated with PID.
* Parenteral treatment
  * Cefotetan 2 g IV q12h OR cefoxitin 2 g IV q6h PLUS doxycycline 100 mg IV/PO q12h for 14 days
  * Clindamycin 900 IV q8h PLUS gentamicin 2 mg/kg loading dose IV or IM followed by 1.5 mg/kg q8h IV or IM and then continue with doxycycline 100 mg IV/PO q12h (especially if TOA present) for a total of 14 days

### Follow-Up

Follow-up examination should be performed within 72 hours to ensure response to therapy.

## DYSMENORRHEA

### Definition and Etiology

* Dysmenorrhea is pain with menstruation.
  * Primary: painful menstruation that occurs within 1 or 2 years of menarche; no evidence of organic pelvic disease.

○ Cramping usually starts 1-4 hours before menstruation and may last 24 hours, although symptoms may begin 2 days earlier and may last up to 4 days.
○ Episodes typically become less severe with increasing age.
• Secondary: defined as menstrual pain resulting from anatomic or macroscopic pelvic pathology (endometriosis, chronic PID, benign uterine tumors, or anatomic abnormalities) and typically occurs in adults.
• Painful menstruation is caused by release of prostaglandins during menstrual flow.

### Treatment
• Mild symptoms: nonsteroidal anti-inflammatory drugs (NSAIDs) or acetaminophen PRN.
• Moderate to severe symptoms: NSAIDs such as ibuprofen 400-600 mg q6-8h or naproxen 250-500 mg q8-12h. These agents are most effective if given before the onset of menses and continued for 2-3 days after.
• Hormonal contraception may be useful if the patient wishes contraception or has pain unresponsive to NSAIDs.

## ABNORMAL UTERINE BLEEDING

### Definition and Etiology
• Abnormal uterine bleeding (AUB) is defined as uterine bleeding that is abnormal in duration, volume, or interval in the absence of pregnancy.
• AUB in adolescents is most often a result of anovulation (cycles become ovulatory on average 20 months after menarche).
• Other etiologies can include structural pathologies, coagulopathy, thyroid dysfunction, polycystic ovarian syndrome (PCOS), infection, hormonal contraception, or very rarely malignancy.

### History and Physical Examination
• Take a thorough menstrual, sexual, and endocrine history.
• On physical examination, look for orthostatic blood pressure changes, tachycardia (indicates severe anemia), hirsutism, thyroid changes, galactorrhea, abdominal/pelvic masses, petechiae, and bleeding gums.
• Consider a pelvic examination if the adolescent is sexually active or has a history suggestive of structural pathology.

### Laboratory Studies
• Order a pregnancy test, complete blood count (CBC), and free thyroxine (free $T_4$)/thyroid-stimulating hormone (TSH).
• Based on the history and physical examination, consider prothrombin time, partial thromboplastin time, platelet function assay, von Willebrand factor testing, pelvic ultrasound, gonorrhea and chlamydia testing (if ever sexually active), and luteinizing hormone, follicle-stimulating hormone, testosterone, and dehydroepiandrosterone sulfate.

### Diagnosis
Differential diagnosis: pregnancy, STD, polyp or other structural cause, foreign body (i.e., retained tampon), bleeding diathesis (von Willebrand disease, idiopathic thrombocytopenic purpura, platelet abnormality, clotting factor deficiency), hormonal causes (anovulation, hypothyroidism/hyperthyroidism, PCOS, late-onset congenital adrenal hyperplasia, exogenous hormones [such as those in oral contraceptive pills, Depo-Provera, Plan B], stress, and excessive exercise).

## Treatment

- Treat underlying disorder if present.
- If AUB is the diagnosis, determine that the patient is hemodynamically stable; if so, consider hormonal therapy to stop the bleeding, oral iron supplementation if anemia is present, and NSAIDs if there is accompanying dysmenorrhea.

## CONTRACEPTION

- The goal of contraception in adolescents is a safe and effective method of preventing pregnancy that is both convenient and reversible.
- Table 10-2 summarizes the most common birth control methods available to adolescents.
- **Absolute contraindications to estrogen-containing hormonal contraception** include history of thromboembolic disease (myocardial infarction, stroke, pulmonary embolism, deep venous thrombosis), pregnancy, breast cancer, exclusive breastfeeding, estrogen-sensitive neoplasias, undiagnosed vaginal bleeding, active viral hepatitis or cirrhosis, major surgery with prolonged immobilization >1 month, symptomatic gallbladder disease, migraine with aura/focal neurologic symptoms, and moderate or severe hypertension (systolic blood pressure >160 mm Hg, diastolic blood pressure >100 mm Hg). The World Health Organization guidelines (see Suggested Readings) contain more information.

## EATING DISORDERS

### Definitions and Diagnostic Criteria

- **Anorexia nervosa (AN)** is a disorder characterized by the pursuit of thinness.
  - Restriction of energy intake relative to requirements, leading to significantly lower body weight in the context of age, sex, developmental trajectory, and physical health. Significantly low weight defined as a weight that is less than minimally normal or, for children and adolescents, less than that minimally expected.
  - Intense fear of gaining weight or becoming fat or persistent behavior that interferes with weight gain, even though underweight.
  - Disturbance in the way in which one's body weight or shape is experienced, undue influence of body weight or shape on self-evaluation, or denial of the seriousness of the current low body weight.
- **ARFID** (avoidant/restrictive food intake disorder) is an eating or feeding disturbance that is characterized by a disinterest in eating or food, which is typically associated with sensory sensitivities or fear of adverse consequences of eating and is associated with a decline in psychosocial functioning. The lack of associated body dysmorphia and pursuit of thinness separates it from AN and bulimia. The disorder is not due to another illness or limited food.
- **Bulimia nervosa (BN)** is a disorder characterized by recurrent episodes of binge eating followed by inappropriate compensatory behaviors.
  - An episode of binge eating is characterized by *both* of the following:
    - Eating, in a discrete period of time (e.g., within a 2-hour period), an amount of food that is definitely larger than most people would eat during a similar period of time and under similar circumstances.
    - A sense of lack of control over eating during the episode (e.g., a feeling that one cannot stop eating or control what or how much one is eating).

**TABLE 10-2** Contraceptive Methods

| Method | Mechanism of action and characteristics | Failure rate | Adverse effects |
|---|---|---|---|
| **No method** | | 85% | |
| **Withdrawal method** | Male withdraws his penis from the vagina prior to ejaculation. Minimizes sperm exposure to vagina | 4-22% | Difficult to do accurately, high failure rates |
| **Rhythm method** | Avoidance of coitus during presumed fertile days<br><br>Ovulation occurs 14 days before menses (assuming 28-day cycle). After ovulation, sperm can survive in the vagina 3-4 days and oocytes up to 24 hr | 6-38% | High failure rates |
| **Barrier/chemical** | | | |
| **Nexplanon (implantable rod)** | Inhibits ovulation by inhibiting the midcycle rise of luteinizing hormone; also thickens cervical mucus and causes endometrial thinning. Approved for 3 years | 0.05% | Menstrual irregularities, acne, insertion/removal problems |
| **Intrauterine device** | Inhibits sperm transport and causes direct damage to sperm and ova, affecting fertilization and ovum transport. Available methods include Skyla (contains progestin, approved for 3 years), Kyleena (contains progestin, approved for 5 years), Mirena, Liletta (contains progestin, approved for 6 years), and ParaGard (copper only, hormone-free, approved for 10 years) | 0.2-0.8% | Menstrual irregularities, dysmenorrhea (particularly with ParaGard), uterine perforation (rare) |

*(Continued)*

**TABLE 10-2** Contraceptive Methods *(Continued)*

| Method | Mechanism of action and characteristics | Failure rate | Adverse effects |
|---|---|---|---|
| Medroxyproges-terone (Depo-Provera) | Same mechanism as Nexplanon | 0.2% perfect use, 3-6% typical use | Menstrual irregularities, weight gain, headache |
| Combined oral contraceptives (COC) | Suppresses ovulation by inhibiting the gonadotropin cycle, changing the cervical mucus and endometrium | 0.3-8% perfect use, 6-18% typical use | Breakthrough bleeding, nausea, breast tenderness, headaches |
| | | | Estrogen-related risk of thromboem-bolism, hypertension, stroke |
| Transdermal patch | Same mechanism as COC<br><br>Releases estrogen and progesterone at controlled rates over 1 week<br><br>Changed weekly for 3 weeks and then patch-free week for withdrawal bleeding | <1% perfect use, 6-8% typical use | Breakthrough bleeding, nausea, breast tenderness, headaches |
| | | | Local site reaction (do not put on breasts), detachment |
| | | | Estrogen-related risks as with COCs |
| | | | May be less effective if weight >90 kg |
| Vaginal ring | Same mechanism as COC<br><br>Releases estrogen and progesterone at controlled rates over 3 weeks, followed by ring-free week for withdrawal bleeding | 0.3% perfect use, 6-8% typical use | Must use backup contraception if out for >3 hr |
| | | | Breakthrough bleeding, vaginitis, estrogen-related risks as with COCs |

**TABLE 10-2** Contraceptive Methods *(Continued)*

| Method | Mechanism of action and characteristics | Failure rate | Adverse effects |
|---|---|---|---|
| Male condom | Mechanical barrier to sperm | 2-18% | Allergic reaction |
| Female condom | Mechanical barrier to sperm | 5-21% | Local irritation |
| Diaphragm (placed intravaginally 1-6 hr before intercourse) | Mechanical barrier to sperm | 6-12% | UTI or vaginal infection |
| Cervical cap (should be used in conjunction with spermicides) | Mechanical barrier to sperm | 16-32% | Irritation |
| Foam or vaginal tablets | Inactivate sperm; should allow 10-15 min to allow the tablets to dissolve | 15-29% | Irritation |
| **Emergency contraception (postcoital)** | Single-dose levonorgestrel (progestin only) therapy now available OTC, taken within 120 hr of unprotected intercourse | Reduces risk of pregnancy by 89-95%, more effective if taken sooner | Spotting, abdominal pain/nausea, may be less effective for those with BMI > 25 |
| | Single-dose ulipristal (brand name Ella), available only by prescription, taken within 120 hr of unprotected intercourse | May be more effective than levonorgestrel EC, particularly closer to the time of ovulation and for women who are overweight/obese | Headache, delayed menstrual cycle, abdominal pain/nausea |
| | Copper IUD insertion within 5 days of unprotected intercourse | Reduces risk of pregnancy by >99% | See IUD adverse effects above |
| | Yuzpe method (use of COC in two divided doses, 12 hr apart) | Reduces risk of pregnancy by 75% | Nausea, vomiting, breast tenderness, headaches |

- Recurrent inappropriate compensatory behaviors to prevent weight gain, such as self-induced vomiting; misuse of laxatives, diuretics, enemas, or other medications; fasting; or excessive exercise.
- The binge eating and inappropriate compensatory behaviors both occur, on average, at least once a week for 3 months.
- Self-evaluation is unduly influenced by body shape and weight.
- The disturbance does not occur exclusively during episodes of AN.
- **Binge Eating Disorder (BED)**
  - Recurrent episodes of binge eating (see above definition).
  - Binge eating episodes are associated with three or more of the following:
    - Eating more rapidly than normal
    - Eating until feeling uncomfortably full
    - Eating large amounts of food when not feeling physically hungry
    - Eating alone because of feeling embarrassed, feeling disgusted, feeling depressed, or feeling guilty afterward
  - Marked distress regarding binge eating is present.
  - Binge eating occurs, on average, at least once a week for 3 months.
  - Binge eating is not associated with recurrent inappropriate compensatory behavior as in bulimia nervosa.
- **Other specified feeding or eating disorder (OSFED) (previously eating disorder, NOS)** is a category of disordered eating behaviors that do not meet the full criteria for other eating disorders. For example
  - All criteria for AN are met, except individual's weight is normal or above normal.
  - All criteria for BN are met, except binge eating and inappropriate compensatory behaviors occur less than once a week and/or for <3 months.
  - All criteria for BED are met, except binge eating occurs less than once a week and/or for <3 months.

## Clinical Presentation

- Anorexia nervosa: weight loss or poor weight gain, amenorrhea, cold hands and feet, constipation, fainting/dizziness/orthostasis, headaches/lethargy, irritability/depression, social withdrawal, poor concentration, and decreased ability to make decisions
- Bulimia nervosa: weight gain, bloating and fullness, guilt/depression/anxiety, and lethargy
- ARFID: failure to meet nutritional and/or energy needs, weight loss, nutritional deficiencies, disinterest in eating/food, reliance on enteral feeds or supplements

## Physical Examination

- Anorexia nervosa and ARFID: bradycardia, loss of muscle mass, and dry skin/hair loss
- Bulimia nervosa: calloused knuckles (Russell sign), dental enamel erosion, and enlargement of salivary glands

## Laboratory/EKG Findings

- Anorexia nervosa and ARFID: electrolyte abnormalities, neutropenia/anemia, increased alanine aminotransferase (ALT)/aspartate aminotransferase (AST), decreased serum glucose, and prolonged QTc
- Bulimia nervosa: increased serum bicarbonate, decreased potassium, prolonged QTc, or other cardiac arrhythmias

## Treatment

*Therapeutic Guidelines*
- Take all concerns seriously.
- Focus on health, not only on weight.
- Use team approach, with mental health provider, dietitian, and primary care physician or adolescent medicine specialist or psychiatrist.
- Follow electrolytes and electrocardiographic (ECG) changes.
- DEXA scan if amenorrheic >12 months.

*Admission Criteria*
- Vital sign instability: temperature <36°C (96.8°F), pulse <50 beats per minute, SBP < 90/50, a drop in blood pressure of 10 mm Hg, or an increase in pulse of >20 beats per minute on standing
- Altered mental status or fainting
- Rapid weight loss (>10% in 2 months or >15% overall) or <80% of ideal body weight
- Potassium <3.0 mmol/L, phosphorus <2.0 mg/dL, or dehydration
- Failure to improve with outpatient management
- Comorbid diagnosis interfering with treatment (i.e., depression, anxiety)
- Unable to eat or drink or uncontrollable binging or purging
- Cardiac arrhythmia or prolonged QTc

## Complications

- Amenorrhea: Restoration of menses occurs with adequate weight gain.
- Cardiac conditions: Abnormal heart contractility, prolonged QT, and ventricular arrhythmias.
- Osteopenia and osteoporosis: Weight gain is the most effective method of increasing bone density.
- Refeeding syndrome: Greatest risk during first few days of refeeding. Administration of glucose causes extracellular phosphate depletion, which limits the ability of the red blood cell to carry oxygen because of decreased levels of 2,3-diphophosphoglycerate. Phosphate depletion can lead to cardiomyopathy, altered consciousness, hemolytic anemia, and death.
- Monitor phosphate and other electrolytes (magnesium and potassium) at least every 24 hours in patients at risk for refeeding when initiating nutritional rehabilitation in an inpatient setting until up to full calories for weight and nutrition restoration.
- May give prophylactic phosphate supplement to prevent phosphorous depletion in an inpatient setting.

## DEPRESSION AND ANXIETY

### Definitions

- Major depressive disorder
  - Depressed mood or loss of interest for at least 2 weeks.
  - Four or more of the following: weight/appetite loss or gain, low energy/fatigue, insomnia or hypersomnia, psychomotor retardation or agitation, worthlessness/guilt, poor concentration/indecisiveness, and suicidality.
  - Distress/impairment in social/occupational/academic functioning.
  - Adolescents may present with irritability.
  - Adolescents may not tell or admit they are depressed.

- Patients feel hopeless, worthless, and helpless.
- School problems, social withdrawal, substance abuse, somatic complaints, and high-risk behaviors should be red flags that a patient may be depressed.
- Persistent depressive disorder (dysthymia)
  - Irritable or depressed mood for most of the day, most days, for at least 1 year, with significant impairment in functioning
  - Two or more of the following: insomnia or hypersomnia, poor appetite or overeating, low self-esteem, helplessness, low energy/fatigue, and poor concentration/indecisiveness
  - No major depressive episode
- Adjustment disorder with depressed mood
  - Emotional symptoms within 3 months of onset of stressor.
  - Distress/impairment in social/occupational/academic functioning.
  - Depressed mood, tearfulness, or hopelessness.
  - Symptoms do not represent bereavement.
  - Once stressor has terminated, symptoms persist for no more than 6 months.
- Generalized anxiety disorder
  - At least 6 months of excessive anxiety and/or worry about events or activities, occurring more often than not.
  - Symptoms are difficult to control and associated with at least one of the following symptoms: irritability, restlessness, easily fatigued, muscle tension, difficulty concentration, or sleep disturbance.
  - Not attributable to another mental disorder, medical condition, or substance use.

## Epidemiology

- The prevalence of major depression and anxiety disorders in adolescents is on the rise.
- Anxiety disorders are the most common mental health disorders in childhood and adolescence. Prevalence among adolescents aged 13-17 is estimated to be between 25 and 37%.
- Past-year prevalence of a major depressive episode (MDE) among U.S. adolescents aged 12-17 was found to be 13.3%, up from 8% in 2007.
- Risk factors: parental history of affective illness, history of abuse, chronic illness, loss through separation or death, medications, coexisting conditions such as attention deficit hyperactivity disorder, or mild mental retardation or learning disabilities.

## Screening

- AAP recommends screening for depression at annual preventive visits from ages 11 to 21.
  - There are a number of validated screening tools for adolescents:
    - Depression-Patient Health Questionnaire (PHQ-2 or PHQ-9), Beck Depression Inventory (BDI), or Kutcher Adolescent Depression Scale (KADS) that may be used.
    - Anxiety-Generalized Anxiety Disorder 7-item scale (GAD-7), Pediatric Anxiety Rating Scale (PARS), Self-Report for Childhood Anxiety Related Emotional Disorders (SCARED).

## Treatment

- Counseling and medications have both been shown to be effective in treating major depression in adolescents, but they are even more effective when used together.

- Treat for at least 6 months after initial episode or 12 months if recurrent episode.
- Selective serotonin reuptake inhibitors (SSRIs) such as fluoxetine, citalopram, escitalopram, sertraline, all show benefit over placebo.
  - Benefits may not be apparent for 4-6 weeks.
  - Response to one SSRI does not predict response to different SSRI.
  - Side effects are few. They may be gastrointestinal (nausea, vomiting, diarrhea, constipation, mouth dryness, appetite change, dyspepsia) or central nervous system related (headache, nervousness, tremor, insomnia, confusion, fatigue, dizziness, decreased libido).
  - There is an FDA **"black box" warning** for SSRIs regarding possibility for increased thoughts of suicide. Overall, the evidence shows that benefits of antidepressant use in depressed adolescents outweigh the risk of this particular side effect, particularly in conjunction with cognitive-behavioral therapy. Patients and their families should be counseled regarding this possible side effect.
  - Principles for treating adolescent depression developed by the Guidelines for Adolescent Depression in Primary Care (GLAD-PC) Working Group, which were published in 2007 and revised in 2018, were endorsed by the American Academy of Pediatrics. Some of the GLAD-PC recommendations for treatment and ongoing management include the following:
    ○ Collaboration with a mental health professional is necessary for patients with moderate/severe depression, coexisting psychosis, and substance abuse or if initial treatment is not successful.
    ○ Practitioners should monitor for adverse events during SSRI treatment, with attempts to adhere to the FDA recommendations for follow-up.
    ○ Involvement of the family/caregivers is necessary in monitoring both response to treatment and adverse events related to medication.
    ○ Regular tracking of outcomes and goals should occur in home, school, and peer settings.
- Tricyclic antidepressants are not recommended in adolescents.
- Major cause of failure is nonadherence.

## SUICIDE IN ADOLESCENTS

- Any patient who talks about suicide should be taken seriously.
- The ASQ (Ask Suicide-Screening Questions) is a brief, 5 question screening tool approved for all ages as a means of evaluating an individual's risk of suicide.

### Epidemiology

- Suicide is the second most common cause of death in adolescents, in whom it represents 15% of all mortality.
- Risk factors include previous suicide attempts, affective disorders, family history or conflict, alcohol and substance abuse, impulsivity, and guns in the home.
- There is often a precipitating factor and a motivation (gain attention, escape, communicate, express love or anger) in addition to preexisting social isolation.

### Treatment

- When adolescents feel depressed, ask about their support system. Ask if they ever thought of hurting themselves, and if so, when and how, if they had a plan, if they would do it again, and if they feel the same way now.

- When patients are suicidal or you are concerned about their safety, you should:
  - Obtain immediate psychiatric consultation
  - Involve the patient's parents and/or support system
  - Contract for safety
  - Consider antidepressant therapy

## ALCOHOL AND DRUG ABUSE

### Definition and Epidemiology

- Commonly abused drugs include alcohol, nicotine, marijuana, amphetamine ("speed") and methamphetamine, cocaine, opioids, methylenedioxymethamphetamine (MDMA; "ecstasy" or "Molly"), lysergic acid diethylamide (LSD), phencyclidine (PCP), prescription drugs (oxycodone, Demerol, methylphenidate), synthetic cathinone ("bath salts"), heroin, "huffing" volatile solvents, and anabolic steroids.
- More than half of adolescents try an illicit drug before the end of high school.
  - At least one-quarter of adolescents have used an illicit drug other than marijuana.
  - It is estimated that 80-90% of adolescents try alcohol by 18 years of age.
- Drugs are widely present and available, even among older elementary and middle school children.
- Regular alcohol and drug use, binge drinking, and related injuries, accidents, and physical consequences are problematic and common.
- The CRAFFT screening tool for alcohol and drug abuse is for the adolescent age group (two or more "yes" answers considered a positive screen).
  - **C:** Have you ever ridden in a CAR driven by someone (including yourself) who was "high" or had been using alcohol or drugs?
  - **R:** Do you ever use alcohol or drugs to RELAX, feel better about yourself, or fit in?
  - **A:** Do you ever use alcohol or drugs while you are ALONE?
  - **F:** Do you ever FORGET things that you did while using alcohol or drugs?
  - **F:** Do your family or FRIENDS ever tell you that you should cut down on your drinking or drug use?
  - **T:** Have you gotten into TROUBLE while using alcohol or drugs?
- Contributing factors can include genetic disposition for alcoholism or substance abuse, parental drug use and role modeling, peer influence, low self-esteem, personality disorders, experiencing abuse or neglect, and depression.

### Treatment

- Recognize and treat addiction as a disease process.
- Encourage family involvement and support. Resources include Alcoholics Anonymous, National Council on Alcoholism and Drug Abuse, and other local resources for formal drug/alcohol abuse evaluation, counseling, and treatment options.

## SUGGESTED READINGS

American Psychiatric Association. Diagnostic and Statistical Manual of Mental Disorders. 5th Ed. Arlington, VA: American Psychiatric Association, 2013.

ASQ Toolkit. Available at https://www.nimh.nih.gov/research/research-conducted-at-nimh/asq-toolkit-materials/index.shtml

Bedsider Birth Control Support Network. Available at web site: www.bedsider.org

Centers for Disease Control and Prevention. STD treatment guidelines, 2015. Available at https://www.cdc.gov/std/tg2015/default.htm

Cheung AH, Zuckerbrot RA, Jensen PS, et al. Guidelines for adolescent depression in primary care (GLAD-PC): Part II. Treatment and ongoing management. Pediatrics 2018;141(3):e20174082.

Committee on Adolescence. Contraception for adolescents. Pediatrics 2014;134(4):e1244–e1256. doi: 10.1542/peds.2014-2299.

English A, Ford CA. The HIPAA privacy policy rule and adolescents: legal questions and clinical challenges. Perspect Sex Reprod Health 2004;36(2):80–86.

Fontham ETH, Wolf AMD, Church TR, et al. Cervical cancer screening for individuals at average risk: 2020 guideline update from the American Cancer Society. CA Cancer J Clin 2020;70:321–346. https://doi.org/10.3322/caac.21628

GLAD-PC Toolkit. Available at www.glad-pc.org

Hatcher RA, et al. Contraceptive Technology. 21th Ed. New York: Ayer Company Publishers, Inc., 2018.

Hornberger LL, Lane MA; Committee on Adolescence. Identification and management of eating disorders in children and adolescents. Pediatrics 2021;147(1):e2020040279. doi: 10.1542/peds.2020-040279.

Johnston LD, et al. Monitoring the Future National Results on Drug Use: 2012 Overview, Key Findings on Adolescent Drug Use. Ann Arbor: Institute for Social Research, The University of Michigan, 2013.

Knight J, et al. Validity of the CRAFFT substance abuse screening test among adolescent clinic patients. Arch Pediatr Adolesc Med 2002;156:607–614.

Medical Eligibility Criteria for Contraceptive Use. 5th ed. Geneva: World Health Organization; 2015. PMID: 26447268.

Meites E, Kempe A, Markowitz LE. Use of a 2-dose schedule for human papillomavirus vaccination—updated recommendations of the advisory committee on immunization practices. MMWR Morb Mortal Wkly Rep 2016;65:1405–1408.

Neinstein LS. Adolescent Health Care: A Practical Guide. 6th Ed. Philadelphia, PA: Lippincott Williams & Wilkins, 2016.

Princeton University Emergency Contraception. Available at web site: www.ec.princeton.edu

Schillie S, Wester C, Osborne M, et al. CDC recommendations for hepatitis C screening among adults—United States, 2020. MMWR Recomm Rep 2020;69(RR-2):1–17.

St Cyr S, Barbee L, Workowski KA, et al. Update to CDC's treatment guidelines for gonococcal infection, 2020. MMWR Morb Mortal Wkly Rep 2020;69:1911–1916.

The Center for Adolescent Health and the Law. Available at web site: www.cahl.org

The Contraceptive Choice Project. Available at web site: www.choiceproject.wustl.edu

Underwood JM, Brener N, Thornton J, et al. Overview and methods for the Youth Risk Behavior Surveillance System—United States, 2019. MMWR Morb Mortal Wkly Rep Suppl 2020;69(1):1–10.

Zuckerbrot RA, Cheung A, Jensen PS, et al.; GLAD-PC STEERING GROUP. Guidelines for adolescent depression in primary care (GLAD-PC): part I. Practice preparation, identification, assessment, and initial management. Pediatrics 2018;141(3):e20174081.

# 11

# Allergic Diseases and Asthma

Alexa Altman Doss, Jeffrey Stokes, Caroline C. Horner, and Lila Kertz

## ALLERGIC RHINITIS

Allergic rhinitis (AR) is self-reported in up to 40% of U.S. children and can have significant effects on quality of life.

### Pathophysiology

- In the early phase, mediators (histamine, tryptase) are released from mast cells when allergen-specific immunoglobulin E (IgE) antibodies are cross-linked by allergens and cause acute mucosal edema, mucous secretion, vascular leakage, and stimulation of sensory neurons.
- In the late phase, recruitment of inflammatory cells (eosinophils, lymphocytes, and basophils) causes persistent inflammation, which may last for days.

### History

- Common symptoms include rhinorrhea, sniffing, nasal congestion, mouth breathing, throat clearing secondary to post nasal drip, sneezing, pruritus, nasal/palatal itching, and cough. Concomitant ocular symptoms often occur (see Allergic Conjunctivitis below).
- Determine whether symptoms are present throughout the year (perennial rhinitis), only during a particular season (seasonal rhinitis), or perennially with seasonal worsening.
- Determine whether symptoms are worse in a specific environment, such as at home with a pet, at daycare, or at school.
- Identify measures that relieve symptoms, such as medication usage and allergen avoidance.
- Inquire about symptoms that suggest asthma (see Asthma below) since 75-80% of children with asthma have concomitant AR.
- Review personal medical history and family medical history for atopic conditions.

### Physical Examination

- Closely inspect the skin, eyes, ears, nose, and throat.
- Many children have dark discoloration below the lower eyelids (allergic shiners) and prominent creases in the lower eyelid skin (Dennie-Morgan lines). A child who frequently rubs his or her nose (allergic salute) may develop a transverse nasal crease (allergic crease).
- Findings on nasal examination include pale, boggy (edematous) turbinates, and clear nasal discharge.
- Mouth breathing may be observed.
- Cobblestoning in the posterior pharynx is a sign of follicular hypertrophy of mucosal lymphoid tissue.

## Evaluation

- Percutaneous skin testing for environmental aeroallergens is sensitive when performed with correct technique and provides prompt information.
- Serum allergen-specific IgE measurements for aeroallergens are an alternative, especially in children with dermatographism, with diffuse eczema, or who cannot discontinue the use of antihistamines or β-blockers.
- Food allergen testing is not recommended for isolated rhinitis symptoms (see Food Allergy below).
- Rhinoscopy to directly visualize the nasal mucosa and upper airway is seldom used in the pediatric population for this diagnosis.
- Differential diagnosis
  - Other common causes of nasal symptoms are nonallergic, including infectious, anatomic/mechanical, or irritant. Symptom overlap may also occur in rhinosinusitis, ciliary dyskinesia, adenoid hypertrophy, and rarely in CSF leak or nasal/sinus tumors.
  - Differentiating AR from recurrent upper respiratory viral infections can be challenging. In the presence of fevers, headache, myalgias, or purulent nasal discharge, an acute viral rhinitis or rhinosinusitis should be considered.
  - Obstructive symptoms and unilateral purulent nasal discharge may suggest a retained foreign body.
  - Mouth breathing and snoring may suggest coexistent adenoidal hypertrophy.
  - Nasal polyps are atypical in childhood allergic rhinitis and should prompt evaluation for cystic fibrosis.

## Treatment

- Avoidance through environmental control
  - For outdoor allergens, limit outdoor activity during peak pollen days (sunny, windy days with low humidity). Close windows and use air conditioning.
  - Although homes cannot be made "allergen free," exposure to major indoor allergens can be reduced.
  - House dust mite avoidance requires multiple interventions for benefit. Measures include changing bedding weekly and washing in hot water (>130°F); placing dust mite impermeable covers on the pillows, mattresses, and box springs; using a high-efficiency particulate air (HEPA) filter vacuum; removing carpeting in the bedroom, and reducing humidity.
  - If the child has allergic symptoms from a pet, removing the pet from the home is ideal. If this option is not feasible, keeping the pet out of the bedroom and restricting the pet to certain areas of the home with HEPA filtration may be helpful.
  - Limiting ambient humidity and water intrusion reduce fungal exposure.
  - Comprehensive pest management strategies are recommended for cockroach allergy.
- Pharmacotherapy (Table 11-1)
  - Intranasal corticosteroids are potent anti-inflammatory agents that relieve rhinorrhea, sneezing, pruritus, and congestion.
    - These agents are indicated for both perennial and seasonal allergic rhinitis.
    - This class is preferred for monotherapy for persistent rhinitis.
    - To optimize benefits, administer daily.
    - Inform patients about proper technique. With the head upright or tilted slightly forward, spray with the nozzle up and outward (away from the septum and

| TABLE 11-1 | Medications Used in the Treatment of Allergic Rhinitis |
|---|---|

**Nasal corticosteroids**

| | |
|---|---|
| Budesonide (Rhinocort Aqua) | <6 years: Not established |
| | 6-11 years: 1-2 sprays each nostril daily |
| | ≥12 years: 1-2 sprays each nostril daily |
| Fluticasone furoate (Sensimist OTC) | <2 years: Not established |
| | 2-11 years: 1-2 sprays each nostril daily |
| | ≥12 years: 1-2 sprays each nostril daily |
| Fluticasone propionate (Flonase) | <4 years: Not established |
| | ≥4 years: 1-2 sprays each nostril daily |
| Mometasone furoate monohydrate (Nasonex) | <2 years: Not established |
| | 2-11 years: 1 spray each nostril daily |
| | ≥12 years: 2 sprays each nostril daily |
| Triamcinolone (Nasacort AQ) | <2 years: Not established |
| | 2-5 years: 1 spray each nostril daily |
| | 6-11 years: 1-2 sprays each nostril daily |
| | ≥12 years: 1-2 sprays each nostril daily |

**Second-generation H1 antihistamines**

| | |
|---|---|
| Cetirizine (Zyrtec) | <6 months: Not established |
| | 6-12 months: 2.5 mg PO daily |
| | 12-24 months: 2.5 mg PO daily or bid |
| | 2-5 years: 2.5-5 mg PO daily |
| | ≥6 years: 5-10 mg PO daily |
| Levocetirizine (Xyzal) | <6 months: Not established |
| | 6 months-≤ 5 years: 1.25 mg PO daily |
| | 6-11 years: 2.5 mg PO daily |
| | ≥12 years: 5 mg PO daily |
| Fexofenadine (Allegra) | <6 months: Not established |
| | 6-23 months: 15 mg PO bid |
| | 2-11 years: 30 mg PO bid |
| | ≥12 years: 60 mg PO bid; 180 mg PO daily |
| Loratadine (Claritin) | <2 years: Not established |
| | 2-5 years: 5 mg PO daily |
| | >5 years: 10 mg PO daily |
| Desloratadine (Clarinex) | <6 months: Not established |
| | 6-11 months: 1 mg PO daily |
| | 12 months to 5 years: 1.25 mg PO daily |
| | 6-11 years: 2.5 mg PO daily |
| | ≥12 years: 5 mg PO daily |

pointed toward the outer portion of the ipsilateral eye). Avoid hard sniffing to prevent excess throat administration.
  ○ Side effects include epistaxis, burning/stinging, and oropharyngeal irritation. Review of proper intranasal administration or temporary discontinuation may resolve these symptoms.
- Antihistamines reduce rhinorrhea, sneezing, and pruritus.
  ○ Second-generation $H_1$ antihistamines (loratadine, desloratadine, cetirizine, levocetirizine, and fexofenadine) are the preferred oral class when antihistamines are used for AR. Second-generation agents are less likely to cross the blood-brain barrier, minimizing sedation. Duration of action allows once daily dosing for most.
  ○ Topical intranasal antihistamines (azelastine and olopatadine) are an initial treatment option for AR. These agents improve congestion more effectively than oral antihistamines and have a favorable safety profile with rapid onset of action. The distinct taste of these medications can limit patient acceptance.
  ○ First-generation $H_1$ antihistamines (hydroxyzine, chlorpheniramine, and diphenhydramine) are not recommended for the treatment of AR. Potential sedation, performance impairment, poor sleep quality, and anticholinergic effects limit their tolerability. Additionally, OTC use of diphenhydramine is not recommended in children <6 years old. The FDA issued an alert in September 2020 warning caregivers of the dangers of the "Benadryl Challenge" where adolescents purposely take large doses of diphenhydramine.
- The leukotriene receptor antagonist montelukast should be reserved for patients with AR who are not treated effectively with or cannot tolerate other allergy medications. A black box warning was issued by the FDA in March 2020 for potential neuropsychiatric events.
- Intranasal ipratropium is an anticholinergic that can be effective when rhinorrhea is the predominant symptom.
- A short (3-7 days) course of oral corticosteroids may rarely be used for severe or intractable symptoms, particularly during the peaks of pollen seasons.
- Topical decongestants (oxymetazoline hydrochloride) are effective for short-term relief of symptoms, such as rhinorrhea and congestion. Limit their use to 3-5 days to avoid rhinitis medicamentosa.
- Oral decongestants are not recommended for maintenance therapy and should be used with caution in children (special caution in patients <6 years of age and with certain conditions such as arrhythmias, hypertension, glaucoma, hyperthyroidism, and other listed conditions).
- Subcutaneous Immunotherapy (SCIT)
  - The exact mechanism of SCIT remains unclear. Reductions in circulating specific IgE and increases in allergen-specific IgG have been observed.
  - Potential benefits of SCIT may include pharmacotherapy reduction, sustained symptom reduction, and asthma prevention in patients with AR.
  - Treatment is individualized and based on identified sensitization to allergens.
  - Immunotherapy requires a multiyear commitment from the caregivers and child.
  - With the known risk of anaphylaxis, SCIT should be prescribed only by physicians trained in allergy and immunotherapy and administered in an office setting equipped to effectively treat reactions.
- Sublingual immunotherapy (SLIT)
  - SLIT products exclusively for grass pollen are approved for children (Grastek ≥5 years, Oralair ≥10 years). Side effects include oral pruritus and throat irritation.

## ALLERGIC CONJUNCTIVITIS

- Allergic conjunctivitis is frequently seen concomitantly with allergic rhinitis (AR).
- Symptoms include watery eyes, itching, redness, and eyelid swelling.
- Pathophysiology is similar to AR and involves the same mediators and inflammatory cells.

### History and Physical Examination

- Allergic conjunctivitis is characterized by acute onset, bilateral involvement, clear watery discharge, and pruritus.
- Examination can reveal bilateral hyperemia and edema of the conjunctivae.
- Red eye is the hallmark of all conjunctivitis, and examination should assess other ocular structures for their contribution.

### Evaluation

- Presence of allergen-specific IgE can be detected by either percutaneous skin testing or allergen-specific IgE (See Allergic Rhinitis above).
- Ocular allergen challenge is sensitive but seldom used clinically.
- Differential diagnosis
  - Bacterial conjunctivitis is characterized by acute onset, thick purulent discharge, minimal pain, and history of exposure. It often occurs as unilateral disease that may subsequently infect the contralateral side.
  - Viral conjunctivitis is characterized by acute/subacute onset, clear watery discharge (often bilateral), and history of recent upper respiratory infection.
  - Keratoconjunctivitis
    - Vernal keratoconjunctivitis has bilateral conjunctival inflammation with the giant papillae on the superior tarsal conjunctiva with ropy mucous discharge. Itching is the most common symptom. Photophobia, foreign body sensation, tearing, and blepharospasm are also reported. Spring time onset is frequent, and children have increased occurrence.
    - Atopic keratoconjunctivitis is bilateral inflammation of conjunctiva and eyelids associated with atopic dermatitis. The most common symptom is bilateral itching of the eyelids, and symptoms are perennial.
    - Both vernal and atopic keratoconjunctivitis are sight-threatening disorders and should prompt immediate referral to an ophthalmologist.

### Treatment

- Identification and avoidance of the identified allergen(s) can be helpful (see AR above).
- Intranasal steroids, oral second-generation $H_1$ antihistamines, and oral leukotriene antagonists can reduce ocular symptoms (as in AR treatment). If ocular symptoms are the main complaint, then topical therapies are preferred.
- Artificial tear substitutes provide a barrier function, wash away allergens, and dilute inflammatory mediators.
- Topical antihistamines with mast cell stabilizing effects (alcaftadine, azelastine, bepotastine, cetirizine, emedastine, epinastine, ketotifen, olopatadine) provide relief of acute symptoms and also prevent symptom development when used prophylactically.
- Mast cell stabilizers (cromolyn, lodoxamide, nedocromil, pemirolast) inhibit mast cell degranulation and release of inflammatory mediators. The need to use them prophylactically and frequent dosing interval may limit their appeal.

- Topical vasoconstrictors (naphazoline, pheniramine) reduce injection but have little effect on pruritus or swelling. Continued use may cause conjunctivitis medicamentosa.
- Topical corticosteroids are tertiary therapy for allergic conjunctivitis and consideration for strong topical steroids should prompt ophthalmology referral. Other indications for ophthalmology evaluation include persistent ocular complaints and consideration for systemic steroids.
- The difficulty of administrating eye drops and the frequency of dosing are the most common limiting factors. Some patients also complain about burning, stinging, and taste.

## ATOPIC DERMATITIS (ECZEMA)

- Atopic dermatitis is a chronic relapsing and remitting inflammatory skin disease characterized by dermatitis with typical morphology and distribution.
- Eczema is a generic term for dry skin, whereas atopic dermatitis is a specific subset of eczema.
- The overall prevalence of atopic dermatitis in the United States is up to 17% among school-aged children, leading to considerable disease-related morbidity, including irritability, secondary skin infections, sleep disturbance, school absenteeism, and poor self-image.

### History

- Age of onset is a consideration, with 45% of affected individuals manifesting atopic dermatitis in the first 6 months of life, 60% by the first year, and 90% by the age of five.
- Pruritus is a cardinal feature of eczema, often described as the "itch that rashes." Scratching leads to further compromise in the skin barrier and augments inflammation.
- Xerosis (dry skin) also involves nonlesional skin.
- (In other conditions, commonly mistaken for atopic dermatitis [seborrheic dermatitis, nummular eczema, and psoriasis], the uninvolved skin is generally healthy.)
- Patients may have a personal and family history of atopy (asthma, allergic rhinitis, food allergy).
- Approximately 70% family history of atopic diseases.
- Exacerbating factors include inhalant allergens (e.g., pet dander, house dust mite) and food allergens (egg, milk, wheat, soy, peanut, tree nuts, shellfish).
- Systemic involvement, with failure to thrive, chronic diarrhea, and/or recurrent infections should prompt consideration of underlying systemic disease, such as immunodeficiency (e.g., Wiskott-Aldrich syndrome, Netherton syndrome, immune dysregulation polyendocrinopathy enteropathy X-linked [IPEX] syndrome, and hyper-IgE syndrome) or malabsorption (e.g., zinc deficiency or cystic fibrosis).

### Physical Examination

- Xerosis
- Morphology of lesions
  - Acute lesions: pruritic papules with excoriation and serous exudation
  - Chronic lesions: lichenified papules and plaques
  - Superficial linear abrasions from scratching
  - Indistinct lesional borders, unlike that of psoriasis

- Areas of involvement. Although atopic dermatitis may appear anywhere on the body, characteristic patterns include:
  - Infants: cheeks, forehead, and extensor surface of extremities
  - Children/adolescents: flexor surface of extremities popliteal and antecubital fossae, and ventral surface of wrists and ankles
  - Atypical areas: diaper region (difficult for child to scratch) and nasolabial folds (commonly involved in seborrheic dermatitis)
- Other physical findings may include:
  - Nipple eczema
  - Ichthyosis, palmar hyperlinearity, keratosis pilaris
  - White dermatographism

## Evaluation

- Diagnosis is based on clinical features. Skin biopsy is not essential for diagnosis.
- Identify factors that exacerbate atopic dermatitis.
- Food allergy
  - One-third of children with moderate to severe atopic dermatitis experience worsening of eczema when exposed to food allergens within about 24 hours. Not typically associated with the classic immediate "allergic" food reaction.
  - Percutaneous skin tests, food-specific serum IgE, and oral food challenges may help identify specific foods.
- Aeroallergen sensitivity
- Infections
  - Bacteria. *Staphylococcus aureus* colonizes (cutaneous, nasal, or both) 80-90% of individuals with atopic dermatitis, potentially leading to superinfection and/or production of superantigens and augmenting cutaneous inflammation.
  - Cutaneous viruses
    ○ Herpes simplex virus (eczema herpeticum). These vesicles and/or individual "punched out" lesions have an erythematous base. Confirm by herpes simplex virus polymerase chain reaction test from a newly unroofed vesicle.
    ○ Molluscum contagiosum
  - *Malassezia sympodialis* (formerly *Pityrosporum ovale*): Consider in individuals with recalcitrant eczema, especially with lesions concentrated on the head, neck, and upper torso. Treatment is oral antifungal therapy (itraconazole).
- Differential diagnosis
  - Dermatologic disease: seborrheic dermatitis, psoriasis, nummular eczema, irritant or allergic contact dermatitis, keratosis pilaris, ichthyosis, lichen simplex chronicus, and Netherton syndrome
  - Infections: scabies, tinea corporis, tinea versicolor, and HIV-associated eczema
  - Metabolic disease: zinc or biotin deficiency and phenylketonuria
  - Immunodeficiency: see earlier discussion
  - Neoplastic disease: mycosis fungoides (cutaneous T-cell lymphoma) and Langerhans histiocytosis

## Treatment

- Limiting exposure to triggers
  - Nonspecific irritants: Wear nonocclusive clothing, and avoid wool or synthetic material.
  - Allergens: Eliminate contact with established allergic triggers (food or aeroallergen) if identified.

- Topical therapy
  - Emollients: Rehydration of the skin is key to stopping the "itch-scratch" cycle by the "soak and seal" method. Daily baths with lukewarm water for 10-20 minutes followed by application of a thick emollient are necessary. Minimize use of soap and products with fragrances.
  - Topical corticosteroids, which are the gold standard of therapy for treatment of acutely inflamed areas
    - Use mild to moderate potency corticosteroids in children (e.g., hydrocortisone 1% ointment and triamcinolone 0.1% ointment, respectively).
    - Use only mild potency corticosteroid on face, genital, and intertriginous areas.
  - Topical calcineurin inhibitors, such as pimecrolimus and tacrolimus.
    - Nonsteroidal topical agents effective in treating atopic dermatitis and are approved for children 2 years of age and older
    - A U.S. Food and Drug Administration "black box" warning for topical calcineurin inhibitors, recommending these drugs as second-line treatment options
  - Topical phosphodiesterase 4 inhibitor, crisaborole, has been approved for use in children 2 years of age and older with mild to moderate atopic dermatitis.
  - Wet-wrap therapy: This involves applying a damp wet layer of cotton dressing (or cotton pajamas) over the topical emollients and then placing a layer of dry clothing above.
- Antimicrobial therapy
  - Topical antiseptics (mupirocin, triclosan, or chlorhexidine) may be applied to open excoriated areas. Intranasal mupirocin may be used to eradicate nasal carriage of *S. aureus* if detected. Neomycin should be avoided because it can cause contact dermatitis.
  - Bleach baths, which may decrease colonization. Add 1-2 cups of household bleach per bathtub (adding a cup of table salt may diminish the stinging sensation). The use of bleach baths is typically twice a week.
  - Systemic antibiotics
    - If there is evidence of bacterial superinfection (e.g., honey-crusted lesions), systemic antistaphylococcal antibiotics are indicated; a 5- to 10-day course is usually sufficient.
    - Prophylactic therapy is not advised because of the emergence of bacterial resistance.
- Systemic corticosteroids: These agents are effective in short courses, but the systemic side-effect profile limits long-term applicability.
- Systemic antihistamines
  - The major therapeutic value of systemic antihistamines resides in the sedative effect of first-generation histamine blockers, which helps minimize scratching and discomfort when used as needed at night. Nonsedating antihistamines are generally ineffective in lessening the pruritus.
  - Topical antihistamines should be avoided because they may cause sensitization and worsen disease.
- Other therapies: ultraviolet light (PUVA), systemic cyclosporine, azathioprine, and immunotherapy
- Dupilumab is an IL-4 receptor subunit monoclonal antibody that has been approved for the use of atopic dermatitis in children with uncontrolled moderate to severe atopic dermatitis 6 years of age and older.

## Special Considerations

- Associated atopic disorders: Atopic dermatitis in early childhood may herald progression toward other allergic conditions. This is known as the atopic march (allergic rhinitis and asthma).

- Prevention
  - No specific prevention policy has demonstrated consistent benefits, including probiotics, moisturizer therapy in infancy, and breastfeeding.
- Natural history: Remission of atopic dermatitis varies depending upon the age of presentation. In children with symptoms starting in the first 2 years of life, 43% had remission by 3 years of age. Severity and atopic sensitization were associated with more significant disease.

## ASTHMA

### Definition

- Asthma is a reversible obstructive lung disease that is characterized by airway inflammation and hyperreactivity with airway mucosal edema, bronchoconstriction, and mucous plugging.
- Clinically, asthma presents with recurrent episodes of wheezing, coughing, chest tightness, shortness of breath, and increased work of breathing.
- Diagnosis is based on history, presence of wheezing, coughing, and increased work of breathing that resolves in response to treatment with bronchodilators and corticosteroids. Many conditions may present with wheezing and must be considered, especially in patients who present with a first episode of wheezing and/or are not responsive to asthma therapy (Table 11-2).

### History

- History of current episode: precipitating factors, onset and progression of symptoms, treatment, and response to treatment
- Chronic history
  - Age of first episode, age at time of diagnosis, and course of the illness over time; typical signs and symptoms as well as precipitating factors (triggers)
  - Medication use: dosage, frequency, route, and schedule of all quick relief and control medications; effect of missed doses of medications; side effects; and adverse reactions. Review inhaled medication administration technique.
  - Assessment of chronic asthma severity (the intrinsic intensity of the disease process) to initiate therapy
    ○ Determine severity by quantifying frequency of daytime symptoms, nighttime symptoms, rescue β-agonist use, and interference with activity.
    ○ See Table 11-3, assessing both domains of impairment (frequency and intensity of symptoms and functional impairment the patient is currently experiencing or

| TABLE 11-2 | Differential Diagnosis for Wheezing Not Responsive to Asthma Therapy | |
| --- | --- | --- |
| **Infection** | **Mass** | |
| Foreign body | Bronchopulmonary dysplasia | |
| Anatomic abnormalities | Congestive heart failure | |
| Allergy | Cystic fibrosis | |
| Sinusitis | Chronic aspiration | |
| Vocal cord dysfunction | Gastroesophageal reflux disease | |

**TABLE 11-3  Classifying Asthma Severity and Initiating Therapy in Children**

### Classifying asthma severity and initiating therapy in children

| Components of severity | | Intermittent Ages 0-4 | Intermittent Ages 5-11 | Persistent Mild Ages 0-4 | Persistent Mild Ages 5-11 | Persistent Moderate Ages 0-4 | Persistent Moderate Ages 5-11 | Persistent Severe Ages 0-4 | Persistent Severe Ages 5-11 |
|---|---|---|---|---|---|---|---|---|---|
| **Impairment** | Symptoms | ≤2 days/week | ≤2 days/week | >2 days/week but not daily | >2 days/week but not daily | Daily | Daily | Throughout the day | Throughout the day |
| | Nighttime awakenings | 0 | ≤2x/month | 1-2x/month | 3-4x/month | 3-4x/month | >1x/week but not nightly | >1x/week | Often 7x/week |
| | Short-acting beta₂-agonist use for symptom control | ≤2 days/week | ≤2 days/week | >2 days/week but not daily | >2 days/week but not daily | Daily | Daily | Several times per day | Several times per day |
| | Interference with normal activity | None | None | Minor limitation | Minor limitation | Some limitation | Some limitation | Extremely limited | Extremely limited |
| | Lung Function • $FEV_1$ (predicted) or peak flow (personal best) | N/A | Normal $FEV_1$ between exacerbations >80% | N/A | >80% | N/A | 60-80% | N/A | <60% |
| | • $FEV_1/FVC$ | | >85% | | >80% | | 75-80% | | <75% |
| **Risk** | Exacerbations requiring oral systemic corticosteroids (consider severity and interval since last exacerbation) | 0-1/year (see notes) | 0-1/year (see notes) | ≥2 exacerbations in 6 months requiring oral systemic corticosteroids, or >4 wheezing episodes/1 year lasting >1 day AND risk factors for persistent asthma | ≥2x/year (see notes) Relative annual risk may be related to $FEV_1$ | ≥2 exacerbations in 6 months requiring oral systemic corticosteroids, or >4 wheezing episodes/1 year lasting >1 day AND risk factors for persistent asthma | ≥2x/year (see notes) Relative annual risk may be related to $FEV_1$ | ≥2 exacerbations in 6 months requiring oral systemic corticosteroids, or >4 wheezing episodes/1 year lasting >1 day AND risk factors for persistent asthma | ≥2x/year (see notes) Relative annual risk may be related to $FEV_1$ |
| **Recommended Step for Initiating Therapy** (See "Stepwise Approach for Managing Asthma" for treatment steps.) The stepwise approach is meant to assist, not replace, the clinical decision making required to meet individual patient needs. | | Step 1 (for both age groups) | Step 1 (for both age groups) | Step 2 (for both age groups) | Step 2 (for both age groups) | Step 3 and consider short course of oral systemic corticosteroids | Step 3: medium-dose ICS option and consider short course of oral systemic corticosteroids | Step 3: consider short course of oral systemic corticosteroids | Step 3: medium-dose ICS option OR step 4 and consider short course of oral systemic corticosteroids |

In 2-6 weeks, depending on severity, evaluate level of asthma control that is achieved.
- Children 0-4 years old: If no clear benefit is observed in 4-6 weeks, stop treatment and consider alternative diagnoses or adjusting therapy.
- Children 5-11 years old: Adjust therapy accordingly.

Key: FEV, forced expiratory volume in 1 second; FVC, forced vital capacity; ICS, inhaled corticosteroids; ICU, intensive care unit; N/A, not applicable

Notes:
- Level of severity is determined by both impairment and risk. Assess impairment domain by caregiver's recall of previous 2-4 weeks. Assign severity to the most severe category in which any feature occurs.
- Frequency and severity of exacerbations may fluctuate over time for patients in any severity category. At present, there are inadequate data to correspond frequencies of exacerbations with different levels of asthma severity. In general, more frequent and severe exacerbations (e.g., requiring urgent, unscheduled care, hospitalization, or ICU admission) indicate greater underlying disease severity. For treatment purposes, patients with ≥2 exacerbations described above may be considered the same as patients who have persistent asthma, even in the absence of impairment levels consistent with persistent asthma.

(Continued)

**TABLE 11-3  Classifying Asthma Severity and Initiating Therapy in Children (Continued)**

| Components of severity | | Classification of asthma severity ≥12 years of age | | | | |
|---|---|---|---|---|---|---|
| | | Intermittent | Persistent | | | |
| | | | Mild | Moderate | Severe | |
| **Impairment**<br><br>Normal FEV₁/FVC:<br>8-19 year 85%<br>20-39 year 80%<br>40-59 year 75%<br>60-80 year 70% | Symptoms | ≤2 days/week | >2 days/week but not daily | Daily | Throughout the day | |
| | Nighttime awakenings | ≤2×/month | 3-4×/month | >1×/week but not nightly | Often 7×/week | |
| | Short-acting beta₂-agonist use for symptom control (not prevention of EIB) | ≤2 days/week | >2 days/week but not daily, and not more than 1× on any day | Daily | Several times per day | |
| | Interference with normal activity | None | Minor limitation | Some limitation | Extremely limited | |
| | Lung function | • Normal FEV₁ between exacerbations<br>• FEV₁ >80% predicted<br>• FEV₁/FVC normal | • FEV₁ >80% predicted<br>• FEV₁/FVC normal | • FEV₁ >80% but <80% predicted<br>• FEV₁/FVC reduced 5% | • FEV₁ <60% predicted<br>• FEV₁/FVC reduced >5% | |
| **Risk** | Exacerbations requiring oral systemic corticosteroids | 0-1/year (see note) | ≥2/year (see note) | | | |
| | | Consider severity and interval since last exacerbation. Frequency and severity may fluctuate over time for patients in any severity category. Relative annual risk of exacerbations may be related to FEV₁. | | | | |
| **Recommended Step for Initiating Treatment** (See "Stepwise Approach for Managing Asthma" for treatment steps.) | | Step 1 | Step 2 | Step 3 and consider short course of oral systemic corticosteroids | Step 4 or 5 and consider short course of oral systemic corticosteroids | |
| | | In 2-6 weeks, evaluate level of asthma control that is achieved and adjust therapy accordingly. | | | | |

Key: EIB, exercise-induced bron-chospasm; FEV₁, forced expiratory volume in 1 second; FVC, forced vital capacity; ICU, intensive care unit

**Notes:**

- The stepwise approach is meant to assist, not replace, the clinical decisionmaking required to meet individual patient needs.
- Level of severity is determined by assessment of both impairment and risk. Assess impairment domain by patient's/caregiver's recall of previous 2-4 weeks and spirometry. Assign severity to the most severe category in which any feature occurs.
- At present, there are inadequate data to correspond frequencies of exacerbations with different levels of asthma severity. In general, more frequent and intense exacerbations (e.g., requiring urgent, unscheduled care, hospitalization, or ICU admission) indicate greater underlying disease severity. For treatment purposes, patients who had ≥2 exacerbations requiring oral systemic corticosteroids in the past year may be considered the same as patients who have persistent asthma, even in the absence of impairment levels consistent with persistent asthma.

From the National Heart, Lung, and Blood Institute, National Institutes of Health. Guidelines for the diagnosis and management of asthma. NIH Publication No. 97–4051, July 1997.

has recently experienced) and risk (the likelihood of asthma exacerbations, progressive decline in lung function or growth, or risk of adverse effects of medications). This classification scheme is most appropriate for patients who are not receiving controller therapy.
- Assessment of asthma control to adjust therapy
  ○ Determine number of school days missed because of asthma; number of previous emergency visits and admissions, including intensive care with or without intubation; prior use of oral corticosteroids, including number of previous corticosteroid bursts and date of last corticosteroid course; and frequency of albuterol usage.
  ○ Use Table 11-4, assessing both domains of impairment and risk, to determine level of asthma control. This approach is most appropriate for patients already receiving controller therapy.
- Environmental history: exposure to allergens (mold, pollen, animals, dust mites, cockroaches) and nonspecific airway irritants (smoke, odors).
- Review of systems
  ○ Focus on allergy; eczema; infection, especially pneumonia, ear, nose, and throat, including otitis media, sinusitis; airway abnormalities; surgery and obstructive sleep apnea; and gastrointestinal, including gastroesophageal reflux, nutrition, and growth.
  ○ Previous testing (e.g., chest radiograph, pulmonary function testing, allergy testing, and sweat test) should be documented.
- Family history: asthma, allergy, eczema, and cystic fibrosis
- Social history to determine barriers to health care, particularly insurance coverage and transportation

## Physical Examination
- A rapid assessment should be initially performed to determine patients requiring immediate attention.
- Assessment should include color, vital signs, oxygen saturation, quality of air exchange, presence of wheezing or crackles, ratio of time spent in inspiration relative to expiration, accessory muscle use, ability to speak in sentences, and mental status.
- See Table 11-5 for a guide to normal respiratory rate by age.

## Laboratory Studies
- A chest radiograph is not routinely required but may be considered during the first episode of wheezing, if the patient is febrile, has marked asymmetry on chest examination, or there is poor response to treatment.
- Pulse oximetry can be used to estimate oxygen saturation.
- Arterial blood gas measurement should be considered in patients in severe distress or with increasing supplemental oxygen requirement. Capillary blood gas measurement is of limited value in evaluation of oxygenation.
- Spirometry is not typically performed in the inpatient or emergency department setting or is it used to establish the diagnosis of asthma; spirometry does demonstrate airway obstruction, as well as reversibility of obstruction.
- Fractional exhaled nitric oxide (FeNO) is a measure of type 2 airway inflammation. It may help to confirm the diagnosis of asthma in patients ≥5 years of age.
- Chest fluoroscopy or bronchoscopy should be considered if the history suggests possibility of foreign body aspiration.

## TABLE 11-4 Assessing Asthma Control and Adjusting Therapy in Children

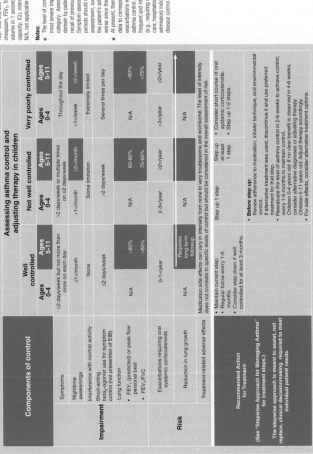

### Assessing asthma control and adjusting therapy in children

| Components of control | | Well controlled Ages 0-4 | Well controlled Ages 5-11 | Not well controlled Ages 0-4 | Not well controlled Ages 5-11 | Very poorly controlled Ages 0-4 | Very poorly controlled Ages 5-11 |
|---|---|---|---|---|---|---|---|
| **Impairment** | Symptoms | ≤2 days/week but not more than once on each day | | >2 days/week or multiple times on ≤2 days/week | | Throughout the day | |
| | Nighttime awakenings | ≤1x/month | ≤1x/month | >1x/month | ≥2x/month | >1x/week | ≥2x/week |
| | Interference with normal activity | None | | Some limitation | | Extremely limited | |
| | Short-acting beta₂-agonist use for symptom control (not prevention of EIB) | ≤2 days/week | | >2 days/week | | Several times per day | |
| | Lung function • $FEV_1$ (predicted) or peak flow personal best • $FEV_1/FVC$ | N/A N/A | >80% >80% | N/A | 60-80% 75-80% | N/A | <60% <75% |
| **Risk** | Exacerbations requiring oral systemic corticosteroids | N/A | 0-1x/year | N/A | 2-3x/year ≥2x/year | N/A | >3x/year ≥2x/year |
| | Reduction in lung growth | N/A | Requires long-term followup | N/A | | N/A | |
| | Treatment-related adverse effects | Medication side effects can vary in intensity from none to very troublesome and worrisome. The level of intensity does not correlate to specific levels of control but should be considered in the overall assessment of risk. | | | | | |
| **Recommended Action for Treatment** (See "Stepwise Approach for Managing Asthma" for treatment steps.) The stepwise approach is meant to assist, not replace, clinical decisionmaking required to meet individual patient needs. | | • Maintain current step. • Regular follow every 1-6 months. • Consider step down if well controlled for at least 3 months. | | Step up 1 step | Step up at least 1 step | • Consider short course of oral systemic corticosteroids. • Step up 1-2 steps. | |

**Before step up:**
- Review adherence to medication, inhaler technique, and environmental control.
- If alternative treatment was used, discontinue it and use preferred treatment for that step.
- Reevaluate the level of asthma control in 2-6 weeks to achieve control; every 1-6 months to maintain control.
- Children 0-4 years old. If no clear benefit is observed in 4-6 weeks, consider alternative diagnoses or adjusting therapy.
- Children 5-11 years old. Adjust therapy accordingly.
- For side effects, consider alternative treatment options.

Key: EIB, exercise-induced bronchospasm; $FEV_1$, forced expiratory volume in 1 second; FVC, forced vital capacity; ICU, intensive care unit; N/A, not applicable

**Notes:**
- The level of control is based on the most severe impairment or risk category. Assess impairment domain by patient's or caregiver's recall of previous 2-4 weeks. Symptom assessment for longer periods should reflect a global assessment, such as whether the patient's asthma is better or worse since the last visit.
- At present, there are inadequate data to correspond frequencies of exacerbations with different levels of asthma control. In general, more frequent and intense exacerbations (e.g., requiring urgent, unscheduled care, hospitalization, or ICU admission) indicate poorer disease control.

| Components of control | | | Classification of asthma control (≥12 years of age) | | |
|---|---|---|---|---|---|
| | | | Well controlled | Not well controlled | Very poorly controlled |
| Impairment | Symptoms | | ≤2 days/week | >2 days/week | Throughout the day |
| | Nighttime awakenings | | ≤2x/month | 1a3x/week | ≥4x/week |
| | Interference with normal activity | | None | Some limitation | Extremely limited |
| | Short-acting beta-agonist use for symptom control (not prevention of EIB) | | ≤2 days/week | >2 days/week | Several times per day |
| | FEV₁ or peak flow | | >80% predicted/personal best | 60-80% predicted/personal best | <60% predicted/personal best |
| | Validated questionnaires | ATAQ ACQ ACT | 0 ≤0.75* ≥20 | 1-2 ≥1.5 16-19 | 3-4 N/A ≤15 |
| Risk | Exacerbations requiring oral systemic corticosteroids | | 0-1/year | ≥2/year (see note) | |
| | | | | Consider severity and interval since last exacerbation | |
| | Progressive loss of lung function | | Evaluation requires long-term followup care | | |
| | Treatment-related adverse effects | | Medication side effects can vary in intensity from none to very troublesome and worrisome. The level of intensity does not correlate to specific levels of control but should be considered in the overall assessment of risk. | | |
| Recommended Action for Treatment (See "Stepwise Approach for Managing Asthma" for treatment steps.) | | | • Maintain current step. • Regular followup at every 1-6 months to maintain control. • Consider step down if well controlled for at least 3 months. | • Step up 1 step. • Reevaluate in 2-6 weeks. • For side effects, consider alternative treatment options. | • Consider short course of oral systemic corticosteroids. • Step up 1-2 steps. • Reevaluate in 2 weeks. • For side effects, consider alternative treatment options. |

*ACQ values of 0.76-1.4 are indeterminate regarding well-controlled asthma.

Key: EIB, exercise-induced bronchospasm; ICU, intensive care unit

### Notes:

- The stepwise approach is meant to assist, not replace, the clinical decisionmaking required to meet individual patient needs.
- The level of control is based on the most severe impairment or risk category. Assess impairment domain by patient's recall of previous 2-4 weeks and by spirometry/or peak flow measures. Symptom assessment for longer periods should reflect a global assessment, such as inquiring whether the patient's asthma is better or worse since the last visit.
- At present, there are inadequate data to correspond frequencies of exacerbations with different levels of asthma control. In general, more frequent and intense exacerbations (e.g., requiring urgent, unscheduled care, hospitalization, or ICU admission) indicate poorer disease control. For treatment purposes, patients who had ≥2 exacerbations requiring oral systemic corticosteroids in the past year may be considered the same as patients who have not-well-controlled asthma, even in the absence of impairment levels consistent with not-well-controlled asthma.

ATAQ = Asthma Therapy Assessment Questionnaire©
ACQ = Asthma Control Questionnaire©
ACT = Asthma Control Test™
Minimal Important
Difference: 1.0 for the ATAQ; 0.5 for the ACQ; not determined for the ACT.

### Before step up in therapy:

— Review adherence to medication, inhaler technique, environmental control, and comorbid conditions.

— If an alternative treatment option was used in a step, discontinue and use the preferred treatment for that step.

From the National Heart, Lung, and Blood Institute. National Institutes of Health. Guidelines for the diagnosis and management of asthma. NIH Publication No. 97-4051, July 1997.

| TABLE 11-5 | Respiratory Rate for Children by Age |
| --- | --- |
| Age | Normal rate |
| <2 months | 60 bpm[a] |
| 2-12 months | 50 bpm |
| 1-5 years | 40 bpm |
| 6-11 years | 30 bpm |
| 12 and older | 20 bpm |

[a]Breaths per minute.

- White blood cell (WBC) count, potassium, and glucose levels may be affected by β-agonists and oral corticosteroids (elevated total WBC and blood glucose, low levels of potassium). Thus, these studies are likely be of little value during an acute exacerbation.
- A nasopharyngeal swab or aspirate may be helpful in identifying viral infection and to guide establishing cohorts of patients within the hospital.
- A sweat chloride test may be performed to evaluate for cystic fibrosis as the cause of chronic symptoms.

### Treatment during Acute Episode

- Oxygen should be administered to maintain oxygen saturation 90% and above.
  - If possible, obtain baseline oxygen saturation in room air before initiating oxygen. Oxygen saturation may drop transiently after albuterol treatments; this is likely due to ventilation-perfusion mismatch and usually resolves in 15-30 minutes.
  - Continuous oximetry is not typically necessary.
  - Check $Spo_2$ with any significant change in respiratory status. As symptoms improve, wean oxygen as tolerated.
- Traditionally, use of inhaled $\beta_2$-agonists has been the preferred treatment of acute symptoms/exacerbation of asthma. However, in 2020, both the Global Initiative for Asthma (GINA) and the National Heart, Lung, and Blood Institute (NHLBI) Asthma Guidelines added the use of inhaled corticosteroids (ICS) combined with formoterol to reverse airflow obstruction quickly in certain patients. It is important to note that while reliever treatment with ICS/formoterol may be recommended, it is not currently approved by the Food and Drug Administration (FDA) for use in this manner. NHBLI distinguishes use of inhaled $\beta_2$-agonists versus ICS/formoterol as follows:
  - In children ages 0-4 years, albuterol is the only recommended reliever medication.
  - In children 5-11 years of age with intermittent or mild persistent asthma, albuterol is the preferred PRN reliever medication. In children ages 5-11 years with moderate persistent asthma, ICS/formoterol for rescue up to 8 puffs/day is the preferred PRN reliever medication. In children aged 5-11 years with severe asthma, albuterol is the preferred reliever medication.
  - In patients ≥12 years of age, with intermittent or mild persistent asthma, albuterol is the preferred PRN reliever medication. In patients ≥12 years of age with moderate asthma, ICS/formoterol is the preferred PRN reliever medication, up to 12 puffs/day. In patients ≥12 years of age with severe persistent asthma, albuterol is

the preferred PRN reliever medication. PRN concomitant ICS and albuterol is an option for patients ages ≥12 years with mild persistent asthma.

- If exacerbation is mild, two to four puffs of albuterol by metered dose inhaler (MDI) may be given with spacer every 20 minutes for 1 hour as initial therapy. Albuterol may also be given via nebulizer.
- During hospitalization, albuterol nebulization treatments (2.5-5 mg) are provided every 1-2 hours and gradually weaned to every 4 hours as the patient's symptoms and status improve.
  - MDI with valved holding chamber may be as effective as nebulized therapy. Administer 8 puffs in place of 5 mg per nebulizer and 2-4 puffs in place of 2.5 mg per nebulizer.
  - Patients whose clinical status tolerates albuterol treatments every 4 hours are usually discharged home.
- Systemic corticosteroids, typically prednisone/prednisolone 2 mg/kg/day (60 mg maximum dose), are given promptly on presentation and typically continued daily for 5 days, typically administered in the morning.
  - Oral dosing is preferred, but intravenous (IV) therapy may be appropriate if the patient is vomiting or intensive care therapy seems likely. If IV Solu-Medrol is necessary, it is recommended to divide dose for every 6-hour administration.
  - Tapering corticosteroids over a longer period of time is recommended for severe exacerbations or if recent (<1 month), course of oral corticosteroids.
- Ipratropium bromide (Atrovent) 0.5 mg may provide additional bronchodilator effect when added to nebulized albuterol treatments during the first 24 hours of the exacerbation. There is no evidence that use after the first 24 hours provides additional benefit.
- Consider magnesium 40 mg/kg/dose (max 2 g) IV for children over 2 years of age with moderate or severe episode. Administer NS bolus 20 mL/kg following magnesium to prevent hypotension.
- Antibiotics have not been shown to be effective when administered routinely for acute asthma exacerbation but may be prescribed for coexisting conditions, such as pneumonia or bacterial sinusitis.
- Medications previously prescribed for control of chronic asthma should be continued during the acute episode to reinforce schedule and technique. If asthma history indicates lack of control with current regimen, see later discussion of Daily Management of Pediatric Asthma for options to optimize home plan to achieve better control.
- Treatments not recommended in the hospital setting include methylxanthine infusions, aggressive hydration, chest physical therapy, incentive spirometry, mucolytics, and sedation.
- Discharge plan after acute episode
  - Patients discharged home from the emergency department may be given a short-term Asthma Action Plan with directions to return to the primary care provider in 3-5 days.
  - Patients discharged home from the inpatient area should be given a home management plan that includes an Asthma Action Plan with quick-relief medicines and control medicines if indicated by chronic severity and an appointment with their primary care physician (see Fig. 11-1).
  - Patients and families should be educated in the use of the Asthma Action Plan and medication administration. Patients may use albuterol MDI with spacer on the day

**Children's**
HOSPITAL · ST. LOUIS
BJC HealthCare

# Asthma Action Plan

## Green Zone: Well

- No signs of asthma
- Able to do normal activities
- No problems while sleeping

- Peak flow above: _____
  (above 80% of best)

★ Rinse mouth after this medicine

Give these medicines every day:

| MEDICINE: | HOW MUCH: | WHEN: |
|-----------|-----------|-------|

## Yellow Zone: Watch Out!

### Early Signs of Asthma:
- Cold symptoms
- Coughing day or night
- Wheezing day or night
- Funny feeling in chest

- My first sign: _____

- Peak flow: _____
  (50-80% of best)

First — give:
- ■ Albuterol      2-4 puffs or 1 nebulizer      1-3 times in first hour

■ Call your Doctor or Nurse if not in Green Zone after first hour.

Next — if asthma is better after first hour, you may give:
- ■ Albuterol      2-4 puffs or 1 nebulizer      every 4 hours as needed

Call your Doctor or Nurse if:
- ■ Albuterol needed more often than every 4 hours.
- ■ Albuterol needed every 4 hours for more than 1 day.

Keep taking other Green Zone medicines.

## Red Zone: EMERGENCY!

### Late Signs of Asthma:
- Tight chest
- Breathing hard or fast
- Using neck or stomach muscles to breathe
- Constant coughing
- Trouble talking or walking
- Vomiting
- Lips or nails blue

- Peak flow below: _____
  (below 50% of best)

First — give *now*:
- ■ Albuterol      6 puffs or 1 nebulizer
- ■ AND call your Doctor or Nurse.

Next — if you cannot reach your Doctor or Nurse *immediately*, give:
- ■ Albuterol      6 puffs or 1 nebulizer
- _____ (oral steroid)
- ■ AND go to the nearest emergency room or call 911.

Patient/Parent/Guardian Signature          Date

RN/MD Signature          Date

Phone number of Doctor or Nurse:
Day: _____
Night: _____

Original 1995. Revised 10/12. Copyright © 2012

**Figure 11-1. St. Louis Children's Hospital Asthma Action Plan.** (Courtesy of St. Louis Children's Hospital.)

of discharge. Patients should have prescriptions and all equipment (e.g., spacers, nebulizer) before discharge.

- It is usually recommended that the patient receive albuterol every 4-6 hours for 1 week or until follow-up appointment.

## Daily Management of Pediatric Asthma

*Control of Asthma*

- The following goals of therapy have been established by the National Heart, Lung, and Blood Institute (NHLBI).
  - Reduce impairment: frequency and intensity of symptoms as well as the functional impairment the patient is currently experiencing (or has recently experienced)
    - Prevent asthma symptoms.
    - Reduce need for inhaled short-acting β-agonist (≤2 days per week).
    - Maintain normal lung function.
    - Exercise and go to school regularly.
    - Meet patients' and families' expectations of and satisfaction with asthma care.
  - Reduce risk: likelihood of asthma exacerbations, progressive decline in lung function or growth, or risk of side effects of medications
    - Prevent recurrent exacerbations and minimize emergency visits or hospital admissions.
    - Prevent loss of lung function and reduced lung growth.
    - Provide optimal pharmacotherapy with no side effects from asthma medication.
- The NHLBI's Stepwise Approach for Managing Asthma should serve as a guideline for decision-making to meet the individual needs of the patient (Fig. 11-2).
- Provide a written Asthma Action Plan that includes medications used daily for control as well as quick relief medications for acute episodes. This plan serves as a guide for self-monitoring and self-management (see Fig. 11-1).
- Severe exacerbations can occur in patients at any level of asthma severity or control. Patients at high risk for asthma-related death require special attention, including intensive education, monitoring, and care. Such patients should be encouraged to seek care early during an exacerbation. Risk factors for asthma-related death include:
- Previous severe exacerbation
- Two or more hospitalizations or three emergency department visits in the past year
- Use of >2 canisters of short-acting β-agonist (SABA) per month
- Poor perception of airway obstruction or worsening asthma
- Low socioeconomic status or inner city residence
- Illicit drug use
- Major psychosocial problems or psychiatric disease
- Comorbidities, such as cardiovascular disease or other chronic lung disease

*Controlling Precipitating Factors (Triggers)*

- Take history to identify factors that precipitate asthma and recommend controls.
- Prioritize based on family's individual situation.
- Give written recommendations to patient and family.
- Allergens
  - For patients who do not have allergies to indoor allergens, environmental interventions are not recommended.
  - For patients with asthma with a specific indoor allergen, verified by clinical history or allergy testing, it is recommended to utilize a multicomponent allergen-specific mitigation intervention.
  - For patients with asthma who are allergic and exposed to pests (i.e., cockroaches or rodents), integrated pest management is recommended.
  - Subcutaneous immunotherapy (SCIT) is recommended for patients who have positive allergy testing, along with worsening asthma symptoms with exposure to the allergens in which they are sensitized; SCIT should not be administered to those with poorly controlled asthma, or those with severe asthma.

## AGES 0-4 YEARS: STEPWISE APPROACH FOR MANAGEMENT OF ASTHMA

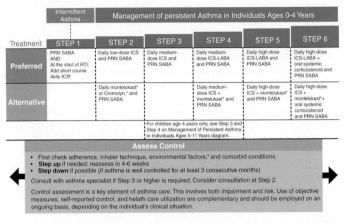

**Abbreviations**: ICS, inhaled corticosteroid: LABA, long-acting beta$_2$-agonist: SABA, inhaled short-acting beta$_2$-agonist: RTI, respiratory tract infection: PRN, as needed

▴ Updated based on the 2020 guidelines.

* Cromolyn and montelukast were not considered for this update and/or have limited availability for use in the United States. The FDA issued a Boxed Warning for montelukast in march 2020.

## AGES 5-11 YEARS: STEPWISE APPROACH FOR MANAGEMENT OF ASTHMA

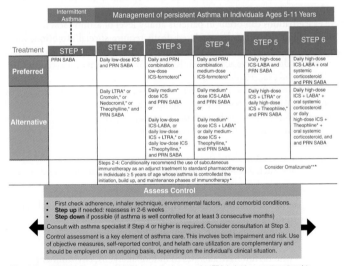

**Abbreviations**: ICS, inhaled corticosteroid: LABA, long-acting beta$_2$-agonist: LTRA, leukotriene receptor antagonist: SABA, inhaled short-acting beta$_2$-agonist

* Updated based on the 2020 guidelines.

* Cromolyn, Nedocromil, LTRAs including montelukast, and Thephyline were not considered in this update and/or have limited availability for use in the United States, and/or have an increased risk of adverse consequences and need for monitoring that make their use less desirable. The FDA issued a Boxed Warning for montelukast in march 2020.

** Omalizumab is the only asthma biologic currently FDA-approved for this age range.

**Figure 11-2. Stepwise approach to management of asthma in children. A.** Ages 0-4 years. **B.** Ages 5-11 years. **C.** Ages 12+ years. (Reprinted from Expert Panel Working Group of the National Heart, Lung, and Blood Institute (NHLBI) administered and coordinated National Asthma Education and Prevention Program Coordinating Committee (NAEPPCC); Cloutier MM, Baptist AP, Blake KV, et al. 2020 Focused updates to the asthma management guidelines: a report from the National Asthma Education and Prevention Program Coordinating Committee Expert Panel Working Group. J Allergy Clin Immunol 2020;146(6):1217–1270, with permission from Elsevier.)

**AGES 12+ YEARS:** STEPWISE APPROACH FOR MANAGEMENT OF ASTHMA

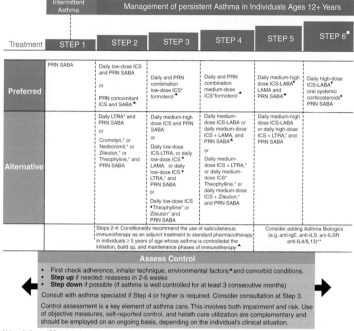

Figure 11-2. (*Continued*)

- Weather. Stay indoors if there is changing weather or poor air quality.
- Colds and viruses. Influenza vaccination annually.
- Irritants. Do not smoke in the house or car. Avoid perfumes and strong odors.
- Exercise. Work out a medical plan to allow exercise. Have quick-relief medicine available during exercise.

## Patient Education

- Individualized education of the patient and family is crucial to successful self-management of asthma.
- Assessment of understanding of the Asthma Action Plan (see Fig. 11-1), correct medication administration technique, and correct use of the peak flow meter (when applicable) should be reinforced at each visit. Reeducate family as needed, especially when changes are made to the management plan.
- Psychosocial issues should be addressed, and patients and families should be referred to support agencies when needed.

## URTICARIA AND ANGIOEDEMA

- Urticaria (hives) are raised, pruritic skin lesions with pale centers that blanch with pressure and are surrounded with erythema.
  - Individual lesions last <24 hours and resolve without leaving any sequelae.
  - Acute urticaria affects approximately 15-25% of people during their lifetime.
- Angioedema is nonpitting, nondependent, asymmetric, localized swelling without overlying erythema.
  - Commonly affected areas are lips, eyelids, tongue, hands, feet, or other highly vascular tissues.
  - Angioedema is generally not pruritic but sometimes causes pain if overlying skin is stretched.
- Urticaria and angioedema can both be caused by release of mediators from mast cells in the skin and subcutaneous tissue.

### Acute Urticaria (With or Without Angioedema)
Episodes of urticaria lasting <6 weeks

*Etiology*
- Multiple mechanisms can activate mast cells. Episodes can be caused by IgE-mediated mechanisms, but a significant proportion is not IgE-mediated.
- Infections: In children, acute urticaria is most commonly caused by an infectious etiology, including respiratory or enteroviruses.
- Idiopathic or spontaneous: No trigger is identified.
- Food: See Food allergy below.
- Insect stings or bites: honeybee, wasp, hornet, yellow jacket, and fire ant. Concerning symptoms related to stings should be evaluated by an allergist.
- Medications: IgE or non–IgE-mediated mechanisms. Most common drugs are antibiotics. Other medications that can cause non–IgE-mediated mast cell degranulation include opiates and nonsteroidal anti-inflammatory drugs (NSAIDs).
- Aeroallergen exposure: Contact with animal dander, trees, grasses, weeds, and inhalation or contact with latex.

*Evaluation*
- The most valuable step is a detailed history and physical examination.
- Percutaneous skin testing or specific IgE is indicated only if clinical history suggests an IgE-mediated cause. The majority of acute urticaria in children does not have features that stipulate testing.
- Specific tests for infectious etiologies suggested by history can be completed only if they will change infectious disease management.

*Treatment*
- Second-generation $H_1$ antihistamines (cetirizine, desloratadine, fexofenadine, levocetirizine, loratadine) are preferred.
- Glucocorticoids are not routinely used. However, a short course of oral glucocorticoids can be considered in episodes that have not responded quickly or completely to antihistamines.
- If an avoidable cause of acute urticaria is identified, the trigger should be avoided.
- If there is concern for systemic symptoms consistent with anaphylaxis, please refer to the Anaphylaxis section below.

## Chronic Urticaria (With or Without Angioedema)

Episodes of urticaria occurring for >6 weeks

### Etiology

* An identifiable cause cannot be determined in the majority of patients with chronic urticaria.
* Prevalence estimate is 0.5-5% in the general population (including adults).
* Types of chronic urticaria include:
  * Chronic spontaneous (idiopathic) urticaria: No identifiable trigger or secondary cause is found.
  * Chronic autoimmune urticaria: Due to presence of autoantibodies against the high-affinity IgE receptor on mast cells.
  * Papular urticaria: Immunologic hypersensitivity to the saliva of the biting insects.
  * Physical urticaria: Triggers may include mechanical (dermatographism and delayed pressure urticaria), thermal (cold- and heat-induced urticaria), exercise/sweating (cholinergic urticaria), vibration, UV radiation (solar urticaria), and water (aquagenic).
  * Others: Muckle-Wells syndrome and familial cold autoinflammatory syndrome may cause urticaria. Autoimmune disorders such as systemic lupus erythematosus should be considered when other features are present.
* Other urticarial disorders include:
  * Urticarial vasculitis: Lesions can last >24 hours, be painful or burning, be non-blanching and leave bruising or hyperpigmentation.
  * Urticaria pigmentosa: This rash of cutaneous mastocytosis is typified by red-brown macules that urticate when scratched.

### Evaluation

* A detailed history and physical examination is critical to identify one of the above forms of disease.
* Special consideration should be given to the duration of each specific wheal. Lesions that last >24 hours could be consistent with urticarial vasculitis or delayed pressure urticaria.
* Challenge tests for physical urticaria include dermatographism (an immediate wheal-and-flare response on stroking the skin), ice cube test (cold urticaria), or pressure testing.
* Consult dermatology for consideration of skin biopsy if there is suspicion for vasculitis or mastocytosis.
* In vitro tests for anti-FcεRI antibodies and histamine release assays for autoimmune urticaria are commercially available. Positive testing identifies a diagnosis but does not change clinical management.
* In the absence of atypical features, laboratory testing is unlikely to yield clinically significant findings in the majority of patients.

### Treatment

* Second-generation $H_1$ antihistamines are first-line therapy (see Acute Urticaria, Treatment).
* If not controlled on second-generation $H_1$ antihistamine therapy, the following options should be considered:
  * Double the dose of second-generation $H_1$ antihistamine as long as not sedated.
  * Add an additional second-generation $H_1$ antihistamine.
  * Add an $H_2$ antihistamine (cimetidine, ranitidine).
  * Add a leukotriene receptor antagonist (montelukast-black box warning for neuropsychiatric events as in the Allergic Rhinitis section).

- Omalizumab (antihuman IgE antibody) monthly is FDA-approved for children ≥12 years of age with chronic urticaria unresponsive to antihistamine therapy.
- Oral glucocorticoids should be reserved for individuals who cannot be controlled with combinations of the above medications and only used in short courses to limit side effects.

## Angioedema (Without Urticaria)

- Angioedema that is unaccompanied by urticaria or pruritus and is not responsive to antihistamine therapy should prompt evaluation for specific underlying causes.
- Hereditary angioedema (HAE), or C1 esterase inhibitor deficiency, is an autosomal dominant condition. The cause is deficiency of C1 esterase inhibitor in 85% and a nonfunctional C1 esterase inhibitor protein in 15% of cases. There are rare cases of HAE with normal C1 esterase inhibitor.
- Acquired C1 esterase inhibitor deficiency is very rare in children and usually associated with B-cell proliferation disorders. The C1q level is reduced in individuals with acquired C1 esterase inhibitor deficiency, but not in HAE.
- Symptoms include recurrent episodes of nonpruritic angioedema. Patients may also have episodes of abdominal pain and laryngeal edema.
- In patients with low clinical suspicion, a C4 level is a good screening test. If the C4 level is reduced, evaluation of C1 esterase inhibitor levels and functional assays should be performed. With high clinical suspicion, the combination of C4 and C1 inhibitor testing is appropriate.
- ACE inhibitors can also cause isolated angioedema, and removal of the offending drug is required.

### Treatment

- Acute management of HAE episodes, besides supportive measures, includes administration of plasma-derived or recombinant C1-esterase inhibitor and bradykinin pathway inhibitors (ecallantide, a recombinant plasma kallikrein inhibitor; icatibant, a synthetic bradykinin receptor antagonist).
- HAE prophylaxis includes replacement C1-esterase inhibitor concentrate and kallikrein inhibitors (lanadelumab and berotralstat in patients ≥12 years). Although available, attenuated androgens cannot be used in prepubertal children or pregnancy, and side effects limit their use in other patients.

## FOOD ALLERGY

### Definition

- Food allergy describes a hypersensitivity reaction to a food protein as a result of an immunologic mechanism. The term adverse food reaction refers to any untoward reaction to a food or food component, regardless of the pathophysiologic mechanism involved.
- Adverse immunologic food reactions are classified as IgE-mediated or non–IgE-mediated, with the majority being IgE-mediated.

### Epidemiology

- Allergy to one or more foods occurs in approximately 6-8% of children and 3-4% of adults in the United States. The majority of food allergic reactions present before 12 months of age.

| TABLE 11-6 | Common Food Allergens |
|---|---|
| Milk | |
| Egg | |
| Peanuts | |
| Soybeans | |
| Wheat | |
| Fish | |
| Tree nuts | |
| Shellfish | |

- Eight foods are responsible for the majority of documented food reactivity in the United States (Table 11-6), although numerous other foods have been shown to trigger allergic reactions.
- Symptomatic food allergy resolves over time in the majority of children with milk, egg, soy, and wheat allergy with the majority of patients able to tolerate these foods by school age. In contrast, allergy to peanuts, tree nuts, and seafood is often lifelong.

## Early Introduction

- In the past, delayed introduction of common allergic foods was recommended, which lead to an increase in the prevalence of food allergy, especially peanut allergy. Early introduction at 4-6 months of age is now recommended and can decrease the risk of developing food allergy.
- The dual allergen exposure hypothesis states that the initial site of allergen exposure plays a role in determining tolerance vs food allergy. Transcutaneous exposure to food allergens bypasses the GI tract and is more likely to lead to allergy. Initial exposure via the GI tract helps promote tolerance.
  - The LEAP study demonstrated a significant reduction in peanut allergy in high-risk infants for developing peanut allergy compared to delayed introduction. High-risk infants include those with moderate-severe atopic dermatitis and/or egg allergy. Based on that study, early instruction of peanut at home is recommended in infants 4-6 months of age who are at low risk. In high-risk infants, referral to allergist is recommended for skin testing.

## Clinical Presentation

As described in Table 11-7, the clinical manifestations of food allergy can vary, depending on the underlying pathophysiologic process.

### IgE-Mediated Food Allergy

- Typical food allergies occur as a result of an immune reaction due to the presence of IgE antibodies to the causative food.
- Symptoms of IgE-mediated food allergy typically occur within 20 minutes of ingestion/exposure but may occur up to 2 hours later.
  - Cutaneous symptoms in the form of acute onset urticaria/rash and/or angioedema are the most common manifestations in IgE-mediated food hypersensitivity reactions. However, skin symptoms may be absent, and their absence is a risk factor for a life-threatening reaction.

| TABLE 11-7 | Characteristics of Adverse Food Reactions Based on Mechanism | |
|---|---|---|
| | **IgE-mediated** | **Non–IgE-mediated** |
| Onset | Rapid in onset, occurring within several minutes to 2 hr after ingestion | Acute and/or chronic symptoms. Acute reaction is delayed in onset by 2-4 hr (for FPIES) |
| Mechanism | Results from mediator release from tissue mast cells and circulating basophils | Multiple mechanisms, including immunologic (e.g., FPIES, eosinophilic gastrointestinal disorders), pharmacologic (e.g., caffeine, histamine), metabolic (e.g., phenylketonuria, lactose intolerance), additives (e.g., MSG, tartrazine), and toxic (e.g., staphylococcal food poisoning) |
| System(s) involved | Cutaneous, gastrointestinal, respiratory, ocular, cardiovascular, and/or multisystem (anaphylaxis) | Usually isolated to the gastrointestinal tract |

- Gastrointestinal symptoms may include nausea, abdominal pain, abdominal cramping, vomiting, and/or diarrhea.
- Respiratory symptoms may include cough, rhinorrhea, sneeze, wheeze, and/or difficulty breathing. Inhalation of food allergens via cooking (e.g., fish) or exposure to airborne particles (e.g., peanut dust) may trigger acute bronchospasm.
- Anaphylaxis resulting from exposure (almost exclusively by ingestion) to food allergens is typically rapid in onset and may lead to death. There is an increased incidence of food-induced anaphylaxis with any of the following risk factors: coexisting asthma; reaction to peanut, tree nut, fish, or shellfish; past allergic reactions with exposure to extremely small amounts of food; and a history of a past food-induced anaphylactic event. Up to 20% of anaphylactic reactions will result in a biphasic reaction, leading to recurrence of symptoms after initial resolution, typically within several hours of the initial anaphylactic event, but may be delayed up to 72 hours later.
- Atopic dermatitis may be exacerbated by consumption of food allergens.
  - Approximately 30-60% of infants with atopic dermatitis have food allergy (see the "Atopic Dermatitis" section).
  - Elimination of the suspected food (following appropriate evaluation, see later discussion) often improves symptoms. Patients are typically able to reintroduce these foods with age and improvement of atopic dermatitis
- Oral Allergy Syndrome (OAS) or Pollen Food Allergy presents as immediate onset of oropharyngeal pruritus and mild edema of the lips and/or tongue in patients with known pollen allergy. Symptoms occur after consuming cross-reactive proteins in fresh, uncooked fruits, vegetables or, less often, peanut, almond, and hazelnut. Cooking, baking, and even briefly microwaving the raw food alters the protein enough to eliminate symptoms. The majority of cases of OAS do not lead to anaphylaxis.

- Apple, pear, cherry, carrot, celery, and potato are cross-reactive with birch pollen.
- Melons and banana are cross-reactive with ragweed pollen.

*Non–IgE-Mediated Food Hypersensitivity*
- Food protein–induced enterocolitis syndrome (FPIES) typically presents in infancy, usually during the first year of life.
  - Acute FPIES symptoms include profuse and repetitive vomiting, often with diarrhea, which may lead to dehydration and lethargy hours after ingestion of offending substance. Milk and soy are the most common causative foods, followed by rice, oat, and sweet potato. Stool contains occult blood, neutrophils, eosinophils, and reducing substances. Tolerance to the food(s) usually occurs by 36 months of age.
  - Chronic FPIES symptoms include intermittent vomiting, chronic watery diarrhea with blood or mucous, weight loss, feeding difficulties, and failure to thrive. These symptoms are usually triggered by the ingestion of milk and/or soy-based formula.
  - Management of these episodes involve fluid resuscitation and supportive care. Ondansetron is commonly prescribed to be available at home in case of accidental exposure. Epinephrine is not effective.
- Food-induced colitis presents with painless rectal bleeding, as in food-induced enterocolitis, but patients are not generally as ill and tend to have appropriate weight gain. Milk and soy are the most common causative foods. Tolerance to the food generally develops by 12-18 months of age.

## Diagnosis: History
- The diagnosis of a food allergy requires a thorough history of the event, which must include the following:
  - The specific food or ingredient thought to provoke the reaction
  - All other food and medication consumed at the same time
  - Quantity of food consumed
  - Method of food preparation, including possibility of cross-contamination with other food
  - Time frame between consumption and reaction
  - Symptoms that occurred on other occasions when the food was consumed, both previously and since the event
  - Intervention administered to resolve symptoms
  - Time frame until resolution of symptoms

## Diagnosis: Skin Testing and Laboratory Studies (IgE-Mediated Food Allergy)
- Once a history of IgE-mediated reactivity has been established, diagnostic testing should be used to confirm the diagnosis. Testing demonstrates the ability to be allergic to a substance and should only be done in accordance with a history of potential allergy. There is no testing for severity of an allergic reaction, only likelihood.
- Epicutaneous skin testing is an excellent way of excluding IgE-mediated food allergies because this approach has a >95% negative predictive value to the common allergenic foods. However, positive skin tests to food (without history of typical IgE-mediated food reaction) have approximately a 50% positive predictive value, reflecting a high prevalence of asymptomatic allergic sensitization.
- Laboratory studies can be used in conjunction with skin testing to confirm a food allergy diagnosis. Food allergen–specific IgE testing uses in vitro testing (e.g., ImmunoCAP system), which has comparable sensitivity and specificity to epicutaneous

testing. These assays provide a quantitative measure of allergen-specific IgE and may provide guidance as to the timing of an oral food challenge (see later discussion).
- Food panels (skin testing and/or blood testing) are not recommended in screening for food allergy. These tests have a high positive predictive value, reflecting a high prevalence of allergic sensitization that may not be a reflection of clinical allergy. Positive results on food panels may result in patients avoiding foods unnecessarily. History suggesting IgE-mediated food reactions should guide specific food testing. Consequently, the diagnosis of IgE-mediated food allergy should not be based only on the presence of food-specific IgE antibodies (by skin testing and/or blood testing), as many people have asymptomatic allergic sensitization to foods of no clinical significance (i.e., they can consume the food without adverse reaction).
- Measurement of specific IgE against specific components of food proteins (i.e., component-resolved diagnostic [CRD] testing) allows for increased accuracy of food allergy (particularly peanut allergy) diagnosis compared with the traditional allergen-specific IgE testing to whole peanut, and it results in a more accurate discrimination between clinically significant food allergy and subclinical peanut sensitization in children who tolerate peanut.
  - Eleven allergen components have been characterized in peanut protein (Ara h 1-11).
  - Ara h 1, 2, and 3 are the most important components associated with clinical reactions to peanut. Among these, **Ara h-2** provides the best correlation with clinically significant peanut allergy.
  - Ara h 8, which cross-reacts with plant proteins, is associated with subclinical sensitization in peanut-tolerant subjects or with oral allergy syndrome, but rarely with clinically significant peanut allergy.

## Oral Food Challenges
- Confirmation of a food allergy may require an oral food challenge, during which the patient consumes the food in question under direct medical supervision, starting with very small quantities and increasing toward a standard portion of the food.
- Oral food challenge is also used to determine the resolution of food allergy.
- Timing of oral challenges may be guided by allergen-specific IgE levels an epicutaneous skin testing results. Allergen-specific IgE levels are trended over time. If levels decreased below a set threshold for the specific food, oral food challenge is offered.
- If an oral food challenge is indicated, the double-blind placebo-controlled method is considered to be the gold standard for the diagnosis of food allergy.
  - A single-blind graded challenge may be appropriate in confirming or refuting histories suggestive of food allergy. Single-blind challenges are particularly useful in young children whose response is not influenced by knowledge of consumption of the suspected food allergen.
- All food challenges should be performed by an allergist in a setting with the personnel and equipment necessary for treatment of a potential anaphylactic reaction.
- When a patient passes an oral food challenge, it is important for the patient to keep this food in their diet regularly as prolonged avoidance in a previously sensitized patient can result in a recurrence of their IgE-mediated food allergy.

## Treatment
- Management of food allergy is based on avoidance of food allergens and preparation for treatment of adverse reactions.
  - Total and strict avoidance of all forms of the food, both as major and minor ingredients, is generally necessary. However, 60-70% of egg and/or milk allergic patients

may tolerate consumption of egg and/or milk-containing baked goods. Potential tolerance to baked egg and/or milk should be established by an oral food challenge.

- IM epinephrine is the first-line therapy for significant acute IgE-mediated food allergy reactions. This medication is lifesaving.
- Immediately available self-injectable epinephrine, such as EpiPen or Auvi-Q, is mandatory for patients with IgE-mediated food allergy. Patients should have two epinephrine autoinjectors with them at all times and two autoinjectors should be kept at school.
- Extensive education regarding use of epinephrine should be provided at each office visit and offered to all caregivers, including day care providers and teachers. A Food Allergy and Anaphylaxis Emergency Care Plan should be available at home, daycare, school, camps, or anytime the food allergic child is away from his or her parent.
- Epinephrine dosing: 0.01 mg/kg/dose, maximum dose, 0.5 mg/dose.
  - Auvi-Q infant: 0.1 mg for patients <15 kg
  - EpiPen Jr or Auvi-Q Jr: 0.15 mg for patients <30 kg
  - EpiPen or Auvi-Q regular: 0.3 mg for patients >30 kg
- Epinephrine should be given to the anterolateral thigh and can be given through clothing.
- Epinephrine doses may need to be repeated every 5-15 minutes.
- Other treatments include antihistamines, corticosteroids, and bronchodilators.
- Educational resources, including instructions for reading ingredient labels and support groups for people with food allergies, should be made available. The Food Allergy Research and Education (FARE) organization (www.foodallergy.org) is an excellent resource.
- Oral desensitization protocols have been shown to increase the threshold of ingested food that causes clinical reaction. Palforzia is a peanut oral immunotherapy product and is the only FDA-approved oral immunotherapy for food allergy. Oral immunotherapy for other common allergenic foods is currently being developed.

## EOSINOPHILIC ESOPHAGITIS

Eosinophilic esophagitis (EoE) is a chronic condition characterized by symptoms of esophageal dysfunction due to inflammation and eosinophils in the esophagus.

### Clinical Presentation

- Patients can present with EoE at any age, though presenting symptoms vary by age.
  - Infants and toddlers: feeding difficulties, vomiting, and poor weight gain
  - School-aged children: abdominal pain, vomiting, reflux, dysphagia, food impaction, anorexia, and early satiety
  - Adolescents: reflux, chest pain, dysphagia, and food impaction
- Coping behaviors are typically seen in school age children and adolescents and include prolonged chewing, increased fluid intake with meals, cutting food into very small pieces, and lubricating foods with condiments. Patients may also avoid textured foods that more commonly cause food impaction.
- Patients with EoE have an increased prevalence of atopic conditions compared to the general population.

### Diagnosis

- Diagnostic criteria include the following:
  - Symptoms related to esophageal dysfunction

- Esophageal eosinophilia on endoscopy biopsy demonstrating >15 eosinophils per high powered field
- Exclusion of alternative etiologies
- During endoscopy, at least two biopsies are obtained from the distal esophagus and proximal or mid esophagus. Eosinophilia is only required from one biopsy site for diagnosis.
- Endoscopic findings include edema/decreased vascular pattern, exudates, linear furrows, rings/trachealization, and strictures. Esophageal rings and strictures are more commonly seen in older adolescent or adult patients.
- There are no laboratory tests specific for the diagnosis of EoE. Approximately 50% of patients with EoE will have peripheral eosinophilia and/or elevated total IgE levels.

## Treatment

- EoE is a chronic, life-long condition. Treatment is aimed at symptomatic and histologic improvement by reducing esophageal eosinophilia and inflammation to prevent esophageal dysmotility and fibrosis.
- The treatment team should be multidisciplinary including an allergist, gastroenterologist, and dietician.
- Patients have three treatment options: food elimination diet, proton pump inhibitors, and swallowed ICS. At this time, there are no FDA-approved medications for EoE, and all medications are off-label use.
- Symptoms can most often be controlled by one treatment modality though some patients require a combination of therapies. Patients can change treatment options at any time.
- Goals of treatment include both symptomatic and histologic improvement. Repeat endoscopies are performed following treatment initiation or after treatment changes to monitor for histologic improvement. EoE is determined to be well controlled when biopsies show <15 eosinophils per high-power field, and patients have symptomatic control. When patients reach symptom control and histologic control with <15 eosinophils per hpf, endoscopies can be performed yearly for surveillance screening as long as the patient maintains on the same treatment regimen. Endoscopies should be performed sooner if symptoms return.

### Food Elimination Diet

- Many families are interested in food elimination diets as this is the only nonpharmacologic treatment option. It is important to acknowledge food elimination diets are significant lifestyle change and some children or adolescents may not be able to adhere to a strict elimination diet.
- Families should meet with a dietician when choosing food elimination to ensure patients will receive appropriate nutrition from other food sources and learn how to read food labels.
- Unfortunately, there is no test to determine a patient's food trigger. Allergy testing including epicutaneous skin testing and food-specific IgE levels have been evaluated, but results do not correlate with EoE triggers. Food elimination diets are initiated based on studies that determined the most common food triggers in all EoE patients and tailored by patient's symptoms and repeat endoscopies.
- Patients can start with a 1, 2, 4, or 6 food elimination diet as below. Patients can add or remove foods based on symptoms and endoscopy results. The greater number of foods eliminated with initiating dietary therapy, the greater chance of remission.
- 1-FED: milk. Thirty-seven percent histological remission rate in children.

- 2-FED: milk and wheat. Forty percent histological remission rate in children.
- 4-FED: milk, wheat, egg, and soy. Sixty-four percent histological remission rate in children.
- 6-GED: milk, wheat, egg, soy, nuts (peanut and tree nuts), and seafood (fish and shellfish). Seventy-three percent histological remission rate in children.

*Proton Pump Inhibitor*
- Proton pump inhibitors are effective in EoE by reducing gastroesophageal reflux symptoms commonly experienced in EoE patients, repairing the esophageal epithelial barrier due to acid exposure, and reducing inflammation.
- Studies have shown a 50-60% clinical and histologic remission with PPI use in children.

*Swallowed Steroids*
- Swallowed ICS are used to coat the esophagus to prevent esophageal inflammation.
- Patients can use fluticasone MDI or budesonide respules. With fluticasone, patients use an inhaler incorrectly to swallow the medication. With budesonide, the vials are mixed with agents such as honey, Splenda, or chocolate syrup to make a viscous liquid that patients swallow.
- Patients should not eat or drink for 30 minutes after taking medication.
- Swallowed steroids are most effective if given twice daily.
- Patients should rinse their mouth after use to prevent thrush as with ICS for asthma.

## ANAPHYLAXIS

Anaphylaxis is an acute, life-threatening allergic systemic allergic reaction that may have a wide range of clinical presentations.

### Etiology
- Lifetime prevalence of anaphylaxis has been estimated at 1.6-5.1%. Children 0-4 years of age have a 3-fold risk of anaphylaxis compared to other age groups.
- The most common causes in children and adolescents are foods and stinging insects. In adults, medications and stinging insects are the most common causes.
  - Most common foods: peanuts, tree nuts, milk, eggs, fish, and shellfish
  - Most common drugs: penicillin, cephalosporins, sulfonamides, and NSAIDs
  - Other medications that have been increasing in frequency are radiocontrast agents, anesthetic agents, and chemotherapeutic and biologic agents.
- Atopy is a risk factor for anaphylaxis to foods, but not other agents. A history of poorly controlled asthma is a risk factor for fatal anaphylaxis. The failure to inject epinephrine appropriately or promptly in the early course of a reaction has been reported as a risk factor for fatal anaphylaxis due to food allergy.

### Pathophysiology
- Onset of anaphylaxis occurs in minutes to several hours following allergen exposure. Degranulation of mast cells and basophils precipitated by the cross-linking between allergen-specific IgE and the allergen releases biochemical mediators such as histamine, leukotrienes, tryptase, prostaglandins, and histamine-releasing factor.
  - Histamine activation of $H_1$ and $H_2$ receptors causes flushing, headache, and hypotension. Activation of $H_1$ receptors alone contributes to rhinorrhea, tachycardia, pruritus, and bronchospasm.

- Delayed anaphylaxis (4 to 12 hours) can occur due to sensitization to galactose α-1,3 galactose (alpha-gal). In areas where the lone star tick is endemic, patients get sensitized to mammalian meat.

## Diagnosis

- Anaphylaxis is highly likely when any one of the following three criteria is fulfilled.
  - (1) Sudden onset of illness (minutes to several hours) with involvement of skin, mucosal tissue, or both (e.g., generalized hives, itching or flushing, swollen lips-tongue-uvula) and at least one of the following.
    - ○ Sudden respiratory symptoms and signs (shortness of breath, wheeze, cough, stridor, hypoxemia)
    - ○ Sudden reduced BP or symptoms of end-organ dysfunction (e.g., hypotonia [collapse], incontinence)
  - (2) Two or more of the following that occur suddenly after exposure to a likely allergen or trigger for that patient (minutes to several hours)
    - ○ Sudden skin or mucosal symptoms and signs
    - ○ Sudden respiratory symptoms and signs
    - ○ Sudden reduced BP or symptoms of end-organ dysfunction
    - ○ Sudden gastrointestinal symptoms (e.g., crampy abdominal pain, vomiting)
  - (3) Reduced blood pressure after exposure to a known allergen for that patient (minutes to several hours)
- Cutaneous manifestations are the most common occurring in 80-90% of cases.
- A serum tryptase level can help with the diagnosis of anaphylaxis, especially if the patient presents with hypotension alone.
  - If anaphylaxis is present, the serum tryptase will be elevated and will peak 1-2 hours after the onset of anaphylaxis and will remain elevated for 4-6 hours.
  - Serum tryptase levels can be normal in mild reactions or in food-induced anaphylaxis.

## Treatment

*Acute Therapy*

- Assess and maintain airway, breathing, and circulation.
- Give intramuscular epinephrine (1:1000 dilution) 0.01 mg/kg in children (maximum dose 0.3 mg) into the anterolateral thigh (preferred) or the deltoid. An epinephrine autoinjector (e.g., EpiPen, Auvi-Q 0.3 mg for children >30 kg, EpiPen Jr, Auvi-Q 0.15 mg for children between 15 and 30 kg, and Auvi-Q 0.10 for children 7.5-15 kg) may be injected through clothing into the anterolateral thigh alternatively. Repeat every 5 minutes as necessary.
- Place the patient in the supine position with elevated lower extremities (or in the left lateral position for vomiting patients).
- Administer supplemental oxygen as needed (6-8 L/min) by face mask or oropharyngeal airway.
- Administer IV saline 20 mL/kg in the first 5-10 minutes if there is hypotension despite epinephrine.
  - If persistent or severe hypotension continues, multiple fluid boluses of 10-20 mL/kg up to 50 mL/kg may be administered over the first 30 minutes.
  - For refractory hypotension after fluid resuscitation and epinephrine administration, dopamine, noradrenaline, or vasopressin may be administered to maintain a systolic blood pressure of >90 mm Hg.

- Administer diphenhydramine at 1-2 mg/kg/dose (up to 50 mg) orally or intravenously. Antihistamine should not be used without epinephrine in anaphylaxis management.
- Ranitidine 1 mg/kg in children (up to 50 mg) orally or intravenously may be added.
- Administer an inhaled $\beta_2$-agonist (albuterol or levalbuterol) for resistant bronchospasm.
- In a patient receiving $\beta$-blockers, consider glucagon 20-30 µg/kg (up to 1 mg in children) injected over 5 minutes intravenously every 20 minutes if initial administration of epinephrine is ineffective. Follow with an infusion of 5-15 µg/min.
- Corticosteroids are not useful acutely, and current data suggest limited usefulness in inhibiting a biphasic or protracted response.
  - Methylprednisolone 1-2 mg/kg (up to 50 mg) may be given intravenously.
  - Oral prednisone 1-2 mg/kg (up to 60 mg) may also be considered.

*Observation*
- Even though the majority of patients who have anaphylactic events respond rapidly to treatment and do not relapse, observation for 4-6 hours postanaphylaxis is suggested because biphasic reactions can occur or the effect of epinephrine may wane. Biphasic reactions vary from <1 to 20% of patients.
- Hospitalization in patients with moderate to severe symptoms is appropriate.

*Discharge and Follow-Up*
- Epinephrine autoinjectors (dosage described in "Treatment" section) with instruction in administration should be prescribed for all patients experiencing an anaphylactic reaction to an allergen present in a community setting. Discharge medications such as diphenhydramine and oral prednisone can be continued for 24-72 hours.
- Education materials should be provided to all patients before discharging home. Patients should be educated about how to avoid the anaphylactic allergen if identified, particularly in food anaphylaxis (resources available from the FARE organization, www.foodallergy.org).
- An anaphylaxis action plan should be formulated. This plan should include the child's name, allergens, parental contact information, when and how to use an epinephrine autoinjector, antihistamine dose, and when to seek emergency help.
- Referral to an allergy specialist should be arranged for a complete evaluation.

## SUGGESTED READINGS

Bernstein J, Lang DM, Khan DA, et al. The diagnosis and management of acute and chronic urticaria: 2014 update. J Allergy Clin Immunol 2014;133(5):1270–1277.

Bielory L, Delgado L, Katelaris CH, et al. Diagnosis and management of allergic conjunctivitis. Ann Allergy Asthma Immunol 2020;124:118–134.

Du Toit G, Roberts G, Sayre PH, et al. Randomized trial of peanut consumption in infants at risk for peanut allergy. N Engl J Med 2015;372(9):803–813.

Dykewicz M, Wallace DV, Amrol DJ, et al. Rhinitis 2020: a practice parameter update. J Allergy Clin Immunol 2020;146(4):721–767.

Expert Panel Working Group of the National Heart, Lung, and Blood Institute (NHLBI) administered and coordinated National Asthma Education and Prevention Program Coordinating Committee (NAEPPCC); Cloutier MM, Baptist AP, Blake KV, et al. 2020 Focused updates to the asthma management guidelines: a report from the National Asthma Education and Prevention Program Coordinating Committee Expert Panel Working Group. J Allergy Clin Immunol 2020;146:1217–1270.

# 12 Child Psychiatry

Andrea Giedinghagen

## INTRODUCTION

- Psychiatric disorders are the most common chronic disorders of childhood: 1 in 5 US children will be seriously impaired by a psychiatric disorder by age 18.
- Many mild psychiatric disorders respond to psychotherapy (ideally with parent/guardian involvement); in other cases, a combination of psychotherapy and medication is indicated. Knowing area providers of evidence-based therapies is invaluable for referral purposes.
- Not all psychotherapy is created equal. Cognitive behavioral therapy (CBT) is a structured, evidence-based therapy for depression and anxiety in children. Dialectical behavioral therapist is a structured, evidence-based therapy that addresses recurrent self-injury, chronic suicidality, and emotional dysregulation.

## ATTENTION DEFICIT HYPERACTIVITY DISORDER

### Definition and Epidemiology

- Attention deficit hyperactivity disorder is primarily marked by difficulties with hyperactivity/impulsivity and modulation of attention. There are three types: predominantly inattentive, predominantly hyperactive/impulsive, and combined type.
- ADHD is the third most frequently diagnosed psychiatric disorder in children. Up to 10% of children in the United States are affected. Median age of diagnosis is 11 years; more severely affected children may be diagnosed earlier, and less severely affected children later.
- Girls are more likely to have inattentive ADHD and thus less likely to be diagnosed than boys (whose hyperactive behavior attracts attention—and gets them treatment).

### Symptoms

- Symptoms must be present for more than 6 months, with some symptoms apparent before 12 years of age. Symptoms must be present in at least two settings (home and school; school and daycare), negatively impact patient's functioning, and not be attributable to another condition.
- **Inattentive ADHD is marked by six or more of the following:**
  - Fails to pay close attention to details (rushes through assignments)
  - Easily distracted (both by external noises/distractors and internal thoughts)
  - Does not listen even when spoken to directly (daydreaming/focused on something else)
  - Does not follow through on tasks/assignments (not due to defiance or not understanding instructions)
  - Difficulty with organization (an always-messy desk, backpack, or room)
  - Avoids tasks requiring prolonged focus (procrastination on projects, putting off homework)

- Frequently loses necessary items (ID cards, phone, homework, gym clothes)
- Often forgetful (of appointments, assignments, or chores)
- **Hyperactive/impulsive ADHD is marked by six or more of the following:**
  - Fidgeting (bouncing leg/kicking chair/tapping pencil, etc.)
  - Difficulty remaining seated when expected (constantly up and about at school)
  - Running or climbing in inappropriate situations (teens may simply feel restless)
  - Acting as if propelled by a motor (always in motion, always buzzing between activities)
  - Difficulty playing quietly (trouble remembering to use "inside voice")
  - Hypertalkativeness (getting in trouble for talking too much at school; hard to interrupt at times)
  - Prematurely blurting answers, or finishing others' sentences
  - Interrupting others (trouble waiting turn to speak, talking over others)
  - Trouble waiting turns (in a game, in line)
- **Combined ADHD is diagnosed when a patient meets criteria for both inattentive and hyperactive presentations.**

## Diagnosis

- History of above symptoms should be supported by questionnaires completed by caregivers and teachers (again, in two or more settings).
- The Vanderbilt ADHD Diagnostic Rating Scale and Connors are both widely used, but the Vanderbilt scale has the advantage of being free.

## Treatment (See Table 12-1)

- Parent management training (PMT) alone is preferred treatment for all presentations of ADHD in children under age 6; it involves teaching parents methods to manage children's disruptive behaviors.
- A combined treatment strategy consisting of PMT and stimulant medication is best for children over 6.
- Methylphenidate is the preferred stimulant for use in children. Start at a low dose of immediate-release formulation after breakfast and after lunch (to minimize chances of stomach upset).
- Titrate to effect in increments of 5-10 mg/week and then choose an extended-release formulation based on desired onset and duration of action (see Table 12-1).
- Move to amphetamine preparation if methylphenidate is ineffective after titration to near-maximal dose, or if side effects are excessive.
- Clonidine and guanfacine are also options, either instead of or to augment stimulant treatment, especially in hyperactive/impulsive ADHD.
- Clonidine can be especially helpful for initial insomnia when given at nighttime.
- Atomoxetine is a selective norepinephrine reuptake inhibitor ideal when other options are contraindicated/ineffective (especially useful when there is comorbid substance abuse).

### *Treatment Side Effects and Contraindications*

- Side effects of stimulants include decreased growth, increased heart rate and blood pressure, decreased appetite, and insomnia. Headaches and stomachaches occur at times as well.
- Side effects of $\alpha$ agonists include hypotension, sedation, fatigue, and constipation.

**TABLE 12-1  Pharmacologic Treatment of ADHD**

| Medication | Dosing | Onset | Duration |
|---|---|---|---|
| **Stimulants** | | | |
| Methylphenidate immediate release (tablets, chewable tablets, and oral solution) | Start: 5 mg bid<br>Avg: 1-2 mg/kg<br>Max: 60 mg/day | 20-30 min | 3-6 hr |
| Methylphenidate extended release<br>Concerta | Start: 18 mg<br>Max: 54 mg (6-12 years)<br>72 mg (13-17 years) | 60-90 min | 10-12 hr |
| Methylphenidate immediate and extended release (30%/70%)<br>Metadate CD[a] | Start: 20 mg/day<br>Max: 60 mg/day | 20-30 min | 8-10 hr |
| Methylphenidate immediate and extended release (50%/50%)<br>Ritalin LA[a] | Start: 20 mg/day<br>Max: 60 mg/day | 20-30 min | 6-8 hr |
| Methylphenidate extended release (chewable tablets and oral solution)<br>QuilliChew ER and Quillivant ER | Start: 20 mg/day<br>Max: 60 mg/day | 20-30 min | 12 hr |
| Mixed amphetamine salts immediate release<br>Adderall | Start: 5 mg/day<br>Avg: 0.5-1 mg/kg<br>Max: 30 mg/day | 30-60 min | 3-6 hr |

| Mixed amphetamine salts extended release<br>Adderall XR | Start: 10 mg/day<br>Avg: 0.5-1 mg/kg/day<br>Max: 30 mg/day | 60-90 min | 10-12 hr |
|---|---|---|---|
| Lisdexamfetamine<br>Vyvanse | Start: 30 mg/day<br>Max: 70 mg/day | 90 min | 10-12 hr |
| **Alpha-agonists** | | | |
| Clonidine immediate release | Start: 0.05-0.1 mg qHS<br>Max: 0.4 mg/day divided | May take days to fully appreciate effect | |
| Clonidine extended release<br>Kapvay | Start: 0.1 mg<br>Max: 0.4 mg/day divided | May take days to fully appreciate effect | |
| Guanfacine immediate release | Start: 0.5-1 mg/qHS<br>Max: 4 mg/day divided | May take days to fully appreciate effect | |
| Guanfacine extended release<br>Intuniv | Start: 1 mg/qHS<br>Max: 4 mg/day | May take days to fully appreciate effect | |
| **Selective serotonin reuptake inhibitor** | | | |
| Atomoxetine<br>Strattera | Start: 0.5 mg/kg (<70 kg)<br>40 mg (>70 kg)<br>Max: 1.2 mg/kg (<70 kg)<br>100 mg/kg (>70 kg) | May take days-weeks to fully appreciate effect on ADHD symptoms | |

<sup></sup>Capsule can be opened and contents sprinkled in applesauce or pudding.

- Side effects of atomoxetine include nausea, dry mouth, decreased appetite, and in rare cases suicidal thoughts.
- Monitor blood pressure, pulse, height, and weight at each visit, and adjust therapy if significant weight loss/growth failure or abnormal vital signs occur.
- Prior to starting stimulants, obtain a personal and family history focusing on cardiac issues: sudden cardiac death, arrythmias, hypertrophic cardiomyopathy, or structural cardiac disease.
- Obtain a personal history of syncope, shortness of breath, chest pain (especially on exertion), or seizures; perform a cardiac examination. Cardiac evaluation and clearance are indicated if abnormalities are present.
- A personal history of psychosis or mania (bipolar disorder) is also a contraindication to starting stimulant therapy or atomoxetine; refer to a child psychiatrist.

## MAJOR DEPRESSIVE DISORDER

### Definition and Epidemiology

- Major depressive disorder (and mood disorders) is the second most frequently diagnosed group of psychiatric disorders among US children.
- The median age of onset is 13 years; roughly 15% of US children are diagnosed with depression or another mood disorder by age 18. Girls are twice as likely to experience depression as boys.
- Depressive disorders are marked by periods of low mood, irritability, decreased pleasure in activities, and impairment in functioning.

### Symptoms

- **Two or more weeks of low or irritable mood (irritability more common in children and teens) and/or decreased interest in usually enjoyed activities, and at least four of the following:**
  - Decreased energy (feeling listless/fatigued)
  - Changes in sleep (too much or too little)
  - Changes in appetite (significantly increased or decreased)
  - Psychomotor agitation (restlessness) or psychomotor retardation (moving slowly enough that others notice)
  - Feeling worthless/down on themselves (younger children may make statements like "No one likes me.")
  - Difficulty concentrating/focusing
  - Recurrent thoughts of death, including thoughts of suicide up to suicide attempts

### Diagnosis

- The United States Preventive Services Task Force recommends regularly screening ALL adolescents for depression.
- Use a screener such as the Patient Health Questionnaire-9 Modified for Adolescents (PHQ-A).

### Treatment (See Table 12-2)

- The standard treatment for moderate to severe depression is a combination of CBT and a selective serotonin reuptake inhibitors (SSRI).
- It takes 4-6 weeks to appreciate a significant difference in depressive/anxious symptoms with SSRI treatment; "not working" after 2-3 weeks is actually "not working yet."
- Titrate at 2- to 4-week increments to effect.

| TABLE 12-2 | Selective Serotonin Reuptake Inhibitors | | | |
|---|---|---|---|---|
| Medication | Starting dose (mg) | Typical dose (mg) | Titration increments (mg) | Maximum dose (mg) |
| Sertraline | 12.5-25 | 50 | 25 | 200 |
| Fluoxetine | 10 | 20 | 10-20 | 80 |
| Escitalopram | 2.5-5 | 10 | 5 | 20 |
| Citalopram | 10 | 20 | 10 | 40 |
| Fluvoxamine | 25 (qHS) | 100 | 25-50 | 300 |

*Treatment Side Effects and Contraindications*
• Prior to SSRI initiation, screen for a personal or family history of bipolar disorder (if present, refer to child psychiatrist).
• Start low and go slow—with preadolescents begin at the lower end of the starting dose range.
• GI upset is the most common early side effect, including nausea and diarrhea.
• In early studies, use of SSRIs in individuals under age 18 was associated with a slightly increased risk of suicidal ideation, but NOT associated with increased risk of completed suicide.
• Patients and families should be advised of the "black box warning" while keeping in mind, THE RISKS OF UNTREATED DEPRESSION ARE MUCH GREATER THAN THE RISKS ASSOCIATED WITH SSRIs.

## ANXIETY DISORDERS

### Definition and epidemiology
• Anxiety disorders are the most diagnosed psychiatric conditions in children and adolescents. Some anxiety is adaptive, but it becomes a disorder when it is excessive and interferes in functioning.
• Anxiety disorders have a mean age of onset of 6 years, and 30% of US children will be affected by an anxiety disorder by age 18.
• Early anxiety symptoms are associated with later mood disorders and suicidal thoughts/attempts.

### Generalized Anxiety Disorder
• Symptoms include frequent worry about a variety of topics over the course of at least 6 months. The worry is difficult to control and accompanied by at least one of the following:
  • Feeling edgy or restless (fidgeting, pacing, difficulty staying still)
  • Feeling tired/fatigued (from being tense all the time)
  • Difficulty concentrating/feeling as if mind is going blank
  • Irritability
  • Muscular tension or soreness (stomachaches and headaches are also common.)
  • Difficulty sleeping (mind racing with worries while trying to get to sleep)

### Social Anxiety Disorder
• Symptoms include marked fear or anxiety in one or more situations in which the child may be observed by others—especially while performing (public speaking,

playing an instrument), or during social interactions (talking to peers at a party). In addition
- The social situation always or almost always creates major distress.
- The child may avoid the situation or endure it with significant anxiety.
- There are panic attacks, or in younger children tantrums/crying, related to the situation.

## Separation Anxiety Disorder

- Separation anxiety can be developmentally appropriate in toddlers; however, it is a sign of disorder when it is developmentally inappropriate (for instance, in a school-age child), is excessive, and causes significant distress or interferes in functioning. It is marked by at least three of the following over a period of at least 1 month:
  - Recurrent, excessive distress or physical symptoms (headache, stomachaches) when anticipating or experiencing separation from attachment figures
  - Persistent and excessive worry about loss of/harm to attachment figures (death, illness, accident)
  - Persistent and excessive worry about being separated from attachment figure (kidnapping, getting lost)
  - Reluctance or refusal to go away from home for fear of separation
  - Reluctance related to or fear of being alone at home or elsewhere without attachment figures
  - Reluctance related to or fear of sleeping away from home or attachment figures
  - Repeated nightmares involving the theme of separation

## Diagnosis

- Diagnosis of anxiety disorders can be made with history alone, or using a tool such as HEADSS.
- Screening questionnaires such as the Generalized Anxiety Disorder questionnaire for adolescents (GAD-7) or the Screen for Child Anxiety Related Disorders (SCARED) can support the diagnosis as well.

## Treatment

- Structured CBT is the treatment of choice for mild to moderate anxiety disorders and for younger children.
- Children with more severe anxiety disorders benefit from a combination of CBT and medication.
- Among children diagnosed with an anxiety disorder, 55% of those treated with an SSRI, 60% of children treated with CBT, and 80% of children treated with a combination experienced significant improvement in symptoms at 12 weeks of treatment.
- One of the primary treatment strategies for anxiety is to avoid avoiding: With support, encourage the child/parents to confront the source of anxiety rather than enabling continued avoidance.
- Initial dosages and titration schedules of SSRIs are the same for anxiety disorders as for major depressive disorders, but anxiety disorders require higher dosages of SSRIs than depressive disorders.

# SUICIDE

## Definition and Epidemiology

- Suicide is the second leading cause of death in US adolescents.
- About 90% of adolescents who attempt or complete suicide have a psychiatric diagnosis.

- Other key risk factors for suicide include a history of impulsivity (especially impulsive aggression), family conflict, a history of maltreatment, LGBTQ+ identity and associated minority stress, a history of prior attempt, access to a gun (or other lethal means), self-injury, and substance abuse.

## Assessment

Use the Columbia-Suicide Severity Risk Screener (C-SSRS) or Ask Suicide Screening Questions (ASQ) to screen all patients. Both are available without cost.

## Treatment

- Anyone who screens at "high risk" or discloses current suicidal thoughts—especially with a plan or desire to act—should be transported by ambulance to an ED for psychiatric evaluation.
- Moderate-risk patients should also participate in safety planning, with parent/guardian involvement; the safety plan should be included in the chart and sent home with the child and the parent/guardian.
- Provide resources to all patients, regardless of screening, including the National Suicide Hotline and Textline: 1-800-273-TALK.

## WHEN TO CONSULT A CHILD PSYCHIATRIST

Consult a child or adolescent psychiatrist when there is:

- Concern for bipolar disorder, or a family history of bipolar disorder, and a child needs medication for a psychiatric condition, as some medications (SSRIs, stimulants) may potentiate mania
- Concern for psychosis (loss of contact with reality), or major impairment in functioning such as school avoidance/failure, frequent or severe tantrums without obvious cause, or repeated running away
- A child at risk of harm to themselves or others (severe aggression, self-harm, or suicidal thoughts)
- A child under five with behavioral symptoms in need of medication management, such as severe ADHD that has not been responsive to behavioral management
- A partial response to medication, or if a child is on more than two psychiatric medications
- A psychiatric condition interfering with treating a medical condition (depression keeping a teen from managing blood glucose in diabetes, or completing pulmonary toilette for cystic fibrosis)

## SUGGESTED READINGS

American Academy of Child & Adolescent Psychiatry. Recommendations for Pediatricians, Family Practitioners, Psychiatrists, and Non-physician Mental Health Practitioners: When to seek consultation or referral to a Child and Adolescent Psychiatrist. Available at https://www.aacap.org/AACAP/Member_Resources/Practice_Information/When_to_Seek_Referral_or_Consultation_with_a_CAP.aspx

American Psychiatric Association. Diagnostic and Statistical Manual of Mental Disorders. 5th Ed. Arlington, VA: American Psychiatric Publishers, Inc., 2013.

Breslin K, Balaban J, Shubkin CD. Adolescent suicide: what can pediatricians do? Curr Opin Pediatr 2020;32(4):595–600.

Cohen E, Mackenzie RG, Yates GL. HEADSS, a psychosocial risk assessment instrument: implications for designing effective intervention programs for runaway youth. J Adolesc Health 1991;12(7):539–544.

Friedman, RA. Antidepressants' Black Box Warning: 10 years later. N Engl J Med 2014;371:1666–1668.

Merikangas K, Hep J, Burstein M, et al. Lifetime prevalence of mental disorders in U.S. adolescents: results from the National Comorbidity Survey Replication—Adolescent Supplement (NCS-A). J Am Acad Child Adolesc Psychiatry 2010;49(10):980–989.

Selph SS, McDonagh MS. Depression in children and adolescents: evaluation and treatment. Am Fam Physician 2019;100(10):609–617.

Siu AL, US Preventive Services Task Force. Screening for depression in children and adolescents: US Preventive Services Task Force Recommendation Statement. Pediatrics 2016;137(3):e20154467.

Southammakosane C, Schmitz K. Pediatric psychopharmacology for treatment of ADHD, depression, and anxiety. Pediatrics 2015;136(2):351–359.

Stanley B, Brown GK. Safety planning intervention: a brief intervention to mitigate suicide risk. Cogn Behav Pract 2012;19(2):256–264.

Walkup JT, Albano AM, Piacentini J, et al. Cognitive behavioral therapy, sertraline, or a combination in childhood anxiety. N Engl J Med 2008;359(26):2753–2766.

# Developmental and Behavioral Pediatrics

Paul S. Simons and Abigail M. Kissel

Developmental and behavioral disorders are the most prevalent chronic medical diagnoses encountered by primary pediatric health care professionals. One in seven children is estimated to have a developmental disability.

An understanding of normal developmental milestones is important because the spectrum of disorders progresses from mild to severe for motor disorders, global cognitive disorders, language/communication disorders, and social/behavioral disorders.

See chart of normal developmental milestones in Appendix B.

## KEY PRINCIPLES UNDERLYING DEVELOPMENTAL-BEHAVIORAL DIAGNOSIS

- **3 primary streams of development**
  - *Motor*
    - Gross Motor
      - Mild—developmental dyspraxia/"clumsy child"/developmental coordination disorder
      - Severe—cerebral palsy, neuromuscular disorder
    - Fine Motor
      - Mild—dysgraphia
      - Severe—cerebral palsy, neuromuscular disorder
    - Oral Motor
      - Mild—speech articulation disorder; drooling, severe tongue-tie
      - Severe—dysarthria/dysphagia
  - *Cognitive (including language and nonverbal processing)*
    - Mild (low average)—slow learner (IQ 80-89)
    - Moderate—borderline (IQ 70-79)
    - Severe—intellectual disability/formerly "mental retardation"—(IQ < 70)
  - *Social/behavioral*
    - Social behavior issues
      - Normal variation/"problem"—shy/slow to warm up temperament or unrealistic parental expectations
      - Mild disorder—socially inappropriate behavior; socially immature; social anxiety
      - Severe disorder—lack of social reciprocity; lack of joint attention; lack of empathy; lack of imaginative play
    - Attentional issues
      - Normal variation/problem—"inattention problem" or "inattentive behavior"
      - Mild disorder—inattention with variable ability to refocus with demand
      - Severe disorder—atypical attention; limited eye contact; perseveration; insistence of sameness; restricted interests; repetitive play/rituals; sensory hypo-/hyper-responsiveness. Some of these signs/symptoms may be behavioral, in addition to attentional.

○ Impulsivity/hyperactivity issues
  – Normal variation/problem—"impulsivity/hyperactivity problem" or "impulsive or hyperactive behavior"
  – Mild disorder—impulsivity; hyperactivity
  – Severe disorder—disinhibition; stereotypic motor mannerisms, manic behavior/mania
• Delay, dissociation, and deviance from a normal developmental trajectory reflect underlying central nervous system dysfunction.
  • The more delayed, dissociated, and deviant the development, the more atypical the behavior should be expected to be.
• There is a spectrum of disorders within each developmental stream.
  • Mild disorders predominate over severe disorders within each stream.
• There is a continuum of developmental-behavioral disorders across streams.
  • Diffuse/global developmental-behavioral dysfunction predominates over more isolated or focal dysfunction. Comorbidities are the rule rather than the exception.

## LEARNING DISABILITIES

### Identifying Children at Risk
• Learning disorders have clear familial components
  • Obtain a detailed family history
• Special circumstances increasing the risk for learning disorders
  • Exposures (prenatal drug/alcohol use, postnatal toxin/lead exposure)
  • Premature infants, especially <32 weeks of gestation
  • Hypoxic events or cyanotic congenital heart disease
  • ACEs (especially four or more or the inclusion of poverty as one)
  • Specific genetic disorders
    ○ Examples:
      – Klinefelter syndrome
      – Turner syndrome
      – Velocardiofacial syndrome
      – Spina bifida with shunted hydrocephalus (visuospatial cognitive skills and math achievement)

### Categories of Neurodevelopmental Problems That Result in Learning Difficulties
• Fine motor/graphomotor problems
• Processing difficulties
  • Visual processing
  • Sequencing
  • Receptive language
  • Expressive language
  • Weak concept formation
  • Slow processing pace
  • Small chunk size
• Organizational difficulties
• Memory difficulties
  • Short-term memory
  • Active working memory
  • Long-term memory

*Learning Disability Subtypes/Comorbidities*
- Multiple learning disabilities
  - Children who have problems in one area of academic achievement often have problems in other areas of academics as well as with social/emotional behaviors.
    - 35-56.7% of children with math learning disorders also had reading learning disorders.
- Learning disability and attention deficit hyperactivity disorder (ADHD).
  - Comorbid learning disabilities account for at least some of the observed academic underachievement in children with ADHD.
  - Secondary attention deficits—attention problems secondary to the underlying learning disorder.
    - It can be very difficult for a student to maintain focus on tasks that are difficult for him or her to understand.
- Nonverbal learning disorders
  - Nonverbal cognitive measures are significantly lower than verbal scores
    - Problem areas can include math computation, organizational skills, higher order math, and science concepts
    - Problems with social perception and social interaction contribute to negative experiences in educational settings

## Interventions and Advocacy
*Federal Laws*
IDEA—Individuals with Disabilities Education Act
- The federal law that makes sure that free and appropriate public education is available for eligible kids and ensures that this includes special education when needed.
  - 0-2—IDEA Part C (Early intervention)
  - 3-21—IDEA Part B (Special Education)
- It is important to know that accommodations are usually changes made for a child in the classroom and fall under a 504, but if special education is needed outside of the classroom, this will fall under an IEP.

*IEP*
- Problem areas are determined by a school completing a Full and Individual Evaluation (FIE), and those qualifying for intervention will be listed in an Individualized Education Program (IEP) plan with stated interventions and improvement measurement goals. Programs must be provided in the least restrictive environment (LRE). Note that this DOES apply to charter schools and does NOT necessarily apply to private schools.
  - Listening comprehension
  - Basic reading skills
  - Reading fluency skills
  - Reading comprehension
  - Mathematics calculation
  - Mathematic problem solving

*Modules*
- *Discrepancy model*
  - Discrepancy between academic achievement and intellectual ability (often a starting point for suspicion of a specific learning disability (SLD)
- *Response to intervention model (RTI)*

- TIER 1—General education or primary prevention
  ○ Administrated to all students
- TIER 2—Secondary Prevention
  ○ Not doing as well as most peers and needs extra help
  ○ Small group tutoring
  ○ School-based problem-solving teams for functional assessment and to manage intervention
- TIER 3
  ○ More intensive, individual programming with progress monitoring
- RTI services must be supported by "scientifically based research… accepted by a peer reviewed journal or approved by a panel of independent experts through a comparably rigorous, objective, and scientific review."
- Failure to show progress with an RTI should prompt FIE and development of more formal IEP if needed.
- *Section 504* of the Rehabilitation Act of 1973
  - Students receiving these services typically have less severe problems than those eligible under IDEA.
  - Accommodations may include
    ○ Extra time to take tests
    ○ Verbal versus written questions or responses
    ○ Adjusting reading level
    ○ Recording of lectures
    ○ Online assignment submission
    ○ Peer tutoring
    ○ Multiple choice versus short essay questions
    ○ Shortened assignments

## SPEECH AND LANGUAGE DEVELOPMENT AND DISORDERS

- Components of speech and language (definition of terms) (Table 13-1)
- Developmental milestones for language (Table 13-2)
  - General rule of thumb for speaking in sentences
    ○ 90% of children use
      – 2-word sentences at age 2
      – 3-word sentences at age 3
      – 4-word sentences at age 4
- WHENEVER speech/language or social problems are being considered an automatic hearing evaluation should be considered.

### Variations in Development

- Forms of language: Phoneme—a speech sound, morphology (how words are formed), Syntax—the rules for combining words in sentences
- Content of language: Semantics—the meaning of words or word combinations
- Function of language: Pragmatics—the broader rules of language use in conversations and socially

### Communication Disorders
*Functional Speech Sound Disorders*
- Phonologic (linguistic aspects of speech production) or articulation (motor aspect) disorder

| TABLE 13-1 | Components of Speech and Language |
|---|---|

| Term | Definition |
|---|---|
| **Speech** | |
| Intelligibility | Ability of speech to be understood by others |
| Fluency | Flow of speech |
| Voice and resonance | Sound of speech. Incorporating passage of air through larynx, mouth, and nose |
| **Language** | |
| Receptive language | Ability to understand language |
| Expressive language | Ability to produce language |
| Phoneme | Smallest units of sound that change the meaning of a word, for example, "map" and "mop" |
| Morpheme | Smallest unit of meaning in language, for example, adding –s to the end of the word to make it plural |
| Syntax | Set of rules for combining morphemes and words into sentences (grammar) |
| Semantics | The meaning of words and sentences |
| Pragmatics | The social uses of language, including conversational skills, discourse, volume of speech, and body language |

From Voigt R, et al. Developmental and Behavioral Pediatrics. Arlington: American Academy of Pediatrics, 2010:203.

- Rule-based errors (phonologic) or substitution, omission, addition, or distortions of phonemes (articulation)
- Many more difficult sounds are not mastered until age 5-6
  - Consonants: j, r, l, y
  - Blends: ie, sh, ch, th, st

Dysarthria

Disorders involving problems of articulation, respirations, phonation, or prosody as a result of paralysis, muscle weakness, or poor coordination (frequently associated with cerebral palsy)

Apraxia/Dyspraxia of Speech

- Problems in articulation, phonation, respiration, and resonance arising from difficulties in complex motor planning and movement.
  - Not due to weakness of the oromotor musculature as seen with dysarthria
  - Lack of association with other oral motor skills, such as chewing, swallowing, or spitting
- Developmental apraxia of speech is differentiated from an expressive language delay in that children with expressive language delay typically follow a normal language trajectory but at a slower pace.
- Acquired apraxia/dyspraxia commonly results from head injury, tumor, stroke, or other problems affecting the parts of the brain involved with speaking and involves loss of previously acquired speech.

| TABLE 13-2 | Developmental Milestones for Language | |
|---|---|---|

| Age | Receptive language | Expressive language |
|---|---|---|
| 0-3 months | Alerts to voice | Cries, social smile |
| | | Coos |
| 4-6 months | Responds to voice, name | Laughs out loud |
| | | Blows raspberries, clicks tongue |
| | | Begins babbling |
| 7-9 months | Turns head toward sound | Says "mama" and "dada" indiscriminately |
| 10-12 months | Enjoys "peek a boo" | Says "mama" and "dada" appropriately |
| | Understands "no" | Waves "bye-bye" |
| | Follows 1-step command with gesture | Begins to gesture |
| | | Shakes head "no" |
| | | 1st word other than mama/dada |
| 13-15 months | Follows 1-step command without gesture | Immature jargoning |
| | | Up to 5 words |
| 16-18 months | Points to 1 picture | Mature jargoning with true words |
| | Points to 3 body parts and to self | Up to 25 words |
| | | Giant words: "all gone, thank you" |
| 19-24 months | Begins to understand pronouns | Up to 50 words |
| | Follows 2-step commands | 2-word sentences |
| | Points to 5-10 pictures | Early telegraphic speech |
| 25-30 months | Understands "just one" | Uses pronouns appropriately |
| | Points to parts of pictures | Uses plural |
| | | Speech is 50% intelligible |
| 3 years | Knows opposites | 250+ words |
| | Follows 2 prepositions | 3-word sentences |
| | | Answer "what" and "where" questions |
| | | Speech is 75% intelligible |
| 4 years | Follows 3-step commands | Answers "when" questions |
| | Points to 4 colors | Knows full name, gender, age |
| | | Tells stories |
| 5 years | Begins to understand left and right | Answer "why" questions |
| | Understand adjectives | Defines simple words |

From Voigt R, et al. Developmental and Behavioral Pediatrics. Arlington: American Academy of Pediatrics, 2010:204.

Voice Disorders
- Variations in pitch, volume, resonances, and voice quality.
- Can be seen in isolation or in connection with a language delay.
- Impaired modulation of pitch and volume can be seen in children with autism spectrum disorders, nonverbal learning disorders, and in some genetic syndromes.
- Velopharyngeal palatal incompetence can cause hypernasal speech and can be a marker of velocardiofacial (22q11 deletion) syndrome.

*Fluency Disorders*
- Interruptions in the flow of speaking
  - Examples—pauses, hesitations, injections, prolongations, and interruptions
- Normal dysfluency is common in early childhood (ages 2.5-4) or occasionally in older children who are nervous or excited.
- Persistent or progressive dysfluency is described as "stuttering."
  - Examples
    ○ Sound prolongations "ca-caaaa-caaaaat"
    ○ Multiple part-word repetitions "ca-ca-ca-cat"

*Language Disorders*
Receptive Language Disorders
- Deficits in language comprehension/auditory processing—recognizing and processing verbal information and sounds.
  - The inattention and distractibility in children with ADHD overlays with "auditory processing disorders"
  - Poor quality acoustic environments; peripheral ear functioning; behavior factors involved in listening; and problems with the cochlea, auditory nerve, brain stem, and cortex can all be involved in causing auditory processing difficulties.
  - Receptive language problems almost always occur in conjunction with expressive delay
Expressive Language Disorder
- Deficits in verbal and written expression—broad spectrum of delays, including developmentally inappropriate short length of utterances, word-finding weakness, semantic substitutions, and difficulty mastering grammatical morphemes that contribute to plural or tense.
  - Signs of Expressive Language Weakness include the following:
    ○ Circumlocutions (using many words to explain a word instead of using the specific term)
    ○ Excessive use of place holders
      – ("um, "uh")
      – Nonspecific words ("Stuff" or "Like")
      – Using gestures excessively, or difficulty generating an ordered narrative
    ○ Decreased speech production in a child who follows multistep commands
Mixed Receptive—Expressive Language Disorder
- May include features of
  - Verbal auditory agnosia (difficulty integrating the phenology of aural information—limited comprehension of spoken language)
  - Phonologic dysfunction—syntactic deficit (extreme difficulty producing language with variable levels of comprehension)
  - Semantic-pragmatic deficit (expressively fluent with sophisticated use of words, but poor comprehension and superficial use of conversational speech)
  - Lexical-syntactic deficit (word finding weakness and hyper order expressive skills weakness)

*Disorders of Pragmatic Language*
- Inability to use language appropriately for social communications
- Commonly seen in children with autism spectrum disorders and children with non-verbal learning disorders
- Social (pragmatic) communication disorder now used for those that struggle with this but do not have identifiable underlying cause (like ASD)

Related Issues
- *Dyslexia*
  - Reading decoding problems with the core problem based on phonological (speech) processing problems—word level problems
- *Dysgraphia*
  - Graphomotor and orthographic processing issues, subword level problems
- *Dyscalculia*
  - While dyscalculia is a math LD, it is highly comorbid with reading/language disorders and visual-spatial problems

## ATTENTION-DEFICIT/HYPERACTIVITY DISORDER

- The most common behavioral disorder of childhood, affecting 8-10% of children.
- Characterized by hyperactivity, poor impulse control, and inattentiveness.
- Twice as common in boys than girls.
- Boys with ADHD tend to have additional EXTERNALIZING issues—ODD, CD.
- Girls with ADHD tend to have additional INTERNALIZING issues—Anxiety, Depression.
- ADHD is a chronic illness, with symptoms that can persist into adulthood. Therefore, it is important that children have a medical home that can coordinate and advocate for their care.
- Diagnosis
  - Hyperactivity
    - Fidgets with hands/squirms in seat
    - "on the go"/"driven by a motor"
    - Talks excessively
    - Difficult to remain seated in classroom settings
  - Impulsivity
    - Often interrupts others
    - Difficulty with turn taking in tasks or conversations
    - Will say or do things without thinking through consequences
    - Invades others' personal space
  - Inattentiveness
    - Often misses details in assignments
    - Difficulty sustaining attention to tasks
    - Difficulty with organization
    - Easily distracted/forgetful
    - Appears to forget concepts they have previously mastered
  - Symptoms must be present before 12 years of age and cause significant impairment in two or more settings. Examples of domains where impairment can be observed include the following:
    - Academic achievement
    - Family relationships
    - Peer relationships

- ○ Self-esteem and self-perceptions
- ○ Accidental injuries
- ○ Overall adaptive functioning
- • Symptoms must also not be explained by a variant of normal developmental behavior or be strictly attributable to another cause—check for anxiety/depression/substance use in teens and trauma/abuse in young children.
- • Treatment
  - • Preschool-aged children: First line of therapy is parent and/or teacher administered behavioral therapy; utilizing medications only if behavioral interventions are unsuccessful or unavailable.
  - • Elementary-aged children and adolescents: Medications (specifically methylphenidates) are first-line therapy, to be used in conjunction with behavioral interventions.
- • Medications
  - • Types (Fig. 13-1)
    - ○ Stimulants (methylphenidates, amphetamine)
    - ○ Alpha 2 agonist (guanfacine, clonidine)
    - ○ Atomoxetine
  - • Generally, start with methylphenidate at lowest dose. Titrate approximately every 1-2 weeks to achieve clinical improvement without side effects. If side effects interfere with achieving optimal dosing, can add an alpha 2 agonist or consider switching medications.
  - • Side effects
    - ○ Stimulants
      - – Appetite loss
      - – Abdominal pain
      - – Headaches
      - – Sleep disturbance
      - – Mood lability and dysphoria in preschool children or when the medication is wearing off in older children
      - – "zoning out"
    - ○ Alpha 2 agonists
      - – Somnolence
      - – Dry mouth
    - ○ Atomoxetine
      - – Somnolence
      - – Decreased appetite
      - – Increase in suicidal thoughts
      - – Reversible liver function abnormalities
  - • Can monitor improvement with standardized forms (e.g., Vanderbilt, ADHD index, SNAP forms)
  - • Which methylphenidate or amphetamine product to use is determined by medication preparation and duration of action.
  - • Combining medications: In some situations, it is best to combine different classes of medications. This achieves lower doses of individual medications (which can lower side effects) while addressing other comorbidities.
    - ○ Stimulants and alpha 2 agonists: best used for patients with disruptive disorders (see section "Disruptive Behavioral Disorders" for more information) or sleep issues
    - ○ Stimulants and SSRI's: can be utilized in patients with anxiety, OCD, and/or depression

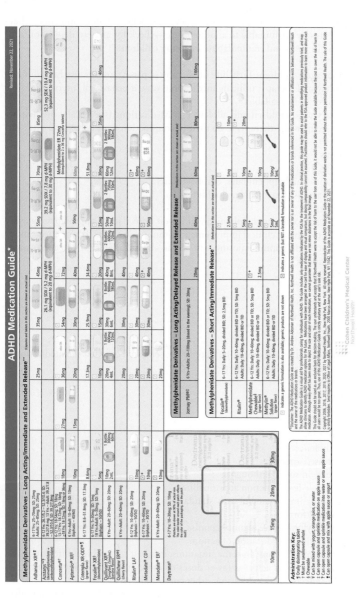

**Figure 13-1. ADHD medication guide.** (Reprinted with permission from Cohen Children's Medical Center Northwell Health. Images no longer actual size due to printing limitations. http://ADHDMedicationGuide.com.)

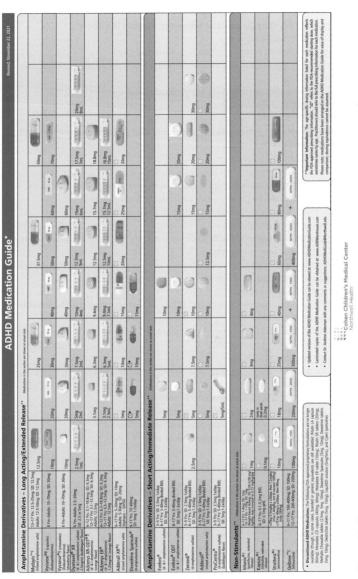

**Figure 13-1.** (*Continued*) (Reprinted with permission from Cohen Children's Medical Center Northwell Health. Images no longer actual size due to printing limitations. http://ADHDMedicationGuide.com.)

## ANXIETY DISORDERS

Anxiety and fear are normal responses to either real or perceived threats. The typical triggers for a child's anxiety and fear evolve as the child matures (Table 13-3).

- **An anxiety disorder may be present when the anxiety is either:**
  - Developmentally inappropriate
  - Inappropriate levels of intensity, duration, or frequency
  - Causes clinically significant impairment in the child's personal, academic, and/or social life.
- **Screening instruments appropriate for primary care**
  - SCARED (readily available online)
  - PHQ-9 (readily available online)
- **Description of specific youth anxiety disorders and potential-associated behavioral and cognitive components**
  - Separation anxiety disorder
    - Developmentally normal from 9 months to approximately 3 years.
    - Excessive anxiety about being apart from caregivers. Can be manifested as:
      - Reluctance/refusal to go to school or separate from caregiver
      - Nightmares and/or constantly wanting to sleep with parents.
      - Various somatic complaints when left alone
      - Fear that some harm will come to either the child or caregivers when separated
    - Symptoms last at least 6 months.
    - Mothers and other caregivers often have a history of anxiety and/or depression and should be screened and referred for treatment if necessary.
  - Generalized anxiety disorder
    - Anxiety that occurs on most days and is not in response to a specific stimulus
    - Activities with possible negative outcomes are avoided.
    - The patient exhibits at least one of the following: restlessness or muscle tension
    - Symptoms last at least 3 months.
  - Specific phobias
    - Excessive and unreasonable fear to a particular stimulus (e.g., flying, animals, blood, heights)
    - Exposure to stimulus provokes anxiety symptoms
    - Child may or may not recognize that anxiety is unreasonable
    - Specific phobia is avoided or tolerated with great distress
    - Symptoms cause significant impairment in child's social, academic, and/or personal life.
    - Symptoms last for at least 6 months.

| TABLE 13-3 | Normal Anxiety Triggers by Developmental Level |
|---|---|
| **Age** | **Anxious triggers** |
| **Infancy/toddlers** | Fear of loss, strangers, separation anxiety |
| **Early childhood (preschool)** | Specific (though not necessarily rational) threats: meteors, end of the world, fires, mythical animals, being kidnapped. |
| **School age** | Domestic animals, death, disease, school anxiety |
| **Adolescence** | Fear of rejection, school performance |

- Social anxiety disorder
  - Excessive fear when exposed to people or situations where a negative evaluation (e.g., embarrassment or humiliation) is possible.
  - The people and situations can be either familiar or novel to the patient.
  - Such situations and people are actively avoided to reduce anxiety.
- **The first line of treatment for anxiety disorders is cognitive behavioral therapy with the addition of a selective serotonin uptake inhibitor, if needed.**
- **Treatment Guidelines for antidepressant agents** (Table 13-4)
  - SSRI's
    - First-line treatment when psychotropic medication intervention (Table 13-5) is needed for the treatment anxiety and depressive symptoms
    - Large margin of safety
    - Side effects
      - Irritability
      - Headaches
      - Appetite changes
      - Constipation or diarrhea
    - Be aware that suicidal ideation can manifest during the early period of medication initiation in children and adolescents with a major depressive disorder. Antidepressants can also unmask manic episodes when given in adolescents with bipolar disorder. Patients must be closely monitored during first few weeks of therapy.

## AUTISM SPECTRUM DISORDERS

### Definition
Behaviorally defined conditions characterized by distinctive impairments in reciprocal social interaction and communication that do not simply reflect associated intellectual disability or a medical condition and by the presence of a restricted, repetitive behavioral repertoire.

### Diagnostic Criteria (Adapted from DSM 5)
- Social communication and interaction—all criteria must be met
  - Deficits in social-emotional reciprocity
    - Unable to have normal back-and-forth conversations
    - Difficulty in sharing of interests or displaying emotions or affect
    - Failure to initiate or respond to social interactions
  - Deficits in nonverbal communications
    - Poorly integrated verbal and nonverbal communications
    - Poor eye contact and use of body language
    - Deficits in the understanding and use of gestures
    - Total lack of facial expressions and nonverbal communication
  - Deficits in developing, maintaining, and understanding relationships
    - Difficulties adjusting behavior in various social settings
    - Difficulties in making friends and cooperative imaginative play
    - Little to no interest in peers.
- Restricted, repetitive behaviors—at least two of the four criteria must be met
  - Stereotyped or repetitive motor movements, use of objects, or speech
    - Simple motor stereotypies—hand flapping, finger mannerisms, spinning
    - Lining up toys or flipping objects
    - Echolalia
    - Idiosyncratic phrases

| TABLE 13-4 | Dosing Guidelines for Antidepressant Agents | | | |
|---|---|---|---|---|
| Type/class | Medication | Initial starting daily dose | Initial target daily dose (serum level)[a] | Maximum daily dose (serum level) | Recommended administration |
| SSRI | Citalopram | 10-20 mg | 20 mg | 60 mg | AM |
| | Escitalopram | 5-10 mg | 10 mg | 20 mg | AM |
| | Fluoxetine | 10-20 mg | 20 mg | 40-80 mg | AM |
| | Paroxetine (i) | 10-20 mg | 20-30 mg | 40-60 mg (ii) | AM or HS |
| | Sertraline | 25-50 mg | 50-100 mg | 150-200 mg | AM |
| SNRI | Duloxetine | 20-30 mg | 40-60 mg | 120 mg (iii) | Daily or BID |
| | Venlafaxine | 37.5-75 mg | 150-225 mg | 375 mg | BID |
| | Venlafaxine XR | 37.5-75 mg | 75-225 mg | 225 mg | Daily |
| Other (iv) | Bupropion | 75 mg | 225-300 mg | 450 mg | TID ≤ 150 mg/dose |
| | Bupropion SR | 100-150 mg | 200-300 mg | 400 mg | BID ≤ 200 mg/dose |
| | Bupropion XL | 150 mg | 300 mg | 450 mg | Daily |
| | Mirtazapine | 7.5-15 mg | 30 mg | 60 mg (v) | HS |

| TCA | Amitriptyline | 25-50 mg | 150-200 mg | 300 mg | HS |
| --- | --- | --- | --- | --- | --- |
| | Clomipramine | 25 mg | 100-150 mg | 250 mg | HS |
| | Desipramine | 25-50 mg | 150 mg (>ng/mL) | 300 mg | HS |
| | Imipramine | 25-50 mg | 150 mg (>ng/mL) (vi) | 300 mg (200-400 ng/mL) (vi) | HS |
| | Nortriptyline | 25–50 mg | 75-100 mg (50-150 ng/mL) | 150 mg (50-150 ng/mL) | HS |

SSRI, selective serotonin reuptake inhibitor; SNRI, serotonin-norepinephrine reuptake inhibitor; TCA, tricyclic antidepressant.

aAntidepressant dosage can be increased every 2-3 weeks as tolerated if remission has not occurred: (i) paroxetine and paroxetine CR have similar side effect profiles, comparable half-lives, and reach steady-state plasma concentrations at similar time intervals, (ii) manufacturer recommended maximum dose for major depressive disorder (MDD) is 50 mg/day, (iii) manufacturer recommended maximum dose for MDD is 60 mg/day, and (iv) trazodone is not included as a treatment option for MDD because therapeutic doses are hard to achieve due to excessive sedation (therapeutic dose 300-600 mg/day). Trazodone may be considered during the acute treatment phase as adjunctive therapy when sedation is desired. (v) Manufacturer recommended that maximum dose is 45 mg/day. (vi) Serum level includes parent drug and active metabolite (imipramine and desipramine, respectively).

From Evidence-Based Best Practices for the Treatment of Major Depressive Disorder in South Carolina. Published February 2008. Available at http://www.sccp.sc.edu/centers/SCORxE/SCORxE Academic Detailing Service. Reproduced with permission.

| TABLE 13-5 | Psychotropic Medication Options for Common Target Symptoms |
|---|---|
| Target symptoms | Medication |
| Aggressive, self-injurious behavior | Risperidone, aripiprazole, ziprasidone |
| Repetitive behaviors | Risperidone, aripiprazole |
| Hyperactivity, inattention | Stimulants (methylphenidates) |
| Sleep disturbances | Melatonin, clonidine, trazodone |
| Anxiety and/or depression | Sertraline, citalopram, escitalopram, fluoxetine |

- Insistence on sameness, inflexibility, and ritualized patterns
  - Extreme distress at small changes (to routine or environment)
  - Difficulties with transitions
  - Rigid thinking patterns
  - Need to take same route or eat same food everyday
- Highly restricted, fixated interests that are abnormal in intensity or focus
- Hyper or hypo-reactivity to sensory input
  - Apparent indifference to pain/temperature (sensory indifference)
  - Adverse response to specific sounds or textures (sensory avoidance)
  - Excessive smelling or touching of objects (sensory seeking)
  - Visual fascination with lights or movement (sensory seeking)
- Symptoms must be present in the early developmental periods.
- Symptoms must cause clinically significant impairment in the child's social, academic, or personal life. Symptoms are graded due to severity.
- Symptoms are not better explained by intellectual disability or global development delay.

## Screening Instruments for Use and/or Diagnosis in Primary Care
- Modified Checklist for Autism (M-CHAT)
- Pervasive Developmental Disorders Screening Test-II Primary Care Screener (PDDST-II PCS)
- Social Responsiveness Scale (SRS)
- Autism Spectrum Screening Questionnaire (ASSQ)
- Social Communication Questionnaire (SCQ)
- Autism Diagnostic Observation Schedule (ADOS2)
- Autism Diagnosis Interview—Revised (ADI-R)
- Childhood Autism Rating Scale (CARS)
- Gilliam Autism Rating Scale—Second Edition (GARS-2)

## Genetic Testing
- Approximately 80% of all cases of autism spectrum disorders are idiopathic, whereas 20% have a known chromosomal, single gene or metabolic etiology.
- 1-3% of children with ASD's will be due to Fragile X, thus it is recommended that Fragile X testing be done during the evaluation of ASD's.
- Chromosomal microarray analysis can be considered if there are signs of major cognitive impairment, dysmorphic features, or a strong family history of developmental delay.
- In girls who have a history of developmental regression, consider testing for Rett syndrome.

- In patients where there is evidence of ataxia, seizures, muscle weakness, hypotonia, or other neurological impairments, testing for disorders of metabolism should be considered.
- Examples of genetic conditions associated with Autism
  - Fragile X
  - Neurofibromatosis
  - Angelman syndrome
  - 22q11 deletion syndrome
  - Williams syndrome
  - Noonan syndrome
  - Cornelia de Lange syndrome
  - Down syndrome

## Complementary and Alternative Medicine (Table 13-6)

- Many families will use alternative therapies for their children with autism.
- Some examples include the following:
  - Chelation of presumed heavy metals
  - Antifungal agents
  - Probiotics
  - Gluten free, casein-free diets
  - Vitamin $B_6$ and magnesium supplementation
  - Auditory and visual integration training
  - Hyperbaric oxygen
  - Chiropractic manipulation
- In general, there is little evidence to support the efficacy of these therapies and some, such as chelation, may be harmful.
- It is important to become familiar with complementary and alternative therapies and discuss with interested families their potential risks, benefits, and efficacy.

## DISRUPTIVE BEHAVIOR DISORDERS

### Definition

Socially disruptive behavior that is generally more disturbing to others than to the person initiating the behavior.

- Problems occur on a continuum, with normal toddler resistance and tantrums at one end and more severe, maladaptive behaviors warranting a medical diagnosis at the other end.
- Treatment generally involves intense behavioral therapy, often involving both child and family.

### Oppositional Defiant Disorder

- A pattern of angry/irritable mood, argumentative/defiant behavior, or vindictiveness
  - Four symptoms from any of the following categories:
    ○ Angry/irritable mood
      – Often loses temper
      – Is often "touchy" or easily annoyed
      – Is often angry and resentful
    ○ Argumentative/defiant behavior
      – Often argues with authority figures

| TABLE 13-6 | Results of Trials of Complementary and Alternative Therapies | |
|---|---|---|
| Therapy | Therapeutic benefit | Major side effects |
| Gluten/casein-free diet | None | None |
| Secretin | None | None, though minor side effects (flushing, vomiting, hyperactivity) were noted |
| Hyperbaric oxygen | None | None noted, but theoretical risk of barotrauma and exacerbation of previous pulmonary disease |
| Vitamin $B_6$ and magnesium | None | None |
| Melatonin | Significant improvements in sleep duration and onset latency | None |

- Often actively defies or refuses to comply with request from authority figures or with rules
- Often deliberately annoys others
- Often blames others for his or her mistakes or misbehaviors
  ○ Vindictiveness
    - Has been spiteful or vindictive at least twice in the past 6 months
- Must last at least 6 months
- Must be exhibited during an interaction with at least one individual who is not a sibling
- Must be associated with distress in the individual or his or her peers or impacts negatively on social, educational, occupational, or other important areas of functioning.
- The behaviors do not occur exclusively during the course of a psychotic, substance use, depressive, or bipolar disorder.

## Intermittent Explosive Disorder
- Recurrent behavioral outbursts representing a failure to control aggressive impulses as manifested by either.
  - Verbal aggression or physical aggression to property, animals or individuals occurring at least twice weekly, on average, for 3 months
  - Three outbursts involving damage or destruction of property and/or physical injury occurring in a 12-month period
- Outbursts are grossly out of proportion to the provocation or to any precipitating psychosocial stressors.
- Outbursts are not premeditated and not committed to achieve some tangible objective.
- Must cause distress of the individual or impairment in occupational or interpersonal functioning or are associated with financial or legal consequences.
- Either chronological or developmental age must be at least 6 years.
- The recurrent outbursts are not better explained by another mental disorder.

## Conduct Disorder

- A repetitive and persistent pattern of behavior in which the basic rights of others or major age-appropriate societal norms are violated, as manifested by the presence of at least 3 of the following 15 criteria in the past 12 months with at least one in the past 6 months.
  - Often bullies, threatens, or intimidates others
  - Often initiates physical fights
  - Has used a weapon that can cause serious physical harm to others (gun, knife, bat, etc.)
  - Has been physically cruel to people
  - Has been physically cruel to animals
  - Has stolen while confronting a victim (e.g., mugging)
  - Has forced someone into sexual activity
  - Has deliberately engaged in fire setting with the intention of causing serious damage
  - Has deliberately destroyed other's property
  - Has broken into someone else's house, building, or car
  - Often lies to obtain goods, favors, or to avoid obligations ("cons" others)
  - Has stolen items of value without confronting a victim (e.g., Shoplifting)
  - Often stays out at night despite parental prohibitions, beginning before age 13 years
  - Has run away from home overnight at least twice or once without returning for a lengthy period
  - Is often truant from school, beginning before age 13 years
- The disturbance causes clinically significant impairment in social, academic, or occupational functioning.
- Subtypes
  - Childhood-onset type: Must show at least one symptom prior to age 10 years.
  - Adolescent-onset type: Show no symptoms prior to age 10 years.
  - Unspecified onset: not enough information to determine whether the first symptom occurred before or after age 10 years.

## PSYCHOEDUCATIONAL TESTING

### Intelligence Testing
- **Kaufman Brief Intelligence Test, Second Edition (KBIT-2)**
  - Verbal, nonverbal, and composite IQ
    - Verbal subtests
      - Verbal knowledge
      - Riddles (measures verbal comprehension, reasoning, vocabulary knowledge, and deductive reasoning)
    - Nonverbal scale—matrices
      - Meaningful and abstract stimuli
- **Stanford Binet for Early Childhood–5**
  - Nonverbal IQ, Verbal IQ, and Full-scale IQ
  - Subtests for both nonverbal and verbal areas
    - Nonverbal fluid reasoning
    - Knowledge (crystallized intelligence)
    - Quantitative reasoning
    - Visual-spatial processing

- ○ Working memory
- Total Factor Index Scores—Sum of verbal and nonverbal scores for each of the five areas
- **Differential Ability Scales–II (DAS)**
  - Frequently used in the early childhood/preschool age
  - 11 core and 10 diagnostic subtests
    - ○ The 11 core items contribute to the general conceptual ability score
    - ○ The diagnostic subtests, measure short-term memory, perceptional abilities, and processing speed
- **Kaufman Assessment Battery for Children–Second Edition (KABC-11)**
  - Five areas assessed
    - ○ Simultaneous processing
    - ○ Sequential processing
    - ○ Planning
    - ○ Learning
    - ○ Knowledge
  - Scores generated
    - ○ MPI
    - ○ Global score
    - ○ Fluid-crystalized index
    - ○ Nonverbal index
- **Wechsler Preschool and Primary Scale of Intelligence–Third Edition (WPPSI-III)**
  - Two age bands
    - ○ 2 years 6 months to 3 years 11 months
    - ○ 4 years to 7 years 3 months
  - Scores reported as *Full-Scale IQ, Verbal IQ, and Performance IQ*
    - ○ 4 core subtests for the younger group
    - ○ 7 core subtests for the older group
- **Wechsler Intelligence Scale for Children–Fifth Edition (WISC-V)**
  - Ages 6 years to 16 years, 11 months
    - ○ 11 subtests—Index Scores
      - – Verbal comprehension
      - – Visual spatial
      - – Fluid reasoning
      - – Working memory
      - – Processing speed
  - *Full-Scale IQ* is produced
  - *General Ability Index* can be computed by using three verbal comprehension subtests and three perceptual reasoning subtests
- **Wechsler Abbreviated Scale of Intelligence (WASI)**
  - Generates a *Verbal IQ, Performance IQ, and Full-Scale IQ*
  - Subtests include Vocabulary, Matrices, Block Design, and Similarities
  - Useful as a screening instrument and used by many school districts to screen for gifted programs

**Additional cognitive tests for assessment of nonverbal abilities**

- **Leiter 3**
  - Age range 3+
  - Measure fluid intelligence
  - Sequential order

- Form completion
- Classification and analogies
- Figure ground
- Matching/repeated patterns
- **Test of Nonverbal Intelligence–4 (TONI-4)**
  - For ages 6+
  - Test for children who have language, hearing, or motor impairment
    ○ Responses require simple pointing or gesture
  - Measure intelligence, aptitude abstract reasoning, and problem solving
  - Uses testing picture book
    ○ Pick items to complete pictures

## Language Testing

- **Clinical Evaluation of Language Fundamentals-5 (CELF-5)**
  - Produces a Core Language Score from the following index scores:
    ○ Receptive Language Index
    ○ Expression Language Index
    ○ Language Content Index
    ○ Language Structure Index
- **Oral and Written Language Scales II (OWLS II)**
  - Produces an Oral Language Composite Score with the following components:
    ○ Listening comprehension
    ○ Oral expression
- **Comprehensive Assessment of Spoken Language-2 (CASL-2)**
  - Produces a General Language Ability Score from the following subscores:
    ○ Receptive vocabulary
    ○ Expressive vocabulary
    ○ Sentence expression
    ○ Sentence comprehension
    ○ Pragmatic language
- **Comprehensive Test of Phonological Processing (CTOPP)**
  - Helps evaluate phonologic processing abilities as a prerequisite to reading fluency
    ○ Dyslexia
    ○ Reading fluency
    ○ Takes 40 minutes to administer

## SUGGESTED READINGS

American Academy of Pediatrics; Rosenblatt AI, Carbone PS. Autism Spectrum Disorders: What Every Parent Needs to Know. American Academy of Pediatrics, 2019.

American Academy of Pediatrics; Wolraich M, Wolraich ML, Hagan JF Jr, Hagan JF Jr. ADHD: What Every Parent Needs to Know. American Academy of Pediatrics, 2019.

American Psychiatric Association. Diagnostic and Statistical Manual of Mental Disorders. 5th Ed. American Psychiatric Publishers, Inc., 2013.

Augustyn M, et al. The Zuckerman Parker Handbook of Developmental and Behavioral Pediatrics for Primary Care. 3rd Ed. Philadelphia, PA: Lippincott Williams & Wilkins, 2010.

Korb D. Raising an Organized Child. American Academy of Pediatrics, 2019.

Voigt R, et al. Developmental and Behavioral Pediatrics. Arlington: American Academy of Pediatrics, 2010.

Wolraich M, et al. Developmental and Behavioral Pediatrics: Evidence and Practice. Philadelphia, PA: Mosby, Inc., 2007.

# 14 Cardiology

William B. Orr and Jennifer N. Avari Silva

## CARDIAC EXAMINATION

### Vital Signs and Inspection

- Heart Rate: varies with age but generally, resting heart rate decreases with age.
  - Table 14-1 lists normal heart rates.
- Blood Pressure:
  - Blood pressure is commonly measured via auscultatory (stethoscope and sphygmomanometer) or oscillometric devices (i.e., Dinamap).
  - Compared to auscultatory methods, blood pressure measurements obtained on oscillometric devices are in general 10 mm Hg higher for the systolic pressure and 5 mm Hg for the diastolic pressure.
  - See Appendix F for blood pressure levels for boys and girls.
  - Orthostatic blood pressure measures are obtained both supine and standing.
  - Orthostatic hypotension is a fall in systolic/diastolic blood pressure of more than 20/10 mmHg within 3 minutes of assuming an upright position.
  - Postural orthostatic tachycardia syndrome (POTS) presents with symptoms associated with an increase in heart rate of ≥30 beats per minute occurring within 10 minutes of standing without a significant decrease in BP.
  - Differential blood pressure between upper and lower extremities occurs in coarctation of the aorta.
  - A complete cardiac examination involves inspection of general appearance, skin color, respiratory effort and rate, and precordial visual inspection.

| TABLE 14-1 | Normal Heart Rates in Children[a] |
|---|---|
| Age | Heart rate (beats/min) |
| 0–1 month | 145 (90-180) |
| 6 months | 145 (105-185) |
| 1 year | 132 (105-170) |
| 2 years | 120 (90-150) |
| 4 years | 108 (72-135) |
| 6 years | 100 (65-135) |
| 10 years | 90 (65-130) |
| 14 years | 85 (60-120) |

[a]Recorded on ECG, with mean and ranges.
*Source*: From Park MK, Guntheroth WG. How to Read Pediatric ECGs, 4th Ed. Philadelphia: Mosby, 2006:46. Copyright Elsevier 2006.

## Auscultation

- Stethoscope anatomy
  - Diaphragm: better for picking up the relatively high-pitched sounds of S1 and S2, the murmurs of aortic and mitral regurgitation, and pericardial friction rubs
  - Bell: more sensitive to the low-pitched sounds of S3 and S4 and the murmur of mitral stenosis
- S1 is produced by closure of the mitral and tricuspid valves in that order. S2 is produced by closure of the aortic ($A_2$) and the pulmonic ($P_2$) valves.
- Physiologic spitting of S2 is the widening of $A_2$ and $P_2$ that occurs by inspiration and disappears on expiration.
- Other heart sounds such as gallops (S3 or S4), clicks, snaps, and rubs are pathologic and should warrant additional evaluation.
- Murmur: See next section.
- Auscultate lung fields.

## Palpation

- Palpated Palpate Precordium
  - Right ventricular heave (lift): volume overload (atrial septal defect) or a pressure overload (large ventral septal defect, pulmonary hypertension, and pulmonary stenosis).
  - Left ventricular heave (lift): aortic stenosis.
  - A thrill (vibration) with grade 4+ murmur is usually pathologic.
  - Palpate abdomen. Hepatomegaly may suggest congestive heart failure.
  - Palpate peripheral pulses. Differential pulses occur in coarctation of the aorta.

## HEART MURMURS

### General Principles

- Heart murmurs are common in children. At least 50% of children will have a murmur noted at some time.
- Murmurs may occur with a history of poor feeding in infants, with activity intolerance or with a family history of congenital heart defects or cardiomyopathy.
- Murmurs can be innocent or pathologic.
- Murmurs should be characterized by the timing (systole/diastolic/continuous), location, radiation, pitch, quality (blowing/harsh/rumbling/musical), shape (crescendo/decrescendo/crescendo-decrescendo/plateau), and intensity (usually on a six-point scale expressed as a fraction, ≥4 must have palpable thrill).
- The intensity (loudness) of a murmur does not necessarily correlate with the severity of the condition. The examination of a child with a murmur should go beyond listening to the murmur.

### Innocent Murmurs

- The vast majority of heart murmurs in childhood are innocent or functional in nature.
- These murmurs occur in the absence of anatomic or physiologic abnormalities of the heart and therefore have no clinical significance.
- The age at onset of innocent murmurs is most frequently 3-8 years.
- Innocent murmurs usually occur during early to midsystole (they are never diastolic), are short in duration, have a crescendo-decrescendo contour, and are usually <3/6 in intensity.

| TABLE 14-2 | Features That May Suggest a Pathologic Murmur |
|---|---|

- All diastolic murmurs
- All holosystolic murmurs
- Late systolic murmurs
- Presence of a thrill

- Innocent murmurs are often louder in the supine position or with fever, anemia, or other conditions that lead to increased cardiac output.
- The venous hum is an innocent continuous murmur best heard in the infraclavicular area. This hum should disappear when the patient is supine or with compression of the neck veins.

### Pathologic Murmurs

- Pathologic murmurs should be suspected when other features of heart disease are present, including poor growth/failure to thrive, tachypnea/tachycardia, and central cyanosis.
- Table 14-2 includes features of murmurs that may be pathologic.
- The timing and location of pathologic murmurs can help narrow the differential diagnosis (Tables 14-3 to 14-8).

### Treatment

- Treatments vary depending on the condition.
- Initiate ABCs if necessary to stabilize the patient.
- If cardiac disease is suspected based on the initial evaluation, seek cardiology consultation before ordering additional tests.

| TABLE 14-3 | Characteristics of Systolic Murmurs along Right Upper Sternal Border | | | |
|---|---|---|---|---|
| Lesion | Timing, quality | Heard best | Transmits to | Comments |
| **Aortic valve stenosis** | Ejection | Second left intercostal space | Neck, left upper sternal border, apex | +/− thrill, ejection click, left ventricular lift, possible single $S_2$ |
| **Subaortic stenosis** | Ejection | — | — | No click |
| **Supravalvular aortic stenosis** | Ejection | — | Back | No click, +/− thrill, associated with Williams syndrome |

| TABLE 14-4 | Characteristics of Systolic Murmurs along Left Upper Sternal Border | | | |

| Lesion | Timing, quality | Heard best | Transmits to | Comments |
|--------|-----------------|------------|--------------|----------|
| **Pulmonic valve stenosis** | Ejection | — | Back | +/− thrill, $S_2$ may be widely split if mild, +/− variable ejection click at 2nd left intercostal space. |
| **Atrial septal defect (ASD)** | Ejection, soft | Second left intercostal space | — | Widely split, fixed $S_2$, +/− diastolic murmur. |
| **Pulmonary artery stenosis** | Ejection | — | Back and both lung fields | $P_2$ may be loud. |
| **Tetralogy of Fallot** | Long ejection murmur | Midleft sternal border or left upper sternal border | — | +/− thrill, single $S_2$. |
| **Coarctation of the aorta** | Ejection | Left interscapular area | — | Pulse and blood pressure disparity. |
| **Patent ductus arteriosus (PDA) in neonates** | High frequency | Left infraclavicular area | — | Bounding pulses. |

| TABLE 14-5 | Characteristics of Systolic Murmurs along Left Lower Sternal Border | | | |

| Lesion | Timing, quality | Heard best | Transmits to | Comments |
|--------|-----------------|------------|--------------|----------|
| **Ventricular septal defect (VSD)** | Regurgitant, harsh, systolic, may be holosystolic | Localized and short if small, muscular | Lower right of sternum, left upper if outflow | May be soft with loud $P_2$ and right ventricular lift if large. |
| **Complete atrioventricular (AV) canal** | Similar to VSD | — | Apical murmur with AV regurgitation, diastolic rumble, may have gallop. | |

*(Continued)*

**TABLE 14-5** Characteristics of Systolic Murmurs along Left Lower Sternal Border *(Continued)*

| Lesion | Timing, quality | Heard best | Transmits to | Comments |
|---|---|---|---|---|
| **Subaortic stenosis with hypertrophic cardiomyopathy** | Ejection | Left lower sternal border or apex, medium pitch | — | +/− thrill, Valsalva increases murmur, squatting decreases murmur. |
| **Tricuspid regurgitation** | Regurgitant systolic | — | — | Multiple sounds: split $S_1$, $S_3$/$S_4$ in Ebstein anomaly. |

**TABLE 14-6** Characteristics of Systolic Murmurs at Apex

| Lesion | Timing, quality | Heard best | Transmits to | Comments |
|---|---|---|---|---|
| **Mitral regurgitation** | Plateau-type blowing | Apex to midprecordium | Left axilla, back | Diastolic rumble if severe. |
| **Mitral valve prolapse** | Midsystolic click with late systolic murmur if mitral regurgitation present | — | | Click moves toward $S_2$ (squatting) and toward $S_1$ (standing). |

**TABLE 14-7** Characteristics of Diastolic Murmurs

| Lesion | Timing, quality | Heard best | Transmits to | Comments |
|---|---|---|---|---|
| **Aortic regurgitation** | Early, decrescendo, high pitched | 3rd left intercostal space | Apex | Short and loud if severe |
| **Pulmonary regurgitation** | Early, medium pitched | 2nd left intercostal space | Along left sternal border | Short and loud if severe |
| **Mitral stenosis** | Mid to late, crescendo low-pitched rumble | Apex | | Soft or loud $S_2$ |

| TABLE 14-8 | Characteristics of Continuous Murmurs | | |
|---|---|---|---|
| Lesion | Timing, quality | Heard best | Comments |
| Patent ductus arteriosus | Louder in systole, machinery | Left mid to upper sternal border | Bounding pulse if large |
| Coronary to right heart fistula | | Left sternal border | Rare cause of murmur |
| Cerebral arteriovenous fistula | Louder in diastole | Infraclavicular | Bruit in head |

## DIAGNOSTIC TOOLS

• The field of cardiology employs a multitude of diagnostic tools.
• Table 14-9 lists some of the most common tools used.

## CONGENITAL HEART DISEASE

• Congenital heart disease is typically divided into four major groups: acyanotic lesions (left-to-right shunts), cyanotic lesions (right-to-left shunt), obstructive lesions, and miscellaneous.

| TABLE 14-9 | Diagnostic Tools and Indications | |
|---|---|---|
| Modality | Types | Description |
| Electrocardiogram (ECG) | 12-Lead, 15-Lead | Graphs the electrical activity (10 sec) of the heart. Helps screen for abnormalities with conduction, depolarization, repolarization, hypertrophy/enlargement, inflammation, and coronary blood flow. |
| Echocardiogram | Transthoracic, transesophageal, fetal, intravascular, stress/exercise | Uses ultrasound to visualize cardiac structures and function in one, two, or three dimension. Also provides Doppler measurements and color mapping of blood flow. |
| Chest plain radiograph | Posteroanterior and lateral views | Provides information about heart size, enlargement of specific cardiac chambers, pulmonary vascular blood flow, lung parenchyma, and bony abnormalities. |

*(Continued)*

**TABLE 14-9** Diagnostic Tools and Indications *(Continued)*

| Modality | Types | Description |
|---|---|---|
| Hyperoxia test | | Uses $PaO_2$ from an arterial blood gas (ABG) to provide insight on the cause of cyanosis. See Newborn with Heart Disease section. |
| Exercise stress test (EST) | Cardiopulmonary exercise test, graded ECG, stress echo, myocardial perfusion (MPI) | Measures parameters of exercise function. Can identify what level (cardiovascular, respiratory, blood, muscle) causes a limitation of exercise performance. Can also identify arrhythmias, ischemia, and valve gradient changes during exercise. |
| Ambulatory blood pressure monitoring (ABPM) | | Obtains multiple awake and asleep blood pressure measurements throughout the day. Helps differentiate pathologic hypertension vs. "white-coat" hypertension |
| Long-term electro-cardiogram monitoring | Holter, event monitor (looping and nonlooping), implantable loop recorder (ILR) | Documents and quantitates the electrical activity of the heart over longer periods of time. See ILR section for more information. |
| Radiologic techniques | MRI, CT | Can provide better-quality images, tissue differentiation, and functional assessment of some cardiac and extracardiac structures. May use contrast. |
| Cardiac catheterization | Diagnostic, Therapeutic | Directly assesses hemodynamics providing the ability to calculate cardiac output, shunts, and resistances. Can use contrast to take direct angiographic images. Can be used for treating certain abnormalities nonsurgically. |
| Electrophysiology study (EPS) | | Provides an intracardiac electrocardiogram identifying conduction abnormalities or sources or arrhythmias. Can ablate certain arrhythmias with radiofrequency or cryotherapy methods. |

**TABLE 14-10** Congenital Heart Disease Lesions

| Acyanotic (Left-to-right shunt lesions) | Cyanotic (right-to-left shunt lesion) | Obstructive | Miscellaneous |
|---|---|---|---|
| Atrial septal defect (ASD) | Truncus arteriosus | Aortic stenosis | Anomalous origin of the coronary artery |
| Ventricular septal defect (VSD) | Transposition of the great arteries | Pulmonary stenosis | |
| Patent ductus arteriosus (PDA) | Tricuspid atresia | Coarctation of the aorta | Cleft mitral valve |
| Atrioventricular septal defect (AVSD) (aka AV canal or endocardial cushion defect) | Tetralogy of Fallot | Interrupted aortic arch (IAA) | Cor triatriatum |
| | Total anomalous pulmonary venous return | | Parachute mitral valve |
| Partial anomalous pulmonary venous return | Single ventricle anatomy (see single ventricle section) | | Pulmonary vein stenosis |

- Many lesions have multiple subtypes that may present as cyanotic or acyanotic making diagnosis and treatment unique and challenging.
- Some of the common congenital heart lesions and their classifications are listed in Table 14-10.

## SINGLE VENTRICLE LESIONS (UNIVENTRICULAR HEART)

- Single ventricle lesions can be any lesions where a biventricular repair is not possible. In order to have a biventricular repair, a heart must have two relatively normal sized ventricles AND two atrioventricular (AV) valves.
- Some of the common heart lesions that require a single ventricle palliation include hypoplastic left heart syndrome (HLHS), mitral atresia, tricuspid atresia, double inlet left ventricle (DILV), and double outlet right ventricle (DORV) with a remote VSD.
- See Chapter 8, Critical Care.
- The type or stages of palliative repair may slightly vary based on the type of univentricular heart lesion.
- The most common palliative surgeries are the modified Blalock-Taussig-Thomas (mBTT) shunt to provide pulmonary blood flow, the bidirectional Glenn (aka superior cavopulmonary anastomosis) done around 3-4 months and the Fontan (aka inferior cavopulmonary anastomosis) done >15 kg around 3-4 years. See Figure 14-1.

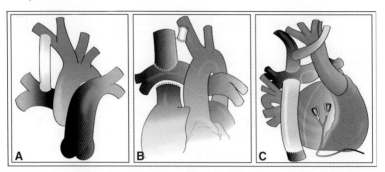

**Figure 14-1. A.** The modified Blalock-Taussig-Thomas (mBTT) shunt consists of an interposition tube graft that connects the subclavian artery to the ipsilateral pulmonary artery. **B.** The bidirectional Glenn shunt consists of an end-to-side anastomosis of the divided superior vena cava to the undivided pulmonary artery. The mBTT is oversewn. **C.** The extracardiac Fontan with pacemaker leads (done on individual need). (Reprinted from Khairy P, Poirier N, Mercier LA. Univentricular heart. Circulation 2007;115(6):800–812.)

## ACQUIRED HEART LESIONS

- The most common acquired heart lesions are usually secondary to either an infection or a rheumatologic process.
- Table 14-11 lists some common acquired heart lesions and where more information can be found.

## ELECTROPHYSIOLOGY

### Electrocardiogram Interpretation
- Electrocardiography is critical in the diagnosis of electrical disorders of the heart. It may serve as a useful screening tool in the evaluation of patients with suspected structural defects or abnormalities of the myocardium.
- Newborns have a large variability in electrocardiogram (ECG) voltages and intervals due in large part to hemodynamic and myocardial adaptations that are needed once the placenta is no longer part of the circulatory system.
- Changes continue, albeit at a slower pace, from infancy through adolescence.
- Algorithms used to interpret ECGs in adults cannot be used in children. This section is a basic, although incomplete, guide to the pediatric ECG.

*Rate*
- The usual recording speed is 25 mm/sec; each little box (1 mm) is 0.04 seconds and each big box (5 mm) is 0.2 seconds.
- With a fast heart rate, count the R-R cycles in 6 large boxes (1.2 seconds) and multiply by 50.
- With a slow heart rate, count the number of large boxes between R waves and divide into 300 (1 box = 300, 2 boxes = 150, 3 boxes = 100, 4 boxes = 75, 5 boxes = 60).
- Table 14-1 lists normal heart rates.

*Rhythm*
- Are the QRS deflections regular? Variation in the heart rate up and down in concert with respirations (sinus arrhythmia) is normal and can be pronounced in young healthy hearts.

**TABLE 14-11** Acquired Heart Lesions

| Lesion | History | Physical examination | ECG findings | Echo findings | Treatment | Comments |
|---|---|---|---|---|---|---|
| **Acute pericarditis (viral)** | Fever, recent viral illness, and pain worse in the supine position, which is decreased by leaning forward | Friction rub | Initial ST segment elevation, PR depression | Normal, pericardial effusion | NSAIDs, colchicine, glucocorticoids | Can cause pericardial effusion |
| **Pericardial effusion/ tamponade** | Similar to pericarditis | Tachycardia, hepatomegaly, Beck triad (distant heart sounds, elevated JVD, hypotension with pulsus paradoxus) | Low-voltage QRS | Fluid between the visceral and parietal pericardium Tamponade: chamber compression from fluid | Based on disease itself (i.e., uremia, collagen disease) Tamponade: pericardial centesis | Fluid may need to be sent to studies. |
| **Myocarditis** | History of URI, chest pain, syncope | May vary with age and severity, signs of CHF in neonates and infants, murmur, irregular rhythm, hepatomegaly | Low QRS voltages, ST-T changes, PR prolongation, prolongation of the QT interval, and arrhythmias | Cardiac chamber enlargement and impaired left ventricle (LV) function | Bed rest, activity limitation, supportive care | Cardiac troponin levels and myocardial enzymes (creatine kinase [CK], MB isoenzyme of CK [CK-MB]) may be elevated. |

*(Continued)*

**TABLE 14-11** Acquired Heart Lesions *(Continued)*

| Lesion | History | Physical examination | ECG findings | Echo findings | Treatment | Comments |
|---|---|---|---|---|---|---|
| **Infective endocarditis** | History of heart defect or recent dental procedure, low-grade fever, and somatic complaints | Murmur, fever, splenomegaly, skin manifestations, embolic or immunologic phenomena | May be normal | Intracardiac mass, abscesses, new valvular regurgitation | Largely in conjunction with I specialist and even CT surgeons | Diagnosis follows the modified Duke criteria. |
| **Kawasaki disease** | See Chapter 30, Rheumatologic Diseases | | | | | |
| **Rheumatic fever** | See Chapter 30, Rheumatologic Diseases | | | | | |

- Irregular QRS pattern suggests the possibility of an atrial arrhythmia. With pauses and narrow QRS, look for evidence of atrial premature contractions with P waves of different appearance and/or axis as compared with sinus beats. The early P wave may not conduct, leading to longer pauses (blocked atrial premature contractions).
- The QRS may be prolonged if conduction down the atrioventricular (AV) node is delayed (aberrant conduction). Wide QRS complexes with pauses may represent premature contractions from a ventricular focus, especially if the T-wave morphology is also altered with the opposite axis.
- Look for a P wave before each QRS at an expected interval, usually between 100 and 150 ms. The P wave should be upright in I and aVF for the typical location of sinus node. The sinus P wave is up in leads I, II, and aVF, pure negative in aVR, and usually biphasic in lead V1—first positive, then negative:
  - Inverted P waves (leads II, III, and aVF) with slower heart rates indicate a low atrial rhythm and are a normal finding.
  - Inverted P waves associated with tachycardias are abnormal and may be ectopic atrial tachycardia or other forms of supraventricular tachycardia (SVT).

*Axis*
- QRS axis is generally simply referred to as axis. However, there is also a P-wave axis and a T-wave axis which also have important implications.
- The QRS axis shows the direction of ventricular depolarization and is assessed using leads I and aVF.
- In children >3 years of age, the usual QRS is between 20 and 120 degrees.
- Left axis deviation can suggest left ventricular hypertrophy or left bundle branch block (LBBB).
- In LBBB, late depolarization in the left ventricle leads to leftward QRS axis and widened QRS with slurred and wide R waves in I, aVL, $V_5$, and $V_6$. Wide S waves are seen in $V_1$ and $V_2$. Q waves may be absent in I, $V_5$, and $V_6$. (Last activated chamber is posterior and leftward).
- Right axis deviation can suggest right ventricular hypertrophy or right bundle branch block (RBBB).
- In RBBB, late depolarization in the right ventricle leads to rightward QRS axis as well as a widened QRS with wide and slurred S in I, $V_5$, and $V_6$. R′ is slurred in aVR, $V_1$, and $V_2$. (Last activated chamber is anterior and rightward).
- Table 14-12 gives the mean QRS axis values by age.

*Intervals and Durations*
- P-wave duration is prolonged >0.1 sec in left atrial enlargement (LAE).
- The PR interval represents atrial depolarization.
- Table 14-13 lists the mean and upper limits of normal PR intervals by age and heart rate.

**TABLE 14-12   Normal QRS Axis Ranges by Age**

| Age | Mean value (range) |
| --- | --- |
| 0-1 month | +110 degrees (+30 to +180) |
| 1-3 months | +70 degrees (+10 to +125) |
| 3 months to 3 years | +60 degrees (+5 to +110) |
| >3 years | +60 degrees (+20 to +120) |
| Adult | +50 degrees (−30 to +105) |

*Source*: From Park MK, Guntheroth WG. How to Read Pediatric ECGs, 4th Ed. Philadelphia: Mosby, 2006:46. Copyright Elsevier 2006.

| TABLE 14-13 | Normal PR Intervals | | | | | | | |
|---|---|---|---|---|---|---|---|---|
| | | | | Age | | | | |
| Heart rate (beats/min) | 0-1 month | 1-6 months | 6-12 months | 1-3 years | 3-8 years | 8-12 years | 12-16 years | Adult |
| <60 | — | — | — | — | — | 0.16 (0.18) | 0.16 (0.19) | 0.17 (0.21) |
| 60-80 | — | — | — | — | 0.15 (0.17) | 0.15 (0.17) | 0.15 (0.18) | 0.16 (0.21) |
| 80-100 | 0.10 (0.12) | — | — | — | 0.14 (0.16) | 0.15 (0.16) | 0.15 (0.17) | 0.15 (0.20) |
| 100-120 | 0.10 (0.12) | — | — | (0.15) | 0.13 (0.16) | 0.14 (0.15) | 0.15 (0.16) | 0.15 (0.19) |
| 120-140 | 0.10 (0.11) | 0.11 (0.14) | 0.11 (0.14) | 0.12 (0.14) | 0.13 (0.15) | 0.14 (0.15) | — | 0.15 (0.18) |
| 140-160 | 0.09 (0.11) | 0.10 (0.13) | 0.11 (0.13) | 0.11 (0.14) | 0.12 (0.14) | — | — | (0.17) |
| 160-180 | 0.10 (0.11) | 0.10 (0.12) | 0.10 (0.12) | 0.10 (0.12) | — | — | — | — |
| >180 | 0.09 | 0.09 (0.11) | 0.10 (0.11) | — | — | — | — | — |

*Source:* From Park MK, Guntheroth WG. How to Read Pediatric ECGs, 4th Ed. Philadelphia: Mosby, 2006:46. Copyright Elsevier 2006.

| TABLE 14-14 | Normal QRS Duration |
| --- | --- |

| Age | 0-1 month | 1-6 months | 6-12 months | 1-3 years | 3-8 years | 8-12 years | 12-16 years | Adult |
| --- | --- | --- | --- | --- | --- | --- | --- | --- |
| Normal (mean in seconds) | 0.05 | 0.055 | 0.055 | 0.055 | 0.06 | 0.06 | 0.07 | 0.08 |
| Upper limit of normal | 0.07 | 0.075 | 0.075 | 0.075 | 0.075 | 0.085 | 0.085 | 0.10 |

*Source*: From Park MK, Guntheroth WG. How to Read Pediatric ECGs, 4th Ed. Philadelphia: Mosby, 2006:46. Copyright Elsevier 2006.

- The QRS duration represents ventricular depolarization. Normal times for depolarization depend on age. A prolonged QRS may indicate bundle branch block, hypertrophy, or arrhythmia.
- Table 14-14 lists the normal QRS durations by age.
- QT Prolongation
  - Long QT syndrome is an important cause of sudden death. Determination of the QT interval is important, especially in patients with syncope or seizures (see "Channelopathies" below).
  - The QT interval is measured in milliseconds (usually in lead II, V5, or V6; do not use leads V1-V3 as there are often U waves in these leads, which can skew measurements) from the start of the QRS complex to the end of the T wave.
  - The U wave, which may occur after the T wave, should be included only if it is at least one-half the amplitude of the T wave.
  - The QT interval is adjusted for heart rate (QTc) by dividing the QT interval (in seconds) by the square root of the *preceding* RR interval (in seconds):
    Bazett formula : $QTc = QT\ interval\sqrt{\left(RR\ interval\right)}$
  - The QTc is usually <0.44 seconds (95th percentile).
  - Patients with long QT syndrome may also have unusual T-wave morphologies, including notched, bifid, or biphasic T waves.

*Voltages and Hypertrophy*
- Before assessing the ECG voltages, make sure the ECG is set on the appropriate standard gain setting, which can be found on the far left of the printed ECG.
- The ECG is only a screening tool for hypertrophy, with high false-negative and false-positive rates, especially in infants. The QRS axis shifts toward the hypertrophied ventricle.
- The QRS voltage will change with hypertrophy and will increase in the same direction as the electrical depolarization and will decrease in leads in the opposite direction.
- In right ventricular hypertrophy, increased R waves may be present in V1 with an increased R/S ratio in V1 and decreased R/S ratio in V6. An upright T wave in V1 between 7 days and 7 years of age is also suggestive of right ventricular hypertrophy.

- In left ventricular hypertrophy, increased R waves may be present in V5, V6, I, II, III, or aVF. The R/S ratio may be decreased in V1 or V2. Inverted T waves in I, aVF, V5, or V6 suggest a "strain" pattern, indicating abnormal repolarization.
- In the setting of bundle branch blocks, the usual criteria for ventricular hypertrophy do not apply.

*ST- and T-Wave Changes*
- J point depression and upward sloping ST segment is normal.
- Flat or downward sloping ST segment with invert T wave is abnormal.
- Pathologic ST change is caused by myocarditis, pericarditis, strain/ischemia/infarction, digoxin toxicity, electrolyte abnormalities.
- Hypocalcemia causes prolonged QTc.
- Hyperkalemia causes tall, peaked T waves.

## ARRHYTHMIA

### General Principles
- Arrhythmias other than sinus abnormalities are uncommon in children.
- Children with congenital heart disease or heart surgery are more likely to have arrhythmias.
- This section presents the basic presentation and therapy of arrhythmias in children, but it is not a complete description.

### Diagnosis
*Clinical Presentation and History*
- Palpitations, syncope, and shock.
- Complaints of heart racing or fluttering.
- Syncope occurring in the midst of exercise.
- Abrupt syncope with no premonitory symptoms.
- Prior history of congenital heart disease or heart surgery.
- Brought on by sudden startle such as alarm clock without preceding symptoms; think long QT syndrome or other channelopathies.

*Physical Examination*
- Possible murmur, irregular rhythm, tachycardia, hypotension, or poor oxygen saturation.
- Edema and poor perfusion in the extremities if in heart failure or shock.
- Possible loss of consciousness.

*Differential Diagnosis: ECG Findings*
- The differential diagnosis of tachycardia starts with determining whether the tachycardia is regular or irregular and the width of the QRS.
- Narrow complex regular tachycardia
  - P before QRS (AKA: long RP tachycardia)
    - Sinus tachycardia
    - Ectopic atrial tachycardia (regular)
    - Persistent junctional reciprocating tachycardia (a slow SVT with inverted P waves in leads II, III, and aVF)

- P within QRS
  - AV node reentry tachycardia: uncommon in children <2 years of age but typical in teenagers
  - Junctional ectopic tachycardia: typically occurs postoperatively, after congenital heart surgery
- P behind QRS: reentry pathway
  - Occurs especially with preexcitation when the patient is in sinus rhythm (Wolff-Parkinson-White [WPW] syndrome)
  - Can present at any age
- More Ps than QRSs
  - Atrial flutter
  - Ectopic atrial tachycardia (regular)
  - Coarse atrial fibrillation ("fib-flutter")
- Narrow complex irregular tachycardia
  - Atrial fibrillation
  - Ectopic atrial tachycardia (irregular)
  - Atrial flutter with variable AV conduction
- Wide QRS complex regular tachycardia
  - Usually ventricular tachycardia
  - **V**entricular > **A**trial depolarizations, which are diagnostic
  - 1:1 **V**entricular and **A**trial depolarizations unusual
  - SVT (any type) with aberrancy or preexisting bundle branch block
  - Antidromic reentry pathway (atrium to ventricle down WPW pathway and ventricle to atrium via AV node)
- Wide complex irregular tachycardia
  - Ventricular fibrillation/fast polymorphic ventricular tachycardia.
  - Torsades de pointes.
  - Atrial fibrillation with WPW. See Figure 14-2A and B showing a patient with WPW and preexcited atrial fibrillation.
  - Ectopic atrial tachycardia, irregular, with aberrancy.

## Treatment (Acute)
*Initial Therapy*
- Do not forget ABCs.
- Assess the hemodynamic status of the patient.
- Attach monitor/defibrillator leads.
- Give oxygen.

*Therapy to Terminate the Arrhythmia*
- Probable narrow complex regular SVT (heart rate usually >220 beats per minute in infants and >180 beats per minute in children):
  - Consider vagal maneuvers but do not delay further treatment.
  - Give adenosine rapid IV push dose of 0.1 mg/kg up to 6 mg followed by rapid flush of NS.
    - Record hard-copy ECG during drug bolus.
  - If the first dose is not effective, repeat using dose of 0.2 mg/kg up to 12 mg (maximum adult [teenager] dose).
- Wide complex tachycardia: unconscious patient who is in shock
  - Use synchronized cardioversion at 0.5-1 J/kg.

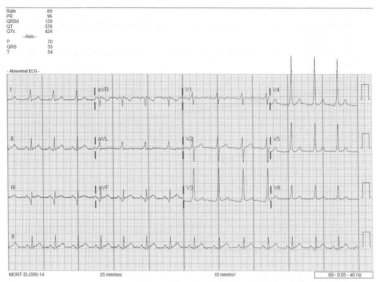

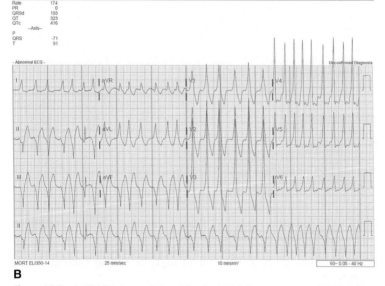

**Figure 14-2. A.** Wolff-Parkinson-White. This is an ECG from a patient with WPW. Note the short PR interval and slurred upstroke of the QRS complex. **B.** Preexcited atrial fibrillation. Patients with WPW can develop atrial fibrillation that is rapidly conducted from the atria to the ventricles via the accessory pathway. This results in an ECG with a wide complex, irregular tachycardia that can often be hemodynamically compromising.

- If not effective, repeat cardioversion with 2-4 J/kg.
- Wide complex, regular tachycardia: awake but unstable patient
  - A trial of adenosine may be considered.

If hemodynamically unstable but awake, consider sedation for synchronized cardioversion but do not delay if the patient is deteriorating.

## IMPLANTED CARDIAC DEVICES

### Insertable Cardiac Monitor (ICM)

- A device that is implanted beneath the skin that can monitor and record heart rhythms.
- Can be programmed to autorecord both brady- and tachyarrhythmias. In addition, the patient has a patient activator that communicates with the device to record the rhythm during a symptomatic episode.

### Pacemaker (PM)

- A system that has the capabilities of pacing the heart for patients with sinoatrial node dysfunction (i.e., symptomatic bradycardia) or atrioventricular node dysfunction (i.e., heart block).
- Pacemaker leads can be placed in the right atrium, right ventricle, or both.
- Leads can be placed via transvenous, epicardial, or hybrid approach.

### Intracardiac Defibrillator

- A system that has the capabilities of a pacemaker but can also defibrillate a patient in ventricular tachycardia or ventricular fibrillation.
- Systems have a defibrillator lead typically placed in the right ventricle.
- Leads can be placed via transvenous, epicardial, or hybrid approach.

### Cardiac Resynchronization Therapy (CRT)

- A system with 3 leads that pace 3 chambers of the heart—right atrium, right ventricle, and left ventricle.
- Leads can be placed via transvenous, epicardial, or hybrid approach.
- Can be a pacemaker only or can have additional capability of a defibrillator.
- Used to treat patients with symptomatic heart failure and a wide QRS complex (>120 ms).

## NEWBORN WITH HEART DISEASE

### General Principles

- The incidence of congenital heart disease in newborns is 5-9 per 1000 live births.
- The development of symptoms at 6-48 hours of age raises the possibility of ductal-dependent cardiac disease.
- Ductal-dependent lesions can be further split into either systemic circulation ductal-dependent lesions or pulmonary circulation ductal-dependent lesions.

### Diagnosis

*Clinical Presentation and History*

- The presentations of congenital heart disease in newborns are presented in Table 14-15.

| TABLE 14-15 | Clinical Presentations of Congenital Heart Disease in Newborns |
|---|---|
| Cyanosis | Because of right-to-left shunts or inadequate mixing of systemic and pulmonary circulations |
| Shock | Usually because of loss of ductal-dependent systemic blood flow in obstructive left heart lesions |
| Congestive heart failure | Presents at different times, usually caused by large left-to-right shunts or poor pump function |
| Murmur | Interpreted in the clinical context |
| Arrhythmia | Usually insignificant unless incessant (prolonged supraventricular tachycardia or congenital complete heart block) |

- Many infants with congenital heart disease are diagnosed prenatally with fetal echocardiography.
  - Newborns without a prenatal diagnosis may have a history of central cyanosis, apnea, tachycardia, tachypnea, hepatomegaly, peripheral edema, or poor feeding. Symptoms from left-to-right intracardiac shunts often develop in the 1st month of life.
  - Peripheral edema or hydrops is less common and suggests long-standing fetal heart failure.
- Pulse oximetry has been endorsed as a valid screening tool in the nursery to identify critical congenital heart disease. Repeated saturations <90% or 90-95% with >3% difference between right arm and leg merits additional evaluation including echocardiogram.

*Physical Examination*
- A basic physical examination and readily available testing should identify most newborns with major congenital heart defects. This screening process allows the timely institution of therapy before a definitive diagnosis is made by consultation with cardiology and echocardiography.
- Special attention should be paid to the presence or absence of murmurs, the nature of S2 sounds (single and loud, fixed split, physiologically split), the character and amplitude of four external pulses and perfusion, and the presence of hepatosplenomegaly.
- Examination findings
  - Bounding right brachial and no femoral pulses: coarctation of aorta
  - Gallop and big liver with murmur: big shunt/congestive heart failure
  - No murmur, symmetric diminished pulses, and shock: ductal-dependent systemic blood flow (e.g., hypoplastic left heart)
- Oxygen saturation in right arm compared with leg
  - Normal: no difference.
  - Leg lower than right arm: differential cyanosis.
    - Ductal-dependent systemic blood flow (coarctation of aorta, interrupted aortic arch, critical aortic stenosis)
    - Pulmonary hypertension with right-to-left shunt at patent ductus arteriosus (PDA)

- Right arm lower than leg: reverse differential cyanosis.
  - Transposition of great vessels (and PDA) with arch obstruction or pulmonary hypertension
- The presence of differential or reverse differential cyanosis by oximetry is diagnostic of right-to-left shunting. However, because of the high affinity of fetal hemoglobin for oxygen, the lack of differential cyanosis by oximetry does not rule out right-to-left shunting (i.e., it is possible to fail a hyperoxia test with $PaO_2$ = 90 mmHg on 100% $FiO_2$ and still have an oxygen saturation >95%).

*Diagnostic Studies*
- ECG
  - Primary arrhythmias (fast or slow): SVT or complete heart block
  - Superior axis (negative in aVF): AV canal or tricuspid atresia
- Hyperoxia test: baseline postductal arterial blood gas (ABG) for $PaO_2$. Give 100% $FiO_2$ for 10 minutes. Draw repeat ABG for $PaO_2$.
- $PaO_2$ > 200 mm Hg: normal
- $PaO_2$ < 200 mm Hg and >150: pulmonary disease
- $PaO_2$ < 70 mm Hg: almost always heart disease
- $PaO_2$ < 30 mm Hg: most often transposition of the great vessels

*Imaging*
- Chest radiograph (exclude major lung disease)
  - Reduced pulmonary blood flow: tetralogy of Fallot or pulmonary atresia
  - Increased pulmonary blood flow: transposition of great vessels or ventral septal defect
  - Hyaline membrane disease appearance in term infant: obstructed total anomalous pulmonary venous connection
  - Recognizable shapes (boot = tetralogy of Fallot; snowman = obstructed total anomalous pulmonary venous connection; egg on a string = transposition of great vessels)
- Echocardiography
  - Often makes a definitive diagnosis
  - Requires significant skill and experience in children; may not be helpful if obtained in a laboratory that scans mostly adults

## Treatment
- See Chapter 8, Critical Care.
- The newborn with cyanosis or shock with suspected heart disease can be stabilized and transported before a definitive anatomic diagnosis is made. It is not necessary to make an exact anatomic diagnosis before deciding to initiate prostaglandin $E_1$ therapy but only to determine that there is a high probability of ductal-dependent congenital heart disease.
- Urgent cardiology consultation is indicated.

*Medications*
- Institution of a continuous infusion of Prostaglandin E1 (PGE1) is usually beneficial. Usual initial doses are 0.05-0.10 mcg/kg/min.

- When the desired effects are achieved, the dose should be decreased to 0.01 mcg/kg/min in steps.
- Supplemental oxygen should be avoided if oxygen saturations are >80-85%.
- Prostaglandin therapy should be avoided in the presence of pulmonary venous obstruction that may occur in total anomalous pulmonary venous connection. This should be suspected if the chest radiograph has a diffuse reticular pattern fanning out from the hilum and obscuring the heart border. Increased pulmonary blood flow from prostaglandin treatment may aggravate pulmonary edema in this setting.

*Nonoperative: Mechanical Ventilation*
- See Chapter 8, Critical Care.
- Intubation with mechanical ventilation should be considered for transportation of neonates on prostaglandin, especially if apnea is noted.
- Mechanical ventilation may also be of benefit for infants in shock by decreasing the work of breathing and thereby decreasing metabolic demands.
- Hyperventilation should be avoided.

## CONGESTIVE HEART FAILURE

### General Principles

- Congestive heart failure in pediatrics is defined as inadequate delivery of oxygen and nutrients to the tissues to meet the metabolic demands of a growing infant or child.
- The most common causes of congestive heart failure vary depending on the age of the patient (Table 14-16).

| TABLE 14-16 | Common Causes of Congestive Heart Failure by Age | | |
| --- | --- | --- | --- |
| **Fetus** | **Newborn** | **Young infant** | **Older child** |
| Tachyarrhythmias | Structural heart disease, especially hypoplastic left heart, critical aortic stenosis and coarctation, and obstructed pulmonary venous return (see "Newborn with Heart Disease" section) | Left-to-right shunts: ventricular septal defects | Cardiomyopathy |
| Anemia— parvovirus | Patent ductus arteriosus in the preterm infant | Coarctation of the aorta | Myocarditis/ pericarditis with pericardial effusion |

## Diagnosis

*Clinical Presentation and History*
- Tachypnea and tachycardia are cardinal symptoms of congestive heart failure.
- With chronic heart failure, infants often have poor feeding, inadequate weight gain, and irritability. Older children often have decreased exercise tolerance, anorexia, and vomiting.

*Physical Examination*
- Surgical scar, murmur, gallop rhythm, muffled heart sounds, tachycardia, tachypnea, or hepatomegaly, which may suggest cardiac disease
- Edema and poor perfusion in extremities

*Diagnostic Studies*
- Laboratory studies
  - In adults, a brain natriuretic peptide (BNP) cutoff value of 100 pg/mL had a sensitivity of 90% and specificity of 76% for identifying those with heart failure.
  - In children, BNP levels can be elevated in patients with cardiomyopathy, left-to-right shunts, and pulmonary hypertension.
- ECG
  - This is used primarily to rule out a tachyarrhythmia.
  - Low QRS voltages and ST-T–wave changes may suggest myocardial or pericardial disease.
- Imaging
  - Chest radiography: important initial test in differential diagnosis that includes cardiac and respiratory disease
    ○ Cardiomegaly or increased pulmonary vascular markings suggest cardiac disease.
  - Echocardiography
    ○ Often makes a definitive diagnosis
    ○ Requires significant skill and experience in children; may not be helpful if obtained in a laboratory that tests mostly adults

## Treatment

- See Chapter 8, Critical Care.
- Management is guided by consultation with a pediatric cardiologist and depends on the etiology of heart failure, hemodynamic status, and clinical symptoms. Specific guidelines are beyond the scope of this text.
- Surgical or catheter-based intervention is usually undertaken for structural heart defects.
- Pharmacologic treatment may include diuretics, systemic vasodilators, β-blockers, and inotropic agents.
- In the emergency department, for patients with probable new congestive heart failure and marked dyspnea, an IV dose of furosemide (Lasix) of 1 mg/kg up to 40 mg can be given while arrangements are made for pediatric cardiology consultation.

## CHEST PAIN

- Chest pain is a common complaint in the pediatric population, but cardiac disease is an uncommon cause of pediatric chest pain (roughly 4% in all pediatric patients presenting to the emergency department with chest pain).
  - Musculoskeletal disorders are the most common identifiable cause of chest pain in children.

- Gastrointestinal causes are suggested by an association with eating or vomiting.
- Pain that awakens a child is more likely to be organic.
- Cardiac causes are especially unlikely in an adolescent with a long-standing history of chest pain.
- Exercise-induced bronchospasm or vocal cord dysfunction should be considered with exertional pain accompanied by difficulty breathing, noisy breathing, wheezing, or cough.

## Diagnosis
*Clinical Presentation and History*
- Chest pain that is seen in patients with known or suspected congenital heart disease, primarily exertional pain, or severe pain of acute onset requires more extensive evaluation.
- History: The following historical information should be sought:
  - History of structural heart disease, especially aortic stenosis
  - Cardiomyopathy/myocarditis: exercise intolerance, family history of sudden unexpected death, murmur, gallop rhythm, hepatomegaly, tachycardia, or tachypnea
  - Tachyarrhythmia: tachycardia preceding the pain, rapid onset, and rapid resolution
  - Pericarditis: fever, recent viral illness, and pain worse in the supine position, which is decreased by leaning forward

*Physical Examination*
- Tenderness on palpation or pain accentuated by inspiration, which suggests a musculoskeletal cause
- Surgical scar, murmur, gallop rhythm, muffled heart sounds, tachycardia, tachypnea, or hepatomegaly that suggests cardiac disease
- Rales, wheezes, or differential breath sounds with pulmonary disease

*Diagnostic Studies*
- Troponin is rarely indicated.
  - Coronary artery disease is rare in children.
  - Troponin levels may be elevated in myocarditis.
- ECG
  - Hypertrophy or T-wave changes may be seen with hypertrophic cardiomyopathy or aortic stenosis.
  - Preexcitation (WPW syndrome) raises the possibility of SVT.
  - Low voltages or ST elevation occurs with pericarditis.
- Chest radiograph: should be considered with more acute presentation or ill-appearing child
  - Cardiomegaly may be present in cardiomyopathy, pericardial effusion, or structural heart disease.
  - Infiltrates, pleural effusion, or pneumothorax suggests respiratory disease.

## Treatment
*Medications*
- Short courses of nonsteroidal anti-inflammatory drugs can be used for musculoskeletal pain.
- β-Agonists and steroids can be used for wheezing or asthma.

*Referrals*
If cardiac disease is suspected based on the initial evaluation, cardiology consultation should be sought before ordering additional tests.

## SYNCOPE

### Definition and Epidemiology

• Syncope, defined as the sudden loss of consciousness and postural tone, occurs at least once in 15-25% of children and adolescents.
• Despite its frequent occurrence, syncope creates significant anxiety for families and caregivers.
• In a study of children presenting to a tertiary care center for syncope, an average of four diagnostic tests was obtained, with an average cost for testing of $1055 per patient. Only 3.9% of the tests were diagnostic.
• Anxiety and depression may be associated with recurrent syncope.

*Etiology*
• Neurocardiogenic (vasovagal) mechanisms cause the vast majority of syncope in children.
• Cardiac causes are uncommon.
• Breath-holding spells are frequently seen in early childhood and are usually classified as pallid or cyanotic (Table 14-17).

### Diagnosis
*Clinical Presentation and History*
• The history before, during, and after the event is most important. Seek history from other observers, such as friends, teachers, and coaches.
• If the event occurred at a sporting event, determine whether the episode/symptoms occurred after participating in an activity (e.g., standing on sidelines) or while engaging in a vigorous activity (suggestive of a cardiac cause).
• Vasovagal-mediated syncope is often characterized by presyncopal symptoms such as dizziness, "head rush," diaphoresis, visual blurring, facial pallor, abdominal pain/nausea, warm or cold sensation, and tachycardia, which last for seconds to minutes.
• There is often a history of positional presyncopal symptoms.
• Loss of consciousness usually lasts for 5-20 seconds, but there may be 5 minutes to several hours of fatigue, weakness, dizziness, headache, or nausea.
• Table 14-18 lists common situations for neurally mediated syncope.
• Seek historical red flags that would suggest a seizure when a child presents with syncope (Table 14-19).
• Seek historical red flags and family history that would suggest a cardiac cause (Tables 14-20 and 14-21).

| TABLE 14-17 Pallid versus Cyanotic Breath-Holding Spell | |
| --- | --- |
| **Pallid** | **Cyanotic** |
| Precipitated by sudden, unexpected, unpleasant stimulus, frequently a mild head injury | Violent crying (temper tantrum) |
| Crying not prominent. | Breath-holding (apnea) in expiration |
| Pallor and diaphoresis are common. | |
| Bradycardia with excessive vagal tone. | |

| TABLE 14-18 | Common Situations for Neurally Mediated Syncope |

- Noxious stimuli such as blood drawing
- Hair combing by someone else
- Shower, hot bath, especially in morning, before breakfast
- Micturition, defecation with Valsalva maneuver
- Hyperventilation
- Standing in line, kneeling in church

| TABLE 14-19 | Historical Red Flags in Syncope That Suggest a Seizure |

- History of seizure disorder
- Shaking of extremities during a syncopal episode
- Drooling, loss of bowel or bladder control during a syncopal episode
- Eyes open during the unresponsive episode.
- Prolonged postictal confusion (mental status recovers promptly in syncope but may be abnormal for a while in seizure)

| TABLE 14-20 | Historical Red Flags That Suggest a Cardiac Cause of Syncope |

- Occurring in the midst of exercise
- Abrupt syncope with no premonitory symptoms
- Prior history of congenital heart disease or heart surgery, especially aortic stenosis or single ventricle
- Brought on by sudden startle, such as by an alarm clock, without preceding symptoms—long QT syndrome
- Acute or subacute history of exercise intolerance between spells—cardiomyopathy, myocarditis

| TABLE 14-21 | Family History That Suggests a Cardiac Cause of Syncope |

- Premature and unexplained sudden death
- Cardiomyopathy
- Arrhythmias, especially long QT syndrome
- Implanted defibrillator
- Congenital deafness (long QT syndrome), seizures

- The most common age at which vasovagal syncope first presents is 13 years, and patients remain at risk of syncope for many years.

*Physical Examination*
- Orthostatic changes in heart rate and blood pressure: vasovagal-mediated syncope.
- Right ventricular heave or loud second heart sound in pulmonary hypertension.
- Systolic murmur in left ventricular outflow tract obstruction. Auscultate for murmur in supine and standing positions to look for dynamic obstruction, suggesting hypertrophic cardiomyopathy.

*Diagnostic Testing*
- Laboratory testing. None is required for cardiac or vasovagal-mediated causes of syncope. If there is concern that a syncopal episode was a seizure, check bedside glucose and electrolyte profile, including magnesium and phosphorus.
- ECG. Perform in all patients. It is inexpensive and a reasonable screen given the low incidence of cardiac disease in children with syncope.
  - Determine corrected QT interval: long QT syndrome.
  - Left ventricular hypertrophy, T-wave abnormalities: abnormal in 80% of patients with hypertrophic cardiomyopathy.
  - Right ventricular hypertrophy: pulmonary hypertension.
  - Preexcitation: WPW syndrome.
  - RBBB with ST elevation in leads $V_1$-$V_3$: Brugada syndrome, a rare cause of ventricular arrhythmias.
  - Complete heart block: rare without a history of congenital heart defect.
- Echocardiography: With atypical history, abnormal cardiac examination, or abnormal ECG, this is usually indicated after consultation with cardiology.
- Tilt table testing: This is not a good screening test because it has 90% specificity but only 60% sensitivity for vasovagal-mediated syncope.

## Treatment
*Behavioral*
- Education and reassurance are usually the only treatment needed for patients with vasovagal syncope. Talk with patients and parents about situations when syncope is common and advise the patients to sit or lie down when they experience presyncopal symptoms.
- A randomized study in adults showed that water before tilt testing enhanced tolerance of upright positioning.
- Increased intake of fluid and salt (pending on resting hypertension) especially before and during physical activity to enhance preload is the primary treatment. Advise the patient to drink enough fluids to make the urine appear clear and to avoid fluids with caffeine. It may be helpful to write a note to allow a water bottle at school and more frequent restroom breaks.
- Isometric maneuvers such as tensing muscles in the arms or legs with prodromal symptoms may decrease the incidence of syncope.

*Medications*
- A number of drugs have been used in patients with recurrent syncope, but data regarding efficacy are limited.
  - Fludrocortisone has been used commonly in children, a small double-blind placebo-controlled trial in children found that patients on a placebo had fewer recurrences as compared with the active treatment group.

- Beta-blockers have proven ineffective in placebo-controlled randomized trials. Smaller studies support the use of selective serotonin reuptake inhibitors. Midodrine (direct vasoconstrictor) may be effective; however, it may cause hypertension (i.e., treatment is worse than the disease).

*Referrals*

If cardiac disease is suspected based on the initial evaluation, cardiology consultation should be sought before ordering additional tests.

## SUDDEN CARDIAC DEATH/SUDDEN CARDIAC ARREST

### Definition and Epidemiology

- By definition, patients that have sudden cardiac death (SCD) die. If they survive, it is called either an aborted SCD or sudden cardiac arrest (SCA).
- The overall incidence of SCA among people aged 0 to 35 years is approximately 2.28 per 100,000 person-years.
- The most common causes of SCD are hypertrophic cardiomyopathy (HCM) or possible (HCM) (43%), coronary artery abnormality (CAA) (17%), myocarditis (6%), channelopathy (3%), MI (3%), other cardiomyopathy (6%), and other (22%).

### Diagnosis

*Clinical Presentation and History*

- Unfortunately, there may be no warning signs that a patient is going to have SCD/ SCA.
- There may be family history of HCM or inherited arrhythmias. Ask questions on family history including SCD, congenital heart disease, cardiomyopathies, or known arrhythmias, known single vehicle car accidents, congenital deafness, SIDS, near drowning, or seizures.
- HCM/LV outflow tract obstruction (LVOTO): Patients may have easy fatigability; dyspnea, palpitations, dizziness, syncope, or anginal pain may be present.
- CAA: may be an incidental finding with no history, angina pain.
- Myocarditis: See Table 14-11. Acquire Heart Lesions.
- Channelopathy: See Channelopathies section below.

*Physical Examination*

- HCM/LVOTO: systolic ejection murmur, LV lift.
- CAA: most likely normal.
- Myocarditis: See Table 14-11. Acquire Heart Lesions.
- Channelopathy: See Channelopathies section below.

*Diagnostic Studies*

- HCM/LVOTO: ECG may show LVH or ST-T changes; echocardiogram is usually diagnostic.
- CAA: ECG will likely be normal if the patient is asymptomatic; echocardiogram is usually diagnostic and may need cardiac CT.
- Myocarditis: See Table 14-11. Acquire Heart Lesions.
- Channelopathy: See Channelopathies section below.

### Treatment

- Treatment for SCA typically follows advanced life support algorithms (PALS).

- Access and early use of AEDs have proven beneficial in out-of-hospital cardiac arrest survival outcomes.
- HCM/LVOTO: activity restriction, beta-blockers, septal myectomy, ICD.
- CAA: Left coronary artery anomalies almost all get surgical correction; right coronary artery anomalies have a lower incidence of SCD, so treatment is less clear.
- Myocarditis: See Table 14-11. Acquire Heart Lesions.
- Channelopathy: See Channelopathies section below.

## Channelopathies

- Specific cardiac ion channel abnormalities predispose patients to arrhythmias and sudden death.
- Long QT syndrome
  - Inherited channelopathy that prolong ventricular repolarization.
  - Prevalence 1:2000 live births.
  - Predisposes patients to syncope (especially with stress) or SCD.
  - Typically manifests as QTc >450 ms in males and >460 ms in females on ECG.
  - Some forms associated with congenital deafness.
  - Treatment: beta-blockers, intracardiac defibrillator (ICD), or left cardiac sympathetic denervation.
  - Figure 14-3A and B shows an ECG of an infant with long QT syndrome.
- Short QT syndrome
  - Inherited channelopathy that shortens ventricular repolarization
  - Incidence low: 0.02-0.1%
  - Predisposes patients to atrial and ventricular fibrillation and SCD
  - Typically manifests as QTc <350 ms for males and <360 ms for females
  - Treatment: ICD
- Brugada syndrome
  - Inherited channelopathy associated with right ventricular conduction delay and ST segment changes in the right precordial leads ($V_1$ and $V_2$).
  - Accounts for as much as 20% of all SCD in patients with structurally normal hearts.
  - Fever can exacerbate arrhythmias in predisposed patients and may unmask ECG changes.
  - Treatment: antipyretics or ICD.
- Catecholaminergic polymorphic ventricular tachycardia
  - Inherited channelopathy related to calcium dysregulation.
  - Predisposes patients to syncope and SCD.
  - Associated with bidirectional ventricular tachycardia, polymorphic ventricular tachycardia, and ventricular fibrillation.
  - Typically symptoms occur with exertion.
  - Treatment: beta-blockers, ICD, or left cardiac sympathetic denervation.

## PREVENTATIVE CARDIOLOGY

- The goal of preventative cardiology is to intervene and modify childhood risk factors and behaviors that could lead to early morbidity and mortality through counseling, intervention, and treatment whenever possible.
- Some of the most targeted risk factors are hypercholesterolemia, hypertension, smoking, and obesity/diabetes, and some interventions to reduce these include low-calorie diets, smoking prevention, increasing physical activity, and weight control programs.

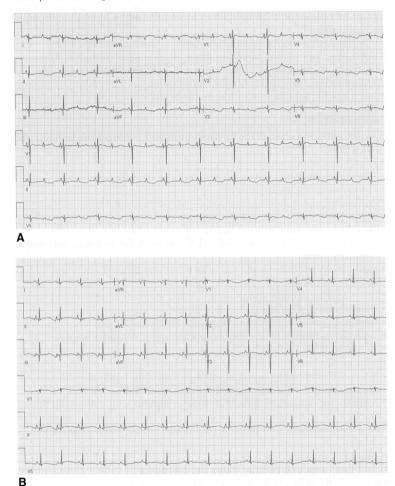

**Figure 14-3. A.** Long QT syndrome. In this infant with long QT syndrome, the QT interval is so prolonged (approximately 700 ms) that there is resultant 2:1 conduction. **B.** As the QT interval slightly shortens, conduction reverts to 1:1, though the QTc remains quite long at approximately 545 ms.

- The American Heart Association has published guideline for the prevention of CV disease.
- Dyslipidemias:
  - Total cholesterol: >170 mg/dL is borderline; >200 mg/dL is elevated.
  - LDL-C: >110 mg/dL is borderline; >130 mg/dL is elevated.
  - TGs: >100 mg/dL is elevated for <10 years; >130 mg/dL is elevated for >10 year.
  - HDL-C: <40 mg/dL is reduced.

• For more information on obesity: See Chapter 1, Primary Care and the Continuity Clinic.

• For more information on diabetes: See Chapter 18, Endocrinology.

• For more information on obesity hypertension: See Chapter 25, Nephrology.

## SUGGESTED READINGS

Bickley LS, Szilagyi PG, Hoffman RM, et al. Cardiovascular system. In: Bates' Guide to Physical Examination and History Taking. Lippincott Williams & Wilkins, 2020.

Chiabrando JG, Bonaventura A, Vecchié A, et al. Management of acute and recurrent pericarditis: JACC state-of-the-art review. J Am Coll Cardiol 2020;75(1):76–92.

Douglas PS, Garcia MJ, Haines DE, et al. ACCF/ASE/AHA/ASNC/HFSA/HRS/SCAI/SCCM/SCCT/SCMR 2011 appropriate use criteria for echocardiography… J Am Coll Cardiol 2011;57(9):1126–1166.

Eindhoven JA, et al. The usefulness of brain natriuretic peptide in simple congenital heart disease-a systematic review. Cardiol Young 2013;23:315–324.

Friedman KG, Kane DA, Rathod RH, et al. Management of pediatric chest pain using a standardized assessment and management plan. Pediatrics 2011;128(2):239–245.

Kemper AR, et al. Strategies for implementing screening for critical congenital heart disease. Pediatrics 2011;128:e1259.

Khairy P, Poirier N, Mercier L-A. Univentricular heart. Circulation 2007;115(6):800–812.

Maisel AS, et al. Rapid measurement of B-type natriuretic peptide in the emergency diagnosis of heart failure. N Engl J Med 2002;347:161–167.

Marino BS, Tabbutt S, MacLaren G, et al. Cardiopulmonary resuscitation in infants and children with cardiac disease: a scientific statement from the American Heart Association. Circulation 2018;137(22):e691–e782.

Newburger JW, et al. Noninvasive tests in the initial evaluation of heart murmurs in children. N Engl J Med 1983;308:61.

Park MK, Guntheroth WG. How to read pediatric ECGs. Vol. 847. Elsevier Health Sciences, 2006.

Park MK, Salamat M. Park's Pediatric Cardiology for Practitioners E-Book. Elsevier Health Sciences, 2020.

Romme JJCM, et al. Drugs and pacemakers for vasovagal, carotid sinus and situational syncope. Cochrane Database Syst Rev 2011;(10):CD004194.

Sheldon RS, Grubb BP, Olshansky B, et al. 2015 Heart Rhythm Society expert consensus statement on the diagnosis and treatment of postural tachycardia syndrome, inappropriate sinus tachycardia, and vasovagal syncope. Heart Rhythm 2015;12(6):e41–e63.

Silva JN, et al. Updates on the inherited cardiac ion channelopathies: from cell to clinical. Curr Treat Options Cardiovasc Med 2012;14:473–489.

Thompson T, Jantzen D, Hasselman T, et al. Comparison of appropriateness and cost of echocardiograms ordered by pediatric cardiologists and primary care providers for syncope." Pediatrics 2021;147:380.

# 15

# Dermatologic Diseases

Lily Chen, Cynthia Wang, and Leonid Shmuylovich

## INTRODUCTION

- Skin disorders are one of the most common problems in pediatrics.
- Never underestimate parental concerns about their child's skin. Unlike many disease processes, the skin is visible and noticeable to parents and others.
- Examination of the skin requires observation and palpation of the entire skin surface under good light. Do not forget to look at the eyes and mouth for mucous membrane involvement.
- Examination should include onset, duration, and inspection of a primary lesion. It is also important to note secondary changes, morphology, and distribution of the lesions.

## NEONATAL DERMATOSES

### Cutis Marmorata

- Transient, blanchable, reticulated mottling that occurs on skin exposed to a cool environment.
- No treatment is necessary. The condition generally resolves by 1 year of age.
- If it persists, consider an evaluation of systemic disease such as hypothyroidism.

### Erythema Toxicum Neonatorum

- Self-limited eruption of scattered erythematous papules and pustules that generally appear in the first few days of life and resolve within several weeks (Fig. 15-1).
- Most common pustular eruption in newborns. Patients are otherwise healthy.
- More commonly occurs in term infants.

### Transient Neonatal Pustular Melanosis

- Rash that is present at birth and characterized by pustules that rupture easily, leaving collarettes of scale and hyperpigmented macules on the neck, chin, forehead, lower back, and shins (Fig. 15-2). New pustules generally do not form after birth.
- Pustules resolve within days, but hyperpigmentation may take months to resolve.
- More common in dark-skinned infants.

### Acne Neonatorum

- Comedones, pustules, and papules on the face that resemble acne vulgaris (Fig. 15-3).
- Develops around 2-3 weeks of age and resolves within 6 months.
- No treatment is usually necessary; wash face with baby soap. In severe cases can develop scarring, referral to a pediatric dermatologist is warranted.
- Distinct from neonatal cephalic pustulosis, which is a self-limited acneiform eruption **without** comedones that typically responds quickly to topical ketoconazole.

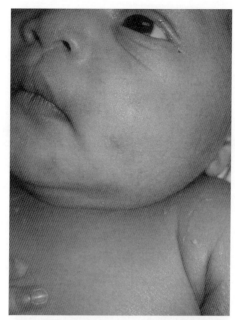

Figure 15-1. Erythema toxicum neonatorum.

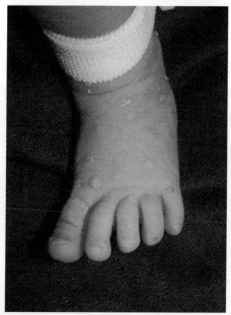

Figure 15-2. Transient neonatal pustular melanosis.

## Milia

- White, pearly, 1-2 mm papules favoring the face (Fig. 15-4) but may occur anywhere. On the palate, they are known as "Epstein pearls."
- May be present at birth.
- Usually resolve without treatment by 2-6 months of age.

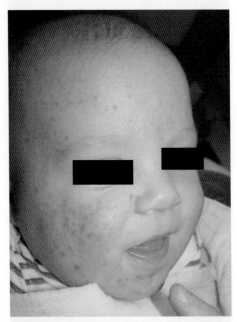

Figure 15-3. **Acne neonatorum.**

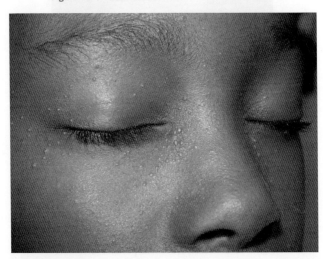

Figure 15-4. **Milia.**

## Miliaria Crystallina

• Tiny, superficial vesicles like "dew drops" favoring the forehead, upper trunk and arms.
• Presents from birth to early infancy.
• Secondary to obstruction of eccrine sweat ducts.
• Resolves without treatment. Prevention consists of avoidance of overheating and limiting excessive swaddling.
• Miliaria rubra consists of erythematous papules, papulovesicles, and pustules in the same distribution after the first week of life in the same distribution and also secondary to obstruction of deeper sweat glands.

## Harlequin Color Change

• Unilateral, blanchable erythema and contralateral pallor that is transient and recurring.
• Presents between 2 and 5 days of life in 10% of healthy newborns.
• Resolves spontaneously. Transient color change lasts from 30 seconds to 20 minutes and can recur multiples times over a period of 24 hours.

## Subcutaneous Fat Necrosis

• Red, circumscribed, firm, rubbery, tender nodules that may become fluctuant favoring the back, buttocks, cheeks, and extremities.
• Presents within the first 4 weeks of life but are not typically present at birth.
• Resolves spontaneously over months, can be associated with early or delayed hypercalcemia.
• Hypercalcemia monitoring recommended for 6 months after appearance of extensive lesions.

## BIRTH MARKS

### Dermal Melanocytosis

• These blue-gray poorly circumscribed macules and patches often occur in lumbosacral area or lower extremities (Fig. 15-5).
• Present at birth and more common in pigmented skin.

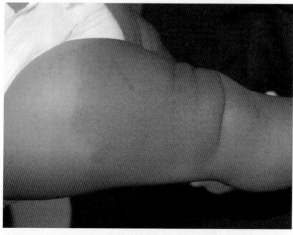

Figure 15-5. Mongolian spots (dermal melanosis).

- Lumbosacral lesions tend to fade during childhood; however, lesions in other locations usually persist.
- Most often an isolated finding, extensive dermal melanosis has been reported with lysosomal storage disorders. No association with melanoma or other skin cancers.

## Café-au-Lait Macules

- These light brown macules or patches (Fig. 15-6) can occur anywhere on the body.
- Most commonly occur in isolation, but multiple lesions can be associated with an underlying syndrome.
  - The presence of six or more macules >0.5 cm in diameter in prepubertal children or >1.5 cm in postpubertal, as well as inguinal or axillary freckling, is suggestive of neurofibromatosis 1.
  - Large, irregular truncal patches may be associated with McCune-Albright syndrome.

## Congenital Melanocytic Nevi

- These brown pigmented macules or plaques may have dark brown or black papules or other irregular pigmentation within the lesions (Fig. 15-7). They may cover large areas of skin and be associated with numerous satellite lesions.
- Lesions are present at birth but may become more noticeable within the first year of life.
- Categorized by predicted adult size:
  - Small (<1.5 cm)
  - Medium (1.5-20 cm)

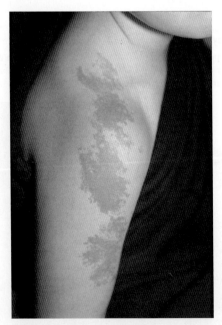

Figure 15-6. **Café-au-lait macules.**

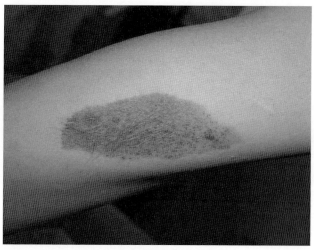

**Figure 15-7.** Congenital melanocytic nevi.

- Large (20-40 cm)
- Giant (>40 cm)
- Small and medium congenital melanocytic nevi have low risk for development of melanoma (<1%). Large and giant lesions have increased risk of melanoma. Large/giant lesions in a posterior axial location also are associated with a risk for neurocutaneous melanosis, which may require MRI evaluation.
- Refer to dermatology for evaluation of concerning lesions, such as ones that are larger, growing/changing, or symptomatic.
- Parents/patients should monitor regularly for concerning signs/symptoms such as focal change in color, growth of nodules, bleeding, pain, or itching.
- Most congenital melanocytic nevi can be managed with close clinical monitoring. Baseline and follow-up photos can be helpful. Excision can be undertaken for definitive management.

## Nevus Sebaceous
- This hairless, yellow-colored plaque tends to have an irregular surface.
- Most commonly located on the scalp (Fig. 15-8), it becomes less prominent after the newborn period but later grows and becomes more papular or verrucous around puberty, when hormone levels increase.
- There is a low risk for development of benign tumors, and order of magnitude lowers risk of malignant tumors within the lesions. Lesions can usually be monitored but may be excised (generally when patients are older) for definitive management.

## Aplasia Cutis Congenita
- Open erosions or healed atrophic scars found most commonly on the scalp and present at birth (Fig. 15-9).
- Consider imaging studies for evaluation of ectopic neural tissue if defect is large, if there is an overlying vascular stain, or if there is presence of "hair collar sign" (hypertrichosis of coarse hair circumferentially at rim of lesion).

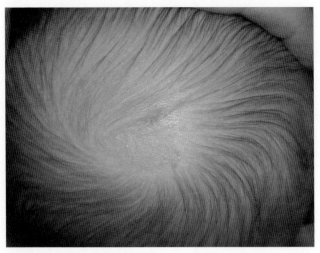

Figure 15-8. **Nevus sebaceous.**

- Small defects often heal on their own, leaving scar tissue. Larger defects may require skin grafting or other surgical interventions.

## Port Wine Stain

- Bright or deep red, well-demarcated macules and patches on the face, classically described as having V1/V2/V3 dermatomal distribution, more recently distribution thought to follow facial embryologic placodes (Fig. 15-10).
- Present at birth and persists. May develop a deeper red hue, thicken and become nodular.

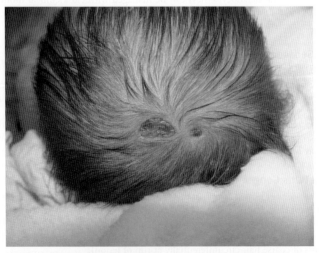

Figure 15-9. **Aplasia cutis congenita.**

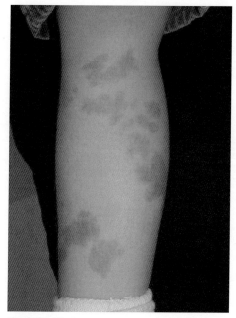

**Figure 15-10. Port wine stain.**

- Caused by somatic GNAQ mutation. If GNAQ mosaicism affects ipsilateral eye or leptomeningeal brain tissue, then it can cause Sturge-Weber syndrome (SWS), a sporadic neurologic disorder where a facial PWS is associated with ipsilateral leptomeningeal/brain and ocular vascular anomalies.
- Lesions affecting forehead/eyelid or hemiface are higher risk for SWS and should be evaluated by ophthalmology for glaucoma shortly after birth and evaluated by neurology given risk of seizure. MRI to evaluate leptomeningeal involvement is typically highest yield at 12 months; low yield and not recommended at birth.
- Pulsed-dye laser treatments can help lighten lesion; typically recurs after treatment.

### Nevus Simplex ("Angel kiss" and "Stork bite")
- Pink-to-red macules and patches found on forehead/glabella, eyelids, philtrum, occiput, and nape (Fig. 15-11).
- Capillary malformation that is present at birth and found in 30-80% of neonates.
- Lesions on the face resolve spontaneously between 1 and 3 years of age. Lesions on the nape of the neck tend to persist.

### Hemangiomas
*Appearance*
- Superficial: bright red, vascular papules, plaques or nodules
- Deep: bluish, subcutaneous, vascular plaques or nodules, sometimes with overlying telangiectases (Fig. 15-12)

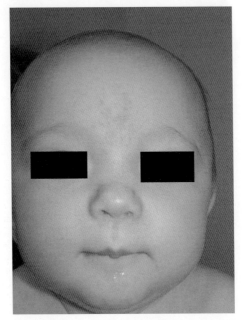

Figure 15-11. Nevus simplex (angel's kiss).

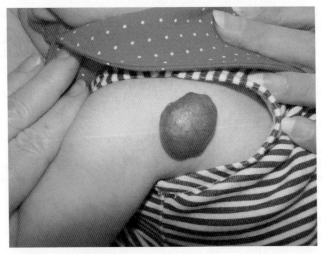

Figure 15-12. Hemangioma.

*Course*

Lesions are minimally present at birth, grow most rapidly during the first 1-3 months of life, grow more slowly for several months, and then involute over years. Most lesions involute by age 5-7 years old.

*Complications and Associations*

- Can disrupt normal anatomy when affecting lips/nose, be cosmetically disfiguring when large on face, affect vision when near or on eyelids, and impact breast development when large and affecting breast buds.
- Ulceration can occur, more likely for lesions on the lip, diaper region, scalp, or skin folds.
- Evaluation for hepatic hemangiomas should be based on signs/symptoms of cardiac failure, independent of cutaneous infantile hemangioma number as previously thought.
- Lower facial or "beard" hemangiomas may be associated with airway hemangiomas. If any concern for noisy breathing, may need ENT evaluation.
- Large, facial, segmental hemangiomas may be associated with a spectrum of extracutaneous anomalies—PHACES syndrome (**P**osterior fossa malformations, **H**emangiomas, **A**rterial anomalies, **C**ardiac defects, **E**ye anomalies, and **S**ternal cleft).
- Large, lower body, segmental hemangiomas may be associated with a spectrum of extracutaneous anomalies—LUMBAR syndrome (**L**ower body segmental infantile hemangiomas with **U**rogenital anomalies, **U**lceration, **M**yelopathy, **B**ony deformities, **A**norectal malformations, **A**rterial anomalies, and **R**enal anomalies).
- Midline lumbosacral hemangiomas may be associated with occult spinal dysraphism.

*Treatment*

- Treatment options include active observation or topical (timolol) or oral beta blockers (propranolol). Choice of treatment is a multifactorial approach as infantile hemangiomas have a wide spectrum of clinical presentations.
- If treating with beta blockers, highest yield to start treatment before 6 months of age.
- Consider referral to dermatology if hemangioma is a threat to vital functions such as vision or airway, has potential for disfigurement (e.g., nasal tip, lip, rapidly growing lesion on face), has high risk for ulceration, or there is concern for extracutaneous involvement.

## ACNE VULGARIS

The etiology of acne is multifactorial. Causes include follicular plugging, increased sebum production, *Cutibacterium acnes* overgrowth, and inflammation.

### Clinical Presentation

- Comedonal: open comedones (blackheads) and closed comedones (whiteheads) (Fig. 15-13A)
- Inflammatory: erythematous, inflammatory papules and pustules
- Cystic: scarring nodules and cysts (Fig. 15-13B)

### Treatment

- General skin care: wash face with soap or acne wash two times per day. Avoid scrubbing and excessive washing.
- Comedonal acne
  - Sample regimen for mild comedonal acne is benzoyl peroxide (BP) 5% wash, clindamycin 1% solution in the morning, and tretinoin 0.1% cream at night.

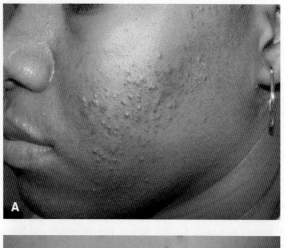

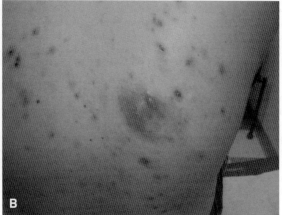

Figure 15-13. **Acne vulgaris. A.** Comedonal acne. **B.** Cystic acne.

- BP and retinoids can be irritating. Advise patients to use only a pea-sized amount for the entire face. Use every other day initially if redness/drying occurs and then increase to daily as tolerance develops.
- BP 2.5% and 5% products are as effective as 10% preparations. BP should not be used at the same time as a topical retinoid.
- Topical retinoids come in a variety of strengths. Start with the least potent for patients with dry or sensitive skin and work up as tolerated.
- Inflammatory acne
  - Consider adding an oral antibiotic (doxycycline) to topical regimen. Oral antibiotics should be continued for 2-3 months minimum.
  - Advise patients to use sunscreen and take with food and a large glass of water to minimize risks of photosensitivity, nausea, and esophagitis, respectively.
- Cystic/nodular or scarring acne

- Refer to dermatologist for possible systemic retinoid therapy (isotretinoin) if inadequate response to above.
- This requires strict contraception in females because the agent is teratogenic.
- For females, consider endocrine workup if early presentation is accompanied by other virilizing signs to look for androgen excess disorder, or if accompanied by hirsutism and irregular periods to look for polycystic ovary syndrome.

## ATOPIC DERMATITIS

### Definition
- This condition is characterized by pruritic, erythematous papules and plaques.
- Secondary changes include lichenification and postinflammatory hyperpigmentation or hypopigmentation.

### Epidemiology
- Strong association with personal or family history of asthma and allergic rhinitis.
- Most eczema improves by 10 years of age.
- Severe, recalcitrant eczematous dermatitis may be associated with immunodeficiencies, including hyper-IgE syndrome, Wiskott-Aldrich syndrome, and severe combined immunodeficiency syndrome.
- Children with eczema are prone to viral superinfection (e.g., herpes simplex virus [HSV], molluscum contagiosum) and colonization with *Staphylococcus aureus*.

### Subtypes
- Infantile
  - From 2 months to 2 years
  - Commonly involves cheeks (Fig. 15-14A), scalp, trunk, and extensor surfaces of the extremities
- Childhood
  - From 2 years to adolescence
  - Commonly involves flexural surfaces, including antecubital, popliteal fossae, neck, wrists, and feet (Fig. 15-14B and C)
- Adolescent/Adult
  - Flexural surfaces; may be limited to hands and/or face
- Nummular
  - Coin-shaped, erythematous, oozing plaques
  - Often occur on hands, arms, or legs (Fig. 15-14D)
- Dyshidrotic
  - Bilateral hand and/or foot dermatitis
  - Intensely pruritic with small vesicles along sides of fingers and toes

### Treatment
- General skin care
  - Limit bathing to 5-10 minutes in lukewarm water up to once daily. Use mild soaps (Cetaphil, Vanicream bar soap) only in small amounts and in the areas necessary.
  - Apply moisturizers at least twice daily including immediately after bathing. Ointments (e.g., petroleum jelly [Vaseline] or Aquaphor) or thick creams (e.g., Eucerin) are more effective than lotions.
  - Avoid products with cocamidopropyl betaine, an ingredient commonly found in products labeled as "baby," which can make eczema worse.

- Emphasizing the chronicity of disease and the need for consistent application of prescribed treatment can improve compliance and outcomes.
- Topical steroids
  - Low strength (e.g., hydrocortisone 1% or 2.5% ointment) can be used for mild to moderate disease. Treat twice daily to affected areas until clear.
  - Mid strength (e.g., triamcinolone 0.1% ointment) can be used for limited amounts of time on more severe, localized areas of disease.
  - High strength (e.g., mometasone or clobetasol ointment) may be needed for severe areas of disease on thicker skin (e.g., hands, ankles). Referral to a pediatric

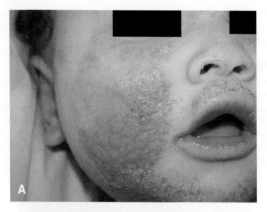

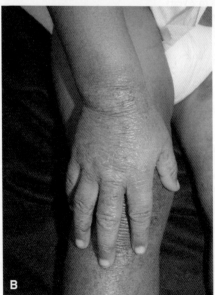

**Figure 15-14. Atopic dermatitis. A.** Infantile eczema with oozing plaques on the cheeks. **B.** Childhood eczema-lichenified plaques with excoriations.

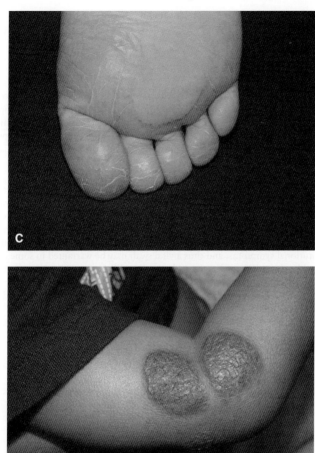

**Figure 15-14.** (*Continued*) **C.** Juvenile plantar dermatosis (foot eczema). **D.** Nummular eczema.

dermatologist may be appropriate if high-strength steroids are required. When skin is improved, patients should be tapered to a lower-strength topical steroid.
- Avoid using topical steroids on the face and intertriginous areas. Risks of topical steroids include skin atrophy, striae, and hypopigmentation (though more commonly hypopigmentation is secondary to eczema and not topical steroid use).
- Topical immunomodulators
  - Topical tacrolimus (0.03% or 0.1%) or topical pimecrolimus (1%) may be useful in limited areas such as the face or body folds, where topical steroids may cause undesirable side effects with prolonged use.

- Antihistamines. Oral diphenhydramine, hydroxyzine, or cetirizine are often useful to control pruritus. These agents may cause sedation, restricting their use to night time.
- Systemic steroids
  - These may be used in short bursts for severe exacerbations.
  - Regular or long-term use is not recommended.
- Systemic anti-inflammatory therapy
  - These may be warranted for children with disease that has been refractory to optimized topical regimens. Traditional options include cyclosporine, azathioprine, mycophenolate mofetil, and methotrexate. Dupilumab, a biologic that inhibits IL-4 and IL-13 signaling, is the only FDA-approved systemic therapy (approved above age 6) and is effective for children with uncontrolled moderate to severe atopic dermatitis.
- Antibiotics
  - Superinfection of eczema is common, with *S. aureus* being the most common pathogen, often requiring oral antibiotics. Consider performing a skin swab for bacterial culture and appropriate antibiotic therapy when a patient has a flare from their baseline, the disease is not improving, and/or when there are oozing/weeping lesions. HSV superinfection can also occur and cause punched out erosions and constitutional symptoms, and thus a viral swab may be warranted in some cases.
  - Dilute bleach baths can decrease colonization. Mupirocin 2% ointment can be used on superinfected lesions and to decolonize the nares.
  - Avoid neomycin/polymyxin/bacitracin (Neosporin) because neomycin and bacitracin are a common cause of contact dermatitis.

## IRRITANT DIAPER DERMATITIS

- Erythematous eroded patches occurring in the diaper area due to moisture and irritation.
- Treatment includes frequent diaper changes, use of thick barrier ointments (e.g., zinc oxide paste), avoidance of diaper wipes given frequent contact allergens ("Water Wipes" are safe alternative), low-strength topical steroids, and/or topical antifungals.

## SEBORRHEIC DERMATITIS

- Characterized by erythematous patches covered by thick, yellow scale.
- "Cradle cap" occurs on the scalp of infants (Fig. 15-15).
  - It is most common at 2-10 weeks and may last for 8-12 months.
  - Treatment involves hydrocortisone 1% ointment. Ketoconazole shampoo can be too drying on infant scalp and is not preferred.
- The adolescent/adult form is characterized by greasy flaking in scalp, eyebrows, nasolabial folds, and chest. Treatment involves the following:
  - Shampoos: sulfur or salicylic acid (T-gel), selenium sulfide 2.5% (Selsun), or ketoconazole 2% (Nizoral) on affected areas, including face and body. Let soak in for several minutes prior to rinsing. Alternate different shampoos.
  - Low-strength topical steroid for 5-7 days if needed.
- Blepharitis is characterized by flaking along eyelids. Treatment involves warm water compresses and baby shampoo eyelid scrubs.

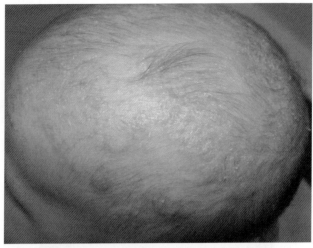

**Figure 15-15.** Seborrheic dermatitis.

## ALLERGIC CONTACT DERMATITIS

- The lesions of allergic contact dermatitis are erythematous papules and vesicles with oozing and crusting. Pruritus may be intense. This is a type IV hypersensitivity reaction.
- Common causes include poison ivy/oak, nickel, cosmetics and fragrances, topical medications, chemicals in diaper wipes, and tape or other adhesives (Fig. 15-16A and B). The distribution often gives clues to the causative agent (e.g., exposed areas for poison ivy, umbilicus for nickel, eyelids and face for nail polish or other cosmetics, buttocks and posterior thigh for toilet seat).
- This may be accompanied by eczematous dermatitis at sites far from initial exposure.
- Treatment
  - Cool water compresses and oral antihistamines for symptomatic relief
  - High-strength topical steroids bid for 5-7 days (avoid face, intertriginous areas)
  - Systemic steroids: 2-3 week taper for severe eruptions
- Referral to a dermatologist for skin patch testing if the condition is recurrent and no causative agent can be identified.

## IMPETIGO

- Erythematous vesicles and pustules that develop into erosions with "honey-colored" crust, most commonly affecting the perioral and nasal regions.
- Superficial skin infection caused by *S. aureus* or group A streptococcus.
- Treat with topical mupirocin 2% ointment or oral antibiotics if extensive. Obtain skin swab for bacterial culture to determine sensitivities.

## TINEA (DERMATOPHYTOSES)

- Fungal infections that are able to invade and multiply within keratinized tissue and are named according to the involved body site, for example, scalp (tinea capitis)

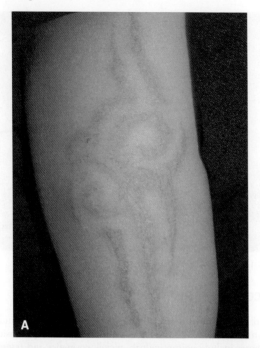

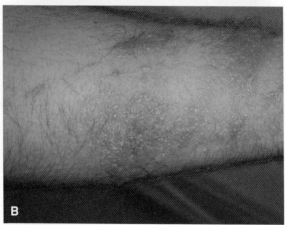

**Figure 15-16. Contact dermatitis. A.** Henna tattoo allergy. **B.** Poison ivy.

(Fig. 15-17A and B), body (tinea corporis) (Fig. 15-18), feet (tinea pedis), groin (tinea cruris), and nails (onychomycosis).
- Occur most frequently in postpubertal hosts except for tinea capitis, which occurs primarily in children.
- Clinical presentation varies based on the causative organism.

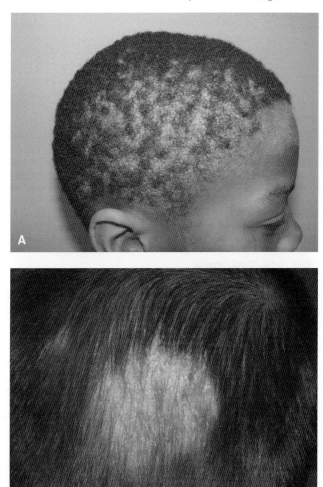

**Figure 15-17. A,B.** Tinea capitis.

- Transmitted via soil, animal, or human contact.
- Diagnosis may be made by clinical appearance, potassium hydroxide treated skin scraping showing branching hyphae, or fungal culture.

## Clinical Presentation

- Tinea capitis: alopecia with or without scale on the scalp most commonly but may also present as black dots due to hair breakage near the scalp or severe pustular reaction with alopecia known as a kerion
- Tinea corporis: erythematous, annular lesions of various sizes on the trunk with central clearing as infection spreads centrifugally from the point of skin invasion

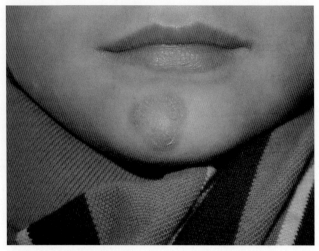

**Figure 15-18. Tinea corporis.**

- Tinea pedis: erythema, hyperkeratosis, scaling, and fissures on plantar surface(s) in a moccasin distribution or erythema, scaling, fissures, and maceration in the web spaces

## Treatment

- Scalp infections: oral systemic therapy such as griseofulvin or terbinafine required as topical therapies are unable to penetrate the hair follicle. May use topical antifungal shampoos in conjunction with systemic therapy to decrease scale and contagiousness.
- Skin infections: topical antifungals (e.g., miconazole, clotrimazole) bid until scaling clears—usually requires weeks of treatment.
- Nail infections: may respond to topical azoles or ciclopirox, but typically requires several months of treatment with oral systemic antifungal (terbinafine).

## WARTS

HPV infection of keratinocytes commonly found in school children with declining prevalence with increasing age.

## Clinical Presentation

- Common warts (verruca vulgaris): hyperkeratotic, papillomatous, exophytic, dome-shaped papules that disrupt skin lines found most commonly on the fingers and dorsal hands (Fig. 15-19A).
- Palmar and plantar warts: hyperkeratotic, endophytic papules with central depression and occasionally black dots representing thrombosed capillaries on palms and soles.
- Flat warts: skin colored to pink-brown, flat topped, relatively smooth papules on dorsal hands, arm, or face.

## Treatment

- About 60% of warts will spontaneously resolve within 2 years.
- Treatment options include active observation, home therapy with OTC salicylic acid, cryotherapy, squaric acid, imiquimod, and intralesional candida antigen.
- Sometimes several different treatments are needed for complete resolution.
- Anogenital warts (Fig. 15-19C) require different treatment methods. These may be caused by autoinoculation or vertical transmission during childbirth, but should prompt consideration of screening for sexual abuse in a child who is not sexually active.

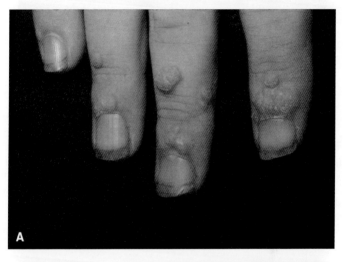

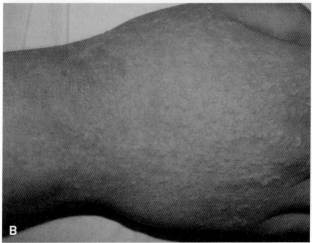

**Figure 15-19. Warts. A.** Verrucae vulgaris. **B.** Flat warts.

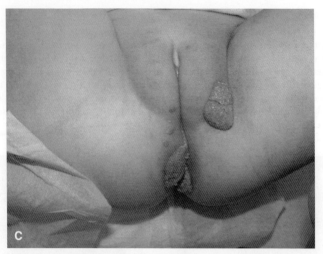

**Figure 15-19.** (*Continued*) **C.** Genital warts (condyloma acuminata).

## MOLLUSCUM CONTAGIOSUM

- Skin colored, smooth, dome-shaped papules with central umbilication caused by a pox virus. May become inflamed, red, and enlarged before resolving (Fig. 15-20).
- Transmitted by contact with an infected person and also thought to travel on water.
- Lesions typically asymptomatic and generally resolve in 6-9 months without intervention.
- Treatment options include observation, tape stripping, and cantharone (blistering agent).

## PYOGENIC GRANULOMA

- Bright red, shiny, dome-shaped papule that bleeds spontaneously or after trauma favoring face and digits.
- Often treated with shave excision and electrocautery of base, recurrence may occur despite treatment.

## SPITZ NEVUS

- Pink, red or pigmented, well-circumscribed, dome-shaped, smooth papule favoring the head, neck, and lower extremities.
- Usually a benign entity, less commonly can have atypical features necessitating excision with conservative margins.
- Diagnosed clinically and/or histologically via biopsy by a dermatologist.

## GRANULOMA ANNULARE

- Pink or red-brown, annular or arcuate dermal plaques without overlying scale favoring dorsal fingers, hands, elbows, feet, or ankles.
- Inflammatory skin disorder of unknown etiology. Treatment options limited.
- Resolves spontaneously but may have a prolonged course of years.

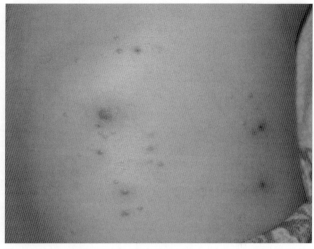

**Figure 15-20. Molluscum contagiosum.**

## LICHEN PLANUS

- Violaceous, flat-topped, polygonal, pruritic papules favoring wrists, back and lower extremities.
- Resolves spontaneously in many cases within 1-2 years.
- Treatment options for focal lesions include topical steroids or topical tacrolimus.

## URTICARIA

- Outbreak of erythematous, raised wheals with individual lesions lasting <24 hours.
- Most commonly idiopathic but can be triggered by upper respiratory infection, drugs, food, or other causes.
- Can be acute (recurring episodes fewer than 6 weeks in duration) or less often chronic (>6 weeks).
- Usually is self-limiting. Treat with nonsedating H1 antagonists first line (often using scheduled daily or bid doses for several months). NSAIDs can exacerbate the condition.
- If associated with anaphylaxis, patients should carry an epi-pen.
- A morphologic subtype of acute urticaria is urticaria multiforme, which is a hypersensitivity reaction consisting of annular polycyclic wheals with dusky centers that can visually mimic erythema multiforme but is clinically distinct.

## ERYTHEMA MULTIFORME

### Clinical Presentation
- Hypersensitivity reaction characterized by acute onset of erythematous papules that evolve into targetoid lesions with dusky centers (Fig. 15-21).
- Previously thought to be on a continuum with Stevens-Johnson syndrome and toxic epidermal necrosis, but now more recently understood to be a distinct presentation that does not progress to these more severe disease processes.
- HSV infection is the most common precipitating factor, although other triggers such as drug exposure are possible.

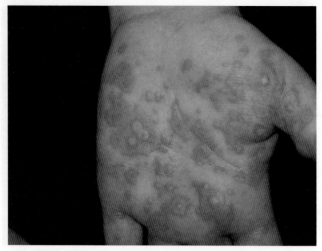

Figure 15-21. **Erythema multiforme with typical target lesions.**

- Classification
  - Erythema multiforme minor: little or no mucosal involvement and systemic symptoms
  - Erythema multiforme major: several mucosal involvement and systemic symptoms (fever, arthralgias, etc.)

## Treatment

- The condition generally self resolves within several weeks without sequelae.
- Antihistamines and topical steroids may provide symptomatic relief.
- Systemic steroids can be considered for severe erythema multiforme.
- Prophylactic acyclovir may be useful to prevent recurrent HSV-related disease.

## STEVENS-JOHNSON SYNDROME AND TOXIC EPIDERMAL NECROLYSIS

### Clinical Presentation

- Stevens-Johnson syndrome (SJS) and toxic epidermal necrolysis (TEN) represent a continuum of severe cutaneous adverse reactions, usually secondary to a medication, that are thought to be caused by cytotoxic T-cell activation leading to keratinocyte apoptosis.
- Prodromal symptoms (fever, malaise, eye irritation, pain on swallowing) are followed a few days later by an eruption of erythematous to dusky macules that progress to blistering and full-thickness epidermal sloughing.
  - Mucosal involvement with erosions and crusting of the oral, ocular, and genital mucosa is prominent.
  - Systemic manifestations are often present and may include fever, lymphadenopathy, hepatitis, and cytopenias.
  - Mortality has been estimated as 0-4% for SJS and 0-17% for TEN.
- Clinically distinct from RIME/MIRM (reactive infectious mucocutaneous eruption)/*Mycoplasma pneumoniae*–induced rash and mucositis), which is secondary

to an infectious etiology, can result in severe mucocutaneous involvement, but typically has limited skin involvement.

- Percent body surface area denuded:
  - <10%: SJS
  - 10-30%: SJS/TEN overlap
  - >30%: TEN
- Almost always secondary to a drug exposure. Look for drugs initiated 7-21 days prior to onset. The most common drug culprits include antibiotics (penicillin, sulfa, doxycycline, sulfonamides, tetracycline), anticonvulsants, and nonsteroidal anti-inflammatory drugs.

## Treatment

- Rapid identification and withdrawal of potential offending medications, as well as supportive care, are the most critical aspects of management. Transfer to an intensive care or burn unit is ideal.
- Replace fluid losses and provide adequate nutrition.
- Administer local wound care. Debridement is not recommended.
- Give antibiotics as needed for superinfection. Avoid prophylactic antibiotics.
- Ophthalmology consultation and ongoing evaluation should be obtained as ocular sequelae can result in blindness.
- Aside from supportive care, many systemic immunosuppressive or immunomodulating therapies have been tried for SJS and TEN. While many centers have historically used systemic steroids and IVIG, cyclosporine and etanercept have been reported in both adult and pediatric case series to have treatment efficacy.

## SUGGESTED READINGS

Canavan TN, Mathes EF, Frieden I, et al. Mycoplasma pneumoniae-induced rash and mucositis as a syndrome distinct from Stevens-Johnson syndrome and erythema multiforme: a systematic review. J Am Acad Dermatol 2015;72(2):239–245.

Conlon JD, Drolet BA. Skin lesions in the neonate. Pediatr Clin North Am 2004;51(4):863–888, vii–viii.

Eichenfield LF, Tom WL, Chamlin SL, et al. Guidelines of care for the management of atopic dermatitis: section 1. Diagnosis and assessment of atopic dermatitis. J Am Acad Dermatol 2014;70(2):338–351.

Hsu DY, Brieva J, Silverberg NB, et al. Pediatric Stevens-Johnson syndrome and toxic epidermal necrolysis in the United States. J Am Acad Dermatol 2017;76(5):811–817.e4.

Krowchuk DP, Frieden IJ, Mancini AJ, et al. Clinical practice guideline for the management of infantile hemangiomas. Pediatrics 2019;143(1):e20183475.

Mallory S, Bree AF, Chern P, et al. Illustrated Manual of Pediatric Dermatology. New York: Taylor & Francis, 2005.

Sabeti S, Ball KL, Burkhart C, et al. Consensus statement for the management and treatment of port-wine birthmarks in Sturge-Weber Syndrome. JAMA Dermatol 2021;157(1):98–104.

Sibbald C, Putterman E, Micheletti R, et al. Retrospective review of drug-induced Stevens-Johnson syndrome and toxic epidermal necrolysis cases at a pediatric tertiary care institution. Pediatr Dermatol 2020;37(3):461–466.

Simpson EL, Paller AS, Siegfried EC, et al. Efficacy and safety of dupilumab in adolescents with uncontrolled moderate to severe atopic dermatitis: a phase 3 randomized clinical trial. JAMA Dermatol 2020;156(1):44–56.

Waelchli R, Aylett SE, Robinson K, et al. New vascular classification of port-wine stains: Improving prediction of Sturge-Weber risk. Br J Dermatol 2014;171(4):861–867.

Zallmann M, Leventer RJ, Mackay MT, et al. Screening for Sturge-Weber syndrome: a state-of-the-art review. Pediatr Dermatol 2018;35(1):30–42.

# 16

# Genetic Diseases

Katherine Abell King, Catherine Gooch,
and Hoanh Nguyen

## DYSMORPHIC FEATURES AND MALFORMATIONS

### Definitions and Epidemiology

- A *dysmorphic feature* is any alteration in the physical structure (morphology) of a person's anatomy.
- A *malformation* is a specific type of structural abnormality caused by an intrinsic (genetic) factor.
  - Major malformations either require surgical intervention or have a significant impact on the patient's health.
    ○ Examples include craniosynostosis, cleft lip and/or palate, congenital heart disease, and omphalocele.
    ○ They occur in up to 3% of all live births.
  - Minor malformations do not have a significant impact on the patient's health.
    ○ Examples include hypertelorism, ear pit or tag, smooth philtrum, transverse palmar crease, and mild soft tissue syndactyly.
    ○ They are not rare in the general population.
- A *deformation* is an abnormal structure caused by an external force during intrauterine development that resulted in abnormal growth or formation.
- A *dysplasia* results from a failure to maintain the intrinsic cellular architecture of a tissue throughout growth and development.

### Etiology

- The pattern of dysmorphic features in a single individual may suggest a named genetic condition (see Table 16-1), such as up-slanting palpebral fissures, epicanthal folds, and a single palmar crease in individuals with Down syndrome.
- There are also nongenetic causes for dysmorphic features. For example, the teratogenic effects of valproic acid can cause a specific constellation of facial features.

### Diagnosis and Evaluation

- Cytogenetics
  - If a patient has at least two major or one major and two minor malformations, a chromosomal microarray analysis (CMA) is indicated. In some cases, a karyotype may be beneficial if there is concern for chromosomal translocations, inversions, or rearrangements.
  - Other indications for CMA include apparently nonsyndromic developmental delay or intellectual disability, and autism spectrum disorders.
- Molecular Sequencing
  - If CMA does not reveal the etiology of the patient's differences, molecular sequencing can be pursued. Depending on the phenotype, this may range from single gene sequencing to panels, to exome, or to genome sequencing.

**TABLE 16-1** Frequently Encountered Genetic Disorders

| Disorder | Selected features | Tests |
|---|---|---|
| 22q11.2 deletion syndrome (also known as DiGeorge or velocardiofacial syndrome) | Congenital heart disease, cleft palate, dysmorphic facial features, intellectual disability, immune deficiency, hypocalcemia, hearing loss, psychiatric disease | FISH/CMA with 22q11.2 deletion |
| Achondroplasia | Disproportionate short stature, rhizomelic limb shortening, macrocephaly, craniocervical junction instability, trident hand, hypotonia | *FGFR3* gene analysis |
| Alagille syndrome | Characteristic facies, paucity of bile ducts, posterior embryotoxon, retinal pigmentary changes, butterfly vertebrae, tetralogy of Fallot | *JAG1, NOTCH2* gene analysis<br>CMA with 20p12 deletion |
| Angelman syndrome | Happy demeanor, ataxia, developmental delay, intellectual disability, dysmorphic facial features, microcephaly, light hair and skin compared to family | Methylation: loss of maternal methylation on 15q11-13, paternal UPD of chromosome 15<br>*UBE3A* gene analysis<br>CMA with maternal 15p11.2 deletion |
| Beckwith-Wiedemann syndrome | Increased growth, hemihyperplasia, omphalocele, macroglossia, neonatal hypoglycemia, embryonal tumor predisposition | Methylation: loss of maternal methylation chr11p15.5, paternal UPD of chromosome 15<br>*CDKN1C* gene analysis<br>CMA with maternal 11p15.5 deletion |
| CHARGE syndrome | Colobomas, heart defects, choanal atresia, growth retardation, genitourinary malformations, ear anomalies, deafness, tracheoesophageal fistula, developmental delay, intellectual disability | *CHD7* gene analysis |
| Cri-du-chat syndrome (also known as 5p minus syndrome) | High-pitched cry, microcephaly, intellectual disability, hypotonia, dysmorphic facial features | CMA with 5p deletion |

*(Continued)*

**TABLE 16-1** Frequently Encountered Genetic Disorders (*Continued*)

| Disorder | Selected features | Tests |
|---|---|---|
| Down syndrome (also known as trisomy 21) | Characteristic dysmorphic features, congenital heart disease, hypothyroidism, duodenal atresia, Hirschsprung, developmental delay, intellectual disability<br><br>Can be difficult to detect in premature infants and neonates | Karyotype<br>Aneuploidy screen<br>Prenatal NIPT |
| Ehlers-Danlos syndrome | Hypermobile type: benign, generalized joint hypermobility, joint pain and dislocations, clinical diagnostic criteria established<br><br>Classical type: generalized hypermobile joints, skin fragility, dystrophic scarring<br><br>Vascular type: small joint hypermobility, skin fragility, atrophic scarring, predisposition to rupture of hollow organs | Hypermobile: no known genetic cause, clinical diagnostic criteria<br>Classical type: *COL5A1, COL5A2* gene analysis<br>Vascular type: *COL3A1* gene analysis |
| Fetal alcohol spectrum disorder | Characteristic facial features (short palpebral fissures, thin upper lip vermillion, smooth philtrum), growth deficiency (height, weight, <10th percentile), CNS involvement (microcephaly, structural brain abnormalities); confirmation of prenatal alcohol exposure not required | Clinical diagnostic criteria |
| Fragile X syndrome | Males with dysmorphic facial features, postpubertal macro-orchidism, autism, developmental delay, intellectual disability, late-onset ataxia, tremor. Females may be variably affected | Fragile X (*FRM1*) gene analysis for abnormal methylation and triplet-repeat expansion |
| Klinefelter syndrome | Males with tall stature, variable learning disabilities, small testes, gynecomastia, infertility | Karyotype<br>Aneuploidy screen<br>Prenatal NIPT |
| Marfan syndrome | Dilation of aortic root, myopia, ectopia lentis, tall, thin build, pectus deformity, joint laxity, long digits, flat feet, characteristic facial features | *FBN1* gene analysis |

| TABLE 16-1 | Frequently Encountered Genetic Disorders (*Continued*) | |
|---|---|---|
| **Disorder** | **Selected features** | **Tests** |
| Neurofibromatosis type 1 | Café au lait macules, neurofibromas, plexiform neurofibromas, axillary/inguinal freckling, optic pathway glioma, Lisch nodules, sphenoid dysplasia | *NF1* gene analysis |
| Noonan syndrome | Short stature, congenital heart disease (pulmonic stenosis), characteristic facial features, broad or webbed neck, mild intellectual disability | Gene panel analysis |
| Osteogenesis imperfecta | Fragile bones, blue sclerae, abnormal teeth, clinical presentation and severity is variable based on type | Gene panel analysis |
| Prader-Willi syndrome | Neonates: feeding difficulty, profound hypotonia<br><br>Children: significant food-seeking behavior leading to obesity, developmental delay, behavioral abnormalities, short stature, hypogonadism | Methylation: loss of paternal methylation 15q11-13, maternal UPD<br><br>CMA with 15q11-13 deletion |
| Rett syndrome | Girls with normal development until around age 18 months, then developmental regression, hand wringing, autism, acquired microcephaly, seizures, intermittent hyperventilation<br><br>Affected males are rare | *MECP2* gene analysis |
| Smith-Lemli-Opitz syndrome | Dysmorphic facial features, microcephaly, cleft palate, 2-3 toe syndactyly, polydactyly, heart defects, hypospadias, intellectual disability, autism, seizures | 7-Dehydrocholesterol<br>*DHCR7* gene analysis |
| Stickler syndrome | Cleft palate, Robin sequence, myopia, retinal detachment, hearing loss, arthritis | Gene panel analysis |
| Treacher Collins syndrome | Dysmorphic facial features, micrognathia, hearing loss, normal intelligence | Gene panel analysis |

(*Continued*)

| TABLE 16-1 | Frequently Encountered Genetic Disorders (*Continued*) | |
|---|---|---|
| **Disorder** | **Selected features** | **Tests** |
| Trisomy 13 (also known as Patau syndrome) | Midline defects, holoprosencephaly, microcephaly, cleft lip or palate, clenched hands, polydactyly, congenital heart disease, hernias, coloboma, microphthalmia, micrognathia | Karyotype<br>Aneuploidy screen<br>Prenatal NIPT |
| Trisomy 18 (also known as Edwards syndrome) | IUGR, clenched hands with overlapping digits, rocker-bottom feet, congenital heart disease, microcephaly, micrognathia | Karyotype<br>Aneuploidy screen<br>Prenatal NIPT |
| Turner syndrome | Females with short stature, webbed neck, coarctation of aorta, premature ovarian failure and infertility | Karyotype<br>Aneuploidy screen<br>Prenatal NIPT |
| VACTERL association | Vertebral anomalies, anal atresia, cardiac malformations, tracheoesophageal fistula, renal and limb anomalies | Diagnosis of exclusion, no known genetic cause |
| Waardenburg syndrome | Hearing loss, heterochromia, white forelock, widely spaced eyes, some types include limb anomalies or Hirschsprung disease | Gene panel analysis |
| Williams syndrome | Dysmorphic facies, supravalvular aortic stenosis, "cocktail party personality," hypertension, hypercalcemia | CMA with7q11.2 deletion |
| Wolf-Hirschhorn syndrome | Microcephaly, dysmorphic facial features with "Greek warrior helmet," poor growth, developmental delay, intellectual disability, hypotonia, hearing loss, seizures | CMA with 4p deletion |

CMA, chromosomal microarray analysis; FISH, fluorescent in situ hybridization; IUGR, intrauterine growth restriction; UPD, uniparental disomy.

- Single gene sequencing should be used when there is high suspicion for a specific disorder, that is, *CHD7* sequencing in suspected CHARGE syndrome.
- Panels are more useful when there are multiple genes that can cause a patient's phenotype. An example of this is epilepsy where there are hundreds of known causative genes.
- When a patient phenotype is very complex and involves multiple organ systems (with a normal CMA), advanced molecular sequencing with exome or genome should be considered. Exome sequencing looks at the molecular sequence of

protein coding genes and genome sequencing looks at the molecular sequencing of almost all genes. Of note, trinucleotide repeat disorders and methylation analysis should be tested for separately as exome and genome may fail to find pathogenic repeats or methylation changes.

- In a patient with multiple malformations, it is also necessary to consider the following studies to detect other occult anomalies:
  - Echocardiogram, abdominal ultrasound (with renal imaging), and neuroimaging study (magnetic resonance imaging [MRI])
  - Ophthalmologic examination and hearing screen (federally mandated newborn screening is sufficient in neonates or infants if there is no clinical concern for hearing loss)
  - Skeletal survey, especially if a patient has short stature or observable bony changes
- Common reasons for referrals for evaluation by medical genetics are presented in Table 16-2.

| TABLE 16-2 Common Reasons for Referral to Medical Genetics |
| --- |

Neurologic
- Seizures
- Autism
- Developmental delay/intellectual disability/developmental regression

Oncology
- Concern for cancer syndrome
- Young age of cancer onset
- Family history of cancer

Endocrinology
- Failure to thrive/short stature

Musculoskeletal
- Concern for connective tissue disorder
- Skeletal dysplasias

ENT
- Hearing loss
- Orofacial clefting
- Craniosynostosis

Cardiac
- Congenital heart disease
- Cardiomyopathy
- Thoracic aortic aneurysm

Genetic
- Known or suspected chromosomal difference
- Known or suspected metabolic disorder
- Family history of genetic disease
- Birth defects

## METABOLIC DECOMPENSATION AS A PRESENTATION OF INBORN ERRORS OF METABOLISM

### Clinical Presentation

- Children with an acute decompensation from an inborn metabolic disease may present with variable and nonspecific symptoms, such as mental status changes that range from fussiness to coma, poor feeding, vomiting, changes in breathing, abnormal movements, seizures, strokes, or liver failure. They may also have chronic conditions, including low tone, global developmental delay, intellectual disability, autism, or cardiomyopathy.
- Children with an underlying metabolic disease and a superimposed acute metabolic stress, such as an infection or trauma, may present with more severe symptoms than expected from the acute stressor alone.
- Patients with an underlying metabolic disease may also experience difficulty recovering from surgery.
- Infants with bacterial sepsis may have an inborn metabolic illness as a predisposing factor, such as the increased incidence of *Escherichia coli* sepsis in patients with galactosemia. Also, a previously healthy neonate who presents with septic symptomatology but no fever or obvious source of infection should have a concurrent metabolic evaluation.

### Laboratory Studies

- To detect a wide range of metabolic disorders, several screening laboratory tests are recommended. If abnormalities are detected, then more definitive studies should be performed.
- For the highest yield, samples should be obtained during an acute illness. Tests to order include the following:
  - Blood tests: point-of-care glucose, comprehensive metabolic panel, blood gas (arterial or capillary), ammonium, complete blood count (CBC) with differential, lactate and pyruvate, serum/plasma amino acids, acylcarnitine profile, quantitative carnitines, and save serum sample.
  - Urine tests: urinalysis (including ketones), reducing substances, organic acids, and save urine sample.
  - Cerebrospinal fluid (CSF) tests: routine studies (cell count, glucose, protein), lactate and pyruvate, amino acids, and save CSF sample.
  - Table 16-3 provides expected laboratory values and other features in common metabolic disorders. Table 16-4 further describes frequently encountered metabolic disorders by category.
- Results of newborn screening tests should be verified.

### Treatment

- If the diagnosis of an inborn metabolic disease is considered, the patient should not receive enteral protein or TPN. Instead, the patient should receive 10% dextrose intravenous (IV) fluids at 1.5-2 times the maintenance rate.
- If a definitive diagnosis is made, then specific and directed therapy can be instituted.
- The appropriate management for an individual with a known metabolic disease depends on the underlying disorder.
  - Patients or their families should be provided with a letter written by their geneticist with management instructions for their specific disorder when they are sick.
  - Contact the geneticist on call for any patient who presents ill to the emergency department, is receiving sedation, or is undergoing a procedure.

| TABLE 16-3 | Metabolic Disorders with Acute Presentation in the First Few Days of Life and Their Key Laboratory and Clinical Features | | | | | | |
|---|---|---|---|---|---|---|---|
| Disorder | Blood gas pH | Urine ketones | Ammonia | Lactate | Glucose | Liver dysfunction | Significant findings |
| MMA/PA | **Low** | **High** | Normal-high | Normal-high | Variable | Normal-hepatomegaly | **Pancytopenia** |
| IVA | **Low** | **High** | Normal-high | Normal-high | Variable | Variable | **Sweaty feet odor** |
| MSUD | Low-normal | Normal-high | Normal-high | Normal-high | Low-normal | Normal | Maple syrup odor |
| OTC deficiency | **Respiratory alkalosis** | **Normal** | **High** | Normal | Low-normal | Variable | Males |
| Galactosemia | Normal | **Normal** | Normal | Normal-**high** | **Low** | Severe | Neonatal *E. coli* sepsis |
| FAOD | Normal-low | **Absent-low** | Normal-high | Normal-high | **Low** | Often normal | Reye-like syndrome |
| Mitochondrial/respiratory chain defects | Normal-low | Normal-high | Normal | **High** | Normal | Hypoalbuminemia | High CSF lactate |

Classic features in **bold**.
CSF, cerebral spinal fluid; FAOD, fatty acid oxidation disorder; IVA, isovaleric academia; MMA, methylmalonic academia; MSUD, maple syrup urine disease; OTC, ornithine transcarbamylase; PA, propionic academia.

| TABLE 16-4 | Clinical Features and Recommended Tests for Frequently Encountered Inherited Metabolic Disorders |
| --- | --- |

| Disorder | Features | Tests |
| --- | --- | --- |
| Amino acid disorders | PKU: fair hair and skin, ID, psychiatric disorders, mousy/musty odor<br><br>MSUD: typically well first few days, leucine intoxication symptoms progressing to coma, ID<br><br>Homocystinuria: thrombosis, ectopia lentis, ID. Poorly evaluated on NBS<br><br>Tyrosinemia I: rapidly progressing acute hepatic failure, anorexia, irritability, hypotonia, severe anemia, thrombocytopenia, renal tubular acidosis. Increased detection by NBS testing includes succinylacetone | NBS, PAA, UOA, UAA, gene analysis<br><br>Homocystinuria: total homocysteine<br><br>Tyrosinemia I: urine succinylacetone, AFP, synthetic liver function test |
| Biotinidase/multiple carboxylase deficiency | Hypotonia, seizures, cutaneous abnormalities (acrodermatitis enteropathica), hearing loss, DD | NBS, enzyme testing, gene analysis |
| Congenital disorders of glycosylation | PMM2-CDG: most common; inverted nipples, lipodystrophy, cerebellar hypoplasia, retinitis pigmentosa<br><br>MPI-CDG: protein-losing enteropathy (chronic diarrhea/FTT) with minimal neurologic involvement. Treatment with oral mannose | Isoelectric focusing for specific types (N-linked disorders), serum O-linked and N-linked glycan profiling; many false positives<br><br>Gene panel analysis |
| Fatty acid oxidation disorders | Most common: MCAD deficiency, VLCAD deficiency, CUD, CPT II<br><br>May present after fasting with hypoketotic hypoglycemia, cardiomyopathy, skeletal myopathy, or Reye-like syndrome | NBS, ACP, quantitative carnitines, uric acid, ammonia, creatine kinase<br><br>Gene analysis |

| TABLE 16-4 | Clinical Features and Recommended Tests for Frequently Encountered Inherited Metabolic Disorders (*Continued*) |
| --- | --- |

| Disorder | Features | Tests |
| --- | --- | --- |
| Fructose 1,6 bisphosphatase deficiency | Hypoglycemia, ketosis, lactic acidosis, liver dysfunction, mental status changes, hypotonia, FTT. Can present without exposure to oral fructose | Lactate, pyruvate, PAA, UAA, uric acid<br><br>Enzyme testing, gene analysis |
| Galactosemia | Hyperbilirubinemia, hepatomegaly, hepatic failure, hypoglycemia, bleeding diathesis, edema, ascites, and congenital cataracts. Potentially lethal in the newborn period | NBS, galactose-1-phosphate level<br><br>GALT enzyme, gene analysis |
| Glycogen storage diseases | Hypoglycemia, lactic acidemia, growth retardation, hyperlipidemia, hyperuricemia<br><br>GSD-I (von Gierke disease):<br><br>Type 1a—hepatomegaly, renomegaly short stature, no response to glucagon (predisposition to hepatic adenomas); type 1b—same 1a also with neutropenia and chronic infections, chronic IBD<br><br>GSD-II (Pompe disease): hypotonia, (massive) cardiomegaly, large tongue, progressive weakness, elevated CPK. NBS available. Also a lysosomal storage disorder<br><br>GSD-V (McArdle disease): muscle weakness and cramping usually with exercise. Second wind phenomenon. Myoglobinuria, elevated CPK | Uric acid, CPK, urine myoglobin, lactate, pyruvate, PAA, UAA, lipid panel, gene analysis<br><br>GSD-II: NBS (some states)<br><br>GSD-V: Forearm exercise test is diagnostic |
| Hereditary fructose intolerance | Require exposure to oral fructose. Symptoms of vomiting, abdominal discomfort, hypoglycemia, FTT, lactic acidosis, aversion to sweets, lack of dental caries | Urine reducing substances, enzyme activity, gene analysis |
| Lysosomal storage diseases | Gaucher: most common, has three types; foam cells on bone marrow | NBS (some states), urine mucopolysaccharide |

(*Continued*)

| TABLE 16-4 | Clinical Features and Recommended Tests for Frequently Encountered Inherited Metabolic Disorders (*Continued*) | |
|---|---|---|

| Disorder | Features | Tests |
|---|---|---|
| | Fabry: X linked, males with median age of onset 9 years, peripheral neuropathy, acro-paresthesias, angiokeratomas, lens/corneal opacities, later renal and cardiac complications chronic lung disease with fibro-sis; females with median age of onset 13 years, fatigue, strokes, renal failure | Urine oligosaccharides<br>Leukocyte lysosomal enzyme panel<br>Brain MRI<br>Gene analysis (especially for females with Fabry) |
| | MPS-I (Hurler): normal at birth w/gradual slowing of development/regression, corneal clouding, dysostosis multiplex, claw hand, mixed hearing loss, macrocephaly | |
| | MPS-II (Hunter): X linked, similar to MPS-I but without corneal clouding. Deafness, coarse features | |
| | Tay-Sachs: regression, onset 6-12 months, hyperacusis, macular cherry red spot, later seizures, blindness | |
| Mitochondrial cytopathies (most common Leigh syndrome, respiratory chain defects, and PDH complex deficiencies) | Most common: Leigh syndrome, PDH complex deficiencies, respiratory chain defects. | Lactate, pyruvate (blood and CSF), PAA, ACP, UOA |
| | Variable symptoms of skeletal myopathy, lactic acidosis, strokes, leukodystrophy, global developmental delay/ intellectual disability, movement disorder, vision impairment/ retinitis pigmentosa/ optic atrophy, hearing impairment, arrhythmias, cardiomyopathy, hepatocellular dysfunction, diabetes, other endocrinopathies, short stature | Muscle biopsy with enzyme analysis.<br>Brain MRI/MRS<br>Gene analysis (mitochondrial DNA, nuclear DNA) |
| | Lactate:pyruvate increased ratio, increased alanine, increased lactate in serum and CSF; MRS with lactate peak; MRI with bilat-eral basal ganglia and brainstem lesions and cerebral atrophy | |

| TABLE 16-4 | Clinical Features and Recommended Tests for Frequently Encountered Inherited Metabolic Disorders (*Continued*) |
| --- | --- |

| Disorder | Features | Tests |
| --- | --- | --- |
| Peroxisomal disorders (degradation of very long chain fatty acids, phytanic acid, others, and steps for plasmalogen and cholesterol biosynthesis) | XL-ALD: X-linked progressive neurodegenerative disorder associated with adrenal involvement. NBS available<br><br>Zellweger syndrome: dysmorphic facies, large fontanelle, feeding difficulties, hypotonia, seizures, cataracts/glaucoma, renal cysts, epiphyseal calcifications | VLCFA<br>Gene analysis (especially for female carriers of XL-ALD) |
| Organic acidurias | Most common: GA1, IVA, MMA, PA. Spectrum of disorders with life-threatening events/metabolic decompensation. Metabolic anion gap acidosis, hyperammonemia, ketosis, hyperglycinemia<br><br>GA1: macrocephaly, acute encephalopathic crises produce dystonia (choreoathetotic movements), basal ganglia stroke, cortical atrophy, ID | NBS, PAA, ACP, UOA, ammonia, quantitative carnitines, gene analysis |
| Urea cycle disorder | OTC deficiency: X linked, most common. Males with hyperammonemia, coma, respiratory alkalosis at birth. Neurologic outcome depends on height and duration of hyperammonemia. Female carriers can have hyperammonemic episodes. Increased urine orotic acid. NBS available in some states | NBS, PAA, ACP, UOA quantitative carnitines<br>Gene analysis (detectable 80-90% of time in OTC) |
| Wilson disease | Progressive neurologic findings, psychiatric disturbance, renal tubular dysfunction, mild or acute hemolysis, and Kayser-Fleischer ring in cornea | Ceruloplasmin<br>Serum copper<br>*ATP7B* mutation analysis |

ACP, acylcarnitine profile; AFP, alpha-fetoprotein; CAN, central nervous system; CPT, carnitine palmitoyl transferase; CUD, carnitine uptake deficiency; CDG, congenital disorder of glycosylation; CPK, creatine phosphokinase; FAOD, fatty acid oxidation disorder; FTT, failure to thrive; GA, glutaric aciduria; GSD, glycogen storage disease; ID, intellectual disability; IVA, isovaleric academia; MCAD, medium-chain acyl-CoA dehydrogenase; MMA, methylmalonic academia; MPS, mucopolysaccharidosis, MRI, magnetic resonance imaging; MRS, magnetic resonance spectroscopy; MSUD, maple syrup urine disease; OTC, ornithine transcarbamylase; PA, propionic academia; PAA, plasma amino acids; PDH, pyruvate dehydrogenase; PKU, phenylketonuria; UAA, urine amino acids; UOA, urine organic acids; VLCFA, very long chain fatty acid; VLCAD, very-long-chain acyl-CoA dehydrogenase.

## GENETIC DISORDERS PRESENTING WITH HYPOGLYCEMIA

Because liver metabolism is a major regulator of glucose homeostasis, many syndromes that involve hepatic dysfunction, including pediatric acute liver failure, can present with hypoglycemia. Examples include defects in gluconeogenesis such as fructose 1,6-diphosphatase deficiency and glycogen storage disease type 1 (see Table 16-4). Similarly, hypoglycemia can be a finding in conditions that result in hyperammonemia such as disorders of fatty acid and organic acid metabolism (see Table 16-3). Congenital hyperinsulinism should also be considered in neonates with persistent hypoglycemia (see Chapter 18).

## GENETIC DISORDERS PRESENTING WITH HYPERAMMONEMIA

### Laboratory Studies

- An evaluation for hyperammonemia is warranted for ammonium >100 μmol/L in neonates or for ammonium >50 μmol/L in children older than 2 months. A single elevated ammonium should be confirmed with a repeat sample.
- Ammonium levels should be drawn arterially or as a free-flowing venous sample, placed on wet ice, and processed immediately.
- Additional studies: comprehensive metabolic panel, urinalysis (including ketones), blood gas if acutely ill, serum/plasma amino acids, urine organic acids and amino acids, acylcarnitine profile, quantitative carnitines, lactate and pyruvate, and creatine kinase.

### Treatment

- The recommended specific treatment depends on the type of disorder. If the patient is acutely ill and the underlying diagnosis is unknown, eliminate oral and parenteral sources of protein and provide adequate fluid (1.5-2 times the maintenance rate) and calories (10% dextrose IV fluids, intralipids).
- After beginning the recommended evaluation for a child with hyperammonemia, the plan for further evaluation and management should be discussed with a geneticist.
- If the levels are significantly elevated and/or rising rapidly, IV arginine and ammonium scavenging drugs, sodium phenylacetate/sodium benzoate (Ammonul), and hemodialysis may be indicated.

## NEWBORN SCREENING

- The state mandated newborn screening test evaluates for many disorders; information on which disorders are screened in each state is available at www.newbornscreening.info.
- For some disorders, the sensitivity relies on the infant eating protein, either breast milk or formula, before testing.
- If an infant is receiving total parenteral nutrition (TPN) at the time of testing, the amino acid analysis is uninterpretable and invalidates testing for certain disorders.
- If an infant has received a packed red blood cell transfusion before obtaining the newborn screening sample, the galactosemia, biotinidase deficiency, and hemoglobinopathy assays are invalid.
- For some disorders, a history of a normal newborn screening result should not preclude sending definitive testing if a specific disorder is clinically suspected.

## Disorders of Fatty Acid Oxidation

- This is a group of autosomal recessive inherited conditions, with reduced activity of enzymes necessary for fatty acid metabolism.
- Infants are especially susceptible to a fasting state, with resulting hypoglycemia and/or acidosis. Symptoms include lethargy, vomiting, seizures, or coma. If untreated, patients can develop liver, heart, kidney, and muscle failure.
- Specific conditions are diagnosed by analyzing the acylcarnitine composition. Newborn screening allows early intervention, including dietary management, which can prevent serious complications.

## Amino Acid and Urea Cycle Disorders

- These metabolic disorders are caused by an inability to metabolize certain amino acids or by the inability to complete the urea cycle to detoxify ammonia, which is a by-product of amino acid metabolism. The buildup of amino acids and/or by-products of amino acid metabolism can cause severe complications.
- Examples of conditions on the newborn screen include phenylketonuria (PKU), maple syrup urine disease, tyrosinemia, homocystinuria, and citrullinemia. Ornithine transcarbamylase (OTC) deficiency is not detected by newborn screening.

## Organic Acidemias

- This group of conditions is due to defective downstream metabolism of amino acids or odd chain organic acids, resulting in specific toxic metabolites that can be found in the blood or urine. The classic presentation is a toxic encephalopathy, but milder forms also exist. Early dietary intervention can prevent serious complications.
- Examples include methylmalonic acidemia, glutaric acidemia type I, and propionic acidemia.

## GENETIC DISORDERS PRESENTING WITH INFANTILE HYPOTONIA

### Etiology

- Hypotonia is a nonspecific sign that may be caused by a wide variety of etiologies.
- Dysfunction in any component of the central or peripheral nervous system can cause hypotonia, including diseases of the muscle, neuromuscular junction, nerves, spinal cord, brain stem, cerebellum, basal ganglia, and cerebrum. Central hypotonia with peripheral spastic hypertonia is highly suggestive of central nervous system (CNS) involvement.

### Clinical Presentation

- Historical features supporting a genetic etiology include family history of neuromuscular disease, parental consanguinity, and a prior affected sibling. However, the absence of these features does not rule out a genetic cause.
- Contractures in the newborn indicate prenatal onset but do not suggest a single, specific diagnosis.
- Additional features that may indicate an underlying syndrome may not be present at a young age or may be difficult to appreciate in the neonate or infant.

### Laboratory Studies

- Several tests are recommended in the evaluation of a child with hypotonia and concern for a genetic disorder.

- Blood tests: methylation studies for Prader-Willi and Angelman syndromes, creatine kinase, aldolase, lactate and pyruvate, serum/plasma amino acids, comprehensive metabolic panel, chromosomal microarray and reflex karyotype, very long-chain fatty acids quantification, *SMN1* gene molecular analysis (if reflexes absent), myotonic dystrophy molecular analysis, and enzyme testing for Pompe disease,
- Urine tests: organic acids. Consider mucopolysaccharidosis screen.
- Other tests: electromyogram, nerve conduction studies, electrocardiogram, echocardiogram, brain MRI, and abdominal and pelvic ultrasound.

## Treatment

- Confirming a genetic diagnosis may affect the treatment regimen and allow parents to more fully understand the child's clinical course.
- Treatment often involves physical therapy and providing methods that support the child, such as splints, braces, or assistive devices. In a few conditions, such as Pompe disease, enzyme replacement therapy is used to treat the underlying disorder and can improve all of the patient's symptoms.

## GENETIC DISORDERS PRESENTING WITH INTELLECTUAL DISABILITY OR GLOBAL DEVELOPMENTAL DELAY

### Definitions

- The term *intellectual disability* applies to children with an IQ < 70 as assessed on standardized testing and significant limitations in both intellectual functioning and in adaptive behavior.
  - A child must be physically and behaviorally capable of participating in the testing for the evaluation to be valid. Thus, the diagnosis of intellectual disability is usually not made until a child is 4-6 years of age, unless a syndromic diagnosis is made in which all affected individuals have intellectual disability (such as Down syndrome).
  - Many individuals with intellectual disability have autism or autistic features.
- The term *developmental delay* is used for young children and infants who are not achieving their developmental milestones within the expected age range. The domains of development include expressive language, receptive language, gross motor, fine motor/problem solving, and social and adaptive skills.
  - If an individual is delayed in one of these domains, he or she has isolated delay in a single domain, and a genetic evaluation is not necessarily indicated.
  - If an individual is delayed in more than one domain, he or she has global developmental delay, and an evaluation for a genetic etiology should be strongly considered unless the cause of the delays is known (neonatal infection, trauma).
  - The degree of delay, or developmental quotient, is calculated by dividing the child's developmental age by the chronologic age. For example, if an 8-month-old infant is rolling, does not have a pincer grasp, and is not yet babbling, the developmental age is 4 months and the child has a developmental quotient of 50%. A developmental quotient can be calculated for each individual domain, and children commonly have variation across the domains. An individual has global developmental delay if he or she has a developmental quotient of 70% or less in two or more domains.
- Finally, the diagnosis of *psychomotor regression* is reserved for individuals who have lost developmental skills. The evaluation for psychomotor regression is beyond the scope of this chapter.

## Initial Evaluation

- In a child with developmental delay, it is essential to rule out a primary medical problem that could explain the delays. For example, any child with language delay should have an audiology evaluation to rule out hearing loss as the underlying pathology.
- An ophthalmology examination may reveal retinal, corneal, or other abnormalities that could lead to a diagnosis even if there is no concern about visual acuity.
- There are many potential causes of developmental delay and learning disability, but unless there is an obvious cause such as hypoxic ischemic encephalopathy or teratogenic exposure, genetic testing should be considered.
- Most genetic workups for developmental delay start with a chromosomal microarray.
- Depending on the presentation, metabolic studies may be considered.
- Molecular sequencing should be used, especially in cases with syndromic features, when a chromosomal microarray is normal. Specific intellectual disability/developmental delay gene panels may be used in more straightforward cases. For cases with a more complex phenotype, exome or genome sequencing may be needed to find a genetic cause of disease.

## Treatment

- Regardless of the etiology, it is important to emphasize that appropriate therapeutic interventions—physical, occupational, speech, and developmental therapies—should be provided to help the child maximize his or her potential.
- In the vast majority of patients, the identification of an underlying genetic etiology does not significantly alter the therapeutic interventions or symptomatic management that the child receives.

## GENETIC DISORDERS ASSOCIATED WITH CONGENITAL HEART LESIONS OR CARDIOMYOPATHY

- Most congenital heart lesions are not pathognomonic for a particular syndrome, but they may provide a clue to the underlying genetic diagnosis. The cardiac lesion may be the only manifestation of a syndrome in some patients.
- Metabolic cardiomyopathies affect the myocardium but do not cause structural anomalies.
  - When a cardiomyopathy is caused by an inborn metabolic disease, it may or may not have associated syndromic features.
- Many times the associated features, such as skeletal myopathy or hepatomegaly, may develop over time, and the absence of these features should not preclude an evaluation for a particular condition.
- If the patient has a cardiac biopsy, it may show evidence of intralysosomal storage of macromolecules (lysosomal storage disease), microvesicular lipid (fatty acid oxidation defect), or abnormal number or appearance of mitochondria (mitochondrial cytopathy).

## Diagnosis and Evaluation

- CMA may be considered in an individual with an isolated congenital heart lesion of unknown etiology. For example, this test can detect 22q11 deletion syndrome, which may present in this way.
- Molecular sequencing can be considered in cases with a normal CMA. Gene panels for congenital heart disease should be considered for all cases with a positive family history or suspected syndromic component.

- For cases with a complex phenotype, especially with a negative panel, exome or genome sequencing may be necessary to find a genetic cause of disease.
- Blood tests recommended for children who present with cardiomyopathy include comprehensive metabolic panel, quantitative carnitines, acylcarnitine profile, ammonium, lactate, pyruvate, serum/plasma amino acids, creatine kinase, aldolase, lipid panel, uric acid, and Pompe disease enzyme analysis, as well as urine for mucopolysaccharidosis screen.

## GENETIC DISORDERS PRESENTING WITH FAILURE TO THRIVE

- There are many genetic causes when children fail to grow as expected. Other causes of failure to thrive such as poor nutrition, familial short stature, and endocrinopathies should be ruled out (see Failure to Thrive under Common Childhood Concerns in Chapter 1).
- Genetic causes of FTT should be suspected when children also present with physical anomalies, dysmorphic features, or developmental delay/intellectual disability.

### Diagnosis and Evaluation

- CMA should be considered as a first-line test in children with failure to thrive. A large percentage of pathogenic deletions and duplications can cause small size, with 22q deletion syndrome being a classic example.
- In some patients, methylation studies should be obtained, as some epigenetic conditions such as Russell-Silver syndrome, Angelman syndrome, and UPD 14 can present with small size.
- Molecular sequencing should be offered when there is a suspicion for a genetic cause of failure to thrive but CMA is normal. There are short stature panels including the most common short stature genes. For cases with a complex phenotype, especially with a negative panel, exome or genome sequencing may be necessary to find a genetic cause of disease.

### Treatment

- Optimal treatment depends on the specific disorder. Some conditions are better suited to human growth hormone therapy than others.
- Many syndromic children will have varied growth patterns and syndrome-specific growth charts should be used once a diagnosis is made.

## ONLINE GENETIC RESOURCES

### GeneReviews

http://www.ncbi.nlm.nih.gov/books/NBK1116/

GeneReviews provides clinical information on selected genetic diseases including presentation, diagnosis, and suggested management. The number of reviews is limited, and there are no reviews of complex traits, such as hypertension. Some general reviews, such as an overview of autism spectrum disorders, are available.

### MedlinePlus

http://medlineplus.gov

This site is maintained by the National Library of Medicine, part of the National Institute of Health, and provides overviews of over 1300 common and rare disorders with a genetic basis, as well as brief information of many genes. The reports provide translations of medical terms, and the language could be appropriate resources for families.

## Online Mendelian Inheritance in Man

http://www.ncbi.nlm.nih.gov/omim

Online Mendelian Inheritance in Man (OMIM) is an annotated bibliography of the vast majority of publications on genetic conditions and the genetic contribution to disease. The database can be searched by disease name, gene, or phenotype. Information on the main page is a cumulative list of data reported in the literature. The clinical synopsis tab links to an outline of disease-specific features.

## American Academy of Pediatrics Committee on Genetics

http://www.aap.org/en-us/about-the-aap/Committees-Councils-Sections/Pages/Committee-on-Genetics.aspx

The American Academy of Pediatrics (AAP) has published management guidelines for a number of relatively common genetic syndromes for the general practitioner. These guidelines include salient features on physical examination, screening parameters, and anticipatory guidance by age for the particular disorder. Because the field of genetics is rapidly changing, these publications may become outdated relatively soon after publication and should not be relied on as the sole tool for the management of patients.

## American College of Medical Genetics (ACMG) Newborn Screening ACTion (ACT) Sheets

http://www.acmg.net/Publications: ACT Sheets and Confirmatory Algorithms

The ACT sheets and the accompanying algorithms are intended to help guide the general practitioner in evaluating abnormal newborn screening results. These sheets provide a brief synopsis of the disorder being screened and guide the physician through the appropriate follow-up procedures. It is strongly recommended that general practitioners also contact the appropriate subspecialist for assistance.

## SUGGESTED READINGS

Jones KL, Jones MC, del Campo M. Smith's Recognizable Patterns of Human Malformation. 7th Ed. Philadelphia, PA: Elsevier, 2013.

Lee B, Scaglia F. Inborn Errors of Metabolism. New York: Oxford University Press, 2015.

Saudubray JM, Baumgartner MR, Walter J. Inborn Metabolic Diseases: Diagnosis and Treatment. Berlin-Heidelberg, Germany: Springer, 2016.

Spranger JW, Spranger JW, eds. Bone Dysplasias: An Atlas of Genetic Disorders of Skeletal Development. 3rd Ed. New York: Oxford University Press, 2012.

Zschocke J, Hoffman GF. Vademecum Metabolicum. 3rd Ed. Friedrichsdorf, Germany: Milupa Metabolics GmbH & Co, 2014.

# 17

# Gastrointestinal Symptoms and Associated Diseases

Elizabeth C. Utterson, Stefani Tica, Robert J. Rothbaum, and David A. Rudnick

## INTRODUCTION

Neonates, infants, toddlers, older children, and adolescents often present with symptoms prompting contemplation of gastroenterological and hepatic disorders. Examples include abdominal pain, vomiting, diarrhea, constipation, gastrointestinal (GI) bleeding, and jaundice. This chapter reviews considerations relevant to medical evaluation and management of such symptoms that the authors have found useful over decades of clinical practice. Comprehensive discussion of clinical presentation, differential diagnosis, evaluation, and management of these symptoms is beyond the space constraints of this chapter. Thus, the considerations here should augment but do not substitute for the clinical judgment of care providers managing individual patients with specific symptoms.

## ABDOMINAL PAIN

- In infants and toddlers, caregivers may attribute crying to abdominal discomfort. Flexing the legs, turning red, spitting up, and passing flatus might be interpreted as supportive evidence. However, excessive crying in the absence of other symptoms or signs (such as vomiting, abdominal distention, hematemesis or hematochezia, fever, or general ill appearance) does not typically originate from an intra-abdominal cause.
- In school age children, functional abdominal pain typically occurs almost daily for at least 3 months, is periumbilical, and may have accompanying nausea or vomiting. Physical examination is repeatedly normal. Anxiety is the most frequent concomitant symptom. The Rome IV criteria for functional GI disorders support symptoms-based diagnosis and allow for judicious use of laboratory testing. Treatment for functional GI disorders works best when approached in a multidisciplinary fashion. Medications options include antispasmodics, tricyclic antidepressants, serotonin selective reuptake inhibitors, and peppermint oil. Dietary treatments include low FODMAP diet. Psychological intervention in the form of cognitive behavioral therapy is often effective with respect to developing or enhancing coping mechanisms. Exercise intervention in the form of aerobic exercise and Pilates or yoga have worked for some patients.
- In older children and adolescents, abdominal pain is often localized to a specific anatomic region, facilitating diagnostic considerations and evaluations. Pain characteristics, frequency, duration, radiation, and accompanying symptoms are readily definable.
  - Right upper quadrant pain: Biliary colic is episodic, often nocturnal, lasts for hours, and then remits. Vomiting may occur.
  - Epigastric pain: Pain from duodenal ulcer disease and pancreatitis occurs in this region, might follow meals, and lasts for hours. Vomiting may occur.

- Left upper quadrant pain: Pancreatitis pain may radiate to this location. Splenic disorders are uncommon in the absence of preexisting splenomegaly.
- Right lower quadrant pain: This is the focus of pain with appendicitis. Ovarian cysts and torsion produce acute pain. Ileal Crohn disease almost always causes more chronic discomfort.
- Left lower quadrant pain: Colonic or ovarian disorders cause pain in this region.
- Findings associated with abdominal pain that increase concern for serious disorders:
  - History
    - Acute onset, for example, duration <1 week
    - Colicky pain with intervening symptom-free intervals
    - Pain localized distant from the periumbilical region
    - Associated symptoms
      - Vomiting, especially bilious emesis
      - Hematemesis, hematochezia or melena
    - Fever
  - Physical examination
    - Tachycardia with or without hypotension
    - Abdominal distention with or without tympany
    - Direct or indirect rebound tenderness
    - Referred pain
    - Hepatosplenomegaly
    - Abdominal mass
- Comprehensive recommendations regarding appropriate supportive and disease-specific management of abdominal pain are beyond the space constraints of this chapter.

## VOMITING

- Definitions
  - Vomiting: forceful expulsion of gastric contents from the mouth.
  - Regurgitation: effortless flow of gastric contents from the mouth (also referred to as infant gastroesophageal reflux [GER], spitting, posseting)
- Physiological GER is common in normal infants. It presents between 1 and 2 months of age, increases over the next few months, and resolves spontaneously. The emesis is gastric contents without blood or bile. GER does not cause excessive crying, poor eating, slow weight gain, apnea, or apparent life-threatening events. If such symptoms or signs are being evaluated, alternative explanations should be sought. Physiological GER requires no intervention (i.e., no dietary change in infant or mother, no suppression of gastric acid, etc.). Multiple studies document the absence of esophagitis or other complications in such infants. Acid suppression may result in increased risk of pneumonia or gastroenteritis.
- Common upper GI diseases associated with vomiting:
  - Pyloric stenosis: Affected infants have repeated emesis of gastric contents, and, occasionally, small amounts of hematemesis. Weight loss can occur. The "olive" is often impalpable. Diagnosis is typically made between 3 and 12 weeks of age.
  - Esophageal disorders: In affected toddlers, vomiting may occur. Eosinophilic esophagitis can present with dysphagia, vomiting, or both. Anatomic narrowing presents with emesis if solid foods cannot traverse the narrowing. Careful history differentiates dysphagia and regurgitation from emesis of gastric contents. Other

than enteric infections, acute gastric and duodenal disorders are uncommon in children without anatomic abnormalities, prior surgery, or ongoing medications.
- Esophagitis from acid and peptic injury most often manifests as heartburn with or without dysphagia. Infectious esophagitis produces acute dysphagia and odynophagia. Herpetic infection elicits fever. Candida infection often creates odynophagia. Either infection can occur in immunocompetent and immunodeficient patients.
- Less common and serious diseases that present with vomiting:
  - Small bowel obstruction due to anatomic abnormality or prior intestinal surgery with adhesions presents with repeated bilious emesis, abdominal pain, and, often, distention with tympany. Urgent evaluation should proceed. Intussusception produces reflex vomiting prior to evolution to obstruction.
  - Posterior fossa tumor: In all children and adolescents, acute onset of daily vomiting with any associated neurologic symptom (headache, irritability, lethargy, ataxia, decreased activity, diplopia) should prompt careful neurologic examination for cerebellar signs of nystagmus, dysmetria, and ataxia. Fundoscopic examination should be attempted and imaging considered. Posterior fossa brain tumors produce vomiting with or without increased intracranial pressure.
  - Caustic ingestion: Acute vomiting, dysphagia, refusal to swallow, and drooling characterize esophageal injury due to caustic ingestion. Oral burns or erosions are often but not always present. Usually, caregivers recognize or witness the event.
  - Esophageal foreign body can present similarly to caustic ingestion, but without evident burns or erosions. A disk battery retained in the esophagus is a medical emergency.
- Important disorders presenting with vomiting by age:
  - Infant vomiting
    ○ Bilious emesis
      – Intestinal malrotation with or without volvulus
        - Malrotation with or without volvulus presents acutely in the first few weeks of life. Abdominal distention and tenderness are often present. Intravascular volume depletion occurs from intraluminal fluid accumulation. Proximal small bowel atresias or stenosis produce a similar clinical picture. Obstructive series may show gasless abdomen or dilated small bowel loops. UGI is diagnostic, demonstrating malposition of the proximal small bowel to the right of the midline and no clear attachment of the ligament of Treitz. Urgent surgical consultation is essential.
      – Meconium ileus
        - This condition produces distal small bowel obstruction and nearly always indicates underlying cystic fibrosis (CF). Examination demonstrates abdominal distention, sometimes with visible bowel loops. Obstructive series shows multiple dilated small bowel loops with air-fluid levels.
      – Hirschsprung disease
        - This is a distal obstructive disorder of the colon. Abdominal distention, delayed passage of meconium, and bilious emesis are hallmarks of the disorder. Obstructive series demonstrates diffuse dilation of small bowel and, possibly, proximal colon. The gold standard for diagnosis is a rectal suction biopsy demonstrating absence of submucosal ganglion cells. Barium enema may help delineate the location of the transition zone and length of aganglionic colon but can also appear normal, especially in the infant <3 months of age.

○ Nonbilious emesis: This occurs with pyloric stenosis. Examination may not show specific findings. Pyloric ultrasound or UGI study shows thickened and elongated pylorus. Therapy includes intravenous rehydration and pyloromyotomy.

- Childhood vomiting
  ○ Bilious emesis
    – Prior abdominal surgery
      - History of prior abdominal surgery should prompt consideration of intra-abdominal adhesions and associated obstruction. Examination shows abdominal distention and tenderness with tympany. Obstructive series demonstrates multiple air-fluid levels in dilated small bowel. Therapy includes nasogastric decompression, intravenous hydration, and serial clinical and radiologic examinations to gauge the necessity of adhesiolysis.
    – Other acquired small bowel obstructions (e.g., intussusception, Henoch-Schonlein purpura [HSP]).
  ○ Nonbilious emesis: Gastroenteritis is the most common cause of acute nonbilious emesis. Many other GI illnesses (e.g., pancreatitis, chole(docho)lithiasis, peptic ulcer disease, and others) have vomiting as a component.

## DIARRHEA

- Acute diarrhea in an otherwise healthy individual is often secondary to self-limited infection. Persistence can also be secondary to infection or other malabsorptive, inflammatory, or secretory conditions. No specific duration consistently separates acute versus chronic diarrhea. Acute infectious diarrhea rarely persists >2 weeks.
- Acute infectious diarrhea
  - The most common viral causes of uncomplicated acute infectious diarrhea in the United States include rotavirus, enteric adenovirus, astrovirus, and norovirus. Symptoms rarely persist >2 weeks in immune competent hosts but can last longer in immunocompromised children.
  - Bacterial causes in the United States include *Campylobacter*, *Clostridium difficile*, *Escherichia coli* species (enterotoxic, mucosa adherent, enterohemorrhagic [e.g., O157:H7]), *Salmonella*, *Shigella*, *Yersinia enterocolitica*, and *Aeromonas* and *Pleisiomonas*. Presentation with acute bloody diarrhea should prompt consideration of bacterial infectious diarrhea. Symptoms generally resolve within 1 week.
  - Shiga-toxin producing enterohemorrhagic *E. coli* O157H7 causes haemolytic uremic syndrome (HUS). Empiric antibiotic therapy increases risk of adverse HUS-related outcome. Aggressive hydration with isotonic IV fluids begun at the time of clinical presentation (i.e., prior to culture-based diagnosis) reduces such risk. Thus, patients with acute bloody diarrhea should (1) have stool cultured by a reliable laboratory capable of identifying the bacterial pathogens listed above; (2) generally not receive empiric antibiotics until *E. coli* O157:H7 has been excluded; and (3) be aggressively hydrated with isotonic IVF until *E. coli* O157:H7 is excluded or the patient's clinical course indicates resolving risk of HUS development or progression.
  - Nonviral, nonbacterial infectious diarrhea in the United States is caused by *Giardia lamblia*, *Cryptosporidium parvum*, *Cyclospora cayetanensis*, and other parasites. Symptoms can persist for weeks, months, or longer. Diagnostic fecal antigen tests for *Giardia* and *Cryptosporidia* are widely available.

- Diagnostic considerations in infants with prolonged diarrhea
  - Persistent infection (see above).
  - Intractable diarrhea of infancy (IDI) represents recurrent episodes of diarrhea and poor weight gain or weight loss, usually in infants <6 months old. Typically, IDI occurs in undernourished infants who suffer acute enteritis and then fail to follow the typical course of spontaneous recovery. Diagnosis is based on physician awareness, appropriate exclusion of alternative explanations, and clinical response to nutritional therapy.
  - Immunodeficiency (e.g., human immunodeficiency virus [HIV], severe combined immunodeficiency [SCID], immunodysregulation-polyendocrinopathy-enteropathy-X linked [IPEX] syndrome, chronic granulomatous disease [CGD], others).
  - Anatomic abnormality (e.g., malrotation).
  - Pancreatic insufficiency (e.g., cystic fibrosis, Shwachman-Diamond syndrome, others).
  - Celiac disease.
  - Cholestasis (i.e., steatorrhea; see Jaundice section).
  - Hirschsprung disease.
  - Other rare causes, for example, congenital chloride diarrhea, congenital sodium diarrhea, neuropeptide-secreting tumors, acrodermatitis enteropathica, autoimmune enteropathy, microvillus inclusion disease, tufted enteropathy, abeta-lipoproteinemia, and others.
- Diagnostic considerations in toddler's, older children, and adolescents with chronic diarrhea
  - Chronic nonspecific diarrhea. High sorbitol intake, for example, apple juice, or high oral fluid intake may exacerbate
  - Lactase deficiency
  - Irritable bowel syndrome
  - Celiac disease
  - Inflammatory bowel disease
  - Cystic fibrosis
  - Hyperthyroidism
  - Factitious
- Initial evaluation and management of chronic diarrhea in nontoxic children
  - Complete history and physical examination (urgent supportive care as needed)
  - Review growth records
  - Examine stool
  - Screening labs: CBC and comprehensive metabolic panel
  - Further evaluation and management based on status, course, and findings

## CONSTIPATION

- Constipation refers to a variable combination of large, hard, painful, or infrequent bowel movements.
- Decreased stool frequency in early infancy, especially if suppositories or enemas have been used to promote stool passage, should prompt consideration of Hirschsprung disease. "Functional constipation" (i.e., stool holding and encopresis) typically presents after 2 years of age. In the general population, Hirschsprung disease is rare, affecting an estimated 1 in 5000 people. Constipation is common, affecting approximately 30% of children.

- Functional constipation, stool holding, and encopresis
  - This condition often includes a behavioral component with cycles of painful defecation and stool withholding.
  - Despite common belief, there is no evidence that oral iron supplementation causes functional constipation.
  - Diagnosis is suggested by palpable stool (scybala) on abdominal examination, digital rectal examination showing mass of hard stool, and fecal soiling apparent on perianal skin or in undergarments. Abdominal plain radiographs are useful in isolated situations such as if the patient will not permit a digital rectal examination. Assessment of fecal retention is reliable only with an experienced pediatric radiologist using a structured scoring system.
  - Treatment includes behavioral modification with encouragement of regular bowel movements and good toiletry habits, laxatives (most commonly polyethylene glycol 3350 [PEG]), and disimpaction. Disimpaction can be accomplished by serial saline enemas or high rate of enteral intake of osmotically active fluids. PEG 3350 solutions can be given as an oral mixture, similar to preparation for colonoscopy. NG infusion of isotonic electrolyte solutions can also be effective. In the patient with distention and marked constipation evident from physical examination, inpatient monitoring of effect may be prudent. Morbidity and mortality has been reported in association with prolonged rectal retention of hypertonic, phosphate containing (e.g., Fleet) enemas, and we now discourage their use.
  - PEG 3350 efficacy and safety for treatment of constipation and preparation for colonoscopy in children have been extensively studied. There is no current systematic evidence showing PEG 3350 causes childhood disease. An NIH sponsored study (1RO1FD005312-01) of the safety of PEG 3350 use in children was previously conducted (outcomes briefly summarized at reporter.nih.gov).
- Hirschsprung disease
  - This is a debilitating and potentially fatal condition. Bowel obstruction results from aganglionosis of a variable length of intestine extending proximally from the rectum. Diagnosis is typically made by 6 months of age, but new diagnoses in older children and adults occur. Approximately 30% of children with Hirschsprung disease have additional congenital anomalies.
  - Typical clinical presentations include neonatal intestinal obstruction, neonatal bowel perforation, delayed passage of meconium, chronic severe constipation, abdominal distension relieved by enema or rectal stimulation, and enterocolitis.
  - Rectal suction biopsy (RSB) is the gold standard test and should be performed in neonates with significant abdominal distension, especially in combination with bilious vomiting, delayed passage of meconium, or bowel perforation. Biopsy should also be considered in other settings (e.g., neonatal bloody diarrhea, delayed passage of meconium (i.e., >24-48 hours after birth), young children with constipation refractory to oral medications). Full thickness biopsy is required for diagnosis is some cases.
  - Management of Hirschsprung disease requires surgery. Prior to surgery, medical management includes rectal decompression, typically with normal saline irrigations through a soft rectal tube, and other support as indicated. Surgical management involves a "pull-through" procedure, typically with the Swenson, Duhamel, or Soave techniques. Whether outcomes are better with one procedure or another has not been established. The individual surgeon's expertise and experience are determining factors.

- Enterocolitis associated with Hirschsprung disease is a potentially fatal complication. It occurs before or after surgery. Clinical features include explosive, malodorous, or bloody diarrhea, abdominal distension, explosive discharge of gas or stool on rectal examination, reduced peripheral perfusion, lethargy, and fever. Abdominal films show multiple air fluid levels, distended bowel loops, saw tooth, irregular mucosal lining, pneumatosis, or absence of air in distal bowel. Recognition remains challenging. Treatment includes bowel rest, nasogastric tube drainage, IV fluids, decompression of dilated bowel with rectal irrigation with normal saline, and broad-spectrum intravenous antibiotics.
- Constipation can also occur as a side effect of medications, with hypothyroidism, and in other clinical settings. Hypothyroidism rarely presents as isolated constipation in children.

## GASTROINTESTINAL BLEEDING

- GI bleeding in pediatrics is potentially serious. Chemical testing (e.g., gastroccult, guaiac) should be done to confirm the presence of blood in vomitus or stool because various ingested substances might be misinterpreted as blood.
- Upper GI (UGI) bleeding refers to a source proximal to the ligament of Treitz and typically presents as hematemesis, coffee ground vomiting, melena, or hematochezia (from rapid transit of blood through the GI tract). Lower GI (LGI) bleeding, that is, bleeding distal to the ligament of Treitz, presents with hematochezia or melena. Occult GI bleeding can present with pallor, fatigue, or microcytic (iron deficiency) anemia.
- Initial evaluation and management should focus on assessment and stabilization of hemodynamic status and evaluation of the magnitude of bleeding. Orthostatic vital sign changes suggest significant blood loss. Patients with signs and symptoms of significant blood loss should be hospitalized. Clinical stabilization generally precedes disease-specific diagnostic evaluations and therapeutic considerations. Patients with suspicion of serious GI bleeding should have large bore IV access secured, fluid resuscitation initiated, and blood sent for type and cross-match. When feasible, an early focused history may inform etiologic consideration.
- Initial labs estimate the extent of bleeding. The hematocrit on the initial CBC might not reflect severity of an acute bleed if compensatory hemodilution has not yet occurred. Microcytosis suggests chronic blood loss. Assessment of the platelet count and PT/PTT should be obtained to assess for contributing coagulopathy. Along with age and presentation (e.g., UGI vs. LGI bleed), additional diagnostics can inform consideration of etiology:
  - Physical examination detecting hepatomegaly or splenomegaly suggests portal hypertension and possible esophageal varices. Laboratory tests may show liver dysfunction and coagulopathy. Low serum albumin could result from liver or inflammatory bowel disease.
  - BUN and creatinine may help with assessment of hydration and consideration of *E. coli* O157:H7-induced HUS.
  - Some clinicians recommend NG tube placement for the evaluation and management of upper GI bleeding. NG tube should be the largest tolerable bore. Initial irrigation with normal saline detects red or dark blood. Continuing irrigations with warm or cold saline do not reduce bleeding. NG tube drainage on low intermittent suction may detect ongoing bleeding from the esophagus or stomach but may not identify duodenal haemorrhage.

- Abdominal obstructive series might suggest obstruction (dilated loops of bowel) or perforation (free air).
- Once stabilized, a complete history and physical should be obtained, which (together with the presentation, course, and findings from initial evaluations) should inform consideration of additional imaging, endoscopic, and other evaluations.
- Empiric acid suppression is often reasonable in the setting of an acute UGI bleed in children or adolescents. Stool culture should be obtained in setting of acute bloody diarrhea (see Diarrhea section).
- Diagnostic considerations are suggested by suspected location, severity of presentation, and age. There is etiologic overlap between age groups.
  - Gross UGI bleed
    - Infant: Large volume bleeding occurs with acute gastritis or gastric ulceration, and coagulopathy (e.g., vitamin K deficiency/hemorrhagic disease of the newborn, other coagulopathy). Lesser bleeding occurs with pyloric stenosis or esophagitis. Swallowed blood from delivery or maternal blood can be regurgitated.
    - Child/adolescent: Large volume hemorrhage may occur with gastritis, gastric ulcer, duodenal ulcer, or esophageal or gastric varices. Rare considerations include vascular malformations (such as hemangiomas or Dieulafoy lesion), tumor, and others. Lesser acute bleeding occurs with esophagitis, most episodes of gastritis, and after repeated emesis (emetogenic gastritis). Vomiting of swallowed blood can occur with oral lesions, epistaxis, or pulmonary hemorrhage.
  - Hematochezia
    - Infant: Small amounts of bleeding in a well-appearing infant may occur with anal fissure, nodular lymphoid hyperplasia, or infant colitis. Anal fissure is visible on external examination. Infant colitis is related to formula protein intolerance in only 40% of infants with blood-streaked stool. In an ill-appearing infant, bleeding may occur with necrotizing enterocolitis, Hirschsprung disease, malrotation/volvulus, intussusception, infectious colitis, and other less common and rare conditions.
    - Child/adolescent: Mild bleeding may indicate anal fissure, hemorrhoid, perianal group A streptococcal infection, solitary rectal ulcer, and retained or sloughed juvenile polyp. In a sicker child, consider intussusception, malrotation/volvulus, HSP, or intestinal ischemia. Intussusception outside the typical age range warrants consideration of a pathological lead point. Other important conditions include infectious colitis, inflammatory bowel disease (ulcerative or Crohn colitis), NSAID-induced intestinal irritation, UGI source with rapid transit, vascular malformation, and multiple others. Meckel's diverticulum may present with bright red bleeding or melena in the older child.
  - Occult GI blood loss with microcytic anemia. Leading considerations include inflammatory bowel disease, celiac disease, multiple juvenile polyps, vascular malformations, and esophagitis.
- Additional comments
  - Urgent endoscopy or colonoscopy is often a consideration at the time of presentation for bleeding. The first step in management is assurance of hemodynamic stability. Intravenous fluids and transfusion of packed red blood cells are initiated. Intravenous octreotide is useful for variceal bleeding. Proton pump inhibitors are often started for upper GI bleeding. Effective upper GI endoscopy requires planning for potential etiologies, clear visualization of mucosa, and stable patient. Effective colonoscopy requires colon preparation. With catastrophic, uncontrollable and

destabilizing bleeding activate surgical consultation and consider arteriography to help localize the anatomic origin.
- Radioisotope tagged red blood cell scans may detect the location of bleeding but depend on a high rate of such bleeding.
- Capsule endoscopy permits imaging (but not biopsy) of small bowel between the duodenum and terminal ileum. Appropriate investigation for risk of capsule retention should be undertaken prior to such study.

## JAUNDICE (HYPERBILIRUBINEMIA)

- Jaundice refers to yellow discoloration of the skin, sclerae, and other mucous membranes and results from elevated serum bilirubin. Hyperbilirubinemia can be conjugated/direct or unconjugated/indirect. The differential diagnoses for direct versus indirect hyperbilirubinemia are distinct.
- All jaundiced infants >2 weeks of age should have a fractionated bilirubin obtained to distinguish direct vs. indirect hyperbilirubinemia. Conjugated hyperbilirubinemia in the newborn period always requires further evaluation and should prompt referral to a pediatric gastroenterologist. Indirect hyperbilirubinemia in the newborn period sometimes requires further evaluation and management.
- Cholestasis refers to reduced canalicular bile flow and primarily manifests as direct hyperbilirubinemia. Prompt identification and diagnostic assessment of neonatal cholestasis is imperative for recognition of disorders amenable to specific intervention and institution of appropriate supportive therapy. Evaluation remains challenging because of diversity of cholestatic syndromes, obscurity of pathogenesis, and overlap of clinical appearance.
- Diagnostic considerations
  - Conjugated hyperbilirubinemia—neonatal and infant
    - Extrahepatic biliary tract obstruction
      - Extrahepatic biliary atresia (BA).
      - Others (e.g., extrahepatic ductal stricture, cyst, or spontaneous perforation, mass). Obstructing gallstones are unusual.
    - Hepatocellular and other intrahepatic disorders (with some examples)
      - Biliary disorders (intrahepatic, e.g., Alagille syndrome, congenital hepatic fibrosis, nonsyndromic bile duct paucity)
      - Drug/toxin (e.g., TPN-associated, medications)
      - Endocrine (e.g., hypopituitarism, septo-optic dysplasia, hypothyroidism)
      - Genetic (e.g., α1-antitrypsin [α1AT] deficiency, progressive familial intrahepatic cholestasis [PFIC: types I and II are characterized by low or normal range serum γGT, type 3 by high γGT], cystic fibrosis)
      - Idiopathic (neonatal hepatitis)
      - Infectious (e.g., sepsis [e.g., *E. coli* UTI], TORCH, hepatitis B, HIV)
      - Metabolic (amino acid, carbohydrate, lipid [bile acid], peroxisomal metabolism)
      - Shock-ischemia
      - Other (less common) causes: bilirubin/bile acid transport disorders (e.g., Dubin-Johnson, Rotor), neonatal hemochromatosis, vascular anomalies
  - Conjugated hyperbilirubinemia—older children and adolescents
    - Disorders of extrahepatic biliary tract obstruction: for example, choledocholithiasis, parasitic infection, choledochal cyst, tumor

- ○ Hepatocellular and other intrahepatic disorders (with some examples)
  - – Biliary disorders (intrahepatic, e.g., Alagille syndrome, congenital hepatic fibrosis, nonsyndromic bile duct paucity)
  - – Endocrine (hypothyroidism)
  - – Immune (e.g., autoimmune hepatitis, primary sclerosing cholangitis, primary biliary cirrhosis)
  - – Infectious (e.g., sepsis, hepatitis A, B, C, E, HSV, EBV, HIV, nontypeable)
  - – Medication/toxin (e.g., TPN [see IV.D.4], medications)
  - – Metabolic/genetic (e.g., α1-AT deficiency, Wilson disease, cystic fibrosis, hemochromatosis, bilirubin/bile acid transport, fatty acid oxidation, mitochondrial, chromosomal anomalies, trisomies)
  - – Miscellaneous (e.g., shock-ischemia, vascular anomalies)
- • Unconjugated hyperbilirubinemia
  - ○ Neonatal and infant: physiological, breast milk, hemolysis, nonhemolytic disease (e.g., congenital hypothyroidism, hemorrhage, hypertrophic pyloric stenosis, Crigler-Najjar)
  - ○ Older children: hemolytic disease, nonhemolytic disease (e.g., Crigler-Najjar, Gilbert's, hepatocellular disease)
- • An additional comment about TPN-associated cholestasis: Long-term TPN is lifesaving in infants and children with intestinal failure. Efforts to mitigate such cholestasis include reduction of soy-based lipid component, substitution with ω-3 based lipids for the soy-based lipid component and avoidance of obesity with associated hepatic steatosis. Further research is needed to define optimal management. Central line infections might also contribute to hepatic dysfunction.
- • Initial evaluation of direct hyperbilirubinemia
  - • First, establish whether the hyperbilirubinemia is direct or indirect:
    - ○ Total and fractionated bilirubin
    - ○ Bilirubin detected in urine (i.e., on a UA) suggests direct hyperbilirubinemia
  - • With direct hyperbilirubinemia, assess for severity of hepatic injury and dysfunction.
    - ○ Markers of injury: serum SGPT/ALT, SGOT/AST, GGT, alkaline phosphatase
    - ○ Measures of dysfunction: PT/INR, albumin, bilirubin, glucose
  - • Severe liver synthetic dysfunction, as demonstrated by coagulopathy, hypoglycemia, or encephalopathy, raises concern for evolving acute liver failure (ALF, see Acute Liver Failure section).
  - • Investigate first for age-specific, specifically-treatable disorders. For example, in infants, consider the following:
    - ○ Blood, urine, other cultures for bacteria, HSV, and enterovirus
    - ○ Review/obtain newborn screen (galactose phosphate uridyl transferase [GPUT] for galactosemia, thyroid function tests); check urine succinyl acetone (for hereditary tyrosinemia I)
  - • Consider imaging and liver biopsy
    - ○ Absence of a gallbladder on U/S is suggestive but not diagnostic of BA. With BA, the hepatobiliary system will not show dilation of components.
    - ○ Intestinal excretion of tracer on biliary scintigraphy can rule out BA but absence of such excretion does not establish the diagnosis. Severe cholestasis is associated with delayed hepatic uptake of tracer.
    - ○ Percutaneous or surgical liver biopsy can help to confirm suspected diagnoses.

- Systematic, organized, comprehensive approach to specific diagnosis
  - In infants, no single noninvasive test is diagnostic of BA. Thus, the diagnosis rests on the presence of particular findings, for example, direct hyperbilirubinemia, and the absence of other explanations, for example, infection or α1-AT deficiency. Prompt investigation for specifically treatable and other common non-BA causes of neonatal/infant cholestasis is important for progression toward a more definitive diagnosis and initiation of management of BA. After idiopathic neonatal hepatitis and BA, α1-AT deficiency is the next most common specific diagnosis. Inborn errors of metabolism often present early in life and are another important consideration.
  - Contemporary, comprehensive next generation DNA-sequencing platforms have been developed and are available for incorporation into differential diagnostic assessments.
  - Further investigations based on course and findings.
- Initial management of direct hyperbilirubinemia
  - Diagnosis-specific therapy as indicated.
  - Supportive care often includes the following:
    - Empiric therapy to optimize growth and development: fat-soluble vitamin supplementation (and monitoring of levels), medium chain triglyceride (MCT)-containing formula for infants
    - Management of pruritus (which is often challenging)
    - Monitoring for portal hypertension (and risk of variceal bleeding)
    - Monitoring for progression of liver disease (consideration of transplantation)
  - If no specific etiology is identified, continue serial clinical re-evaluation of status.
- Initial evaluation and management of indirect hyperbilirubinemia. This topic has been the subject of previously published reviews.

## ACUTE LIVER FAILURE

- ALF is rare, serious and sometimes fatal. Prior experience showed that approximately half of all children with ALF recover without liver transplantation, and that ALF is the indication in 10% of all liver transplants.
- ALF in children is caused by specific infectious, toxic, metabolic, immune-mediated, ischemic, and other etiologies, and prior experiences have also shown that approximately half of all pediatric cases are idiopathic.
- The clinical presentation may include nausea, vomiting, lethargy, anorexia, and fever as well as jaundice, pruritus, purpura, and encephalopathy
- Diagnosis is based on recognition of signs, symptoms, and laboratory findings of severe liver injury in patients without previously known liver disease. Such findings include jaundice with direct hyperbilirubinemia, coagulopathy with prolonged PT/INR, encephalopathy, and liver-based hypertransaminasemia. Encephalopathy may be difficult to recognize in infants and young children.
- Specific interventions exist for some ALF etiologies, including sepsis, acetaminophen-induced (see VII.F), metabolic (e.g., hereditary tyrosinemia type I) and genetic (e.g., Wilson's) diseases, neonatal hemochromatosis, autoimmune, and certain other conditions. All affected patients should receive supportive care in a tertiary or quaternary care facility with intensive care and liver transplantation capabilities. Such care includes serial clinical and laboratory evaluations, efforts to maintain perfusion, oxygenation and electrolyte balance, avoidance of sedative and hepatotoxic medications,

avoidance of interruption of dextrose infusion, monitoring for complications of cardiovascular, respiratory, neurological, hematological, renal and infectious complications, and early consideration of liver transplantation. Outcomes (i.e., transplant-free recovery, liver transplantation, and death) are difficult to reliably predict and depend in part upon regenerative recovery of the liver. Declining serum transaminases may be a promising sign in association with improvement in liver synthetic function but represent a worrisome finding if associated with increasing bilirubin and worsening coagulopathy.

• Acetaminophen-induced hepatotoxicity is the leading specific etiology of ALF in children (10-15%). Both acute intentional and chronic unintentional (therapeutic misadventure) presentations occur. The Rumack-Matthew nomogram estimates the risk of hepatotoxicity after single acute ingestion. Acetaminophen-induced hepatotoxicity results from depletion of hepatocellular glutathione stores. Early *N*-acetylcysteine (NAC) administration, which repletes glutathione, is highly effective for treating acute acetaminophen-induced ALF when given in a timely manner and should be provided to all patients with acetaminophen-induced ALF according to established dosing regimens.

• A recently published NIH-funded placebo-controlled clinical trial tested intravenous NAC in pediatric patients with non–acetaminophen-induced ALF. The results did not support broad use of NAC in non–acetaminophen-induced pediatric ALF. Another recently published NIH-funded study from the same group found that incorporating diagnostic test recommendations into electronic medical record order sets available at admission reduced the percentage of indeterminate diagnoses and correlated with reduced liver transplant without increased mortality in these subjects.

## SUGGESTED READINGS

Apley J, Naish N. Recurrent abdominal pains: a field survey of 1,000 school children. Arch Dis Child 1958;33(168):165–170. doi: 10.1136/adc.33.168.165.

Boyle JT. Gastrointestinal bleeding in infants and children. Pediatr Rev 2008;29(2):39–52. doi: 10.1542/pir.29-2-39.

Fawaz R, Baumann U, Ekong U, et al. Guideline for the Evaluation of Cholestatic Jaundice in Infants: Joint Recommendations of the North American Society for Pediatric Gastroenterology, Hepatology, and Nutrition and the European Society for Pediatric Gastroenterology, Hepatology, and Nutrition. J Pediatr Gastroenterol Nutr 2017;64(1):154–168. doi: 10.1097/MPG.0000000000001334.

Gordon M, Naidoo K, Akobeng AK, et al. Cochrane review: osmotic and stimulant laxatives for the management of childhood constipation (Review). Evid Based Child Health 2013;8(1):57–109. doi: 10.1002/ebch.1893

Heuckeroth RO. Hirschsprung disease—integrating basic science and clinical medicine to improve outcomes. Nat Rev Gastroenterol Hepatol 2018;15(3):152–167. doi: 10.1038/nrgastro.2017.149.

Holtz LR, Neill MA, Tarr PI. Acute bloody diarrhea: a medical emergency for patients of all ages. Gastroenterology 2009;136(6):1887–1898. doi: 10.1053/j.gastro.2009.02.059.

Hyams JS, Di Lorenzo C, Saps M, et al. Functional disorders: children and adolescents. Gastroenterology 2016;S0016-5085(16)00181-5. doi: 10.1053/j.gastro.2016.02.015.

Keating JP. Chronic diarrhea. Pediatr Rev 2005;26(1):5–14. doi: 10.1542/pir.26-1-5.

Kleinman RE, Goulet OJ, Mieli-Vergani G, et al., eds. Walker's Pediatric Gastrointestinal Disease: Physiology, Diagnosis, Management. 6th Ed. Raleigh, NC: People's Medical Publishing House, 2018.

Kramer RE, Lerner DG, Lin T, et al.; North American Society for Pediatric Gastroenterology Hepatology, Nutrition Endoscopy Committee. Management of ingested foreign bodies in children: a clinical report of the NASPGHAN Endoscopy Committee. J Pediatr Gastroenterol Nutr 2015;60(4):562–574. doi: 10.1097/MPG.0000000000000729.

Lauer BJ, Spector ND. Hyperbilirubinemia in the newborn. Pediatr Rev 2011;32(8):341–349. doi: 10.1542/pir.32-8-341.

Lee WM, Squires RH Jr, Nyberg SL, et al. Acute liver failure: summary of a workshop. Hepatology 2008;47(4):1401–15. doi: 10.1002/hep.22177.

Narkewicz MR, Horslen S, Hardison RM, et al.; Pediatric Acute Liver Failure Study Group. A learning collaborative approach increases specificity of diagnosis of acute liver failure in pediatric patients. Clin Gastroenterol Hepatol 2018;16(11):1801–1810.e3. doi: 10.1016/j.cgh.2018.04.050.

Neidich GA, Cole SR. Gastrointestinal bleeding. Pediatr Rev 2014;35(6):243–253; quiz 54. doi: 10.1542/pir.35-6-243.

North American Society for Pediatric Gastroenterology, Hepatology & Nutrition. Clinical Guidelines & Position Statements. Available at https://naspghan.org/professional-resources/clinical-guidelines/. *(This website contains links to clinical guidelines and position states by the North American Society for Pediatric Gastroenterology, Hepatology and Nutrition (NASPGHAN), including those referenced here as well as other topics.)*

Pashankar D, Schreiber RA. Jaundice in older children and adolescents. Pediatr Rev 2001;22(7):219–226. doi: 10.1542/pir.22-7-219.

Rosen R, Vandenplas Y, Singendonk M, et al. Pediatric gastroesophageal reflux clinical practice guidelines: joint recommendations of the North American Society for Pediatric Gastroenterology, Hepatology, and Nutrition and the European Society for Pediatric Gastroenterology, Hepatology, and Nutrition. J Pediatr Gastroenterol Nutr 2018;66(3):516–554. doi: 10.1097/MPG.0000000000001889.

Rudolph JA, Squires R. Current concepts in the medical management of pediatric intestinal failure. Curr Opin Organ Transplant 2010;15(3):324–329. doi: 10.1097/MOT.0b013e32833948be.

Smith CH, Israel DM, Schreiber R, et al. Proton pump inhibitors for irritable infants. Can Fam Physician 2013;59(2):153–156.

Squires RH Jr. Acute liver failure in children. Semin Liver Dis 2008;28(2):153–166.

Squires RH, Dhawan A, Alonso E, et al.; Pediatric Acute Liver Failure Study Group. Intravenous *N*-acetylcysteine in pediatric patients with nonacetaminophen acute liver failure: a placebo-controlled clinical trial. Hepatology 2013;57(4):1542–1549. doi: 10.1002/hep.26001.

Suchy FJ, Sokol RJ, Balistreri WF, et al., eds. Liver Disease in Children. 5th Ed. Cambridge, UK: Cambridge University Press, 2021.

Tabbers MM, DiLorenzo C, Berger MY, et al.; European Society for Pediatric Gastroenterology Hepatology, Nutrition, North American Society for Pediatric Gastroenterology. Evaluation and treatment of functional constipation in infants and children: evidence-based recommendations from ESPGHAN and NASPGHAN. J Pediatr Gastroenterol Nutr 2014;58(2):258–274. doi: 10.1097/MPG.0000000000000266.

# 18 Endocrinology

Ana María Arbeláez, Carine Anka, Katherine Burgener, Samuel Cortez, Jennifer May, and Stephen Stone

## DIABETES MELLITUS

### Definition

- Diagnostic criteria are (1) based on laboratory measurements, symptoms of diabetes mellitus (DM) and random plasma glucose of $\geq 200$ mg/dL, (2) fasting ($\geq 8$ hours), plasma glucose of $\geq 126$ mg/dL, (3) a 2-hour plasma glucose of $\geq 200$ mg/dL on an oral glucose tolerance test in the absence of acute illness, or (4) $HbA_{1c} \geq 6.4\%$.
- Asymptomatic children should receive a provisional diagnosis of diabetes and have confirmatory testing with repeat testing on a different day.
- Patients with fasting blood glucose of 100-125 mg/dL with symptoms of diabetes should have an oral glucose tolerance test (1.75 g/kg glucose, up to maximum of 75 g).
- The most common forms of diabetes are type 1 and type 2 diabetes; however, other forms including genetic or drug-/disease-induced forms exist.

#### Type 1 Diabetes Mellitus

- Autoimmune disease resulting from destruction of pancreatic β-cells.
- Characterized by absolute insulin deficiency.
- Classic clinical symptoms are polyuria, polydipsia, and weight loss.
- Urgent referral of all patients with new-onset type 1 diabetes for initiation of insulin therapy and intensive education.
- Wearing medic alert bracelets by patients with this diagnosis is important.
- Patients with type 1 diabetes mellitus (T1DM) are at risk for other autoimmune conditions and require regular screening.

#### Type 2 Diabetes Mellitus

- Characterized by peripheral insulin resistance, impaired regulation of hepatic glucose production, and inadequate compensatory insulin secretory response, eventually leading to β-cell failure.
- Risk factors are obesity, family history, and polycystic ovarian syndrome (PCOS).
- Increased incidence in Native American, African American, Hispanic, and Asian children at a lower body weight.
- Screening should be done in children at high risk for type 2 diabetes with a fasting plasma glucose and $HbA_{1c}$ every 1-2 years beginning at age 10 or after onset of puberty.

### Treatment

#### Insulin Regimens

- There are different types of insulin preparations (Table 18-1).
- Insulin is the first-line treatment for all patients with T1DM and for those with type 2 diabetes mellitus (T2DM) with severe hyperglycemia or an $HbA_{1c} > 8.5\%$ or ketosis.

| TABLE 18-1 | Time Course of Action of Human Insulin Preparations |

| Insulin | Onset | Peak | Maximum |
| --- | --- | --- | --- |
| Lispro (Humalog®)/aspart (Novolog®)/glulisine (Apidra®) | <15 min | 30-90 min | 4-6 hr |
| Regular | 30 min | 2-3 hr | 6-8 hr |
| NPH | 2-4 hr | 6-10 hr | 14-18 hr |
| 70/30 70 NPH/30 regular | 30-60 min | Dual | 14-18 hr |
| Glargine U-100 (Lantus®/Basaglar®) | 2 hr | None | 24 hr |
| Degludec (Tresiba) | 1-2 hr | None | >40 hr |
| Glargine U-300 (Toujeo®) | | | |

- Suggested starting daily dosages for subcutaneous (SC) insulin at diagnosis, which are based on patient requirements:
  - <3 year = 0.3-0.4 U/kg/day
  - 3-6 year = 0.5 U/kg/day
  - 7-10 year = 0.6-0.8 U/kg/day
  - 11-14 year = 0.8-1 U/kg/day
  - >14 year = 1-1.5 U/kg/day
- Basal bolus regimen—preferred insulin regimen in children. Can be given as multiple injections or via pump:
  - Allows for greater glycemic control and greater flexibility.
  - Basal insulin dose is started as ½ of the total daily dose: once daily dose of glargine (Lantus or Basaglar) or twice daily dose of detemir (Levimir).
  - Degludec (Tresiba) is a longer acting basal insulin (approximately 36 hours); conversion is 80% of the glargine dose.
  - Remaining total daily dose is given with short-acting insulin (lispro or aspart) with meals—based on carbohydrate intake.
  - Continuous subcutaneous insulin infusion (insulin pump): Give 90% of the basal insulin dose used on multiple SC injection over 24 hours. Mealtime boluses of short-acting insulin are given via the pump based on carbohydrate intake and pre-meal blood glucose values. With only short-acting insulin present in the pump, disruption of insulin delivery can be associated with ketosis and even diabetic ketoacidosis in a period of several hours; equivalent glycemic control can be obtained with basal bolus insulin and insulin pump with good adherence.
  - Twice-daily injections: to be considered if poor adherence or if unable to count carbohydrates. Patients on this regimen should have fixed meal times and carbohydrate intake. Dose is started as ⅔ total dose is given in AM: It is broken as ⅓ of calculated dose is lispro or aspart, and ⅓ NPH. The other ⅓ of the total dose is given in PM: and broken as ½ of the calculated dose as lispro or aspart, and ½ neutral protamine hagedorn (NPH).

*Insulin Pumps*
- Insulin pumps are an alternative method of delivering insulin to patients instead of multiple daily injections.
  - Insulin pumps deliver insulin via a cannula inserted below the skin.
  - Most insulin patients using an insulin pump use rapid-acting insulin (i.e., lispro or aspart) only.

- The pump delivers a constant supply of rapid-acting insulin (basal rate).
- The user delivers a larger (bolus) dose of insulin to cover for meals and snacks.
- Advantages of an insulin pump include assistance with dose calculations, more precise insulin doses, convenience, and decreased insulin injections.
- Insulin pumps can break or malfunction. Thus, patients should receive training on how to use and troubleshoot an insulin pump prior to starting one.
- Patients who do not regularly monitor their blood glucose are not appropriate for an insulin pump.

*Insulin Dose Adjustment*
- Glargine or basal insulin
  - The goal of basal insulin is to suppress hepatic gluconeogenesis, thus maintaining the blood glucose steady while fasting (i.e., overnight).
  - Compare blood glucose at bedtime to prebreakfast; if rising, increase the basal insulin; if falling, decrease the basal.
  - In general, small adjustments (5-15%) are appropriate.
- Insulin to carbohydrate ratio (ICR)
  - ICR specifies the number of grams of carbohydrate that 1 unit of rapid acting insulin will cover.
  - Can roughly calculate as 500/total daily insulin dose.
  - To calculate carbohydrate dose divide total carbohydrate consumed by ICR. For example, an ICR of 10, or a ratio of 1:10, means that one unit of insulin will cover 10 grams of carbohydrate. For example, if a person with an ICR ratio of 1:10 eats 30 grams of carbohydrate, they will require three units of insulin to cover this meal.
  - To adjust ICR, monitor blood sugar from one meal to the next, or 4 hours after a mealtime. If preprandial blood glucose is high after eating, decrease number in ICR; if low, increase number in ICR. It has an inverse relationship.
  - If preprandial blood glucose goes high after eating, decrease ICR; if low, increase ICR.
- Insulin sensitivity factor (ISF) (aka. correction factor)
  - ISF specifies how many mg/dL the blood glucose will drop in response to 1 unit of short acting insulin.
  - Can roughly calculate as 1800/total daily insulin dose if measuring blood glucose in mg/dL.
  - To calculate blood sugar correction dose subtract current blood glucose from target blood glucose. This also has an inverse relationship.
  - To adjust ICR, monitor blood glucose. If blood glucose is above target and stays above the target after a correction, lower the number in the ISF, if it goes from high to low, then increase number in ISF.
- Target blood sugar
  - Target for what blood sugar ISF calculation is based on.
  - This can be individualized based on the patients' age and risk for hypoglycemia. Many patients are set at 120 mg/dL. Tightly controlled patients may use 100 mg/dL, whereas younger patients may be as high as 180 mg/dL.
- Alternative (sliding scale)
  - This combines the ISF and target together in a single calculation based on a range. You still need to account for the ICR. For example, add 1 unit for every 50 mg/dL > 150 mg/dL.

*Metformin*
- First line of treatment for adolescents with T2DM without ketosis.
- Start most patients on 500 mg once to twice daily, and as tolerated may advance to 1000 mg bid.

- Most common side effect is stomach upset; make sure to give with meals.
- Discontinue in patients who have lactic acidosis or receiving IV contrast.

*Blood Glucose Monitoring*

It should be done before meals, bedtime, or if symptoms of low blood glucose occur. Middle-of-the-night (2 AM) glucose levels should be obtained at the onset of therapy with changes of PM or basal insulin doses.

*Continuous Glucose Monitors*

- Continuous glucose monitors (CGM) are an alternative method to monitoring blood glucose compared to fingerstick measurements.
  - They work by inserting a small sensor into the subcutaneous tissue.
  - They send blood glucose information to a receiver every 5-15 minutes, not only displays the blood glucose but also provides trend arrows indicating if the blood glucose is going up, down, or staying steady.
  - Depending on the brand and model, some need to be calibrated. Some are accurate enough that they can replace fingerstick readings for insulin doses.
  - Patients should be educated that there is a 15- to 20-minute delay in the CGM reading compared to the blood glucose. Thus, patients are encouraged to verify low blood sugar levels with a fingerstick measurement.
- Closed-Loop Technology
  - The latest advancement in insulin pump and CGM technology is to integrate these devices together, allowing for real-time adjustments of insulin delivery. Current models will actively adjust basal insulin delivery. However, the patient still needs to bolus for meals. This is called hybrid-closed-loop. More advanced closed-loop systems are currently under investigation.

*Dietary Recommendations*

- Caloric requirements:
  - Up to age 10: 1000 kcal + 100 kcal/year
  - After age 10: for females: 45 kcal/kg/day; for males: 55 kcal/kg/day
- Tight dietary control is best achieved when patients count carbohydrates.
  - 1 carbohydrate unit = 15 g of carbohydrate
- Carbohydrate goals (general guidelines for grams of carbohydrate per meal):
  - <8 years: 40-60 g
  - 9-12 years: 60-80 g
  - >12 years: 80-100 g

*Monitoring*

- If BG ≥ 300 mg/dL or patient vomiting, he or she should check urine for ketones.
- Hemoglobin (Hgb) $A_{1c}$ levels provide estimate of an average of blood glucose levels over the 3 months preceding measurement (Table 18-2). Monitor every 3-4 months. Target HbA$_{1c}$ in children is ≤7.5% but may be individualized.
- In patients with type 1 diabetes screening for autoimmune thyroid disease (TSH) and celiac disease (TTG IgA, with total IgA) should occur after diagnosis and again approximately every 2 years.
- Microalbumin, eye examination, and monofilament examination annually in T1DM with ≥5 year duration or once in puberty and in all T2DM starting at diagnosis.
- Lipids:
  - T1DM: every 5 years from 8 to 18 years old and annually after 18 years
  - T2DM: annually after diagnosis
  - Goal LDL < 130 mg/dL

| TABLE 18-2 | Hemoglobin $A_{1c}$ Values and Corresponding Blood Glucose Levels |
|---|---|
| **Hemoglobin $A_{1c}$ (%)** | **Average blood glucose (mg/dL)** |
| 4-6 | Nondiabetic |
| 6 | 120 |
| 7 | 150 |
| 8 | 180 |
| 9 | 210 |
| 10 | 240 |

## Hypoglycemia and Diabetes

- Hypoglycemia is the most common complication of diabetes management and is the limiting factor of adequate glycemic control.
- Symptoms are shakiness, sweatiness, nervousness, headache, irritability, confusion, and seizures.
- Patients with recurrent hypoglycemia are more likely to experience hypoglycemia unawareness and thus may require an insulin dose adjustment.
- Treat mild-to-moderate hypoglycemia with 15 g of fast-acting sugar, such as 4 oz juice or glucose tablets. Recheck blood glucose 15 minutes later.
- Treat severe hypoglycemia (loss of consciousness or seizures) with glucagon 1 mg intramuscularly (if <20 kg, give 0.5 mg intramuscularly) or give intranasal glucagon (Baqsimi).
- Hypoglycemia unawareness is the lack of hypoglycemic symptoms and adequate responses to hypoglycemia. This may develop in young patients or those with recurrent hypoglycemia or after exercise. Will resolve with hypoglycemia avoidance.

## DIABETIC KETOACIDOSIS

Diabetic ketoacidosis (DKA) is characterized by serum glucose >200 mg/dL, ketonemia (>3 mmol/L) or ketonuria, dehydration, and serum pH < 7.3 or serum bicarbonate <15 mEq/L.

### Etiology

- T1DM: new onset, insulin omission, illness
- T2DM: severe illness, traumatic stress, or use of some antipsychotic agents

### Clinical Presentation

- Patients with a range of symptoms that may be present with mild-to-severe DKA: vomiting, deep-sighing respirations (Kussmaul) with acetone odor, abdominal pain, and somnolence or loss of consciousness
- Those with new-onset DM or ongoing poor glycemic control including history of polyuria, polydipsia, polyphagia, nocturia, and weight loss

### Laboratory Studies

- Rapid assessment: blood glucose and urine ketones
- Initial studies: basic metabolic profile (BMP), venous blood gas, complete blood count (CBC), Hgb $A_{1c}$, urinalysis, electrocardiogram (ECG) if potassium is abnormal, blood and urine culture if temperature >38.5°C or signs of infection:

- Anion gap (mEq): (Na − [Cl + HCO$_3$]); normal: 8-12
- Corrected Na: Na + [(glucose − 100)/100] × 1.6
- Plasma osmolarity: 2(Na) + Glucose/18 + blood urea nitrogen/2.8
  ○ Patients with DKA have plasma osmolarity >300 mOsm/L.

## Treatment (Fig. 18-1; Table 18-3)

### Mild Diabetic Ketoacidosis or Ketosis
- Characteristics: pH > 7.3, HCO$_3$ > 15 mmol/L, and moderate-to-large ketones.
- Often, outpatient treatment is appropriate.
- Monitor BG and ketones every 2 hours from insulin dose. Repeat dosing if ketones persist moderate or large.

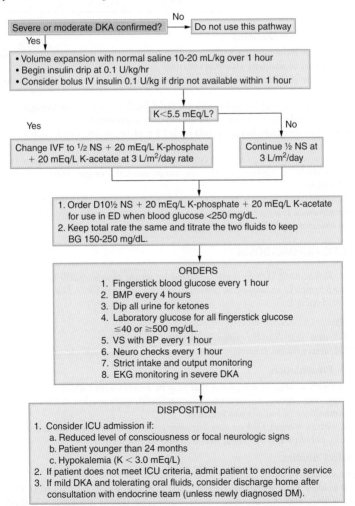

Figure 18-1. **Algorithm showing the management of diabetic ketoacidosis (DKA).**

**TABLE 18-3** Summary of DKA Management

1. If appears dehydrated/vomiting—consider NS bolus (initial 10 mL/kg).
2. Labs
   a. If pH > 7.3, bicarbonate >15 mEq/L: consider SQ insulin (see Sick Day Management).
   b. If pH < 7.3, bicarbonate <15 mEq/L, anion gap >12: Insulin drip (see below).
3. Insulin drip
   a. Regular insulin: 0.1 U/kg/h (1 U/mL)
   b. IVF: 2-3 L/m²/day
      i. Do not give K until serum K < 5.5 mEq/L and pt have voided.
      ii. ½NS + 20 mEq/L K$_{acetate}$ + 20 mEq/L K$_{phos}$ (substitute KCl if K$_{phos}$ is not available).
      iii. D10½NS + 20 mEq/L K$_{acetate}$ + 20 mEq/L K$_{phos}$ (substitute KCl if K$_{phos}$ is not available).
      iv. Start with all ½NS—when BS < 250-300 mg/dL or falling by >100 mg/dL per hour then changed to 50% ½ NS + 50% D10½NS.
      v. Target BS while on insulin drip 150-250 mg/dL.
4. Monitoring
   a. Dstick, neurochecks q1h
   b. BMP q4h
   c. Give Lantus early (while still on insulin drip).

**Consider PICU Admission for:**
1. VBG pH < 7.10
2. Bicarbonate <5 mEq/L
3. K < 3.0 mEq/L
4. Age <3 year
5. Concern for cerebral edema (Table 18-4)

**Signs of Cerebral Edema:**
1. Mental status changes
2. Severe headache
3. Recurrence of vomiting after initial improvement
4. Cushing triad
5. Papilledema
6. Fixed or dilated pupil(s)
7. Focal neurologic signs

**Initial treatment for Cerebral Edema:**
1. Decrease IVF rate
2. Mannitol 0.5-1 g/kg
3. Head CT after treatment

**Quick Conversion Formulas:**
1. 1 kg = 2.2 lb
2. BSA = [4 × *weight (kg)* + 7]/[90 + *weight (kg)*]

- Give additional short-acting insulin (lispro and aspart) every 2-3 hours:
  - Moderate ketones: usually 5-10% of total daily dose
  - Large ketones: usually 10-20% of total daily dose
- If blood sugar is <150 mg/dL, it may be necessary to give additional sugary drinks to bring the blood sugar up before additional insulin.
- Increase oral fluid intake to compensate for increased urinary losses and help clear ketones.
- If patient is on an insulin pump and unable to clear ketones, give additional bolus of short-acting insulin by SC injection and change the pump site.

- If concomitant hypoglycemia results from gastrointestinal (GI) disease, consider SC glucagon rescue therapy with 1 unit (10 μg)/year of age, starting at 2 units and up to 15 units (150 μg).
- If patients are unable to clear ketones, or they have labored breathing, confusion, or lethargy, refer them to the emergency department for further care.

*Moderate Diabetic Ketoacidosis*
- Characteristics include persistent emesis, high levels of ketones, pH 7.2-7.3, and $HCO_3$ 10-15 mEq/L.
- Experienced centers can manage moderate DKA in the emergency department or short-stay unit.
- Intravenous (IV) hydration is often necessary.
- Start 0.1 U/kg/hr regular IV insulin drip with hourly BG monitoring until anion gap closes. If unable to start drip consider giving 0.1 U/kg short-acting insulin every 2-3 hours, or 10-20% of total daily dose, or regular insulin q2-4h or 2 times usual BG correction dose.
- Admit if not resolving after 3-4 hours (i.e., anion gap not closing and/or unable to take oral fluids), if newly diagnosed, or if the ability of caregivers is questionable.

*Severe Diabetic Ketoacidosis*
- Characteristics include high levels of ketones, pH < 7.1, $HCO_3$ <10 mEq/L, pH < 7.2, or mild-to-moderate DKA along with other organ system impairment, such as altered mental status, impaired renal function, or respiratory distress.
- Admit for therapy and intensive monitoring (fingerstick blood glucose q1h, BMP q4h, dipstick of all urine for ketones, vital signs with blood pressure q1h, neurology checks q1h, strict input/output).
- Consider intensive care unit admission if patient has reduced level of consciousness or focal neurologic signs, age <24 months, or a potassium level <3.0 mg/dL.

*Hyperglycemic Hyperosmolar Syndrome*
- Hyperglycemic hyperosmolar syndrome (HHS) is a rare acute complication of diabetes, which is more common in T2DM.
- Consider this diagnosis if very high glucose, in the absence of ketosis.
- HHS has a high incidence or mortality.

## Other Therapeutic Strategies
*Intravenous Hydration*
- Simple hydration frequently causes a 180-240 mg/dL drop in glucose.
- Volume expansion (first phase [if poor perfusion or hypotension]): normal saline (NS) 10-20 mL/kg over 1 hour and then reassess volume status.
- Rehydration (second phase): ½NS plus potassium acetate plus potassium phosphate (see later discussion) at 3 L/m$^2$/day:
  - Decrease to 2.5 L/m$^2$/day if there are concerns about the risk of cerebral edema.
  - When blood glucose is <250 mg/dL, change to D5½NS. (Have D10½NS + potassium acetate + potassium phosphate available for use when blood glucose <250 mg/dL. Keep the total rate the same and titrate the two fluids to keep blood glucose from 150 to 250 mg/dL.)

*Potassium Replacement*
- Once urine output is established and potassium is <5.5 mEq/L, start potassium administration.

- Potassium level falls with correction of acidosis, decreased blood glucose, and initiation of insulin.
- Add potassium 30-40 mEq/L to IV fluids as potassium phosphate, potassium acetate, and/or potassium chloride (i.e., ½NS + 20 mEq/L, potassium phosphate + 20 mEq/L potassium acetate at 3 L/m²/day).

*Intravenous Insulin*
- Volume expansion should be initiated before insulin administration.
- Initiate the insulin drip at 0.1 U/kg/hr.
- If the blood glucose is <150 mg/dL and the patient remains acidotic, **do not stop the insulin drip, but increase the dextrose**. If the acidosis is resolving (pH > 7.3, $HCO_3$ > 15 mEq/L), the insulin infusion rate can be reduced to 0.08 or 0.05 U/kg/hr, especially if 10% dextrose is required to keep glucose above 150 mg/dL.
- Change to SC insulin when patient is able to take oral fluids, the pH is >7.25, or $HCO_3$ is >15 mEq/L, and the anion gap has closed. Consider administration of PM glargine during treatment of DKA (while insulin drip is running) to facilitate discontinuation of insulin drip at the appropriate time and guarantee basal insulin onboard after discontinuation of the drip. Basal insulin should be given at least 1-2 hours before stopping the insulin infusion.

*Cerebral Edema*
- This is the most common cause of death during DKA in children (0.4-1% of cases).
- Anticipate cerebral edema in the first 24 hours after initiation of treatment. Always have mannitol available during the first 24 hours in patients with severe DKA.
- Symptoms are change in affect, altered level of consciousness, irritability, headache, equally dilated pupils, delirium, incontinence, emesis, bradycardia, and papilledema (Table 18-4).
- Treatment
  - Cerebral edema is a medical emergency and immediate intervention is necessary.
  - Cerebral edema is a clinical diagnosis. Brain computed tomography (CT) is not indicated before treatment or to establish diagnosis; however, consider CT to evaluate for thrombosis or infarction in addition to cerebral edema.

| TABLE 18-4 | Cerebral Edema Diagnostic Criteria | |
|---|---|---|
| **Diagnostic criteria** | **Major criteria** | **Minor criteria** |
| Abnormal response to pain | Altered mental status/fluctuating LOC | Vomiting |
| Decorticate or decerebrate posture | Sustained HR deceleration (not due to sleep or improved intravascular volume) | Headache |
| Cranial nerve palsy | | Lethargy |
| Abnormal neurologic respiratory pattern (such as Cheyne-Stokes) | Age-inappropriate incontinence | Hypertension, diastolic BP > 90 |
| | | Age <5 years |

From Muir AB, Quisling RG, Yang MC, Rosenbloom AL. Cerebral edema in childhood diabetic ketoacidosis: natural history, radiographic findings, and early identification. Diabetes Care. 2004 Jul;27(7):1541-6. Copyright and all rights reserved. Material from this publication has been used with the permission of American Diabetes Association.

- Mannitol 0.5-1 g/kg IV push over <30 minutes.
- Decrease IV infusion rate to 2-2.5 L/m$^2$/day.
- Consider hyperventilation and dexamethasone.

## HYPOGLYCEMIA

- There is a normal process during fasting to maintain fuel supply to the brain.
- Normal fasting adaptation includes (1) hepatic glycogenolysis (when glycogen stores are depleted: >4-8 hours fast in infants and >8-12 hours fast in children), (2) hepatic gluconeogenesis, and (3) hepatic ketogenesis.
- Hypoglycemia does not represent a single entity but is a defect in these major adaptive pathways.

### Definition
- Clinical hypoglycemia is defined as the presence of Whipple triad: (1) signs and symptoms of hypoglycemia, (2) documented low BG, and (3) resolution with carbohydrate intake.
- A plasma glucose level below 50-60 mg/dL is recognized as the glycemic threshold for evaluation of hypoglycemia after 48 hours of life.

### Clinical Presentation
- Infants: cyanotic spells, apnea, respiratory distress, refusal to feed, subnormal temperature, floppy spells, myoclonic jerks, somnolence, and seizures.
- Children: tachycardia, anxiety, irritability, hunger, sweating, shakiness, stubbornness, sleepiness, and seizures.
- Infants and children often cannot recognize or communicate symptoms and recurrent hypoglycemia may blunt symptoms and hormonal responses.

### History
- Infants considered at risk of hypoglycemia and who require glucose monitoring: neonates with symptomatic hypoglycemia, neonates who had perinatal stress, congenital syndromes (such as Beckwith-Wiedemann), abnormal midline facial malformations or microphallus, family history of a genetic form of hypoglycemia, large-for-gestational-age birth-weight, prematurity or postmaturity, infant of diabetic mother.
- A good history is crucial when evaluating hypoglycemia.
- Key information: age of patient, gestational age and birth weight (for infants), length of the fasting period, triggering event (e.g., fructose ingestion), glucose infusion rate (GIR), perinatal history, comorbidities (e.g., liver disease, midline defects, etc.), and potential ingestion of glucose lowering medications.

### Laboratory Studies
- Newborn infants who are at increased risk for the development of either acute or persistent hypoglycemia glucose should be screened at birth and then prefeed for 24-48 hours until blood glucose is stable (>50 mg/dL at <48 hours of age or >60 mg/dL at >48 hours of age).
- An actual laboratory blood glucose measurement, not a glucometer result, to confirm true hypoglycemia is very important.
- The critical sample to diagnose the underlying cause generally must be obtained during a hypoglycemic episode or during a formal fast. This sample is obtained

when blood glucose levels fall below 50-60 mg/dL depending on age of the infant:
- Samples for plasma glucose, insulin, C-peptide, ketones or β-hydroxybutyrate, lactate, serum HCO3, free fatty acids, cortisol, growth hormone, and plasma ammonia are obtained (use mnemonic: PICKLE).
- Urine for ketones is also obtained immediately following the hypoglycemia.
- In patients who are being worked up for hypoglycemia, also obtain blood for plasma total and free carnitine, urinary organic acid profile, and plasma acylcarnitine profile (always do so before a diagnostic fast).
- During a normal response to a blood glucose level below 50 mg/dL, the insulin level should be undetectable (<2 μU/mL), β-hydroxybutyrate increased (>2 mmol/L), lactate reduced (<1.5 mM), free fatty acids increased (>1.5 mmol/L), and counterregulatory hormones increased.

## Evaluation (Fig. 18-2)

*Transient Hypoglycemia of Infancy: Transient Neonatal Hyperinsulinism*
- *Infants of diabetic mothers*
  - This manifests as transient hypoglycemia as a result of hyperinsulinemia following chronic exposure to elevated blood glucose in utero. Infants are usually macrosomic, and the hypoglycemia can last 3-7 days.
  - Treatment consists of frequent feeds or, if needed, supplemental IV glucose at 5-10 mg/kg/min.
- Intrauterine growth retardation and perinatal stress
  - This can be manifested as hypoglycemia and usually persists for >5 days of life. Insulin levels may be inappropriately elevated.
  - Treatment involves frequent feedings, or most infants are responsive to diazoxide (5-15 mg/kg/day).

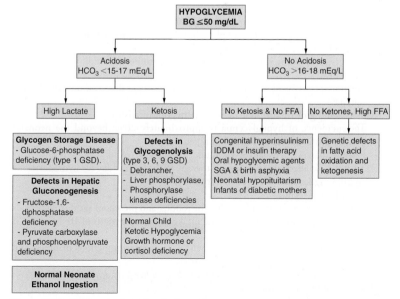

Figure 18-2. **Diagnostic algorithm for hypoglycemia.**

- Infants taking β-blockers, which cause hypoketotic hypoglycemia because of suppression of lipolysis

*Persistent Hypoglycemia of Infancy or Childhood*
- *Hypoglycemia with lactic acidosis*: inborn errors of metabolism
  - Glycogen storage disease type 1 (glucose-6-phosphatase deficiency).
    - ○ Infants can develop hypoglycemia on day of life 1, although because of frequent feeds, this can go undiagnosed for months. Fasting tolerance is usually very short (2-4 hours).
    - ○ Associated conditions include lactic acidemia, tachypnea, hepatomegaly, hyperuricemia, growth failure, hypertriglyceridemia, and neutropenia.
    - ○ Treatment consists of frequent carbohydrate feeds, uncooked cornstarch (>1 year of age), limited fructose and galactose intake, and granulocyte-macrophage colony–stimulating factor.
  - Defects in hepatic gluconeogenesis (fructose-1,6-diphosphatase deficiency).
    - ○ Patients usually develop hypoglycemia after fasting for 8-10 hours or after fructose ingestion.
    - ○ Associated conditions include lactic acidemia and hepatomegaly.
  - Galactosemia (galactose-1-phosphate uridyl transferase deficiency).
    - ○ This usually presents with jaundice without hepatomegaly and neonatal *Escherichia coli*–related sepsis.
    - ○ Later on in life, patients can develop hepatomegaly, cataracts, developmental delay, ovarian failure, and Fanconi syndrome.
    - ○ Treatment consists of galactose-restricted diet.
  - Other causes of hypoglycemia with lactic acidosis: alcohol ingestion or rubbing alcohol.
  - Normal newborns. Infants have poor ability to make ketones and gluconeogenesis in first 24 hours of life.
- *Hypoglycemia with ketosis*
  - Inborn errors of metabolism: glycogen storage disease types 3, 6, and 9 (debrancher, liver phosphorylase, and phosphorylase kinase deficiencies respectively).
    - ○ Fasting tolerance is usually 4-6 hours.
    - ○ Patients can present with failure to thrive, hepatomegaly, cardiomyopathy, and myopathy.
    - ○ Treatment consists of frequent feedings, low free sugar diet, and uncooked cornstarch.
  - Cortisol and growth hormone deficiency (hypopituitarism).
    - ○ The incidence of hypoglycemia is approximately 20%; beyond the neonatal period, this is usually associated with ketosis.
    - ○ Fasting tolerance is usually 8-14 hours.
    - ○ Treatment is adequate replacement therapy (8-12 mg/m$^2$/day for hydrocortisone and 0.3 mg/kg/week for growth hormone).
  - Ketotic hypoglycemia.
    - ○ This occurs more commonly during the toddler and preschool age during periods of intercurrent illness, with poor oral intake or fasting periods of 10-12 hours. It is a diagnosis of exclusion.
    - ○ Treatment involves frequent carbohydrate intake during periods of illness and avoidance of a prolonged overnight fast.
- *Hypoglycemia without acidosis (no ketosis; no elevated free fatty acids):*
  - Congenital hyperinsulinism.

**Diangostic criteria for hyperinsulinism (HI)**

| | Diagnostic of HI[a] | Suggestive of HI |
|---|---|---|
| Glucose | <50 mg/dL (after first 48 hr of life) | <65 mg/dL (after first 48 hr of life) |
| Beta-hydroxybutyrate | <1.1 mmol/L | <2 mmol/L |
| Free fatty acids | <0.5 mmol/L | <1.5 mmol/L |
| Insulin[b] | Detectable | Detectable |
| Glucagon stimulation test (0.03 mg/kg to max of 1 mg, IV or IM. Measure glucose at 0, 15, 30 min) | BG increase of 30 mg/dL within 30 min | BG increase of 30 mg/dL within 30 min |

- The most common cause of persistent hypoglycemia of the newborn.
- Time of onset, clinical features, fasting tolerance (0-6 hours), and therapy depend on the severity and type of disease or mutation. Patients usually are large for gestational age and do not present with failure to thrive.
- Patients usually have high glucose requirements (10-30 mg/kg/min).
- Patients respond to a glucagon stimulation (0.03 mg/kg to a maximum of 1 mg IV) with an increase in glucose >30 mg/dL within 15-30 minutes.
- Different types include the following:
  ○ Recessive mutations of potassium channel genes (SUR 1, Kir6.2). Patients are unresponsive to diazoxide. Treatment is subtotal pancreatectomy (98%); if hypoglycemia persists after surgery, consider medical management with octreotide or 10-20% dextrose enteral infusion. Avoid octreotide in neonatal period due to risk of necrotizing entercolitis.
- Dominant mutation of potassium channel genes. Treatment is subtotal pancreatectomy (98%); if hypoglycemia persists after surgery, consider medical management as described above. Approximately 50% of children with diffuse HI require additional medical management after near-total pancreatectomy.
  ○ Focal hyperinsulinism: focal loss of heterozygosity for maternal 11p and expression of paternally transmitted potassium channel mutations of either SUR 1 or Kir6.2. Treatment is focal resection; patients are unresponsive to diazoxide.
  ○ Dominant mutations of glutamate dehydrogenase: hyperinsulinism hyperammonemia syndrome. Treatment is diazoxide.
  ○ Dominant mutations of glucokinase. Treatment is diazoxide.
  ○ Recessive mutations of short-chain acyl-CoA dehydrogenase (SCHAD): abnormal metabolites in acylcarnitine profile and urine organic acids. Treatment is diazoxide.
- Neonatal hypopituitarism. Clinical features associated with this condition are midline defects, microphallus, cholestatic liver dysfunction, and jaundice.
- Furtive insulin or oral insulin secretagogue administration is characterized by hypoglycemia with high insulin levels but low C-peptide. When this is suspected, social work should be involved in evaluation of the case.
- Post-Nissen dumping syndrome occurs in some infants following surgery for reflux disease.
  - Treatment consists of frequent feedings, and inhibitors of gastric motility as well as acarbose may be useful.

- *Hypoglycemia without acidosis (no or abnormally low ketosis but high free fatty acids)*
  - Fatty acid oxidation and ketogenesis defects. Patients do not present in the neonatal period because fasting tolerance is 12-16 hours. The first episode is usually triggered by nonspecific illness.

## Treatment
- The goal is to keep blood glucose above 70 mg/dL after a 7-hour fast and between meals.
- Specific therapies include the following:
  - Dextrose: IV 0.2 g/kg bolus (2 mL/kg of 10% dextrose), followed by 10% dextrose continuous infusion (5 mL/kg/hr of 10% dextrose is approximately a GIR of 8 mg/kg/min in a newborn). Adjust rate to keep BG 70-150 mg/dL.
  - Glucagon (only if insulin induced): 0.5 mg SQ or IV if <20 kg or 1 mg SQ or IV if >20 kg. Nausea and emesis are common side effects.
  - Diazoxide: 5-15 mg/kg/day divided into 2-3 doses. Start with 10 mg/kg/day. Side effects: fluid retention and congestive heart failure.
  - Octreotide: 5-15 µg/kg/day and may increase up to 50 µg/kg/day SQ divided in 2 doses (8 AM, 2 PM + enteral dextrose). Second dose typically needs to be higher; or q6h equivalent doses (+/− enteral dextrose) or via continuous SQ infusion. Tachyphylaxis is a common problem. It can also cause suppression of other hormones such as glucagon, cortisol, growth hormone, and thyroid-stimulating hormone.
  - Uncooked cornstarch (glycogen storage disease type 1): 1-2 g/kg/dose in older infants (>6 months old).
  - Carnitine (for CPT1 defect): 100 mg/kg/day divided in 3-4 doses.

## ADRENAL INSUFFICIENCY

Adrenal insufficiency may be primary (as a result of disorder of the adrenal gland) or secondary (as a result of congenital anomalies or acquired insults to the hypothalamus or pituitary).

### Etiology
- Primary acute adrenal insufficiency: Waterhouse-Friderichsen syndrome (septicemia with subsequent bilateral adrenal infarcts), infection (tuberculosis, histoplasmosis, cytomegalovirus, HIV), medications (ketoconazole).
- Primary chronic adrenal insufficiency: autoimmune (polyglandular autoimmune syndrome, Addison disease), congenital adrenal hyperplasia (CAH), congenital adrenal hypoplasia, Wolman disease (lysosomal storage disease that includes calcification of the adrenals), adrenoleukodystrophy, congenital unresponsiveness to ACTH.
- Secondary adrenal insufficiency: isolated ACTH deficiency, radiation, craniopharyngioma, septooptic dysplasia, and iatrogenic (chronic steroid therapy). Traumatic, hemorrhagic, or autoimmune.
- Insults to the pituitary are associated with ACTH deficiency, as well as deficiencies of growth hormone, LH, FSH, and TSH.

### Clinical Presentation
- Signs
  - General: weight loss, hypotension/shock, vitiligo
  - Primary adrenal insufficiency only: hyperpigmentation of extensor surfaces, hand creases, gingival, lips, areola, scars

- Symptoms: weakness, fatigue, anorexia, nausea, vomiting, salt craving, postural dizziness.
- Laboratory abnormalities include hyponatremia (90%), hyperkalemia (60%) if primary adrenal insufficiency; hypercalcemia, metabolic acidosis, anemia, lymphocytosis, eosinophilia, and azotemia may also be present. Hyperkalemia is not evident with any adrenal insufficiency.

## Screening and Diagnosis

- Random plasma cortisol levels are not very useful except in infants, in patients in shock, or during a crisis if treatment is emergent.
- Initial diagnostic procedures could include 8 AM serum cortisol, ACTH, and electrolytes.
    - An early morning serum cortisol value >11 µg/dL (300 nmol/L) makes it unlikely that the patient has clinically important hypothalamic-pituitary-adrenal insufficiency.
    - An early morning serum cortisol value <3 µg/dL (80 nmol/L) makes adrenal insufficiency very likely if the patient has presumed normal circadian rhythmicity.
    - Low cortisol with high ACTH levels supports primary adrenal insufficiency.
    - If the patient's condition permits waiting to initiate therapy, perform an **ACTH stimulation test** with cosyntropin. If suspicion of primary adrenaline sufficiency: 250 µg IV, and monitor plasma cortisol levels at time 0, 30, and 60 minutes. If suspicion of secondary adrenal insufficiency, perform a low-dose 1-µg cosyntropin test. A serum cortisol value of ≥18 µg/dL (497 nmol/L) at 30 or 60 minutes indicates a normal response. However, this value may vary depending on the laboratory assay used.
- Dexamethasone can be given if emergent therapy is necessary and ACTH stimulation testing can be performed shortly thereafter.

## Treatment

### Acute Adrenal Crisis

- Rapid IV volume expansion with 20 mL/kg NS or $D_5NS$ if there is concomitant hypoglycemia.
- Close monitoring of electrolytes and blood glucose.
- Hydrocortisone at 50 mg/m² IV bolus; then 50 mg/m²/day divided in q4-6h.
- If no IV or diagnosis established: dexamethasone 1 mg/m² IV or IM.

### Chronic Adrenal Insufficiency

- Physiologic replacement (hydrocortisone 6-12 mg/m²/day PO divided in q8h; the best dose is the lowest the patient can support without symptoms).
- If suspecting mineralocorticoid deficiency, give fludrocortisone 0.1 mg/day PO in primary adrenal insufficiency. Increase dose if needed.
- Stress dosing.
- Minor illness (nausea, emesis, fever). Triple total daily corticosteroid dose and divide three times daily or give hydrocortisone 30-50 mg/m²/day IV for 48 hours or until symptoms resolve. Patients should have injectable corticosteroid available and be instructed in intramuscular use for emesis or emergencies (dexamethasone 1 mg/m²/day) or Solu-Cortef (50 mg/m² per dose).
- Major stress (severe illness, general anesthesia, bone fracture). Give hydrocortisone 50-100 mg/m²/day IV divided in q6-8h.
- Decreasing from stress to physiologic doses can be done at any rate followed by careful slow decreases in steroids below physiologic doses because of concern of adrenal insufficiency.

- The patient should receive stress dosing during times of illness if below stress dosing or off of steroids until an ACTH/cosyntropin (Cortrosyn) test verifies adrenal sufficiency.
- A MedicAlert bracelet must be worn by a patient with this diagnosis.
- Postoperatively (for pituitary lesions). A cortisol value >8 µg/dL 24 hours after stopping dexamethasone or hydrocortisone is reassuring. The patient will still need an ACTH/cosyntropin stimulation test 1 month after surgery.

*Corticosteroid Potencies*

The relative potencies of corticosteroids vary (see Table 18-5).

## CONGENITAL ADRENAL HYPERPLASIA

- CAH is the most common cause of genital ambiguity in the newborn.
- It has autosomal recessive inheritance.
- It is caused by deficiency in one of the enzymes of the corticosteroid biosynthetic pathway (Table 18-6).
  - Most common enzyme deficiency is 21-hydroxylase.
  - The primary defect is the inability to synthesize adequate cortisol, and steroids distal to the missing enzyme resulting in excessive corticotropin-releasing hormone and ACTH, causing the adrenal glands to become hyperplastic.
  - Increased trophic hormone stimulation leads to excessive adrenal androgen production (androstenedione), which is peripherally converted to testosterone, leading to virilization.
  - Steroidogenic defects that interrupt aldosterone synthesis result in an inability to maintain sodium balance, and if not diagnosed promptly, this can lead to hyponatremic dehydration, shock, and death that typically presents at 7-10 days of life.
- Newborn screening is available for 21-hydroxylase deficiency (Fig. 18-3).
  - Most states perform routine screening by assay of 17-hydroxyprogesterone (17-OHP) obtained by heel puncture at 2-4 days of life. Screening before 24 hours of life leads to a high false-positive rate.
  - Assays vary widely, and 17-OHP levels can be affected by gestational age, severe illness, and stress.
  - If ambiguous genitalia, decreased alertness, poor weight gain, or highly elevated 17-OHP is evident on screening, the infant should be immediately referred to a pediatric endocrinologist and admitted. An elevated 17-OHP on screening should be confirmed with a laboratory serum 17-OHP, and electrolytes should be followed until diagnosis of CAH is excluded.

| TABLE 18-5 | Relative Potencies of Systemic Corticosteroids | | |
|---|---|---|---|
| Drug | Glucocorticoid activity | Mineralocorticoid activity | Biologic half-life (hr) |
| Hydrocortisone | 1 | 1 | 8-12 |
| Prednisone/ prednisolone | 4 | 0.3 | 18-36 |
| Methylprednisolone | 5 | 0 | 18-36 |
| Dexamethasone | 25-40 | 0 | 36-54 |
| Fludrocortisone | 10-15 | 125 | 18-36 |

**TABLE 18-6 Enzyme Defects and Phenotype of Congenital Adrenal Hyperplasia**

| Enzyme deficiency | Female phenotype | Male phenotype | Treatment | Diagnostic labs | | | |
|---|---|---|---|---|---|---|---|
| | | | | 17-OHP | K | Na | Others |
| **21-OH deficiency (90%)** | | | | | | | |
| Classic salt-wasting | Virilized/ambiguous genitalia | Normal genitalia/ salt-losing crisis at 1-2 weeks old | GC, MC; NaCl in infants | ↑ (usually >2000 ng/ dL) | ↑ | ↓ | Acidosis, decreased glucose |
| Classic simple virilization | Virilized/ambiguous genitalia | Phenotypically normal | GC, ±MC | ↑ (usually >2000 ng/ dL) | N | N | |
| Nonclassic | Premature adrenarche, irregular menses, advanced bone age | Premature adrenarche, advanced bone age | GC | Modest ↑ on ACTH stimulation | N | N | |
| **11β-OH deficiency (5%)** | Hypertension, hypokalemia, virilization | Hypertension, hypokalemia (not as neonate) | GC, treat hypertension | | ↓ | N | ↑ DOC |
| **17α-OH deficiency (1%)** | Hypertension, absence of adrenarche/puberty | Hypertension, ambiguous genitalia | GC, sex steroids, treat hypertension | | ↓ | N | ↓ sex steroids, cortisol, ↑ DOC |

21-OH, 21-hydroxylase; 11β-OH, 11β-hydroxylase; 17α-OH, 17α-hydroxylase; 17-OHP, 17-hydroxyprogesterone; DOC, deoxycorticosterone; N, normal; GC, glucocorticoids (hydrocortisone 10-20 mg/m²/day divided tid); MC, mineralocorticoids (fludrocortisone typically 0.1 mg daily); NaCl, sodium chloride supplements typically 1-2 g or 17-34 mEq of sodium daily.

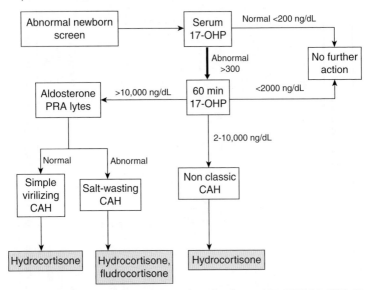

**Figure 18-3. Diagnostic and treatment algorithm for 21-OH CAH.** (17-OHP, 17 hydroxyprogesterone; PRA, plasma renin activity; CAH, congenital adrenal hyperplasia).

- Therapeutic monitoring.
  - Patients should have close monitoring with a multidisciplinary team.
  - Serial monitoring of 17-hydroxyprogesterone and androstenedione levels.

## GLUCOCORTICOID EXCESS (FIG. 18-4)

- Cushing disease is the most frequent cause of hypercortisolism. Caused by ACTH-secreting adenoma or rarely by ectopic ACTH-secreting tumor, which drives the adrenal cortisol production.
- It may also be caused by Cushing syndrome, which refers to the autonomous cortisol secretion or exogenous exposure to corticosteroids. Etiologies include adrenocortical adenoma, adrenocortical carcinoma, McCune-Albright syndrome, and multiple endocrine neoplasia 1, or due to exogenous steroid intake.
- Most sensitive indicators of glucocorticoid excess are excessive weight and impaired linear growth.
- Other clinical manifestations include moon face, dorsocervical fat pad ("buffalo hump"), obesity, hypertension, thinning of the skin, violaceous striae, bruising, and hirsutism.
- Initial evaluation to confirm hypercortisolism is 24-hour urinary-free cortisol (in excess of 70-80 $\mu$g/m$^2$ in children with suspicion of glucocorticoid excess) or salivary cortisol at 2300 hours (normal concentration is <0.28 $\mu$g/dL) or an overnight 1 mg dexamethasone suppression test can also be performed as an outpatient study. Dose should be given orally at 2300 hours and measure 0800 serum cortisol. Level $\geq$1.8 mg/dL is suspicious of hypercortisolism.
- Repeat testing If clinical suspicion is high and all tests are negative.
- After confirming hypercortisolism, it is important to detect the source.

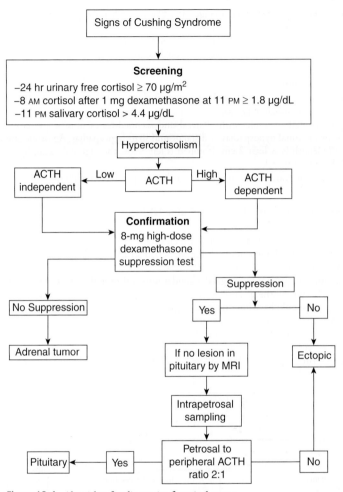

**Figure 18-4. Algorithm for diagnosis of cortisol excess.**

## AMBIGUOUS GENITALIA

### Definition

- A disorder of sex development (DSD) occurs when there is incongruence between a child's external genitalia, his or her gonads (ovaries or testes), and his or her chromosomal sex (XX—female or XY—male).
- This incongruence often manifests as external genitalia that are neither overtly male nor female, termed ambiguous genitalia.

### History

- Maternal history—virilization before or during pregnancy, amniocentesis results, medications (androgens-progestins endocrine disrupters, phenytoin)

- Family History—parental consanguinity, relatives with ambiguous genitalia, primary amenorrhea, early death, or stillbirth
- Discordance between genital appearance and a prenatal karyotype
- Electrolyte abnormalities, jaundice, hypoglycemia

## Physical Examination

- Apparent female genitalia with an enlarged clitoris and/or posterior labial fusion, and/or an inguinal/labial mass.
- Apparent male genitalia with bilateral undescended testes, and/or a microphallus, and/or proximal hypospadias or distal or mid shaft hypospadias. A normal stretched penile length is at least 2 cm. If gonad is felt below the inguinal canal, ligament is likely to be a testicle.
- Dysmorphic features, midline defects, other congenital anomalies.

## Differential Diagnosis (Figs. 18-5 and 18-6)

*Management*

- Initial labs may include karyotype, including FISH with SRY probe, ultrasound of the pelvis/abdomen to check for Mullerian structures, electrolytes, and CAH 6 Cortrosyn screen.
- The child should not be assigned a gender until a thorough evaluation by a specialist has been performed.
- The child should have long-term management by a multidisciplinary team: endocrinology, urology, psychology, genetics, and social work.
- The family must be well informed on the diagnosis and play an active role in the gender decision for the child.
- Long-term support should be offered to all patients with DSD and their families

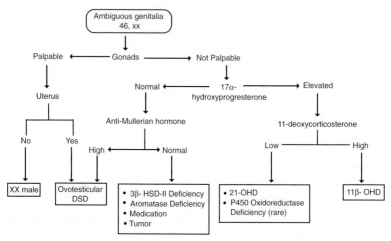

**Figure 18-5. Algorithm for diagnosing disorder of sexual differentiation (DSD) in 46xx with ambiguous genitalia.** (11β-OHD: 11β-hydroxylase deficiency, 3-HSD-II 3b-hydroxysteroid dehydrogenase deficiency).

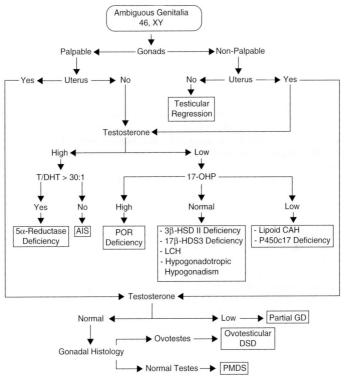

**Figure 18-6. Algorithm for diagnosing disorders of sexual differentiation (DSD) in 46xy with ambiguous genitalia.**

## TRANSGENDER HEALTH

### Definitions

- Sex: designation of a person at birth as either "male" or "female" based on his or her anatomy (genital and reproductive organs) and biology (chromosomes and hormones).
- Gender identity: a person's internal sense of self. It may be male, female, somewhere in between, a combination of both, or neither.
- Gender expression: reference to the external manifestation of a person's gender identity. This may include choices in clothing, hairstyle, speech, and mannerism.
- Gender dysphoria: defined as clinically significant distress related to an incongruence between an individual's gender identity and the gender assigned at birth.
- Transgender: a person whose gender identity differs from the sex that was assigned at birth.
- Cisgender: People whose gender identity and gender expression align with their assigned sex at birth.

### Epidemiology

- Accurate estimates of the United States transgender population have been challenging to acquire due to lack of data collection in population-based surveys.

- Recent studies suggest that the prevalence of a self-reported transgender identity in children, adolescents, and adults ranges from 0.5% to 1.3%.

## Primary Care Considerations

- Significant health disparities exist for the transgender population and stem from a number of sources like insufficient provider training in health care needs specific to transgender individuals.
- Primary care providers can promote a sense of safety and inclusion by identifying unisex bathrooms; exhibiting posters and brochures about transgender health concerns; and posting a public statement of nondiscrimination, including gender identity options on registration forms and other materials (not just male or female).
- Home: It is important to assess for family awareness of and support for the adolescent's current gender identification. Parental support is positively associated with higher life satisfaction and fewer depressive symptoms among transgender adolescents.
- School: A nationwide internet survey in the United States found that transgender youth were at higher risk for bullying or harassment compared to their cisgender peers.
- Sexual health: If the patient is on cross-sex hormones, it is important to remind him or her that while a side effect may be infertility, such therapies should not be relied upon for contraception. Furthermore, testosterone is contraindicated in pregnancy and may have adverse effects on a developing fetus.
- Mental health: Transgender adolescents were at two to three times greater risk of depression, anxiety, and suicidal ideation. About 56% of youth who identified as transgender reported previous suicidal ideation, and 31% reported a previous suicide attempt, compared with 20% and 11% among matched youth who identified as cisgender, respectively. These findings highlight the importance of assessing mood and suicidal ideation during visits with these patients.

## Gender-Affirming Care

- *Social affirmation* includes reversible changes to one's gender expression, such as name or pronoun changes or changing one's clothing or appearance.
- *Legal affirmation* includes legally changing the name and gender identifier on all identification and legal documents.
- *Medical affirmation* involves administration of sex steroids to induce the desired physical changes that match the patient's gender identity.
- *Surgical affirmation (gender-affirming surgery)* involves irreversible procedures to achieve the desired physical changes that align the patient's gender identity.

### Medical Affirmation

- Both the Endocrine Society and World Professional Association for Transgender Health (WPATH) offer recommendations on the medical management of transgender adolescents.
- Medical professionals have an ethical responsibility to help adolescents appropriately weigh the pros and cons of medical interventions.
- Puberty suppression
  - Pubertal onset in particular is accompanied by intense anxiety and distress.
  - Gonadotropin-releasing hormone (GnRH) analogs are safe, reversible medications that pause pubertal development.
  - GnRH can be initiated when patients reach Tanner stage 2 or at any subsequent point throughout puberty.
  - GnRH relieves the distress of pubertal development in an adolescent who is experiencing gender dysphoria.

- Gender-Affirming Hormone Therapy (GAHT)
  - According to the Endocrine Society guidelines, cross-sex hormones can be initiated around age 16 years.
  - Feminizing treatment for male-to-female individuals consists of using an estrogen or antiandrogen alone or a combination of the two with a potential progestin adjunct.
  - Masculinizing treatment consists mainly of testosterone. Several formulations are available, including intramuscular injections, transdermal patches, and gels.
  - Not all patients will desire the same degree of transition, and their medication regimen should reflect the goals of the patient.

## DIABETES INSIPIDUS

### Definition
- Central diabetes insipidus is due to insufficient vasopressin (antidiuretic hormone [ADH]). Nephrogenic diabetes insipidus is due to or renal unresponsiveness to vasopressin.
  - These cause a syndrome of polyuria and polydipsia, and potentially electrolyte abnormalities such as hypernatremia, which are characteristic of diabetes insipidus (DI).
  - With an intact thirst mechanism, copious water drinking ($>2$ L/m$^2$/day) may maintain normal osmolality. However, problems with thirst mechanism or insufficient water intake leads to hypernatremic dehydration.

### Etiology (Table 18-7)

*Clinical Presentation and Laboratory Studies*
- Clinical characteristics: polyuria, polydipsia (water intake $>2$ L/m$^2$/day)
- Urine osmolality $<300$ mOsm/kg and serum osmolality $>300$ mOsm/kg, urine specific gravity $<1.005$
  - Serum sodium and serum osmolality are usually normal or slightly elevated in children with uncomplicated DI and free-water access.

| TABLE 18-7 | Etiology of Diabetes Insipidus |
|---|---|

**Central causes**
   Congenital: autosomal dominant, DIDMOAD
   Trauma/injury: injury to the sella turcica, intraventricular hemorrhage
   Surgery: pituitary—hypothalamic surgery/neurosurgical
   Tumors: craniopharyngioma, germinoma
   Infection: tuberculosis, meningitis, Listeria
   Infiltrations: sarcoidosis, Langerhans histiocytosis
   Wolfram syndrome: diabetes insipidus, diabetes mellitus, optic atrophy, deafness (DIDMOAD)

**Nephrogenic causes**
   Electrolyte disturbances; hypokalemia, hypercalcemia
   Nephrocalcinosis
   Congenital: X-linked recessive
   Chronic renal failure, polycystic kidney disease
   Drugs: demeclocycline, lithium

| TABLE 18-8 | Water Deprivation Test | | | | | |
|---|---|---|---|---|---|---|
| Condition | Urine osmolality (mOsm/kg) | Plasma osmolality (mOsm/kg) | Specific gravity | Urine:plasma osmolality ratio | Urine volume | Weight loss |
| Normal/psycho-genic polydipsia | 500-1400 | 288-291 | 1.010 | >2 | Decreased | No change |
| Diabetes insipidus | <300 | >300 | <1.005 | — | Increased | ≥5% |

- Water deprivation test: used to confirm the diagnosis of DI (Table 18-8)
  - Begin the test in the morning after 24 hours of adequate hydration and after patient empties his or her bladder.
  - Weigh the patient and give no fluid until completion of test.
    - Measure weight and urine volume and specific gravity hourly.
    - Check urine and serum osmolality and serum sodium every 2 hours.
  - Terminate the test if weight loss approaches 3-5% of initial body weight or if orthostatic hypotension, serum osmolality >300, serum sodium >145, or if urine osmolality >600 ×2 or >1200.
- Vasopressin test: used to differentiate between a nephrogenic and central etiology (Table 18-9)
  - Give vasopressin 0.05-0.1 U/kg subcutaneously at the end of water deprivation test after measuring vasopressin level.
  - Monitor urine output, concentration, and water intake (water intake is limited to documented output during deprivation test) for an additional 2 hours.
  - After 2 hours, an increase in urine osmolality over 50% above baseline gives diagnosis of central DI, whereas a rise of <10% above baseline gives diagnosis of nephrogenic DI.
  - If central DI is confirmed, obtain pituitary MRI.

### Treatment
*Central Diabetes Insipidus*
- Provide fluid replacement with hypotonic solutions to reduce driving up urine output.
- 1/4 NS with additives is a good maintenance fluid.

| TABLE 18-9 | Vasopressin Test | | |
|---|---|---|---|
| Condition | Urine osmolality | Urine volume | Fluid intake |
| Central diabetes insipidus | >600, or increase by 50% | Decreased | Decreased |
| Nephrogenic diabetes insipidus | <300, or no increase | No change | No change |

- Those with nonintact thirst mechanisms should be restricted to about 1 L/m²/day of fluid if they are taking desmopressin (DDAVP).
- May correct water deficit with free enteral water or D5W via IV.
- Monitor status.
  - Formula to correct free-water deficit: if Na 145-170 mEq, 4 mL × (current sodium − desired sodium) × weight (kg) × 0.6/24 hours or 48 hours; if Na ≥170 mEq, 3 mL × (current sodium − desired sodium) × weight (kg) × 0.6/24 hours or 48 hours
- Administer vasopressin drip after surgery or if the patient is NPO or clinically unstable.
  - Start at 0.2 mU/kg/hr and titrate up every 30 minutes based on UOP, specific gravity, and serum sodium level.
  - 1.5 mU/kg/hr usually achieves twice normal vasopressin needed for maximal antidiuretic effect.
  - It has a very short half-life (5-10 minutes).
  - Stop drip if Na < 140 mEq/L or UPO < 1 mL/kg/hr.
  - It is important to restrict the patient to 1 L/m²/day of IV fluids when continuous vasopressin is administered to prevent hyponatremia.
  - DDAVP: Aim to maintain sodium level 140-150 mEq if thirst is not intact and 135-145 mEq for intact thirst. Titrate to allow 1-2 hours of breakthrough urine output (2-3 mL/kg/hr) with specific gravity <1.005 per day. DDAVP is available in the following forms:
    ○ Subcutaneous: most potent (4 μg/mL).
    ○ Intranasal: 10-fold less potent than subcutaneous (10 μg/mL).
    ○ Oral: 100- to 200-fold less potent than subcutaneous (0.1-mg, 0.2-mg tablets).
    ○ Buccal: diluted inhaled DDAVP (1-5 μg per dose) most commonly used in infants who require much smaller doses.
    ○ Thiazide diuretics are another treatment option in infants.

*Nephrogenic Diabetes Insipidus*
- Thiazide diuretics
- Nonsteroidal anti-inflammatory drugs
- Amiloride

## SYNDROME OF INAPPROPRIATE ANTIDIURETIC HORMONE (SIADH)

Vasopressin (ADH) level is inappropriately high despite low serum sodium and osmolality.

### Etiology
Meningitis, encephalitis, pneumonia, tuberculosis, AIDS, mechanical ventilation, brain trauma, head trauma, neurosurgery, prolonged nausea, vomiting, ethanol intoxication, pregnancy, medication side effects

### Clinical Presentation
- Hyponatremia (serum sodium <135), in the setting of euvolemia or hypervolemia with decreased urine output and inappropriately concentrated urine (urine Osm > 100 mOsm/kg and urine sodium >30 mEq/L).
- Diagnosis cannot be made in the setting of hypothyroidism, adrenal insufficiency, renal insufficiency, or diuretic use.

## Treatment
- Fluid restriction to 0.8-1 L/m²/day.
- Other therapies such as demeclocycline or vasopressin receptor antagonists may be tried in special cases.

## TRIPHASIC RESPONSE (AFTER PITUITARY STALK TRANSECTION)

### Usually Post–Central Nervous System (CNS) Surgery or Head Injury
- Initial DI (occurring within the first few hours) followed by syndrome of inappropriate secretion of ADH (SIADH) phase (lasting up to 5-10 days), followed finally by central DI disorder
- Occurs after an acute injury to neurohypophysis without transection of the septum (basal skull fracture or status-post transection of the stalk during CNS surgery)

### Treatment
- Restrict fluids to 0.8-1 L/m²/day of ½NS plus 5% dextrose.
- Replace output in excess of 40 mL/m²/hr with mL/mL of 5% dextrose plus water, max 120 mL/m²/hr.
- Monitor strict input/output charts and electrolytes regularly.

## CEREBRAL SALT WASTING

- Increased urinary salt loss secondary to increased secretion of natriuretic peptides.
- Occurs in the setting of CNS disease.
- Difficult to differentiate from SIADH; however, patients are typically intravascularly volume depleted.

### Etiology
Brain tumors, head trauma, hydrocephalus, neurosurgery, cerebral vascular accidents, brain death

### Clinical Presentation
Hyponatremia (serum sodium <135) in the setting of hypovolemia, excessive urine output, elevated urinary sodium excretion (often >150 mEq/L)

### Treatment
Restoring intravascular volume with sodium chloride, patients often need hypertonic (3%) saline infusion to correct hyponatremia.

## HYPOTHYROIDISM

- Primary (thyroid gland dysfunction: elevated thyroid-stimulating hormone [TSH], low free thyroxine)
  - Congenital.
  - Atrophic autoimmune thyroiditis: serum positivity for thyroid peroxidase antibodies.
  - Hashimoto thyroiditis: goiter, positive serum thyroid peroxidase antibodies, and thyroid-stimulating hormone-binding inhibitory immunoglobulin (TBII), more common in Turner syndrome.

- Familial: Pendred syndrome, which consists of goiter and eighth nerve deafness, is an autosomal recessive disorder in the *SLC26A4* gene.
- Iodine deficiency: presents with a goiter.
- Treatment for hyperthyroidism or radiotherapy of neck for lymphoma, leukemia.
- Drugs: amiodarone, iodine-containing medication.
- Secondary (low TSH and normal or low free thyroxine)
  - Pituitary or hypothalamic disease

## CONGENITAL HYPOTHYROIDISM

### Epidemiology and Etiology

- This condition occurs in 1 in 4000 births.
- Thyroid dysgenesis/agenesis, hypoplasia, ectopic presence (75%).
- Dyshormonogenesis (10%): may resolve; usually organification defect.
- Transient hypothyroidism (10%): maternal thyroid antibodies, iodine deficiency/excess.
- Hypothalamic-pituitary TSH deficiency (5%).

### Clinical Presentation

- No symptoms (most infants)
- Possible symptoms
  - Wide cranial suture, delayed skeletal maturation
  - Umbilical hernia
  - Prolonged jaundice
  - Hypotonia, puffy hands and feet, macroglossia
  - Hoarse cry
  - Goiter (dyshormonogenesis; transient only)

### Laboratory Studies

- Newborn screening protocols should be done after 24 hours of life.
  - If the screen is abnormal, obtain serum TSH and free thyroxine ($T_4$).
- Presume disease if after 2 days of life, the serum TSH is >20-25 mU/L in a well-term infant. TSH peaks at delivery and remains elevated for 2-5 days, which stimulates the rise of $T_4$ 2- to 6-fold. $T_4$ remains elevated for several weeks.
- Sick or very premature infants must be evaluated with free $T_4$ and TSH.
- For low $T_4$ and normal TSH, consider thyroid-binding globulin deficiency versus hypothalamic/pituitary disturbance (TSH/TRH deficiency).

### Treatment

- Institute treatment as soon as the diagnosis is confirmed to optimize neurologic development.
- Give thyroxine treatment orally 10-15 µg/kg/day (starting dose usually 37.5 µg once daily). For term infants with Down syndrome, start at a low dose of 25 µg once daily.
- Monitor TSH and free $T_4$ 2 weeks after initiation of treatment and then every 2 weeks until TSH is normal.
  - Test every 3 months in first year of life.
  - Test every 4 months between 1 and 3 years old.
  - Test every 6 months until growth is complete.
  - Test 4-6 weeks after dose is changed.

- Aim for free T4 in upper end of normal.
- There is decreased absorption of thyroxine with soy formula, iron supplements, calcium supplements, and proton pump inhibitors.

## ACQUIRED HYPOTHYROIDISM

### Clinical Presentation
- Growth deceleration (one of earlier markers)
- Delayed ossification
- Dry skin; dry, brittle, thin hair
- Cold intolerance
- Low energy
- Constipation
- Proximal myopathy, ataxia, slow reflexes
- Headache, precocious puberty, and galactorrhea (seen in pituitary disease)
- Possible hypercalcemia, hypercholesterolemia, and hyperprolactinemia

### Laboratory Studies
- Obtain a thyroid function test.
- If TSH is low or normal in light of a low free $T_4$, then investigate for pituitary disease.

### Treatment
- For infants, use 10-15 µg/kg/day of thyroxine orally (starting dose usually 37.5 µg once daily).
- In 6 to 12 months consider starting dose of: 6 to 8 mcg/kg/dose once daily, in 1 to 5 years: 5 to 6 mcg/kg/dose once daily, 6 to 12 years: 4 to 5 mcg/kg/dose once daily, >12 years with incomplete growth and puberty: 2 to 3 mcg/kg/dose once daily, Adolescents with growth and puberty complete 1.75 mcg/kg/dose once daily.
- For infants and children with Down syndrome, consider starting thyroxine dose of 25 µg once daily.
- It is necessary to assess if a patient is taking their medications when reviewing abnormal thyroid function tests while on therapy.
- Monitor TSH and free T4 4-6 weeks after initiating therapy or adjust dose by 12.5 to 25 mcg/day every 4 to 6 weeks as needed.

## HYPERTHYROIDISM

### Etiology
- Graves disease (most common cause in childhood)
  - Diffuse toxic goiter, proptosis, and pretibial myxedema
  - Female > male
  - HLA B8, DW3 association
  - Thyroid-stimulating antibody present
  - May have other autoimmune association: vitiligo, DM type 1, idiopathic thrombocytopenic purpura, rheumatic fever, Addison disease
- Solitary nodule/adenoma (fine-needle aspiration or biopsy warranted to rule out cancer): Plummer disease, toxic uninodular goiter
- De Quervain thyroiditis: acute disease with tender goiter and elevated total triiodothyronine ($T_3$)
- Subacute thyroiditis: viral origin (mumps, coxsackievirus, adenovirus)
- Riedel thyroiditis: dense thyroid fibrosis, including the neck vessels and trachea

- Tumors: ovarian tumors, choriocarcinoma, hydatidiform mole
- Transient neonatal: secondary to transmission of stimulating antibodies in maternal Graves disease, lasts 6-12 weeks

## Clinical Presentation

- General symptoms and signs
  - Increased appetite, short attention span
  - Hyperactivity
  - Tachycardia, palpitation, dyspnea
  - Goiter
  - Smooth skin, increased sweating, tremor
  - Hypertension, cardiomegaly, atrial fibrillation
  - Eye signs: exophthalmos, lid retraction, lid lag, impaired convergence
- Thyroid storm
  - Acute onset
  - Presenting symptoms: tachycardia, high-grade fever, hypertension, restlessness
  - Progression to delirium, coma, and death if not treated rapidly
- Neonatal hyperthyroidism
  - Classically born premature
  - Intrauterine growth retardation
  - Goiter, exophthalmos, microcephaly
  - Irritable, hyperalert, with possible tachycardia, tachypnea, hyperthermia, hypertension

## Laboratory Studies

- Free or total $T_4$ and $T_3$ elevated
- TSH decreased
- Thyroid-stimulating immunoglobulin (TSI) and/or TBII positive
- Increased radioactive iodine uptake

## Treatment

*Medications*

- Antithyroid medication
  - Propylthiouracil (PTU) currently has a black box warning due to increased hepatotoxicity. Only use during pregnancy and thyroid storm.
  - Methimazole delivered as once-daily dosing (0.25-1.0 mg/kg/day). Do not use in women of childbearing age because of teratogenicity. Side effect: Hepatotoxicity, agranulocytosis, patient develops fever, pharyngitis, or jaundice. Stop the medication and measure WBC, AST, ALT. These labs should also be monitored regularly.
- Symptomatic control with propranolol or atenolol
- Radioactive iodine ablation (need to discontinue antithyroid medication 7-10 days prior).
- Thyroid storm: high-dose PTU, propranolol, and potassium iodide if needed; antipyretics

*Surgery*

- Subtotal thyroidectomy

## GOITER

- An enlargement in the thyroid gland

## Etiology

- Congenital.
- Colloid goiter (prepubertal girls, euthyroid).
- Iodine deficiency.
- Graves or Hashimoto disease.
- Thyroiditis.
- Multinodular (McCune-Albright syndrome).
- Thyroid neoplasm (rare in children, the most common is papillary). It is important to exclude coexisting pathology such as multiple endocrine neoplasia syndrome before a surgical procedure particularly if medullary carcinoma.

## Diagnosis

- The child may be hypo-, hyper-, or euthyroid.
- Assess goiter for size and consistency. Determine whether it is diffuse or nodular.
- Additional investigations include thyroid ultrasound, neck CT, and fine-needle aspiration of the gland if single prominent thyroid nodule present.

## Treatment

- Monitor status regularly if the child is nonsymptomatic from the goiter.
- If goiter compromises airway or feeding, then consider surgical removal.
- Some endocrinologists prefer using thyroid medication in euthyroid patients to reduce the size of the goiter.

## SHORT STATURE

- Disturbances of growth are most common presenting complaints in the pediatric endocrine clinic.
  - Fetal growth is dependent on maternal factors (placental sufficiency, maternal nutrition, etc.), insulin-like growth factor-2 (IGF-2), and insulin.
  - Growth in late infancy and childhood is dependent on growth hormone/IGF-1 axis and thyroid hormone. Growth is more rapid during infancy—up to 20 cm per year in 1st year of life, 12 cm/year in 2nd year, and 8 cm per year in 3rd year. It is common to see shifts in the growth curve in the first 18 months when children are adjusting to their genetic potential growth isopleth. During childhood, growth rate is fairly constant at approximately 2 inches (approximately 5 cm) per year.
  - Pubertal growth is dependent on sex hormones as well as growth hormone/IGF-1 axis and the thyroid gland. There is a mild deceleration in growth velocity before initiation of pubertal growth spurt.
- Abnormal growth and stature: criteria
  - Child's growth curve is crossing isopleths after 18 months old.
  - Child's growth rate is <2 inches or <5-7 cm/year after age 3.
  - Height is <2 standard deviations (SDs) (4 inches/10 cm) below from midparental height.
  - Height is <2 SDs mean height of children of same sex and chronologic age (e.g., height <3rd percentile on growth chart).
- If poor weight gain and lack of nutrition is the problem without affecting height velocity, it is unlikely to be an endocrine cause and patient may warrant a GI evaluation instead.

## Etiology (Fig. 18-7)

- Normal growth patterns that can look like a growth disorder
  - Genetic (familial) short stature. Children have normal growth velocity, normal timing of development and puberty, and bones fuse at the appropriate age. Height is short because of a short mother and/or a short father. Bone age (BA) = chronologic age (CA).
  - Constitutional delay of growth and puberty. Children have normal growth velocity, delayed timing of puberty, and delayed BA. There is a family history of late bloomers. Anticipate a less robust growth spurt BA < CA.
- Primary growth failure
  - Chromosomal disorders such as Turner syndrome, Down syndrome, Noonan syndrome, Russell-Silver syndrome, Prader-Willi syndrome, and pseudohypoparathyroidism
  - Skeletal dysplasias such as hypochondroplasias, achondroplasias, osteogenesis imperfecta, and Albright hereditary osteodystrophy
- Secondary growth failure
  - Prenatal onset
    ○ Maternal hypertension, fetal alcohol syndrome, and congenital infections.
    ○ Small for gestational age (SGA). Infants are born with weights below the 10th percentile for their gestational age. Russell-Silver syndrome is one of the many syndromes that includes SGA and postnatal growth failure.

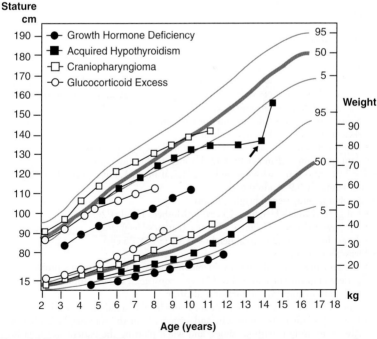

**Figure 18-7. Patterns of different endocrine causes of growth abnormalities.** Arrow in figure indicates time of initiation of thyroid hormone replacement.

- Postnatal onset
  - Endocrine, such as hypothyroidism, growth hormone deficiency, growth hormone resistance (Laron dwarfism), and glucocorticoid excess (iatrogenic or endogenous)
  - Nonendocrine, such as renal failure, renal tubular acidosis, malabsorption, cystic fibrosis, celiac disease, and Crohn disease

## History

- Physical history
  - History of changes in growth pattern and onset of puberty
  - History of chronic illnesses
  - Prenatal exposures to toxins, drugs, or alcohol; use of other medications (e.g., steroids, psychostimulants)
  - History of prematurity; weight for gestational age, and catch-up growth
- Social history
  - History of adoption and ethnic background
  - History of child abuse or neglect, which may give information supportive of psychosocial dwarfism
- Family history
  - History of pubertal development. Age of menarche in mother and age of physical changes or cessation of growth in father may give information that supports the diagnosis of constitutional growth delay.
  - Family history of chronic diseases (e.g., inflammatory bowel disease, neurofibromatosis, mental retardation, calcium problems, renal disease). The child's symptoms of these diseases are very important.

## Physical Examination

- Abnormal facial features, shortening of fourth or fifth metacarpals, cognitive impairment, and skin lesions may be suggestive of genetic disorders.
- Arm span and upper-to-lower segment (U/L). Determination of the arm span and U/L ratio (lower segment is the measurement from the symphysis pubis to the floor) is useful to determine the etiologies of short stature. Examples:
  - Short arm span or small legs and normal trunk (increased U/L ratio) may indicate skeletal dysplasia or hypothyroidism.
  - Long arms and decreased U/L ratio may indicate hypogonadism.
  - Arm span longer than height may also suggest abnormal spine growth.
- The U/L ratio varies with age and race: 1.7 at birth, 1.4 at 2 years, 1 at 10 years, approximately 0.9 at adulthood.
- Calculating midparental height (in cm).
  - For girls: (Father's Height − 13 cm) + (Mother's Height)/2
  - For boys: (Mother's Height + 13 cm) + (Father's Height)/2
  - Target height is midparental height ± 2 SD (1 SD = 5 cm).
- Measurement of growth.
  - The growth curve is the most valuable instrument for assessing the problem. The pattern of growth of a normal child is very consistent, and deviations in the process may warrant concern and further evaluation.
  - Obtain length (lying down) up to age 2 and height (standing) onward.
  - It is important to be consistent and systematic in the way height is obtained. Always measure it without shoes, and when plotting the patient in the growth

curve, be as accurate as possible regarding the actual age of the child. Be sure to correct for genu recurvatum or leg length asymmetries when obtaining the measurements. Do not forget that pediatric patients do not shrink, so if unsure of your measurement, remeasure the patient again.
- It is strongly recommended that you use the metric system. The tendency to round off numbers becomes problematic when an inch is the measure.
- Bone age: gives a level of bone maturation based on centers of ossification and closure of epiphyses.
- Up to an age of 2 years, a hemiskeletal bone age (Elgenmark method) is more accurate; after that, obtain a left hand/wrist radiograph using the method of Greulich and Pyle.

## Laboratory Studies
- General screening tests: CBC with differential, ESR/CRP, celiac screening, BMP, urinalysis, bone age, free $T_4$ and TSH, prolactin (postpuberty), IGF-BP3, IGF-1 (>4 years of age)
- Specialized tests: karyotype, growth hormone stimulation test; dexamethasone suppression test
  - Growth hormone stimulation test
    - There is no gold standard test for the diagnosis of growth hormone deficiency.
    - Growth hormone stimulation tests are needed because of the pulsatile nature of growth hormone release. A growth hormone level by itself is meaningless in the evaluation of short stature. Provocative agents include clonidine, L-dopa, arginine, insulin, glucagon, and growth hormone–releasing hormone.
    - Up to 25% of normal children fail any given stimulation test, so it is important to consider the rest of the clinical picture and document abnormal results using two different agents to classify a patient as growth hormone deficient. It is considered a pass if the stimulation test has a peak growth hormone response >7-10 ng/mL.

## Treatment (Growth Hormone Therapy)
- Food and Drug Administration–approved indications for the use of growth hormone.
  - Growth hormone deficiency
  - Turner syndrome
- SHOX deficiency.
  - Renal insufficiency
  - Prader-Willi syndrome
  - SGA
  - Idiopathic short stature (predicted target height: girls, <4′ 11″; boys, <5′ 3″)
- Effectiveness: best response in the first year of therapy.
- Administration and dosage.
  - Give as an SC injection starting at 0.3 mg/kg/week given 6-7 day/week.
  - For patients with Turner syndrome, give 0.35 mg/kg/week.
- Cost: expensive (approximately $52,000 per inch of growth).
- Potential adverse effects: slipped capital femoral epiphysis, glucose intolerance/diabetes, pseudotumor cerebri, scoliosis. Some individuals with short stature will not respond to growth hormone.

## PUBERTAL DEVELOPMENT

### Definitions

- Puberty is the stage when primary and secondary sexual characteristics develop, and growth is completed. Pubertal changes are a consequence of increased gonadotropins and sex steroid secretion.
- Adrenarche: increased adrenal androgen that causes sexual hair and typically occurs at approximately the same time as puberty. However, in some disorders, this may occur prematurely, independent of puberty.
- Gonadarche: increased gonadal activity resulting from a pubertal gonadotropin-releasing hormone (GnRH)-stimulated luteinizing hormone (LH) response or elevated estradiol.
- Pubarche: development of sexual hair.
- Thelarche: onset of breast development.
- Menarche: onset of menstrual periods.
- Pubertal gynecomastia: palpable or visible breast tissue in at least one-third to one-half of boys during puberty. It may coincide with the onset of puberty and presumably occurs due to imbalance between androgens and estrogens, and it occurs before testosterone levels have reached adult levels. It lasts about 6-18 months. Enlargement typically is <4 cm in diameter.
- Typical sequence of puberty.
  - Girls: breast development, initiation of growth spurt, pubic hair, and, lastly, menarche.
    ○ Around 15% of girls have pubarche prior to thelarche.
  - Boys: testicular growth, followed by pubic hair development, and finally the peak growth spurt.

### History

- Access for time of onset of pubertal changes such as presence of breasts, vaginal discharge, growth of pubic, axillary, or facial hair, and evidence of a growth spurt
  - Other signs and symptoms (neurologic) for CNS abnormalities, headaches, visual changes
- Medication or exposure history
- Ages at which parents underwent puberty; height of the biologic parents

### Physical Examination

- Tanner stages are used to grade pubertal progression, including breast development, testicular size, and pubic hair progression (see Appendix D). Breast and pubic hair progression is determined by a comparison method with the Tanner stages.
- The size of the testes is determined by using an orchidometer.
  - The Prader orchidometer consists of a set of ellipsoids encompassing the range of testicular volume from infancy to adulthood (1-25 mL) to use for direct comparison with the patient's testes.
  - A volume of 4 mL closely correlates with the onset of pubertal development. A volume of 4-6 mL corresponds to Tanner II, 8-10 mL to Tanner III, 12-15 mL to Tanner IV, and 20-25 mL to Tanner V.
- In girls, assess the vaginal mucosa for estrogen exposure (pink color, thickened mucosa, mucoid secretions).
- It is also very important to plot the patient's height and weight on a growth curve to determine any degree of growth acceleration and growth potential of the patient.

## PRECOCIOUS PUBERTY

- Classically defined as the premature onset and rapid progression of sexual development (i.e., breast development, testicular enlargement), with concomitant pubertal levels of hormones and inappropriate acceleration of skeletal age.
- Before age 8 in Caucasian girls (before 7 in African American or Hispanic girls). Before age 9 in boys.

### Etiology

- Central precocious puberty (CPP) (GnRH dependent)
  - Idiopathic (95% in girls)
  - CNS abnormalities (most common cause in males)
  - Lesion (e.g., hamartoma)
  - Disorder (e.g., cerebral palsy)
  - Neurofibromatosis
- Peripheral-Precocious Pseudopuberty (PPP) (GnRH independent)
  - Congenital virilizing adrenal hyperplasia
  - McCune-Albright syndrome (peripheral precocity + fibrous dysplasia of bone + café-au-lait macules)
  - Tumors (e.g., ovarian granulosa cell tumor, Leydig cell tumor, adrenal adenoma/adenocarcinoma, human chorionic gonadotropin-secreting tumor)
  - Ovarian cysts
  - Exogenous sex steroids (e.g., estrogen or testosterone cream, oral contraceptives)
  - Primary hypothyroidism
  - Familial testotoxicosis

### Diagnosis

*Initial Testing*

- Gonadotropin elevation with LH predominance in the pubertal range is consistent with CPP.
- Plasma ultrasensitive estradiol levels and testosterone levels at time of obtaining gonadotropins, respectively, in girls and boys are helpful on making this diagnosis.
- A GnRH analogue stimulation test (leuprolide) in which gonadotropins are measured at intervals following injection of GnRH can be used to diagnose CPP. If an LH peak of >5 IU/L is present, it is consistent with a pubertal response.
- Bone age will eventually show an acceleration.

*Imaging*

- Brain magnetic resonance imaging (MRI) should be performed in all boys with CPP or girls in which cause is unexplained.
- Pelvic ultrasound provides information on uterine and ovarian size and hormonal stimulation, as well as possible ovarian cyst or tumor.

### Treatment

- Treat the underlying cause if there is one (e.g., tumor, hypothyroidism, CAH).
- In other cases, GnRH therapy can be used to pause centrally mediated pubertal development, to avoid growth impairment, and to try to reach maximum growth potential.
- Monitor response to treatment with LH, FSH, (testosterone or estradiol) several months after initiating treatment.

- In conditions with autonomous gonadal steroid production, such as McCune-Albright syndrome or testotoxicosis, adjunct therapy with aromatase inhibitors, estrogen receptor antagonists, spironolactone, or ketoconazole has been used.

## PREMATURE ADRENARCHE

- The presence of adrenarche before age 9 for boys and 8 for girls
- This can be differentiated from true puberty by the presence of adrenarche (sexual hair) without the presence of testicular enlargement or breast development.

### Etiology

- Idiopathic, benign (most common)
- True central precocious puberty
- Congenital adrenal hyperplasia
- Adrenal or gonadal androgen secretory tumors
- Exogenous androgen exposure

### Diagnosis

- Bone age
- 17-OH Progesterone level (to rule out CAH)
- Dehydroepiandrosterone sulfate (DHEAS) (to exclude adrenal tumor)
- Free and total testosterone

### Treatment

- Treatment is geared to treating the underlying disorder if present.
- If no underlying disorder is present, then reassurance is appropriate.

### Benign Premature Thelarche

- Bilateral or unilateral breast development between 6 and 24 months of life
- Not associated with other signs of sexual development or bone age advancement
- This is usually self-limiting and regress after a few months thus, reassessment and observation at 6 months is appropriate

## DELAYED PUBERTY

- This is defined as lack of pubertal changes by age 13 in girls and 14 in boys.
- Patients should also have an endocrine evaluation if >5 years have elapsed between the first signs of puberty and completion of genital growth in boys or menarche in girls (or if no menarche by 16 years).

### Etiology

- Delayed
  - Constitutional delay of growth and maturation (most common cause)
  - Hypothyroidism
  - Chronic illness and malnutrition
- Central (low gonadotropins)
  - Intracranial pathology: craniopharyngioma, prolactinoma, empty sella
  - Congenital conditions: genetic syndromes such as Kallmann syndrome (isolated gonadotropin deficiency with anosmia), Prader-Willi syndrome, Bardet-Biedl syndrome, CHARGE, septooptic dysplasia
  - Acquired conditions: cranial radiation, autoimmune disease, sickle cell, hemosiderosis

- Gonadal (high gonadotropins)
  - Genetic syndromes: Turner syndrome, Klinefelter syndrome, androgen insensitivity, 5α-reductase deficiency, mixed gonadal dysgenesis, vanishing testis
  - Acquired conditions: autoimmune, mumps, orchitis, chemotherapy, surgery, gonadal torsion, radiation

## Diagnosis

- There is no reliable test to differentiate between those with normal late puberty (constitutional delay of growth and maturation) and those who have actual disorders preventing puberty.
- Therefore, all patients with no signs of puberty by 14 years of age, without a family history of late puberty, should have an evaluation, which should include the following:
  - Free $T_4$ and TSH (to exclude hypothyroidism)
  - LH and FSH (to exclude primary gonadal failure, elevated LH and FSH would indicate this)
  - Smell test (to exclude Kallmann syndrome)
  - Head MRI (to exclude intracranial pathology)
  - Testosterone or estradiol level
  - Prolactin (to exclude prolactinoma)
  - Bone age

## Treatment

- Focus should be on treating the underlying cause first if one is identified.
- Treatment of primary gonadal failure as a cause of delayed puberty in males typically involves the administration of testosterone IM injections (50-100 mg) on a monthly basis at gradually increasing doses or gradually increasing oral estrogen replacement for girls orally or by transdermal patch.
- Measure response in boys through testosterone levels to determine correct dose.

## CALCIUM METABOLISM

- Serum calcium circulates in the ionized form; representing 50% of total serum calcium. Of the remainder 40% circulate bound to albumin or globulin.
- Serum calcium is regulated within close limits by several factors:
  - Vitamin D [1,25 (OH)2-D]: induced in response to PTH, hypophosphatemia, and hypocalcemia
    - Increases absorption of calcium and phosphorus from small intestine
    - Facilitates action of PTH on distal tube to increases retention of calcium and decreases retention of phosphorus
  - PTH: secreted in response to a decrease in serum ionized calcium or elevated phosphorus concentration; also in response to calcitriol and magnesium
    - Increases renal calcium absorption and decreases reabsorption of phosphorus
    - Mobilizes calcium from skeleton by transforming osteoblast to osteoclast
    - Increases renal 1α-hydroxylation of 25(OH)-D
  - Calcitonin: secreted from parafollicular cells in the medulla of thyroid gland
    - Decreases serum calcium by inhibiting action of osteoclast on bone, and restoring calcium into bone
    - Antagonizes the effect of PTH on bone and kidney; no effect on intestine

- Magnesium
  - Necessary for secretion of PTH (in states of hypomagnesemia, hypocalcemia may develop)

## HYPOCALCEMIA

### Etiology

- Parathyroid Dysfunction/hypoparathyroidism:
  - Alteration in Ca sensing
    - Autosomal dominant hypocalcemia: activating mutation to calcium receptor
  - Hypoparathyroidism
    - Inappropriately low or normal PTH in the setting of a low calcium
    - Parathyroid agenesis/dysfunction: familial, AD, AR, X-linked recessive (e.g., San-jad-Sakati, Barakat, Kenny-Caffey, Di-George)
    - Acquired hypoparathyroidism
      - Autoimmune: isolated or autoimmune polyendocrinopathy
      - Mitochondrial disease: Kearns-Sayre
      - Infiltrative processes: Wilson, hemochromatosis
      - Granulomatous disorders
      - Radiation exposure/postsurgical
      - Idiopathic
    - Abnormal PTH secretion: hypomagnesemia or critical illness
    - Peripheral resistance to PTH: pseudohypoparathyroidism, pseudopseudohypo-parathyroidism, loss of function mutation to PTHR1: Blomstrand chondroplasia
- Vitamin D abnormalities
  - Vitamin D deficiency: 25-hydroxyvitamin D level <20 (deficient), <30 (insuf-ficient)
    - Etiology: nutritional deficiency, inadequate sun exposure, liver disease: impaired 25(OH)D production. Iatrogenic: that is, phenobarbital: increased turnover to inactive metabolites
  - Vitamin D resistance:
    - Hydroxylase deficiency or vitamin D receptor dysfunction: VDDR types I & II
- Alteration in organs involved in calcium homeostasis
  - Renal failure causes hyperphosphatemia: excess phosphate complexes with calcium; or lack of calcitriol production impairs intestinal calcium absorption.
  - Intestinal malabsorption.
  - Hungry bone syndrome.
- Other causes
  - High phosphate load: tumor lysis, rhabdomyolysis, etc.
  - Acute illness: for example, pancreatitis
  - Drugs: furosemide, calcitonin, bisphosphonate

### Signs and Symptoms

- Can be asymptomatic if long standing.
- Neuromuscular irritability, muscle cramps, weakness, lethargy, paresthesia of the extremities and in most severe situation convulsions and/or laryngospasm.
- Lengthening of QTc interval on ECG.
- Chronic hypocalcemia: calcification of basal ganglia, cataract formation, poor teeth enamel formation.

- Chvostek sign: twitching at the angle of the mouth after tapping of facial nerve below zygomatic arch.
- Trousseau sign: carpopedal spasm when blood pressure cuff is inflated 15 mm Hg above systolic blood pressure, for 2-5 minutes.
- In pseudohypoparathyroidism, there is peripheral resistance to PTH despite apparent normal functioning PTHR1 receptors so patients will present with hypocalcemia, hyperphosphatemia, elevated PTH levels, no concomitant increase in calcitriol level, or increased renal phosphaturia. Some patients may present with short stature, obesity, round face, subcutaneous ossifications, short 4th and 5th metacarpal bones known as Albright hereditary osteodystrophy.

## Biochemical Evaluation

Monitor serum calcium, albumin, ionized calcium (in the setting of low albumin, acidosis, alkalosis), magnesium, phosphate, PTH, 25(OH)D, 1,25(OH)2D, urine measurements of calcium, phosphate, and creatinine (in conjunction with serum measurements) (Fig. 18-8).

## Management of Acute Hypocalcemia

*In Symptomatic Patients*
- Monitoring ECG.
- Calcium gluconate 10%: 2 mL/kg administered slowly over 10 minutes to avoid cardiac conduction problems.
- Repeat dose every 6-8 hours.
- Phosphate and bicarbonate infusions should never be given concomitantly to prevent calcium salt precipitation.
- Central IV access is preferable; extravasation of calcium causes severe chemical burns and skin damage.
- To maintain normocalcemia; continuous IV infusion of calcium (20-80 mg Ca/kg/24 hours).

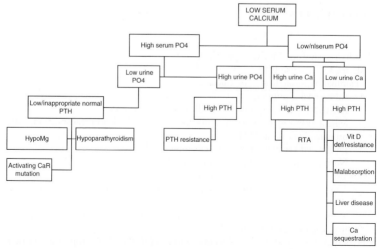

**Figure 18-8.** Diagnostic algorithm of hypocalcemia.

- Continuous infusion preferable over bolus in cases of good IV access; large fraction of calcium content in bolus is lost in urine.
- Titrate infusion to achieve a low normal serum calcium.
- Correct hypomagnesemia when present: $MgSO_4$ (50% solution) 25-50 mg Mg/kg IV or IM every 4-6 hours. Maintenance dose of 30-60 mg Mg/kg/day oral or continuous infusion if needed.

*In Asymptomatic Patients*
- Treat underlying cause.
- Oral therapy should be first line of treatment.
- Calcium supplements: calcium carbonate (40% Ca), calcium citrate (21% Ca), calcium gluconate (9.4% Ca), calcium glubionate (6.6% Ca).
- Dose of oral calcium: 25-100 mg Ca/kg/day divided every 4-6 hours.
- Regular monitoring of calcium, phosphorus, and urine calcium/creatinine.

## Management of Chronic Hypocalcemia

- Treat underlying cause.
- Calcium supplements to achieve serum calcium that doesn't cause symptoms, avoid hypercalcemia and excessive hypercalciuria.
- Aim for serum calcium levels in low normal range ~ 8.5-9 mg/dL to limit hypercalciuria.
- Addition of thiazide diuretic limits hypercalciuria.
- Correction of underlying hypomagnesemia.
- Calcitriol: 10-50 ng/kg/day: hypoparathyroidism, renal failure, liver disease, defects in 1-α-hydroxylase function.
- In case of intestinal malabsorption, consider calcidiol 1-3 μg/kg/day.
- Phosphate binders are not required usually.
- Regular monitoring of calcium, phosphorus, and urine calcium/creatinine.
- In case of vitamin D deficiency: 1000-4000 international units of vitamin D3 daily. Monitor 25-hydroxyvitamin D level 2-3 months after starting treatment.

## HYPERCALCEMIA

### Etiology
- Parathyroid dysfunction/hyperparathyroidism
  - Altered Ca2+ sensing
    ○ Familial hypocalciuric hypercalcemia
      – Autosomal dominant
      – Inactivating mutation in one of alleles coding for CaR
      – Mild asymptomatic hypercalcemia, increased renal calcium reabsorption, inappropriately normal PTH
      – Diagnosed incidentally on lab screening
      – Normal appearance of parathyroid gland
    ○ Neonatal sever hyperparathyroidism
      – Homozygous for inactivation mutation or heterozygous for a very severe inactivation mutation
      – Manifestations of hyperparathyroidism, hyperplasia of parathyroid gland that may require surgical removal
  - Hyperparathyroidism: hypercalcemia with elevated or inappropriately normal PTH; 80% adenomatous changes and other subset show generalized hyperplasia.

- ○ Primary hyperparathyroidism
  - – Sporadic forms
  - – Multiple endocrine neoplasia types I and IIa
  - – Tc-99 (Sestamibi) scan confirms the diagnosis.
- ○ Secondary/tertiary hyperparathyroidism: longstanding stimulation of parathyroid gland in response to chronic hypocalcemia in hyperplastic changes with concomitant increase in PTH secretion
  - – Renal failure, renal tubular acidosis
  - – Chronic therapy for hypophosphatemic rickets
- • Excessive PTH receptor activity
- ○ Jansen syndrome
  - – Mutation of PTH receptor causing it to be constitutively active
  - – Hypercalcemia, metaphyseal dysplasia, and other skeletal finding consistent with hyperparathyroidism
  - – Undetectable PTH levels because parathyroid responds appropriately to hypercalcemia
- • Vitamin D excess
  - • Nutritional or therapeutic: increase intestinal calcium absorption and hypercalcemia, increase phosphate absorption and appropriately suppressed PTH
  - • Granulomatous disorders: unregulated expression of 1-α-hydroxylase in monocytic cells leading to production of 1,25(OH)2D (i.e., sarcoidosis, tuberculosis, leprosy)
- • Immobilization
  - • Prolonged for more than 2 weeks results in decreased bone accretion and increased resorption, initially noted as hypercalciuria; when persistent frank hypercalcemia
- • Malignancy
  - • Rare in children
  - • Can be due to metastases to bone with concomitant dissolution of mineral content
  - • Can be due to production of lytic factors by original tumor that promote calcium mobilization (PTHrP, IL6, TNF, prostaglandin)
- • Excess thyroid hormone: disproportional stimulation of osteoclast function causing bone resorption and hypercalcemia
- • Other causes
  - • Drugs (thiazide, lithium)
  - • Vitamin A excess: osteoclast-mediated bone resorption
  - • High calcium load: milk alkali syndrome
  - • Hypophosphatemia
  - • Adrenal insufficiency, pheochromocytoma, and vasoactive polypeptide-secreting tumors' mechanisms not well defined
- • Infancy and neonates
  - ○ Williams syndrome
    - – Transiently during infancy in 15%.
    - – Unknown etiology; mildly elevated calcitriol and calcidiol have been reported.
    - – Resolve before 1st year of life; hypercalciuria persists.
  - ○ Subcutaneous fat necrosis
    - – Neonates, often premature with traumatic birth or critical illness with poor perfusion.
    - – Subcutaneous fat undergoes necrosis, significant infiltration by mononuclear cells.
    - – Etiology unknown, excessive prostaglandin E production, and mononuclear-derived calcitriol were mildly elevated in some cases.

## Signs and Symptoms

- Aymptomatic
- Failure to thrive arrest in weight gain and linear growth
- Mild hypercalcemia (12-13.5 mg/dL)
  - Generalized weakness, anorexia, constipation, and polyuria
- Severe hypercalcemia (>13.5 mg/dL)
  - Nausea, vomiting, dehydration and encephalopathic features with coma and seizure
  - Respiratory distress, apnea, and hypotonia in neonates

## Physical Examination

- Typically normal.
- When not dehydrated, hypertension may be noted.
- Shortened QTc on ECG.
- Chronic hypercalcemia: calcification in skin, kidney, SQ tissue, cardiac arteries, and gastric mucosa.

## Biochemical Evaluation

Similar to evaluation in hypocalcemia (Fig. 18-9)

## Management of Hypercalcemia

When hypercalcemia is severe or patient is symptomatic (cardiac, gastrointestinal, or CNS dysfunction)

- Provide adequate hydration, preferably normal saline at 3 L/m² for the first 24-48 hours.
- Loop diuretic (furosemide) 1 mg/kg every 6 hours.
- If it doesn't respond to these initial measures
  - Calcitonin (blocks bone resorption) 4 U/kg SQ every 12 hours; efficacy diminishes with continuous administration due to tachyphylaxis.
  - Bisphosphonate (inhibit osteoclast action) etidronate 7.5 mg/kg/day or pamidronate 0.5-1 mg/kg/dose given as single-dose IV infusion.
  Additional management options are determined by the etiology of hypercalcemia.

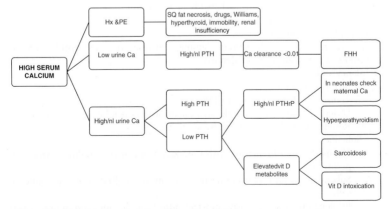

Figure 18-9. **Diagnostic algorithm of hypercalcemia.**

- Glucocorticoids-prednisone—1 mg/kg/day: inhibits both 1-α-hydroxylase activity and intestinal Ca absorption in cases of excess vitamin D ingestion or activity, and reduces interlukin-1-β production in JRA
- Surgical resection
  - Of affected gland in cases of adenoma
  - Three and one-half glands in cases of 4-gland hyperplasia or secondary hyperparathyroidism
  - Total parathyroidectomy with autotransplantation of minced parathyroid gland for patients with MEN

## SUGGESTED READINGS

American Diabetes Association. Standards of medical care in diabetes. Diabetes Care 2020;44(Suppl 1).

Brook C, Clayton P, Brown R. Clinical Paediatric Endocrinology. 7th Ed. Chichester, UK: Wiley Blackwell, 2019.

Guss C, Shumer D, Katz-Wise SL. Transgender and gender nonconforming adolescent care: psychosocial and medical considerations. Curr Opin Pediatr 2015;27(4):421–426.

Lifshitz F. Pediatric Endocrinology. 5th Ed. New York, NY: CRC Press, 2006.

Link to Pediatric Endocrine Society Clinical Practice Guidelines. Available at: https://pedsendo.org/society-topic/care-guidelines/

Radovick S, MacGillivray MH. Pediatric Endocrinology: A Practical Clinical Guide. 3rd Ed. New York, NY: Springer Science & Business Media, 2018.

Sarafoglou K, Hoffmann G, Roth K. Pediatric Endocrinology and Inborn Errors of Metabolism. 2nd Ed. New York, NY: McGraw Hill Companies, 2017.

Sperling M, ed. Pediatric Endocrinology. 5th Ed. Elsevier Health Sciences, 2020.

Hembree WC, Cohen-Kettenis PT, Gooren L, et al. Endocrine treatment of gender-dysphoric/gender-incongruent persons: an endocrine society clinical practice guideline. J Clin Endocrinol Metab 2017;102(11):3869–3903.

# 19 Hematology and Oncology
Sima Bhatt and Melanie Fields

## FEVER AND NEUTROPENIA

### General Principles
- Absolute neutrophil count (ANC) <1500/μL is defined as neutropenia.
  - Risk of infection increases dramatically with severe neutropenia (ANC < 500/μL).
- Differential diagnosis
  - Congenital neutropenia: severe congenital neutropenia, cyclic neutropenia, reticular dysgenesis, autoimmune neutropenia, Shwachman-Diamond syndrome, Fanconi anemia
  - Acquired neutropenia: malignancy, chemotherapy, radiation, aplastic anemia (autoimmune), infection (viral, bacterial sepsis), and hypersplenism
- Laboratory evaluation: complete blood count (CBC), blood cultures (including each lumen of venous access device)
  - Only 30% of patients have positive blood cultures.
    - The most common organisms are *Streptococcus* spp., *Staphylococcus epidermidis, Pseudomonas aeruginosa, Escherichia coli, Klebsiella pneumoniae, Staphylococcus aureus*, methicillin-resistant *S. aureus, Enterococcus faecalis, Campylobacter jejuni, Candida albicans*, and vancomycin-resistant *Enterococcus.*
  - Obtain urine culture if the patient has hematuria or symptoms of a urinary tract infection (UTI).
- Treatment: Immediately start a broad-spectrum antibiotic, such as cefepime.
  - Alternate lumens if more than one is present.
  - For patients allergic to penicillin/cephalosporins, alternatives include meropenem, imipenem, or aztreonam.
  - Add vancomycin (dosing per age and renal function) after 48 hours of persistent fever.
    - Start vancomycin immediately for unstable patients, patients with acute myeloid leukemia (AML) on chemotherapy (at risk for α-streptococcal sepsis), signs of sinus infection (also consider fungal coverage), cutaneous breakdown, or history of prior gram-positive infection.
  - Add antifungal therapy, amphotericin B or voriconazole, if fever lasts for >5 days.
  - For signs of sepsis (e.g., hypotension), consider adding an aminoglycoside.
  - Continue trimethoprim-sulfamethoxazole (TMP-SMX) prophylaxis.
  - For oncology patients with fever, neutropenia, and negative blood culture results, continue antibiotic therapy until the patient is afebrile for 24 hours and has a rising ANC.
    - If an oncology patient has a positive blood culture, he/she should complete a 7- to 10-day course of antibiotics (choice of antibiotic depends on sensitivity analysis of the isolated organism) after the first negative blood culture and should not be discharged until afebrile for a minimum of 24 hours with a rising ANC.

○ Evaluate patients with tachypnea, low $O_2$ saturation, and fever for *Pneumocystis jirovecii* infection.
  – Lung signs are often minimal.
  – Chest radiograph may show diffuse interstitial disease.
  – Definitive testing includes bronchoalveolar lavage.
  – Treatment includes glucocorticoid pulses and high-dose TMP-SMX.

## ONCOLOGIC EMERGENCIES

### Superior Vena Cava Syndrome/Superior Mediastinal Syndrome

- Clinical presentation: cough, hoarseness, dyspnea, orthopnea, wheezing, stridor, chest pain, upper body or facial swelling, plethora and cyanosis of the face and neck, and diaphoresis.
- Differential diagnosis depends on the location of the mass causing the syndrome.
  - Posterior mediastinum: neuroblastoma, paraganglionic masses, and primitive neuroectodermal tumor (PNET)
  - Anterior/superior mediastinum: T lymphoma, teratoma, thymoma, and thyroid masses
- Because of risks of anesthesia, the diagnosis should be established using the least invasive means possible.
  - Check serum α-fetoprotein and human chorionic gonadotropin to differentiate germ-cell tumors from lymphomas.
  - Use spiral computed tomography (CT) to differentiate calcification in neuroblastoma.
  - Use peripheral smear in the case of lymphoblastic lymphomas.
- Treatment
  - Low risk: biopsy, then treatment
    ○ Symptomatic patients should be monitored in the intensive care unit (ICU).
  - High risk: empiric therapy of prednisone 40 mg/m²/day divided four times a day and/or radiotherapy should be given.
    ○ As soon as the patient has been stabilized, the lesion should be biopsied to improve diagnostic yield.

### Pleural/Pericardial Effusion

- Thoracentesis: Send for protein content, specific gravity, cell count, lactate dehydrogenase (LDH), cytology, culture, and other biologic/immunologic assays.
- Tamponade: Chest radiograph shows water bag cardiac shadow, and electrocardiogram (ECG) shows low-voltage QRS.
- Treatment: Pericardiocentesis may relieve cardiac symptoms, but the underlying etiology must ultimately be treated.

### Massive Hemoptysis

- Differential diagnosis: invasive pulmonary aspergillosis (incidence with hemoptysis is 2-26%), metastatic disease, toxicity from therapy, coagulopathy (disseminated intravascular coagulation [DIC]), and thrombocytopenia.
- Diagnosis involves chest radiography and chest CT after stabilization.
- Treatment involves lying on same side as hemorrhage to prevent collection in the normal lung, transfusion with platelets, RBCs, fresh frozen plasma (FFP) and cryoprecipitate as needed, and volume resuscitation.

## Neutropenic Enterocolitis (aka Typhlitis)

- Inflammation of the bowel wall, most commonly of the terminal ileum and cecum, in a neutropenic patient.
- Signs and symptoms are abdominal pain in setting of severe neutropenia, fever, and either diarrhea or paralytic ileus.
  - Monitor closely for an acute, surgical abdomen because these patients are at a high risk for perforation.
- Diagnose with abdominal ultrasound or CT scan.
- Treatment
  - Broad-spectrum antibiotics to cover gram-negative enterics and anaerobes.
  - Bowel rest/decompression.
  - Consider treatment with G-CSF and irradiated granulocytes.
  - Surgical intervention is reserved for patients with bowel perforation or other dire complications.

## Hemorrhagic Cystitis

- Painless blood in the urine (microscopic more common than macroscopic) secondary to chemotherapy (most commonly cyclophosphamide or ifosfamide)
  - Prevention: vigorous hydration during and after chemotherapy treatment, and mercaptoethane sulfonate (Mesna)
- Diagnosis: urinalysis, ultrasound (boggy, edematous bladder wall), cystoscopy
  - BK virus or adenovirus infection should be considered in hematopoietic stem cell transplant (HSCT) patients
- Treatment
  - Stop radiation treatment/chemotherapy.
  - Hydration.
  - Transfusion to correct low platelets and coagulopathy.
  - Consult urology for bladder irrigation with cold saline via catheter or cystoscope to remove blood clots.

## Altered Consciousness

- Differential diagnosis: metastatic disease, sepsis/DIC, primary central nervous system (CNS) infection (fungal, bacterial, or viral encephalitis), metabolic abnormality, leukoencephalopathy, intracranial hemorrhage, cerebrovascular accident (CVA), oversedation, hypercalcemia, hyperammonemia because of hepatic dysfunction
  - Chemotherapy induced
    - Ifosfamide may cause symptoms of acute somnolence, neurologic deterioration, seizure, and coma.
      - Patients are at higher risk with poor renal clearance, which leads to a buildup of the toxic metabolite chloroacetaldehyde.
    - Other therapeutic agents to consider: carmustine, cisplatin, thiotepa, high-dose cytarabine (Ara-C), amphotericin, interleukin-2, trans-retinoic acid.

## Cerebrovascular Accident (Stroke)

- Differential diagnosis: cerebral arterial/venous thrombosis as a result of inherited thrombophilia or chemotherapy (L-asparaginase), intracranial hemorrhage, sepsis/DIC, and radiation therapy–induced vascular occlusions
  - The most common cause of stroke within the hematology/oncology patient population is sickle cell disease (SCD) (discussed below).

- Diagnose with magnetic resonance imaging (MRI) and CT (most helpful if concerned for hemorrhage)
  - The MRI may need to be repeated in 7-10 days to evaluate full extent of infarct.
  - Treatment: Consider corticosteroids, mannitol, FFP (± antithrombin III concentrate in patients with L-asparaginase-induced CVA), and platelets depending on etiology and symptoms.

## Seizures

- Differential diagnosis: metastatic disease, CVA, infection, chemotherapy (intrathecal methotrexate, Ara-C, busulfan, etc.), syndrome of inappropriate secretion of antidiuretic hormone/hyponatremia (vincristine, cyclophosphamide, etc.)
- Laboratory evaluation: consider electrolyte evaluation, anticonvulsant drug levels, EEG, CT with and without contrast, MRI, and cerebrospinal fluid (CSF) analysis
- Treatment
  - Seizure safety precautions (roll patient on side in case of vomiting, move patient to safe environment, remove all items from mouth) and monitor vital signs to provide supplemental $O_2$ as needed
  - Anticonvulsant therapy to acutely stop seizure activity
    - Lorazepam (Ativan): 0.05-0.1 mg/kg IV push over 2 minutes (max dose 4 mg).
    - Diazepam (Valium): Administer per rectum. Dosing dependent on age and weight.
  - Monitor closely for respiratory depression with these medications.
  - Address underlying problem (e.g., infection).

## Spinal Cord Compression

- Symptoms: back pain (local or radicular) occurs in 80% of cases.
  - Any patient with cancer and back pain should be considered to have spinal cord compression until proven otherwise.
- Evaluation: spine radiographs (diagnosis confirmed by plain radiographs in <50% of cases), bone scan, and MRI (with and without gadolinium)
  - If patients are not ambulatory, they should undergo emergent MRI (or myelography).
- Treatment: dexamethasone bolus dose of 1-2 mg/kg IV immediately, followed by MRI

## Hyperleukocytosis

- White blood cell (WBC) count >100,000/µL
- Signs and symptoms: hypoxia, dyspnea, blurred vision, agitation, confusion, stupor, cyanosis
- Treatment: hydration, alkalinization, allopurinol or urate oxidase (rasburicase), leukapheresis, and/or hydroxyurea
  - Transfuse RBCs with caution (keep Hb <10 g/dL to minimize viscosity)
- Complications: death, CNS hemorrhage, thrombosis, pulmonary leukostasis, metabolic derangements (hyperkalemia, hypocalcemia/hyperphosphatemia), renal failure, gastrointestinal hemorrhage

## Tumor Lysis Syndrome

- Cell lysis resulting in the triad of hyperuricemia, hyperkalemia, and hyperphosphatemia, which can then cause secondary renal failure and symptomatic hypocalcemia
  - May trigger DIC, especially in patients with high tumor burdens

- Risk factors: bulky abdominal tumors (e.g., Burkitt lymphoma), hyperleukocytosis, increased uric acid and LDH levels, poor urinary output
- Laboratory studies: CBC, serum electrolytes, calcium, phosphorus, uric acid, urinalysis, LDH, prothrombin time/partial thromboplastin time (PT/PTT)
  - Consider D-dimer, fibrinogen, and fibrin degradation product (FDP) if concerned for DIC
- Imaging: ECG for hyperkalemia, ultrasound to rule out kidney infiltrations or ureteral obstruction
- Treatment
  - Hydration: $D_5W$ + 40 mEq/L $NaHCO_3$ at 3000 mL/m²/day.
  - Avoid potassium in IV fluid.
  - Allopurinol: 10 mg/kg/day or 300 mg/m²/day (divided tid, maximum of 600 mg/day), or urate oxidase (Rasburicase) 0.15 mg/kg IV once (subsequent dosing dependent on uric acid levels).
    - Test for glucose-6-phosphate dehydrogenase (G6PD) deficiency prior to giving urate oxidase in males of African or Mediterranean descent.
  - Monitor serum electrolytes, phosphorus, calcium, uric acid, and urinalysis (DIC profile if needed) multiple times per day until laboratory values stabilize.
  - Consider dialysis if the patient is symptomatic from electrolyte derangements and/ or the patient's electrolytes cannot be normalized.
  - For hyperkalemia, stop all potassium infusions, Kayexalate (1 g/kg PO with 50% sorbitol), calcium gluconate for cardioprotection only, insulin (0.1 unit/kg + 2 mL/kg of 25% glucose), and albuterol nebulizer therapy for temporary palliation.

## Hypercalcemia

- Symptoms: anorexia, nausea, vomiting, polyuria, diarrhea resulting in dehydration, gastrointestinal/renal impairment, lethargy, depression, hypotonia, stupor, coma, bradycardia, and nocturia.
- Risk factors: paraneoplastic syndrome, hyperleukocytosis, and tumor lysis syndrome.
- Treatment: Note that a serum calcium level <14 mg/dL may respond to loop diuretics alone (see later discussion).
  - Pamidronate
  - Hydration with normal saline (three times maintenance) and loop diuretics
  - Glucocorticoids (prednisone 1.5-2 mg/kg/day): requires 2-3 days to work

## HEMATOPOIETIC STEM CELL TRANSPLANT ISSUES

### Sinusoidal Obstructive Syndrome

- Capillary endothelial inflammation of the liver leading to third spacing of fluids.
- Clinical presentation usually occurs in the first 30 days post-BMT, while the greatest risk is within the first 10 days post-BMT.
  - Hepatomegaly right upper quadrant pain, jaundice (usually hyperbilirubinemia without any other liver function abnormalities until end stage), ascites/weight gain, and platelet consumption
- Risk factors: preexisting hepatitis, antibiotic usage before treatment (vancomycin, acyclovir), age >15 years, CMV seropositive, female sex, pretreatment radiation to abdomen, intensive conditioning (single-dose total body irradiation [TBI], use of busulfan), and second BMT.

- Treatment is primarily supportive including diuretics, renal replacement therapy, and blood product transfusions as needed (platelets, FFP, cryoprecipitate).
  - Defibrotide, a single-stranded polydeoxyribonucleotide with antithrombotic properties, is the only pharmacologic therapy available.

## Fluid Management

BMT patients are fluid restricted starting 12-24 hours infusion of stem cells at 1500/$m^2$/day until engraftment occurs.

## Infection

- The threshold for suspecting infection in children undergoing transplant is very low. Any change in clinical status should alert a provider to the possibility of infection.
- Prophylactic antibiotics may be used when ANC is <500/$\mu$L, for patients early post-HSCT (first 100 days) and/or patient with active graft versus host disease (GVHD).
- Consider the addition of vancomycin and amphotericin, respectively, at 24 and 48 hours of continued fevers.
- Drug interaction of antifungals, such as voriconazole, with immunosuppressants, such as cyclosporine A and tacrolimus, should be considered when adding or adjusting medications.

## Vaccination

- Vaccinations are resumed in HSCT recipients 6-12 months posttransplant.
- Inactivated influenza vaccine can be offered as early as 4 months posttransplant.
- Live vaccines should be avoided until patients are at least 24 months posttransplant, off immunosuppression, and without active GVHD.

## Graft versus Host Disease

- GVHD occurs in recipients of allogeneic transplants when donor lymphocytes recognize and attack the "foreign" host cells.
- Acute GVHD occurs 20-100 days after BMT.
  - Symptoms: dermatitis (rash), hepatitis, cholestasis, colitis (diarrhea)
  - Prophylaxis to prevent GVHD may include a calcineurin inhibitor like cyclosporine (target range of 250-350 ng/mL) or tacrolimus (target range of 8-14 ng/mL), and posttransplant methotrexate or cyclophosphamide
  - Treatment: glucocorticoids (first line), steroid refractory GVHD (ruxolitinib for patients >12 years)
- Chronic GVHD occurs 100 or more days after HSCT.
  - Symptoms: sicca syndrome with thickened skin, lichen planus and/or papules, cholestatic jaundice, colitis (diarrhea) and eye lesions (dry eyes)
  - Treatment: glucocorticoids, calcineurin inhibitors, ibrutinib, azathioprine, mycophenolate, thalidomide, psoralen ultraviolet A (PUVA) (skin), hydroxychloroquine, and pentostatin

## ACUTE LYMPHOBLASTIC LEUKEMIA

- Epidemiology: Acute lymphoblastic leukemia (ALL) is the most common cancer in pediatrics.
- Clinical presentation: ALL presents with increased or decreased WBC with low platelets and/or hemoglobin (2 or more cell lines affected).

- Signs and symptoms: low-grade fever, fatigue, pallor, bone pain, night sweats, mucosal bleeds, petechiae, generalized lymphadenopathy, hepatomegaly, and/or splenomegaly
  - Retinal hemorrhage or leukemic infiltrates may be seen on fundoscopy.
- Risk assessment: age <1 year and >10 years, male sex, WBC > 50,000/µL at diagnosis, CNS disease, unfavorable cytogenetics, and pretreatment with glucocorticoids
  - Presence of trisomy +4, +10, +17, or t(12;21)(p13;q22) (*ETV6/RUNX1*) in the leukemia cells confers a favorable prognosis.
  - Presence of the Philadelphia chromosome [t(9;22)(q34;q11)] (*BCR/ABL*), Ph-like fusions (CRLF2/JAK and ABL-class fusions), iAMP21, hypodiploidy (<44 chromosomes) or translocations involving the mixed lineage leukemia (*MLL*) gene on 11q23 confer a poor prognosis.
- Classification: Types of ALL are differentiated by surface markers.
  - Precursor-B ALL is the most common and is CD19+ and CD20+, often with CD10+.
  - T cell: CD4+, CD8+, and TdT+.
  - Burkitt or mature B cell: surface immunoglobulin and CD20+.
- Treatment lasts approximately 2 years
  - Therapy starts with a 28-day induction cycle.
    - Prednisone, vincristine, and asparaginase
    - Adriamycin or daunorubicin is added for four-drug induction therapy in high-risk patients.
  - If the child is in remission at end of induction, he/she receives consolidation therapy, interim maintenance, and delayed intensification for approximately 24 weeks.
  - Maintenance therapy follows and typically involves daily oral 6-MP, weekly oral methotrexate, and an oral corticosteroid pulse, vincristine, and intrathecal methotrexate once every 12 weeks.
  - Children with CNS leukemia receive additional intrathecal therapy and occasionally radiation therapy.

## ACUTE MYELOBLASTIC LEUKEMIA

- AML has a poor prognosis when compared to ALL.
- Classification of AML is determined by surface markers (Table 19-1).

| TABLE 19-1 | Surface Markers for Acute Myeloblastic Leukemia | | | | |
|---|---|---|---|---|---|
| Marker | M1/M2 | M3 | M4/M5 | M6 | M7 |
| CD11b | | + | ++ | | |
| CD13 | | + | ++ | + | + |
| CD14 | | | ++ | | |
| CD15 | + | ++ | ++ | | |
| CD33 | ++ | ++ | ++ | ++ | ++ |
| CD34 | ++ | + | + | + | + |
| CD41 | | | | | ++ |
| CD42 | | | | | ++ |

- Risk assessment is determined by cytogenetics and response to induction therapy.
  - Presence of t(8;21)(q22;q22), inversion of chromosome 16, *NPM1* mutation or CEBPα mutation confers a favorable prognosis.
  - Presence of t(15;17)(q22;q21), which is characteristic of acute promyelocytic leukemia (APL), confers a favorable prognosis.
  - Presence of *FLT3* mutations, monosomy 5, monosomy 7, 5q-, or 11q23 abnormalities confers a worse prognosis.
  - Residual disease (bone marrow or extramedullary) at the end of induction confers a worse prognosis.
- Treatment is of shorter duration (approximately 6 months) but entails more intense chemotherapy compared with ALL.
  - Various chemotherapy combinations exist, but the mainstays of treatment are anthracyclines (e.g., daunorubicin, mitoxantrone, or idarubicin) and Ara-C.
  - Induction recovery and clinical remission is followed by courses of consolidation therapy.
  - Siblings are tested for human leukocyte antigen (HLA) matching for potential matched sibling allogeneic HSCT if a patient has a poor response to induction therapy or has high-risk cytogenetics.
    - Patients without a matched sibling are usually offered chemotherapy only if they have a complete remission after induction therapy.
    - Matched, unrelated donor transplant is considered at the time of relapse, or in the case of resistant leukemias, because of the risks associated with unrelated donor transplant.
  - AML therapy is associated with prolonged and severe neutropenia, and AML patients have a high risk of gram-positive sepsis, such as α-streptococcal and staphylococcal infections. Therefore, patients require antimicrobial prophylaxis during periods of neutropenia.

## NON-HODGKIN LYMPHOMA

- Non-Hodgkin lymphoma (NHL) encompasses >12 neoplasms.
- It is the most frequent malignancy in children with AIDS; thus, HIV screening should be performed in all children with NHL.
- Lineage category information is presented in Table 19-2.
- Clinical presentation depends on classification and grade.
  - Low grade: Painless, diffuse peripheral lymphadenopathy (LAD) seen primarily in older adults.
  - Intermediate grade: Painless peripheral LAD is the most common, but localized extranodal disease is also seen (e.g., GI and bone).
    - Median age is 55 years, but this type of NHL is also common in children and young adults.
  - High-grade lymphomas are most commonly seen in children and young adults.
    - Lymphoblastic lymphoma most commonly presents with mediastinal involvement, which manifests as shortness of breath, dyspnea, wheezing, stridor, dysphagia, and head/neck swelling.
    - Approximately two-thirds of patients with lymphoblastic lymphoma are male.
  - Small non–cleaved cell lymphoma (SNCCL)/Burkitt/non-Burkitt is also usually considered a childhood disease but has a second peak after 50 years of age.
    - Burkitt lymphoma commonly presents in the abdomen and GI tract (approximately 80%).

| TABLE 19-2 | Classification of Non-Hodgkin Lymphoma |
| --- | --- |

| Lineages (immunophenotype/genotype) | Median survival (years) |
| --- | --- |
| B lineage (nodal) | |
| Low grade: | |
| Small lymphocytic | 5.5–6 |
| Lymphoplasmacytic/lymphoplasmacytoid | 4 |
| Follicular small cleaved cell | 6.5–7 |
| Follicular mixed small cleaved/large cell | 4.5–5 |
| Intermediate grade: | |
| Follicular large cell | 2.5–3 |
| Diffuse small cleaved/mixed small and large | 3–4 |
| Intermediate lymphocytic/mantle cell | 3–5 |
| High grade: | |
| Diffuse large cell lymphoma | 1–2 |
| Immunoblastic | 0.5–1.5 |
| Small non–cleaved cell | 0.5–1 |
| T lineage: | |
| Lymphoblastic | 0.5–2 |
| Peripheral T-cell lymphoma | 1–2 |
| Primary extranodal lymphoma (classified by site; most are B-cell and MALT lineages) | |

- ○ Non-Burkitt lymphoma presents in the bone marrow and with peripheral LAD.
  - ○ Presentation in the right lower quadrant is common and can be confused with appendicitis.
- Diagnosis: physical examination, CBC, serum electrolytes with liver function studies, LDH, uric acid, chest radiograph, chest/abdomen/pelvis CT, bilateral bone marrow aspiration/biopsy, CSF analysis
  - Also consider a bone scan, MRI for bone marrow involvement, and/or positron emission tomography (PET) scan.
- Treatment of NHL is dependent on pathologic subtype and stage.
  - Therapy of Burkitt lymphoma is usually short (around 4-6 months), whereas T-cell lymphomas require treatment for a longer duration period, with emphasis on CNS prophylaxis.
    - ○ The addition of rituximab (anti-CD20) to the therapeutic protocol has improved outcomes.
    - ○ Patients with Burkitt lymphoma are at high risk for tumor lysis syndrome.

## HODGKIN LYMPHOMA

- Hodgkin lymphoma (HL) is characterized by a pleomorphic lymphocytic infiltrate.
  - Reed-Sternberg (RS) cells are multinucleated giant cells, which are the malignant cells of HL.

- Epidemiology: There is a bimodal age distribution, with an early peak in the mid-late 20s and a second peak after 50 years of age.
  - Most cases outside of the United States, and approximately one-third of cases in the United States, are associated with Epstein-Barr virus (EBV) in RS cells.
- Clinical presentation: painless and firm adenopathy that spreads contiguously
  - Supraclavicular and cervical lymphadenopathy is common, with mediastinal involvement seen in approximately two-thirds of patients.
  - Primary subdiaphragmatic disease is rare (approximately 3% of patients).
  - Screen for systemic symptoms, including fever >38°C for 3 consecutive days, drenching night sweats, or unexplained weight loss of 10% or more in the 6 months preceding admission.
    - "A" after stage designation denotes a lack of systemic symptoms, while a "B" denotes the presence of these systematic symptoms.
  - Generalized pruritus and ethyl alcohol–induced pain in lymph nodes are rare symptoms, but pathognomonic for Hodgkin disease.
- Diagnosis: physical examination for lymphadenopathy and hepatosplenomegaly, CBC (autoimmune thrombocytopenia and autoimmune hemolytic anemia are commonly associated with Hodgkin disease), LDH, ESR, uric acid, renal and hepatic function tests, neck/chest/abdomen/pelvic CT, and PET scan (more commonly used)
  - Bilateral bone marrow aspirate and biopsy should be obtained in patients with stage III–IV disease, with B symptoms, and at relapse.
- Therapy commonly involves cycles of multiagent chemotherapy (adriamycin, bleomycin, vinblastine, dactinomycin, brentuximab vedotin, and others). In some cases, external beam radiation is utilized. Checkpoint inhibitors like pembrolizumab are increasingly utilized for the treatment of Hodgkin lymphoma.

## WILMS TUMOR

- The most common renal tumor seen in children.
- Primary presentation is most frequently an abdominal mass that does not cross the midline (in contrast to neuroblastoma, which often crosses midline).
  - Most commonly unilateral, but can occur in both kidneys
- Diagnosis: chest (to assess for metastasis)/abdomen/pelvis CT, CBC, and evaluation of kidney and liver function.
- Histology (embryonal vs. anaplastic) and staging of tumor are important in determining the treatment regimen, which consists of chemotherapy and radiation therapy.
- Ten percent of Wilms tumors are associated with malformation syndromes:
  - Denys-Drash syndrome (*WT1* mutation on chromosome 11): a disorder affecting the kidney and genitalia, often involving ambiguous genitalia, nephropathy, and Wilms tumor
  - Sporadic aniridia (11p13 region → *PAX6* gene ): absence of the iris
  - WAGR syndrome (11p13 region deletion *WT1* suppressor gene product and *PAX6* gene): **W**ilms tumor, **A**niridia, **G**enitourinary anomalies, mental **R**etardation
  - Beckwith-Wiedemann syndrome (*IGF2, CDKN1C, H19, KCNQ1, KCNQ1OT1* mutations on chromosome 11): a cancer predisposition syndrome associated with macroglossia, organomegaly, midline abdominal defects (e.g., omphalocele, umbilical hernia, divarication of recti), gigantism, neonatal hypoglycemia, and ear pits or grooves
  - Hemihypertrophy (may be a clinical variant of BWS as a result of incomplete penetrance of *LIT1* epigenetic mutations): asymmetric overgrowth syndrome

## NEUROBLASTOMA

- Tumors that arise from primitive sympathetic ganglion cells and can secrete catecholamines.
- Neuroblastoma is most frequently diagnosed in children <5 years of age, with a peak around 2 years.
- Clinical presentation: palpable abdominal mass, fever, anemia, diarrhea, hypertension, Horner syndrome, cerebellar ataxia, and opsoclonus/myoclonus
  - Metastatic disease is often evident at presentation, which can manifest as bone pain, proptosis and periorbital ecchymosis from retrobulbar metastasis, skin nodules, or a blueberry muffin rash.
- Diagnosis: chest/abdomen/pelvic CT, bone scan, MIBG scan, bilateral bone marrow aspiration/biopsy, urine vanillylmandelic acid (VMA) and homovanillic acid (HVA), LDH, histologic examination of palpable lymph nodes.
- Therapy depends on patient age, tumor staging, and other factors but may include a combination of chemotherapy, surgical excision, radiation therapy, autologous BMT, and immunotherapy.

## OSTEOSARCOMA

- Tumors that arise from the bone and are able to produce immature bone or osteoid.
- Epidemiology: peak incidence is in the second decade of life, during the adolescent growth spurt.
- Clinical presentation: pain and palpable mass over the involved bone that has been present for many months
  - Occurs in the metaphyseal region of long bones, most commonly in the distal femur and proximal tibia
- Diagnosis: plain radiographs and MRI of the affected area, chest CT, bone scan to assess for metastatic disease and biopsy by an orthopedic surgeon specializing in orthopedic oncology
  - Radiographic findings are variable, but commonly include periosteal new bone formation (lifting of cortex to form Codman triangle), soft tissue masses, and ossification of the soft tissue in a radial or "sunburst" pattern.
  - Lesions can be osteosclerotic (approximately 45%), osteolytic (approximately 30%), or mixed sclerotic/osteolytic (approximately 25%).
  - From 15% to 20% of patients have detectable metastatic disease (>85% have pulmonary metastases) at presentation portending a poor prognosis.
- Treatment: surgical excision with wide margins, in addition to neoadjuvant chemotherapy pre- and postsurgery.

## RHABDOMYOSARCOMA

- Soft tissue malignancy of skeletal muscle origin.
- Clinical presentation: The most common primary sites for rhabdomyosarcoma to arise include the head and neck (e.g., parameningeal, orbit, pharyngeal), genitourinary tract, and the extremities, but masses can also arise in the trunk, intrathoracic, and gastrointestinal tract (liver, biliary, and perianal/anal).
- Diagnosis: imaging of the primary tumor (modality depends on location), evaluation for metastasis (bone scan, chest CT and/or bone marrow biopsy), CBC, LDH, uric acid, evaluation of kidney and liver function.
- Treatment: surgical resection with chemotherapy and radiation therapy.

## EWING SARCOMA

- Ewing sarcoma refers to tumors of either bone (Ewing tumor of bone) or soft tissue (extraosseous Ewing; "classic Ewing"), derived from primitive pluripotent cells of neural crest origin (postganglionic parasympathetic autonomic nervous system).
  - PNET is considered to be a more differentiated form of this entity and can occur as a primary tumor of bone or soft tissue.
- Clinical presentation: pain, palpable mass, pathologic fracture, and fever that have been present for months.
- Diagnosis: radiograph of bone, MRI of primary tumor, bone scan, chest CT for lung metastases, LDH, urine VMA/HVA (to distinguish from neuroblastoma), and bilateral bone marrow aspiration/biopsy.
  - Radiographic findings usually show a destructive lesion of the diaphysis, with cortex erosion and multilaminar periosteal reaction (i.e., "onion peel").
- Treatment: surgical resection with chemotherapy and radiation therapy.

## RETINOBLASTOMA

### Hereditary Variant

- Positive family history is found in 6-10% of patients; however, 30-40% of "sporadic" cases may be hereditary.
- Mean age at diagnosis is 14-15 months.
- Disease is usually bilateral/multifocal, distant to the first tumor, which contrasts the past belief that these second primary tumors only develop within the radiation field.
- There is a high risk of developing secondary nonocular tumors, such as osteosarcoma.
- Treatment is a combination of cryotherapy and chemotherapy.
- Genetic counseling of parents and child regarding risk to progeny is essential.

### Nonhereditary Variant

- Negative family history
- Mean age at diagnosis is 23-27 months.
- Disease is always unilateral/unifocal.
  - Note that 15% of patients with unilateral tumors may have hereditary disease.
- There is no increased risk of secondary nonocular tumors.

## ANEMIA

- There is a decrease in oxygen carrying capacity secondary to a decreased quantity of RBCs and hemoglobin.
  - Classification is based on decreased or disordered production of RBCs, intrinsic RBC abnormalities (hemoglobinopathies, enzyme deficiency, RBC membrane defects), or extrinsic destruction (Fig. 19-1).
- Patient and family history are essential to the diagnosis.
  - Past medical history of recent infections (e.g., hepatitis-induced aplastic anemia), trauma, transfusion, blood loss (e.g., GI blood loss and menstrual cycle), medications (e.g., medications that cause bone marrow suppression, NSAIDs that cause GI blood loss), and neonatal history of hyperbilirubinemia (e.g., congenital hemolytic anemia, such as hereditary spherocytosis [HS], hereditary elliptocytosis [HE], or G6PD deficiency).

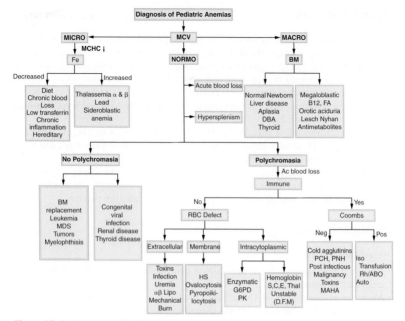

Figure 19-1. **Diagnosis of pediatric anemias.**

- Dietary history of the patient and mother (if the patient is an infant)
  - Quantity of cow's milk is essential after the age of 1 year if concerned about iron deficiency anemia.
  - Determine if the patient has any symptoms of pica.
- Sex must be considered in the diagnosis of X-linked diseases, such as G6PD deficiency.
- Family history of anemia, jaundice, gallstones, splenomegaly, surgeries, or transfusions
  - Consider race and heritage when assessing hemoglobinopathies (Hb S, Hb E, β-thalassemia, and α-thalassemia).
- Laboratory evaluation: Initial evaluation includes a CBC, reticulocyte count, and an evaluation of the peripheral smear.
- Decreased or disordered production: serum iron panel containing total serum iron, total iron-binding capacity and circulating transferrin receptor, ferritin, serum lead, serum $B_{12}$, RBC folate, serum creatinine, erythropoietin, bone marrow biopsy/aspirate and infectious work-up
- Hemoglobinopathy evaluation: hemoglobin electrophoresis
- Enzymatic deficiency: G6PD deficiency, RBC enzyme panel
- RBC membrane defects: osmotic fragility test
- Extrinsic destruction: direct Coombs, bilirubin panel, LDH, and serum haptoglobin
- Treatment is dependent on etiology:
- Iron deficiency: Oral iron supplementation to be continued for 3 months after normalization of hemoglobin, or IV iron repletion

○ The field is moving away from two-three times daily dosing of oral iron supplementation as newer studies show decreased iron absorption with such regimens due to spikes in hepcidin after the initial daily dose.
• G6PD: Avoid oxidant drugs or exposure.
• Thalassemia: chronic transfusion therapy or HSCT.
• Aplastic anemia: immunosuppression or HSCT.

## SICKLE CELL DISEASE

• Includes multiple genotypes, all of which include at least one copy of HbS (amino acid glutamine substitution for valine in the sixth position of the beta globin gene): examples include Hb SS, Hb SC, Hb Sβ$^0$-thalassemia, Hb Sβ$^+$-thalassemia.
• HbS pathologically polymerizes into chains in its deoxygenated state, distorting RBC shape into a sickled form. In addition to having altered rheology that obstructs the microcirculation, sickled RBCs hemolyze, leading to intravascular clotting, endothelial activation, and inflammation in all organ systems.

### Febrile Illness in Children with SCD
• Due to functional asplenia (or surgical if the patient has undergone splenectomy), patients with SCD are at risk for sepsis and bacteremia. Most commonly, the offending organism is *Streptococcus pneumoniae*.
• Due to this risk, children with SCD are prescribed daily prophylaxis with penicillin upon diagnosis. Prophylaxis stops at the age of 5 years unless the patient has undergone splenectomy or has a history of invasive pneumococcal infection. Furthermore, patients with SCD receive immunization with both the conjugate 13-valent vaccine and the 23-valent polysaccharide vaccine.
• History and physical examination should include vital signs with peripheral $O_2$ saturation, evaluation for signs of infection, pulmonary examination for crackles, wheeze and/or retraction, spleen size compared to baseline as documented in outpatient records, and neurologic examination.
• Laboratory and imaging studies to consider include CBC with differential, reticulocyte count, type and screen, blood culture, nasopharyngeal swab for viruses, chest plain radiographs, and urinalysis and urine culture (if symptomatic).
• Treatment: ceftriaxone.
• Substitute meropenem if patient has a cephalosporin allergy.
• Observe patient for 1 hour after ceftriaxone administration with repeat vital signs and assessment if not planning on admission as there are reports of severe ceftriaxone-induced hemolysis in patients with SCD.
• The presence of a focus of infection (e.g., otitis media) or viral symptoms does not alter urgency of administration of parental antibiotics, or preclude bacteremia or sepsis.
• Admit for any of the following:
  • Toxic appearance, including respiratory distress
  • Children <2 years of age
  • History of bacteremia or sepsis
  • Temperature >39°C
  • If the patient has any of the following laboratory parameters: hemoglobin <5 g/dL, reticulocyte count <5%, WBC > 30,000/μL or <5000/μL, platelet count <150,000/μL

- Evidence of severe pain, aplastic crisis, splenomegaly or splenic sequestration, acute chest syndrome, stroke, or priapism
- Unable to follow up in clinic, communication challenges (e.g., lack of contact information/phone number) or history of poor outpatient follow-up
- Inpatient management of SCD patients with fever
  - Laboratory studies and imaging include CBC and reticulocyte counts daily until patient stabilizes, blood culture q24h with fever, chest plain radiographs for any worsening of respiratory status, and an active type and screen with the blood bank
    - Consider urinalysis and urine culture, abdominal ultrasound, liver function tests, amylase/lipase, imaging of bones/joints and/or lumbar puncture (LP) if indicated.
  - Treatment: cefotaxime or ampicillin and sulbactam
    - Discontinue prophylactic penicillin while giving broad-spectrum antibiotics.
    - Pain control as needed with ibuprofen and PO/IV opioids.
    - Maintain $O_2$ saturation $\geq 92\%$ *or* at patient's baseline value ($SpO_2$ often does not correlate with $PO_2$ and central $SaO_2$ in patients with SCD).

## Acute Chest Syndrome

- ACS is defined as a new infiltrate on chest radiograph, in addition to one of the following: chest pain, fever, cough, tachypnea, or wheezing. An oxygen requirement is not required for the diagnosis of ACS.
  - The pathophysiology of ACS remains unclear
    - *Chlamydia pneumoniae* and *Mycoplasma pneumoniae* are the most common infectious causes for ACS.
    - Pulmonary fat embolism has also been implicated as an etiology.
- ACS is the most common cause of death in patients with SCD.
- Laboratory evaluation includes daily CBC and reticulocyte counts until patient has clinically stabilized and type and screen.
- Treatment: IV cephalosporin (cefotaxime or ampicillin and sulbactam) and an oral macrolide antibiotic (azithromycin)
  - Supplemental $O_2$ to maintain saturations $\geq 92\%$ or at baseline.
  - Incentive spirometry q2h while awake, and strongly consider more aggressive airway clearance with EzPAP.
  - Provide adequate pain control with ibuprofen and PO/IV opioids to limit splinting.
  - Consider scheduled albuterol if patient has history of asthma, and/or there are signs of reactive airway disease or wheezing on examination.
  - Transfusion of 10 mL/kg of RBCs to improve oxygen carrying capacity in patients with a supplemental oxygen requirement or hemoglobin below baseline
    - All transfused blood should be matched for C, E and K antigens.
  - Exchange transfusion for decline in clinical status (e.g., increasing respiratory distress, worsening radiographic findings, continued decline in hemoglobin after simple transfusion).
  - Glucocorticoids (prednisone) pulse can be considered for those with a reactive airway component to their disease.
    - Consider glucocorticoids carefully as there is an increased risk of intracranial hemorrhage and vasoocclusive pain in patients with SCD who receive glucocorticoids.
  - Maintenance IV fluids at 1500 mL/m$^2$/day.

## Acute Splenic Sequestration

- Red blood cells are trapped in the spleen, resulting in an acutely enlarging spleen with a drop in hemoglobin by at least 2 g/dL and a normal (or elevated) reticulocyte count (consider an aplastic crisis if the reticulocyte count is decreased).
  - Often associated with mild to moderate thrombocytopenia.
  - Can progress quickly, leading to death from hypovolemic shock within hours.
  - Due to the life-threatening nature of this disease complication, parents receive education and instruction to regularly monitor spleen size at the time of diagnosis of SCD.
- Monitoring includes vital signs with blood pressure q2h, pulse oximetry, and serial abdominal examinations q1-2h (location of spleen should be marked on the patient's abdomen with each examination).
- Laboratory evaluation: CBC may be obtained multiple times in a 24-hour period depending on the patient's clinical status.
- Treatment
  - Packed red blood cell (PRBC) transfusion of 5-10 mL/kg for Hb < 5-6 g/dL. In severe cases, urgent initiation of transfusion before inpatient admission may be lifesaving.
    - Transfusion releases the sequestered red blood cells, resulting in a larger-than-expected increase in hemoglobin after a single transfusion.
    - All transfused blood should be matched for C, E and K antigens.
  - Antibiotics if febrile (as described under treatment of febrile illness in SCD).
  - $O_2$ to keep saturation ≥92% or at patient's baseline.
  - Provide adequate pain control with ibuprofen and PO/IV opioids.
  - Incentive spirometry q2h.

## Aplastic Crisis

- Acute illness associated with hemoglobin below patient's baseline and a substantially decreased reticulocyte count (often <1%)
  - Most commonly caused by parvovirus B19 infection, which infects approximately 50% of children with SCD by the age of 10 years.
- Laboratory evaluation: daily CBC and reticulocyte counts until patient has clinically stabilized, type and screen, and a parvovirus PCR or serologic testing
- Treatment
  - RBC transfusions for symptomatic anemia or Hb < 5 g/dL with no evidence of erythroid recovery
    - All transfused blood should be matched for C, E and K antigens.
    - Multiple transfusions may be necessary.
    - Avoid transfusion of Hb > 10 g/dL.
  - Appropriate isolation per hospital guidelines for possible parvovirus infection

## Acute Stroke

- Historically, approximately 10% of patients with Hb SS have an overt stroke, defined as an acute and persistent neurologic deficit associated with an infarct on imaging, by the age of 20 years.
- Examination: A complete neurologic examination, including the NIH stroke scale.
- Laboratory evaluation: CBC with differential, reticulocyte count, type and screen, hemoglobin electrophoresis to determine % of HbS, PT, PTT, serum electrolytes, serum calcium, and glucose.

- Imaging evaluation: MRI and magnetic resonance angiography of the brain without sedation.
  - If a MRI brain is not immediately available, CT *without* contrast to exclude intracranial hemorrhage should be performed prior to intervention, with the MRI afterward.
  - Sedation for imaging purposes should only be performed if the imaging results will significantly alter the planned intervention.
- Treatment: If the patient does not receive chronic transfusion therapy, he/she should undergo an emergent exchange transfusion to decrease % HbS <30%, while maintaining the hemoglobin at approximately 10 g/dL.
  - Consider a simple RBC transfusion of 10 mL/kg if patient's hemoglobin is ≤ 8.5 g/dL and the exchange is not available within 2 hours.
  - If the patient receives chronic transfusion therapy, his/her % HbS will most likely be <50%. Consult with a hematologist regarding the appropriate intervention.
  - All transfused blood should be matched for C, E, and K antigens.
  - IV tissue plasminogen activator (tPA) is not recommended for children with SCD < 18 years of age.
- Monitoring: Neurologic checks q1h and vital signs every 15 minutes for at least the first hour, including close monitoring of blood pressure and continuous pulse oximetry. These patients often require ICU admission secondary to their requirement for close monitoring.
- Seizure therapy as needed.

## Pain/Vasoocclusive Crises

- Physical examination: A complete examination should be performed with emphasis on hydration status, evidence of infection, lung examinaton (>50% of patients with ACS are initially admitted for a VOC), spleen size, penis, and a complete neurologic examination.
- Laboratory evaluation: daily CBC and reticulocyte counts until patient has clinically stabilized, and type and screen and creatinine on admission
  - Consider a chest radiograph if the patient has fever, tachypnea, cough, chest pain, or an abnormal lung examination.
  - Consider transaminases, amylase, lipase and abdominal ultrasound to rule out cholelithiasis, cholecystitis, hepatopathy and pancreatitis in patients with upper quadrant, abdominal pain.
- Treatment: a combination of IV fluids, NSAIDs, opioids and supportive care
  - IV fluids: maintain euvolemia
  - NSAIDs
    - May consider use of ketorolac for a maximum of 5 consecutive days instead of ibuprofen
      - Recommend ensuring a normal creatinine prior to starting ketorolac, and close monitoring of urine output and renal function.
    - Scheduled motrin, or home NSAID, after completing 5 days of ketorolac
  - Opioid
    - Patients with SCD should have a home pain plan to manage vasoocclusive episodes, which include an NSAID (most often motrin) and opioid (most often hydrocodone/acetaminophen or oxycodone).
    - If a patient is admitted for a vasoocclusive crisis, then that patient has failed PO opioids at home and/or in the emergency department, supporting the need to transition to IV opioid therapy to adequately control pain.

- For patients <7 years or developmentally unable to understand patient-controlled analgesia (PCA), consider scheduled intermittent dosing of IV morphine or a continuous infusion of morphine without the PCA. Dosing should be titrated for the patient's clinical status.
- For patients ≥7 years and developmentally able to understand PCA, consider a continuous infusion of morphine with a PCA. Dosing should be titrated for the patient's clinical status.
- Consider hydromorphone or fentanyl if the patient has a morphine allergy or has uncontrolled pain with morphine
- Monitor patients receiving opioid therapy closely for the following:
  - Respiratory depression with a continuous pulse oximeter.
  - CNS depression with scheduled neurologic checks.
  - Constipation: Treat with stool softeners as needed.
  - Itching: Treat with nalbuphine hydrochloride or a low-dose infusion of naloxone.
- The IV opioids should be weaned each day as the pain crisis improves, with the goal of transitioning to an oral pain regimen. Oral pain medications should be given 30 minutes to 1 hour prior to stopping the IV medication. The patient is then discharged to continue their oral pain regimen (scheduled) for the first 24 hours after discharge.

○ Consider consultation of anesthesia/pain service for lidocaine infusion as adjunctive pain treatment
  - Subanesthetic ketamine infusion should be considered for hospitalized patients with vasoocclusive pain that is refractory to opioids if appropriate expertise and infrastructure is available.

○ Supportive care: application of heat to affected area and physical activity to increase blood flow to affected bone and muscles
  - Daily physical therapy if possible.
  - Ice packs should not be utilized in patients with SCD.
  - Maximize nonpharmacological therapies, such as massage, transcutaneous electrical nerve stimulation (TENS), yoga and etc.

○ All patients admitted with vasoocclusive pain should use incentive spirometry during hospitalization to decrease the risk of developing acute chest syndrome.

○ Red blood cell transfusion should not used as treatment for an acute vasoocclusive crisis unless there is another indication for transfusion.

## Priapism

- Vasoocclusive crisis in the cavernous sinus of penis, leading to prolonged and persistent erection in young adolescent males
- Treat pain as previously described.
- Start IV fluids.
- Consult urology for cavernous sinus irrigation.
  ○ Preoperative transfusion will be required prior to sedated procedure.

## Immunizations and Prophylactic Medications

- Patients with SCD are functionally asplenic secondary to recurrent vasoocclusive episodes in the splenic sinusoids leading to ischemia, fibrosis, and atrophy of the spleen. This process results in increased susceptibility to encapsulated organisms (*Streptococcus* spp., pneumococcus, *Salmonella*, and *Meningococcus*).

- Penicillin prophylaxis is given to prevent infection and continued until the child is at least 5 years old. Prophylaxis with penicillin is continued indefinitely if the patient undergoes surgical splenectomy or has a history of invasive pneumococcal infection.
  - Children <3 years of age: penicillin VK 125 mg PO bid
  - Children >3 years of age: penicillin VK 250 mg PO bid
- Immunization per guidelines for patients with functional asplenia
  - Children > 6 years should have received at least one dose of PCV13 (conjugate 13-valent pneumococcal vaccine)
  - Recommend vaccination with PPSV23 (23-valent polysaccharide pneumococcal vaccine) and meningococcal vaccines (including serogroup B) per current guidelines

## Primary Disease Modification in Sickle Cell Disease

- Hydroxyurea is a once daily, oral ribonucleotide reductase inhibitor that causes an increase in fetal hemoglobin in patients with SCD, while also decreasing inflammation and endothelial activation by reducing the number of leukocytes and expression of adhesion molecules.
  - Hydroxyurea as primary disease modification should be considered in all patients with Hb SS or Hb Sβ°-thalassemia patients that are >9 months of age, with the goal of ultimately reducing long-term disease complications.
  - Hydroxyurea is usually continued during hospitalization unless there is evidence of drug toxicity, such as neutropenia, thrombocytopenia, or reticulocytopenia.
- Chronic transfusion therapy can be used to suppress hemoglobin S while increasing total hemoglobin and oxygen carrying capacity. Transfusions can be provided as scheduled simple transfusions, manual exchange transfusions, or erythrocytopheresis. Primary and secondary stroke prevention are the most common indications for chronic transfusion therapy.
  - Extended red cell antigen profiling is strongly recommended over ABO/RhD typing, at a minimum profiling C/c, E/d, K, Jk$^a$/Jk$^b$, Fy$^a$/Fy$^b$, M/N and S/s.
  - Complications of chronic transfusion therapy that must be considered and monitored for include hemosiderosis/iron overload requiring chelation therapy, alloimmunization, delayed hemolytic transfusion reactions, and infection and thrombosis with central venous catheters.
- Crizalizumab is a monoclonal antibody targeting p-selectin that is administered as a monthly outpatient infusion.
  - Approved for use in children 16 years and older to reduce vasoocclusive crises.
- Voxelotor is a daily oral medication that reversibly binds to hemoglobin, stabilizing the hemoglobin in the oxygenated state and inhibiting polymerization.
  - Approved in children with SCD aged 4 years and older.
- L-Glutamine is an essential amino acid that is involved in reducing oxidative stress in the red blood cell. The Endari formulation has FDA approval for twice daily, oral administration to reduce vasoocclusive episodes in SCD.

## WORKUP FOR BLEEDING

- Screening tests: CBC with platelet count, platelet function analysis (PFA-100), protime (PT), activated partial thromboplastin time (aPTT), thrombin time (TT), fibrinogen level, and FDPs

| TABLE 19-3 | Abnormal Screening Tests in Various Hemorrhagic Disorders |
|---|---|

| Disorder | Platelet count | PFA-100 | aPTT | PT | TT | Fibrinogen |
|---|---|---|---|---|---|---|
| Thrombocytopenia | X | | | | | |
| Platelet dysfunction | | X | | | | |
| Hemophilia | | | X | | | |
| Factor VII deficiency | | | | X | | |
| Dysfibrinogenemia | | | | | X | |
| Hypofibrinogenemia | | | | | X | X |
| DIC | X | X | X | X | X | X |

- Abnormal platelet number: immune thrombocytopenic purpura (ITP), bone marrow suppression (e.g., secondary to medication or infection), bone marrow replacement (e.g., leukemia), bone marrow failure, von Willebrand disease (vWD) type IIb
- Normal platelet number, but abnormal PT or PTT: factor deficiency (Table 19-3)
  ○ Consider mixing studies
    – Normal control plasma is added to a patient's plasma and incubated.
    – Correction of prolonged PT or PTT suggests deficiency of coagulation factor.
    – Noncorrection of PT or PTT suggests the presence of inhibitors to coagulation.
- Normal platelet number and abnormal TT: Dysfibrinogenemia
- Normal platelet number and PT/PTT, abnormal PFA-100: platelet dysfunction (acquired or congenital), (Table 19-4) or von Willebrand disease
- Abnormal platelets, PT, aPTT, fibrinogen, TT: DIC, liver disease
- Normal platelets, PT, aPTT: possibly FXIII deficiency, $\alpha_2$-antiplasmin

## DISSEMINATED INTRAVASCULAR COAGULATION

- Exposure of tissue factor causing concomitant activation of the coagulation and fibrinolytic cascades with resultant microvascular thromboses, consumptive coagulopathy, and microangiopathic hemolytic anemia. Thus, patients may experience bleeding, thrombosis, or both.

| TABLE 19-4 | Platelet Aggregation Responses in Inherited Platelet Function Disorders |
|---|---|

| | Storage pool disease | Glanzmann thrombasthenia | Bernard Soulier disease |
|---|---|---|---|
| Collagen | ↓ | ↓↓ | N |
| ADP | ↓ | ↓↓ | N |
| Epinephrine | ↓ | ↓↓ | N |
| Arachidonic acid | N | ↓↓ | N |
| Ristocetin | N | N | ↓↓ |

- DIC is always secondary to another process causing endothelial damage and exposure of tissue factor, such as sepsis or malignancy.
- Laboratory evaluation: platelet count is low; PT and PTT are prolonged; fibrinogen is <100 mg/dL; D-dimer is >2 µg/mL; clotting factors II, V, VIII, antithrombin III, and protein C are usually low; and microangiopathic hemolytic anemia is seen on peripheral smear.
- Treatment
  - Treat the underlying cause.
  - Supportive care with transfusion of platelets, FFP, and cryoprecipitate as needed. See Transfusion Principles section for doses.
  - Heparin therapy has shown no benefit.

## HEMOPHILIA AND COAGULATION FACTOR DEFICIENCIES

- Factor VIII deficiency (hemophilia A) and factor IX deficiency (hemophilia B)
  - Laboratory studies show a prolonged aPTT that corrects with 50:50 mixing and a normal PT. Factor VIII or IX will be decreased.
    ○ Baseline factor levels primarily dictate disease severity
      – Severe hemophilia: <1% factor activity.
      – Moderate hemophilia: between 1%and 5% factor activity.
      – Mild hemophilia: >5% factor activity.
      – Of note, factor IX is decreased at birth. Factor activity levels must be interpreted with consideration of normal values for age.
    ○ Send CBC, PT, PTT, factor VIII, and factor IX from the cord blood in a baby with suspected hemophilia (mom is a known carrier) and attempt to avoid a heel stick. Do not perform an arterial stick.
    ○ Consider a head ultrasound after delivery if laboratory values suggest hemophilia.
  - Defer circumcision and nonessential procedures in newborns with hemophilia until appropriate factor replacement can be arranged.
  - Patients with hemophilia should still receive vitamin K at delivery and all normally scheduled immunizations. Pressure should be applied for 5 minutes after each injection.
  - Treatment of factor VIII deficiency
    ○ Each unit of factor VIII per kilogram raises blood factor activity level approximately 2%.
    ○ Dose factor VIII (units) = U/dL desired rise in plasma fVIII × Weight (kg) × 0.5.
    ○ The half-life of factor VIII is 12 hours. Frequency and duration of repeated dosing depend on the location and severity of the bleeding.
    ○ Mild to moderate bleeding: factor VIII 25-30 U/kg IV
      – Desmopressin (DDAVP) can be used in lieu of factor VIII infusion in patients with mild hemophilia if they have previously shown a response to DDAVP
        - IV—0.3 µg/kg IV once
        - Nasal spray—150 µg/spray: <50 kg: 1 spray, >50 kg: one spray each nostril
    ○ Severe, life threatening: factor VIII 50 U/kg IV, followed by repeated infusions of 20-25 U/kg IV q12h or a continuous factor infusion.
    ○ Surgical patients: 50 U/kg IV; usually requires repeat administration q6-12h for a total of 10-14 days or until healed.
    ○ Therapy for oral bleeding: aminocaproic acid (Amicar) 100 mg/kg PO q6h or tranexamic acid (antifibrinolytic agents).

   – These are insufficient to treat hemarthroses or hematuria.
- Treatment of factor IX deficiency
  - Each unit of factor IX per kilogram raises blood factor activity level approximately 1%.
  - Dose factor IX (units) = U/dL desired rise in plasma fVIII × Weight (kg) × 1.5.
  - The half-life of factor IX is 18-24 hours. Frequency and duration of repeated dosing depend on the location and severity of the bleeding.
  - Mild to moderate bleeding: factor IX 40 U/kg IV.
  - Severe, life threatening: factor IX 80 U/kg, followed by 40 U/kg q24h or a continuous factor infusion.
  - Therapy for oral bleeding: aminocaproic acid or transexamic acid (antifibrinolytic agents).
    – These are insufficient to treat hemarthroses or hematuria.
- Factor XI deficiency (hemophilia C)
  - Rare autosomal recessive disorder (e.g., Ashkenazi Jews, Noonan syndrome)
  - Treatment: replacement with factor XI concentrate or FFP infusion
- Factor XIII deficiency
  - Autosomal recessive inheritance
  - Often presents with umbilical cord bleeding (80% with homozygous deficiency) and intracranial hemorrhage (33%)
  - Diagnosis: measurement of factor XIII activity or urea solubility test, where clot stability is assessed in 5 M urea
    - PT and PTT will be normal
  - Treatment: replacement with recombinant factor XIII or purified, plasma-derived factor XIII concentrate
    - Cryoprecipitate or FFP infusions can be used if one of the factor XIII products is not available.

## VON WILLEBRAND DISEASE

- Autosomal-dominant inheritance for type 1 and 2 subtypes
- Presents with symptoms of mucosal bleeding, such as bruising and recurrent epistaxis
- Laboratory evaluation: PFA-100, PT, aPTT, vWF antigen and ristocetin cofactor activity, vWF multimer levels, factor VIII levels and blood type
- Type 1 (70-80% of patients with vWD)—quantitative deficiency
  - Reduced vWF antigen and ristocetin cofactor activity with a platelet-dependent vWF activity/vWF:antigen ratio > 0.7
    - Normal vWF multimers and factor VIII
  - Treatment: DDAVP (0.3 µg/kg IV or 150 µg/nostril q12-24h) and/or vWF concentrate (e.g., Humate-P, Alphanate, Vonvendi)
- Type 2A (10-12% of patients with vWD)—qualitative defect
  - Reduced vWF antigen and ristocetin cofactor activity with a platelet-dependent vWF activity/vWF:antigen ratio <0.7 and reduced number of high molecular weight multimers resulting in a severe deficiency of cofactor activity
    - Normal factor VIII
  - Treatment: factor VIII/vWF concentrate (e.g., Humate-P, Alphanate, Vonvendi)
- Type 2B (3-5%)
  - A gain of function mutation in the *vWF* resulting in increased binding of vWF to platelets, forming aggregates with increased clearance

- Reduced vWF antigen and ristocetin cofactor activity with a platelet-dependent vWF activity/vWF:antigen ratio <0.7 with reduced platelet count (bleeding severity often correlates with severity of thrombocytopenia)
  - Possibly reduced number of high molecular weight multimers
  - Normal factor VIII
- Diagnosis with targeted genetic testing is recommended
  - Increased ristocetin-induced platelet aggregation with low dose ristocetin stimulation due to the gain of function mutation was historically used for diagnosis.
- Treatment: factor VIII/vWF concentrate (e.g., Humate-P, Alphanate, Vonvendi)
  - DDAVP is contraindicated in type 2B von Willebrand disease.
- Type 2N (1-2%)
- vWF cannot bind to factor VIII, which leads to accelerated clearance of factor VIII.
- Reduced vWF antigen and ristocetin cofactor activity with low factor VIII levels.
  - Normal high molecular weight multimer levels.
  - Consider this diagnosis if a patient has "mild hemophilia" and a family history with affected males and females.
- Diagnosis with either vWF:factor VIII binding assay (assessing von Willebrand factor's ability to bind to recombinant factor VIII in vitro) or targeted genetic testing.
- This subtype has an autosomal recessive inheritance, making proper diagnosis even more essential to ensure appropriate genetic counseling.
- Types 2M and 3 are rarely seen and require the care of a hematologist.

## THROMBOCYTOPENIAS

- Differential diagnosis by age of presentation
  - In newborns
    - Genetic disorders: thrombocytopenia with absent radii (TAR), Wiskott-Aldrich syndrome, osteopetrosis, or inborn errors of metabolism
    - Immune-mediated destruction of platelets: neonatal alloimmune thrombocytopenia, maternal ITP, maternal systemic lupus erythematosus (SLE), maternal hyperthyroidism, maternal drugs, maternal preeclampsia, neonatal alloimmune thrombocytopenia
    - Nonimmune mediated (probably related to DIC): asphyxia, aspiration, necrotizing enterocolitis, hemangiomas (Kasabach-Merritt syndrome), thrombosis, respiratory distress syndrome, hemolytic uremic syndrome, heart disease (congenital/acquired)
    - Hypersplenism
  - In older children
    - Decreased production: amegakaryocytic thrombocytopenia, myelodysplasia, aplastic anemia, leukemia
    - Increased destruction: ITP, DIC, sepsis, HUS, hypersplenism, drugs

### Idiopathic (Immune) Thrombocytopenic Purpura

- Immune-mediated platelet destruction and impaired production with a peak age of diagnosis of 2-4 years of age
  - ITP can be a primary disorder or secondary to another condition (e.g., primary immunodeficiencies, Evan syndrome, autoimmune disorders such as SLE).

- Acute ITP is most often a self-limited disease that usually resolves within months regardless of whether therapy is given in >60% of patients that are younger than 20 years.
- Chronic ITP is defined as disease that persists for longer than 12 months.
- On examination, the child is clinically well with bruising and petechiae
  - Mucosal bleeding most often occurs in ITP. Severe bleeding is uncommon and occurs in approximately 20% of children. Less than 1% of children have intracranial hemorrhage.
  - A palpable spleen is appreciated in approximately 10% of cases.
- Treatment
  - Acute ITP
    ○ Observation alone for those without bleeding.
    ○ For patients with non–life-threatening bleeding, guidelines recommend prednisone for 5-7 days over anti-D globulin (WinRho, used in Rh+ patients only) or intravenous immune globulin.
  - Chronic ITP: Thrombopoietic receptor agonists are recommended prior to rituximab or splenectomy per current guidelines. Trialing rituximab is recommended prior to splenectomy. Immunization is required prior to splenectomy with post-splenectomy antibiotic prophylaxis.

## THROMBOCYTOSIS

- Platelets are acute phase reactants.
- Most cases of thrombocytosis are secondary (e.g., acute infection, asplenia).
- Primary thrombocytosis (e.g., essential thrombocythemia) is rare in pediatric populations.

## HYPERCOAGULOPATHY

- Aside from clots associated with central venous catheters, spontaneous clots in veins and arteries may arise in children with cancer, congenital heart disease, infection, nephrotic syndrome, following surgery or TPN, obesity, SLE, liver disease, SCD, critical illness, or in those with a genetic predisposition for thrombosis.
- Laboratory evaluation: CBC, PT, aPTT, antithrombin III, proteins C and S, factor V Leiden gene mutation, prothrombin gene 20210 mutation, factor VIII level, and lipoprotein A levels. Measurement of antithrombin III, protein C, and protein S should not occur with an acute thrombosis, as levels may be falsely abnormal (low). *MTHFR* gene mutation and homocysteine levels are rarely tested. Hematology should be consulted to help determine the need for evaluation for an underlying predisposition for blood clots.
- Imaging (ultrasound, magnetic resonance venography, CT angiogram, etc.) is required for diagnosis and monitoring of the clot.
- Treatment: Thrombosis is most commonly managed with low molecular weight heparin (LMW heparin) at 1 mg/kg SC q12h in pediatrics.
- Activated factor Xa levels should be checked 4 hours following the second dose.
- The desired therapeutic level for the treatment of a thrombosis is 0.6-1 U/mL.
- IV unfractionated heparin infusions can be used in critically ill patients with rapidly changing clinical status and/or with potential need for surgical intervention.
- Oral anticoagulants, such as warfarin and direct oral anticoagulants (DOACs, e.g., dabigatran, rivaroxaban) can be used in select patients. Consultation with a hematologist can provide guidance in choosing the most appropriate anticoagulant, and how best to monitor treatment.

- Thrombolytic therapy with tissue plasminogen activator, which converts plasminogen to plasmin, and thrombectomy is considered for severe, life or limb-threatening thromboses.

## TRANSFUSION PRINCIPLES

### Packed Red Blood Cells
- After consideration of etiology of anemias and clinical status, transfuse for hemoglobin (Hb) ≤ 7 g/dL or symptomatic anemia.
- Transfuse 10-15 mL/kg PRBCs over 2-4 hours with an expectation that the hemoglobin will rise approximately 1-1.5 g/dL if there is not ongoing loss (Table 19-5).

### Platelets
- Transfuse for platelets ≤10,000/μL or symptomatic thrombocytopenia in the setting of decreased production.
  - Do not transfuse for idiopathic thrombocytopenia (ITP) or autoimmune destruction unless requiring an emergent surgical procedure.
- Transfuse 10-20 mL/kg of platelets (Table 19-6).
  - Round to unit volume to minimize waste.
  - There are few indications (e.g., trauma, acute hemorrhage in the operating room, massive transfusion protocol) that require transfusion of more than a single unit of platelets. Consider discussing with hematology and/or transfusion medicine if requiring multiple units per day.
  - Fever, sepsis, amphotericin administration, splenomegaly, alloantibodies, ongoing blood loss, hemolytic uremic syndrome, thrombotic thrombocytopenic purpura, clot formation, and necrotizing enterocolitis can explain a poor response to transfusion.

### Fresh Frozen Plasma
- FFP contains clotting factors, immunoglobulin, and albumin.
- Transfuse 10-20 mL/kg.
  - FFP does not need to be screened for CMV.
- The patient may also require parental vitamin K for production of their own clotting factors

### Cryoprecipitate
- Contains fibrinogen, vWF, and other high molecular weight factors
- One unit is 10-15 mL.
- Transfuse approximately 1 U/5 kg

### Transfusion Reactions
- Allergic reactions are characterized by urticaria, angioedema, bronchospasm, hypotension, and anaphylaxis that occur during or within 4 hours of a transfusion.
  - **Stop infusion** and administer
    - ○ Diphenhydramine for treatment of pruritus and hives
    - ○ Epinephrine for severe reactions (anaphylaxis, bronchospasm, hypotension, shock)
    - ○ Fluids for hypotension
    - ○ Albuterol for bronchodilation
    - ○ Narcotics (meperidine) for rigors
    - ○ Acetaminophen for fever

**TABLE 19-5  Recommendations for Transfusion of RBCs**

| | Leukoreduced | Irradiated | CMV negative | CMV untested | Sickledex negative | Minor antigen compatible |
|---|---|---|---|---|---|---|
| NICU patients | X | X | X[a] | | | |
| Immunosuppressed | X | X | | X | | |
| Solid organ transplant | X | X | | X | | |
| ALLOgeneic BMT | X | X | X[b] | X | | |
| AUTOlogous BMT | X | X | | X | | |
| SCD | X | | | X | X | X |

[a]CMV seronegative products given if the patient is <4 months old and was ≤1500 g at birth.
[b]Patient should receive CMV untested products if he/she is CMV seropositive.

| TABLE 19-6 | Recommendations for Transfusion of Platelets | | | |
|---|---|---|---|---|
| | Leukoreduced | Irradiated | CMV negative | CMV untested |
| Solid organ transplant | X | X | | X |
| ALLOgeneic BMT | X | X | X[a] | |
| AUTOlogous BMT | X | X | | X |

[a]Patient should receive CMV untested products if he/she is CMV seropositive.

- ○ Glucocorticoids for moderate to severe reactions (urticaria, fever, chills, diaphoresis, and pallor)
- Consider excluding IgA deficiency in patients with a history of anaphylactic transfusion reactions.
- Acute hemolytic reaction
  - These are most often immune-mediated reactions (primarily from ABO incompatibility) that result in intra- or extravascular hemolysis characterized by a spectrum of symptoms ranging from fever, chills, diaphoresis, abdominal pain, and/or hemoglobinuria, to hypotension, acute kidney injury/renal failure, DIC, and/or shock.
  - **Stop infusion with change in vital signs and monitor patient closely for evolution of these symptoms.**
  - Send patient's blood sample and transfusion bag to blood bank to type and crossmatch to determine if there is serological incompatibility.
  - Treatment is supportive care.
- Delayed transfusion reaction is characterized by anemia, hyperbilirubinemia, and abdominal pain that occurs 3-10 days after the transfusion.
  - The risk for this type of reaction is highest in those with a history of red blood cell transfusion resulting in alloimmunization; however, the antibody has since become undetectable. The patient then has an amnestic immune response and hemolysis of the incompatible red blood cells.
  - Symptoms include jaundice, fever, chills, pain, hypertension, and hemoglobinuria.
  - Confirm with Coombs test.
  - Treatment is supportive care and attempting to avoid further transfusion.
- Febrile nonhemolytic reactions are characterized by fever, chills, diaphoresis, and rigors.
  - These reactions are caused by preinflammatory cytokines and/or interaction between patient antibodies and donor antigen on the transfused cells.
  - **Stop infusion.**
  - This is a diagnosis of exclusion, so patient samples must be sent for Coombs testing and a septic transfusion reaction should be considered.
  - Treat with acetaminophen and narcotics (meperidine) for rigors.
  - Glucocorticoids may also help.

## SUGGESTED READING

Orkin SH. Nathan and Oski's Hematology and Oncology of Infancy and Childhood. 8th Ed. Philadelphia, PA: Elsevier Saunders, 2015.

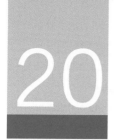

# Primary Immunodeficiencies
Maleewan Kitcharoensakkul

## DEFINITION

Primary immunodeficiencies (PIs) are heterogeneous diseases characterized by impairment in the development and function of the immune system. Individuals with PIs can present with severe or recurrent infections and/or immune dysregulation leading to atopy, autoimmunity, lymphoproliferation, or malignancy.

## CLASSIFICATION

- There are at least 400 distinct genetically identified PIs listed in the 2019 International Union of Immunological Societies (IUIS) phenotypical classification.
- PIs can be classified into ten groups of disorders based on the parts of the immune system primarily involved. Examples of diseases in each group are listed in Table 20-1.
- This chapter focuses on the PIs that typically present with susceptibility to infection. Other PIs listed in Table 20-1 more commonly have autoimmune/autoinflammatory manifestations or are associated with bone marrow failure syndromes.

## PREVALENCE

- The prevalence of PIs varies geographically and is thought to be underestimated.
- Approximately 1 in 500 people is affected by one of the known PIs.
- Primary antibody deficiencies and combined immunodeficiencies (CIDs) are the most common PIs diagnosed in both children and adults.

## WARNING SIGNS OF PIs IN CHILDREN

The Jeffrey Modell Foundation (JMF) has developed a list of warning signs for PIs. The presence of two or more of these warning signs should trigger an evaluation for PI.

- Four or more new ear infections within 1 year
- Two or more serious sinus infections within 1 year
- Two or more months on antibiotics with little effect
- Two or more pneumonias within 1 year
- Failure of an infant to gain weight or grow normally
- Recurrent deep skin or organ abscesses
- Persistent oral thrush or fungal infection of the skin
- Need for intravenous antibiotics to clear infections
- Two or more deep-seated infections, such as septicemia
- A family history of PIs

**TABLE 20-1** Groups of PIs

| Group of disorders | Examples of diseases |
|---|---|
| Immunodeficiency affecting cellular and humoral immunity | Severe combined immunodeficiency |
| | Combined immunodeficiency |
| Syndromic cellular immunodeficiencies | 22q11 deletion (DiGeorge) syndrome |
| | Wiskott-Aldrich syndrome |
| | Ataxia-telangiectasia |
| | NEMO deficiency syndrome |
| | Hyper IgE syndromes |
| Predominantly antibody deficiencies | Agammaglobulinemia |
| | Common variable immunodeficiency |
| | Specific antibody deficiency |
| | Selective IgA deficiency |
| Congenital defects of phagocyte number and function | Congenital neutropenia syndromes |
| | Chronic granulomatous disease |
| | Leukocyte adhesion deficiency |
| Complement deficiencies | Deficiency in C1q, C1r, C1s, C2-C9 |
| Defects in intrinsic and innate immunity | Mendelian susceptibility to mycobacterial disease (MSMD) |
| | Defects in toll-like receptors and their pathways |
| Diseases of immune dysregulation | Immunodysregulation, polyendocrinopathy, enteropathy, X-linked (IPEX) syndrome |
| | STAT3 gain-of-function |
| | Autoimmune, polyendocrinopathy, candidiasis, ectodermal dystrophy (APECED) |
| | Autoimmune lymphoproliferative syndrome (ALPS) |
| Autoinflammatory disorders | Monogenic causes of periodic fever syndromes |
| | Type I interferonopathies |
| Bone marrow failure | Fanconi anemia |
| | Dyskeratosis congenita |
| Phenocopies of inborn errors of immunity | Diseases associated with somatic mutations or with autoantibodies |
| (Conditions resemble PIs and are not due to germline mutations) | |

Other warning signs of PIs in children:

- Infection with atypical mycobacteria
- Complications from a live vaccine
- Nonhealing wounds
- Granulomas
- Unexplained fevers
- Early-onset autoimmunity such as inflammatory bowel disease (IBD)
- Autoimmunity with multiple organ involvement
- Persistent dermatitis in infants
- Evans syndrome (a combination of autoimmune hemolytic anemia [AIHA] and immune thrombocytopenia)
- Early-onset or recurrent hemophagocytic lymphohistiocytosis

## APPROACH TO THE PATIENT WITH A POSSIBLE PI

Most patients with PI present with recurrent or chronic infections. History and focused examination can guide evaluation and diagnosis.

### History
- Infection history, including age at onset of infection, type of infectious agents, sites of infection, severity of infection, requirement for intravenous antibiotic to clear infection, complications of infection, frequency of infection, and the most recent episode of infection. Of note, practitioners should recognize that young children who are immune competent may have up to 8 episodes per year of upper respiratory tract infections.
- History that may suggest immune dysregulation
  - Autoimmune disorders, including cytopenias, hepatitis, and enteropathy
  - Chronic lung diseases
  - Endocrine disorders, including type I diabetes, adrenal insufficiency, and thyroid disorders
  - Skin conditions, including vasculitis, psoriasis, eczema, vitiligo, urticaria, chilblains, and granulomas
  - Allergic disorders, including atopic dermatitis
  - Chronic joint symptoms
  - Ocular involvement, such as uveitis
  - History of hemophagocytic lymphohistiocytosis, lymphoproliferative disorders, or childhood-onset malignancy
- Past medical history
  - Prior medical conditions and/or treatments that can affect the immune system, including chemotherapy, steroid use, and chronic illnesses
  - Other risk factors associated with recurrent illnesses, including daycare attendance, passive smoke exposure, asthma, cystic fibrosis, asplenia, and malnutrition
- Developmental history
  - Developmental delays, including speech delay, are associated with some PIs.
- Immunization history
  - Complications from live vaccines.
  - Type of pneumococcal vaccine (pneumococcal 13-valent conjugate vaccine or Prevnar vs. pneumococcal polysaccharide or Pneumovax) is needed to interpret the result of vaccine titers.

- Family history
  - Family members with diagnosed PIs, childhood death, recurrent/severe/atypical infections, autoimmunity, lymphoproliferative disorders, allergic disorders, or malignancy
  - History of consanguinity
- Medications
  - Immunosuppressive medications can be associated with acquired immunodeficiency and can affect interpretation of lab results.

## Examination

Physical examination in these children is necessary to identify sources of infection, organ involvement, and dysmorphic features associated with genetic syndromes and certain PIs.

- Examination findings that may suggest PIs:
  - Poor weight gain
  - Dysmorphic features
  - Skin: rashes, erythroderma, petechiae, poor wound healing, telangiectasia, granulomas
  - Hair abnormalities
  - Head and neck: nasal polyps, absence of tonsils, gingivitis, conical teeth, candidiasis, enlarged lymph nodes
  - Respiratory: wheezing or other signs of asthma or chronic lung disease
  - Abdomen: hepatosplenomegaly
  - Neurologic: ataxia, neuropathy
  - Extremities: arthritis, limb anomalies, clubbing of fingers

## Initial Laboratory Screening for PIs

Laboratory testing for PIs depends on clinical suspicion and usually can be guided by the type and severity of infections and presence/absence of immune dysregulation, Tables 20-2 and 20-3. Measurement of IgG subclass levels is **not** routinely recommended as a part of an initial evaluation for PIs, as these levels change over time and treatment depends on the presence or absence of specific antibody responses to antigens. Testing for genetic mutations is not included in typical screening labs ordered by general practitioners, but genetic testing can be helpful in complex patients or after a PI diagnosis has been made by clinical testing; these results are necessary for genetic counseling and can potentially identify targeted therapies for certain PIs. Patients with abnormal labs or who continue to have recurrent/severe/atypical infections or other symptoms concerning for immune dysregulation should be referred to an immunologist for further evaluation.

## PRESENTATION, EVALUATION, AND TREATMENT OF PIs

PIs that typically present with susceptibility to infections discussed in this chapter include (1) immunodeficiencies affecting cellular and humoral immunity (CIDs), (2) syndromic cellular immunodeficiencies, (3) predominantly antibody deficiencies, (4) phagocytic disorders, (5) complement deficiency, (6) defects in intrinsic and innate immunity, and (7) diseases of immune dysregulation.

**TABLE 20-2** Clinical Features of Common PIs

| Disorder | Viral infections | Bacterial infections | Fungal infections | Inflammatory complications |
|---|---|---|---|---|
| Combined immunodeficiency | Adenovirus, CMV, EBV, rotavirus, norovirus, etc. | Any | Candida PJP | Skin and GI inflammation in Omenn syndrome |
| Primary antibody deficiencies | Enterovirus in XLA | Encapsulated bacteria, S. aureus, Mycoplasma | — | Both hematologic and organ-specific autoimmunity in CVID and XLA |
| Phagocytic disorders | — | S. aureus, Serratia, Klebsiella, E. coli, Burkholderia, Salmonella | Aspergillus Candida Nocardia | GI and GU inflammation in CGD |
| Complement deficiencies | — | Neisseria Other encapsulated bacteria | — | Increased risks of autoimmune disease in deficiency of early complement component |

| TABLE 20-3 | Initial Screening Labs for PIs |
|---|---|
| **Suspected PIs** | **Initial labs** |
| Combined immunodeficiency | CBC and differential |
| | Flow cytometry to enumerate T, B, and NK cells |
| | Serum immunoglobulin levels (IgG, IgA, IgM, IgE) |
| | Specific antibody levels to protein antigens and polysaccharide antigens |
| | If initial labs are abnormal or there is a high index of suspicion for combined immunodeficiency, consider proliferation assays to mitogens and antigens, as well as proliferation assay to anti-CD3 |
| Primary antibody deficiency | Serum immunoglobulin levels (IgG, IgA, IgM, IgE) |
| | Specific antibody levels to protein antigens and polysaccharide antigens |
| | CBC and differential |
| | If initial labs are abnormal, consider sending flow cytometry to enumerate B cells and its subsets, and checking albumin level to evaluate for protein loss |
| Phagocytic disorders | CBC and differential |
| | Examination of blood smear to evaluate morphology |
| | Measurement of neutrophil oxidase function by DHR flow cytometry |
| | Flow cytometry for adhesion molecules |
| | Bone marrow biopsy may be indicated in selected patients |
| Complement deficiencies | CH50 and AH 50 (if abnormal, this should be repeated since the accuracy of testing relies on quality of samples) |
| | Level or function of individual complement components |

## Immunodeficiency Affecting Cellular and Humoral Immunity (Combined Immunodeficiency)

This group of PIs primarily affects T cells. However, B-cell function is also impaired because B cells require accessory signals from helper T cells for induction of specific antibody responses.

### Severe Combined Immunodeficiency

- Severe combined immunodeficiency (SCID) is characterized by a complete absence of specific immunity due to severe dysfunction of T cells with varying function of B and NK cells. If left untreated, most patients will succumb to life-threatening infections within the first 2 years of life.

- Causes: Several different genetic mutations, including *IL2RG, ADA, RAG1, RAG2, ADA,* and *IL7R.*
- Clinical manifestations: Prior to the implementation of newborn screening, SCID patients typically presented with life-threatening complication of common viral pathogens, persistent mucocutaneous candidiasis, opportunistic infections, chronic diarrhea, or severe complications due to live vaccines.
  - Omenn syndrome is a unique clinical manifestation of SCID involving diffuse erythroderma, hepatosplenomegaly, elevated eosinophil count, and elevated IgE levels.
- Labs: Since 2019, all newborns in the United States have been screened for SCID by T-cell receptor excision circle (TREC) assay. TREC is a marker of thymic output that is very low or absent in all SCID patients regardless of their genotypes. It is a highly sensitive test. False-positive results may be seen in patients with primary or acquired thymic defects, conditions associated with loss of T cells, or congenital heart defects.
  - When newborn screen is positive for possible SCID or patients have clinical symptoms concerning of SCID, further workup includes complete blood count (which may show lymphopenia, although normal absolute lymphocyte count does not exclude SCID), enumeration of lymphocyte subsets by flow cytometry (typically naïve CD4+ T cells <200 cells/mcl), and chest plain radiographs (which may show absent thymic shadow) should be considered. Once SCID diagnosis is confirmed by flow cytometry of lymphocyte subsets, genetic testing should be pursued.
- Treatment: SCID is considered a medical emergency due to patients' susceptibility to life-threatening infections. Hematopoietic stem cell transplant (HSCT) can be a curative treatment for patients with SCID, and outcomes depend on the patient's age and infection status at the time of transplant. While awaiting transplant, patients should receive antimicrobial prophylaxis and immunoglobulin replacement therapy and should avoid receiving any live vaccines.
  - Other available treatment options for SCID depend on the causative genetic defect, including enzyme replacement therapy for adenosine deaminase (ADA) deficiency, gene therapy (through clinical trials) for ADA deficiency and X-linked SCID, or thymic transplant.

*Combined Immunodeficiencies*
- CIDs are characterized by T-cell defects that are less severe than SCID and thus may present later in childhood. This group of disorders includes hyper-IgM syndrome and activated phosphoinositide 3-kinase δ syndrome (APDS), which are discussed in more detail below, as well as several others. Treatment with HSCT may not be indicated in some patients, depends on the defects and their clinical manifestations.
- **Immunodeficiency with hyper-IgM (HIGM) syndrome**
  - HIGM syndrome is characterized by an inability to switch the production of IgM isotype to IgG, IgA, or IgE isotypes.
  - Causes: Defects in genes involved in immunoglobulin class switch recombination or somatic hypermutation. Both X-linked recessive (CD40L) and autosomal recessive (CD40) defects have been described.
  - Clinical manifestations: Patients often present with recurrent bacterial infections, *Pneumocystis jirovecii* pneumonia (PJP), or infections from *Cryptosporidium* species. A subset of patients also develops autoimmune cytopenia (most commonly neutropenia) or organ-specific autoimmunity.
  - Labs: Normal to increased serum IgM level with decreased levels of IgG, IgA, and IgE.

• Treatment: HSCT is the only curative treatment for HIGM syndrome.
• **Activated phosphoinositide 3-kinase δ syndrome (APDS)**
  • APDS is characterized by autosomal-dominant mutations that increase the activity of the PI3Kδ pathway leading to recurrent respiratory tract infections and lymphoproliferation.
  • Causes: Heterozygous gain-of-function mutations in PI3KCD or PI3KR1.
  • Clinical manifestations: Recurrent bacterial infections, severe/persistent herpesvirus infections, and lymphoproliferation. Autoimmunity is also seen in 20-30% of patients.
  • Labs: Progressive T- and B-cell lymphopenia, decreased number of naïve T cells, and hypogammaglobulinemia.
  • Treatment: Immunoglobulin replacement therapy, antimicrobial prophylaxis, and consideration of mTOR inhibitors or selective PI3Kδ inhibitors for treatment of immune dysregulation.

## Combined Immunodeficiencies with Associated or Syndromic Features

• This group encompasses PIs associated with distinguishing clinical features that might influence or guide the diagnostic approach. These diseases include DiGeorge syndrome, Wiskott-Aldrich syndrome, ataxia telangiectasia, and other DNA repair defects, NEMO syndrome, and hyper-IgE syndromes.
• **DiGeorge syndrome (DGS)**
  • DGS is characterized by cardiac defects, thymic hypoplasia, and hypocalcemia. DGS patients usually have mild-to-moderate immunodeficiency, characteristic facial features, and language delay.
  • Causes: Chromosome 22q11.2 microdeletion is the leading cause of DGS (approximately 90% of cases).
  • Clinical manifestations: DGS patients can have recurrent respiratory tract illnesses resulting from their T-cell deficits and/or structural abnormalities. They also have an increased incidence of certain autoimmune diseases, such as juvenile idiopathic arthritis and autoimmune cytopenia.
  • Labs: Usually mild-to-moderate T-cell lymphopenia (T-cell count 500-1500 cells/μL), hypogammaglobulinemia, and poor antibody responses.
  • Treatment for immunodeficiency: T-cell count typically improves during the first year of life, and one-third of DGS patients produce a normal number of total T cells by the end of their first year of life. Generally, patients with complete DiGeorge phenotype with CD3+ T cells <50 cells/μL require thymic transplant, antimicrobial prophylaxis, and avoidance of live vaccines. For partial DiGeorge syndrome, live vaccines are generally allowed after 1 year of age if labs show CD8+ T cells >300 cells/μL, CD4+ T cells >500 cells/μL, normal or near normal proliferative response to mitogen and tetanus, and presence of antibodies to killed vaccine antigens.
• **Wiskott-Aldrich syndrome (WAS)**
  • WAS is characterized by immunodeficiency, microthrombocytopenia, and severe eczema. WAS patients also have an increased risk of autoimmune disorders and lymphoid malignancies.
  • Causes: X-linked pathogenic variant of *WASP* gene.
  • Clinical manifestations: Patients have increased susceptibility to various pathogens, including herpesvirus, bacteria, fungi, and PJP. Excessive bleeding after circumcision can be an early diagnostic sign of WAS.

- Labs: Thrombocytopenia associated with small platelet volumes, T-cell lymphopenia, and low IgM levels (with high IgA and IgE levels) may be present. Patients classically have poor responses to polysaccharide antigens.
- Treatment for immunodeficiency: HSCT is the most reliable curative treatment for WAS. Splenectomy may be indicated in patients with refractory thrombocytopenia, but this is associated with an increased risk of septicemia. Gene therapy for WAS has been successfully reported, but long-term outcomes are unknown.
- **Ataxia telangiectasia (A-T)**
  - A-T is a rare autosomal recessive disorder characterized by progressive neurologic impairment, oculocutaneous telangiectasias, immunodeficiency, radiation hypersensitivity, predisposition to malignancies, and premature aging.
  - Causes: Biallelic variants of *ATM* genes.
  - Clinical manifestations: Ataxia is often the earliest clinical manifestation of A-T and becomes obvious after 5 years of age. A-T patients can have recurrent upper and lower respiratory tract infections, but severe viral and systemic bacterial infections are uncommon. Patients can develop noninfectious cutaneous granulomas following the MMR vaccine.
  - Labs: Elevated alpha-fetoprotein levels, moderate lymphopenia, low immunoglobulin levels (particularly IgA), and impaired antibody responses and lymphoproliferative responses to mitogens and antigens.
  - Treatment for immunodeficiency: Some patients may benefit from prophylactic antibiotics and/or immunoglobulin replacement therapy. Careful monitoring and managing other risk factors for infections (such as aspiration) is recommended.
- **NEMO deficiency syndrome**
  - NEMO deficiency syndrome is characterized by defects of NF-κB activation that lead to ectodermal dysplasia and immunodeficiency.
  - Causes: Hypomorphic variant in the *IKBKG* gene causes X-linked anhidrotic ectodermal dysplasia with immunodeficiency in males. The autosomal-dominant form is caused by a gain-of-function variant in the *IKBA* gene.
  - Clinical manifestations: Patients are susceptible to recurrent pyogenic, mycobacterial, and serious viral infections. A subset of patients also develops inflammatory and autoimmune conditions such as colitis, AIHA, and arthritis.
  - Labs: Elevated IgM or IgA levels and low IgG and IgE levels may be present. Patients with NEMO syndrome usually have no response to the conjugated or polysaccharide pneumococcal vaccine.
  - Treatment for immunodeficiency: Immunoglobulin replacement and prophylactic antibiotics should be considered, and HSCT is a consideration in patients with a severe clinical phenotype. Vaccination with BCG vaccine is contraindicated.
- **Hyper-IgE syndromes (HIES)**
  - HIES are characterized by elevated serum IgE levels, eczema, and recurrent infections.
  - Causes: In addition to loss-of-function mutation of *STAT3* (Job syndrome) and DOCK8 deficiency, there are at least six other genetic defects that can lead to features of HIES.
  - ***Dominant-negative mutations in STAT3 (STAT3 LOF, or Job syndrome)***
    - Clinical manifestation: Recurrent pneumonia, eczema, boils, chronic mucocutaneous candidiasis, dysmorphic facies, connective tissue and skeletal abnormalities, vasculopathy, and elevated IgE level.
    - Treatment: Antimicrobial prophylaxis against staphylococcal infections and treatment of disease-associated complications are recommended in patients with

STAT3 deficiency. HSCT may reduce frequency and severity of infections and pulmonary complications in selected patients.

- **DOCK8 Deficiency**
  - Clinical manifestations: Eczema, recurrent bacterial pneumonia and skin infections, cutaneous viral infections from HPV, HSV, zoster, and molluscum, chronic cryptosporidium infection, vasculitis, and malignancy. DOCK 8 deficiency is considered a combined immunodeficiency affecting both T- and B-cell functions.
  - Treatment: HSCT can be curative in DOCK8-deficient patients.

## Predominantly Antibody Deficiencies

- Predominantly antibody deficiencies can be broadly classified into six different phenotypes based on the presence or absence of hypogammaglobulinemia, antibody responses to vaccines, and B-cell counts (Table 20-4). These disorders have certain features in common:
  - Patients often develop recurrent infections at 6-9 months of age, coinciding with a nadir period of prenatally acquired immunoglobulins, but some patients have onset of symptoms at a later age.
  - Infections include recurrent acute respiratory tract infections, bacterial infections from encapsulated organisms, and severe bacterial infections such as septic arthritis, osteomyelitis, meningitis, septicemia, and enterocolitis.
  - Patients can present with immune dysregulation, such as autoimmune cytopenias, IBDs, granulomatous inflammation, chronic lung diseases, bronchiectasis, autoimmune thyroiditis, and vitiligo.
  - Evaluation for patients with suspected primary antibody deficiencies should include immunoglobulin levels (IgG, IgA, IgM, and IgE) and vaccine titers (protein antigens such as tetanus and diphtheria, as well as polysaccharide antigens such as pneumococcus).
  - Treatment often involves patient and family education, initiation of antibiotic prophylaxis and/or immunoglobulin replacement therapy, and prompt response to acute infections. Chronic immunosuppressive therapy may be indicated for the treatment of noninfectious complications.

### Agammaglobulinemia

- Agammaglobulinemia is characterized by a severe reduction of all serum immunoglobulin isotypes with absent circulating B cells.
- Causes: X-linked (*BTK*), autosomal recessive (*IGHM, IGLL1, CD79a, CD79b, BLNK, PIK3R, PIK3CD, TCF3,* and *SLC39A7*), and rarely autosomal-dominant (*TCF3,* and *TOP2B*) forms of the disease have been described.
- Clinical manifestations: Patients usually became symptomatic by 6-12 months of age with increased susceptibility to infections as described above. They also can develop meningoencephalitis from enteroviruses and complications from live polio vaccines.
- Treatment: In addition to standard therapy with immunoglobulin replacement, hematopoietic cell transplantation and gene therapy have been attempted in patients with X-linked agammaglobulinemia.

### Common Variable Immunodeficiency

- Common variable immunodeficiency (CVID) is characterized by a significant reduction of IgG, IgA, and/or IgM, along with poor or absent vaccine responses. B-cell counts can be low or normal. CVID is one of the most common symptomatic PIs, but other PIs must be excluded before making the diagnosis.

**TABLE 20-4** Screening Lab Results in Predominantly Antibody Deficiencies

| Disease | Immunoglobulin levels | | | Vaccine response | B-cell count |
|---|---|---|---|---|---|
| | IgG | IgA | IgM | | |
| Agammaglobulinemia | Absent | Absent | Absent | Absent | Very low-absent |
| Common variable immunodeficiency | Low | Normal or low | Normal or low | Low | Normal or low |
| Hypogammaglobulinemia | Low | Normal | Normal | Normal | Normal |
| Specific antibody deficiency | Normal | Normal | Normal | Low to polysaccharide vaccines | Normal |
| Selective IgA deficiency | Normal | Absent | Normal | Normal | Normal |
| Transient hypogammaglobulinemia of infancy | Low | Normal or low | Normal or low | Normal | Normal |

- Causes: The majority of CVID cases have no identified genetic defects.
- Clinical manifestations: Recurrent infections, as well as autoimmune/inflammatory features such as enteropathy, immune-mediated lung disease, granulomatous inflammation, bronchiectasis, liver dysfunction, and organomegaly.
- Treatment: Immunoglobulin replacement, prophylactic antibiotics, and careful monitoring and treatment of disease-associated complications.

*Specific Antibody Deficiency*
- Specific antibody deficiency (SAD) is characterized by recurrent infections and impaired antibody response to polysaccharide antigens with intact protein antibody response, as well as normal immunoglobulin levels and IgG subclasses in patients over 2 years old.
- Causes: The genetic defects of SAD are unknown.
- Clinical manifestations: Patients usually present with recurrent bacterial infections of the upper and lower respiratory tract. Atopic diseases may also be increased.
- Labs: Establishing a diagnosis of SAD relies on assessing antibody response to the pneumococcal polysaccharide vaccine. (A normal response to pneumococcal vaccines is a response to 50% or greater of serotypes for patients under 6 years of age, and a response to 70% or greater of serotypes for patients over 6 years of age. Generally, postvaccination titers of $\geq 1.3$ µg/mL, or a two-fold rise compared to prevaccination titers, is considered an adequate response.)
- Treatment: Antibiotic prophylaxis is recommended for patients with mild clinical phenotype, and they may benefit from additional immunization with conjugate pneumococcal vaccines. In patients with severe phenotype or failure to respond to antibiotic prophylaxis, immunoglobulin replacement should be considered.

*Selective IgA Deficiency (sIgA Deficiency)*
- Selective IgA deficiency is characterized by a serum IgA level of <7 mg/dL and normal levels of IgG and IgM in patients older than 4 years. It is the most common primary antibody deficiency, but at least two-thirds of patients with sIgA deficiency are asymptomatic.
- Causes: The genetic defects of sIgA deficiency are unknown.
- Clinical manifestations: Symptomatic patients usually present with recurrent sinopulmonary infections or gastrointestinal diseases. A subset of patients may progress to CVID, and there are reports of increased prevalence of autoimmune and allergic diseases. Anaphylactic reactions to blood products have also been reported in patients with sIgA deficiency, but the majority can receive blood products without reactions.
- Treatment: Clinicians should reassure patients that the majority of individuals with sIgA deficiency are healthy and live normal lives. Antibiotic prophylaxis is considered only in patients with continued infections despite management of underlying conditions. Immunoglobulin therapy does not replace IgA, and it is rarely indicated in sIgA deficiency.

*Transient Hypogammaglobulinemia of Infancy*
- Transient Hypogammaglobulinemia of Infancy (THI) is characterized by IgG levels <2 standard deviations below the mean for age-matched controls with possible involvement of IgA, and less frequently IgM. Levels spontaneously return to normal, usually by 2-3 years of age.
- Causes: Unknown.
- Clinical manifestations: Most patients with THI are asymptomatic.
- Labs: Clinicians should ensure that the patients have normal specific antibody response and normal lymphocyte subsets.

- Treatment: Observation and reassurance. A small subset of patients may require antibiotic prophylaxis for recurrent respiratory tract infections; immunoglobulin replacement is rarely indicated.

## Phagocyte Disorders

- Phagocyte defects can lead to neutropenia and/or poor neutrophil function.
- Neutropenia can be classified as primary or acquired (see review in Chapter 19). Congenital neutropenia syndromes are a group of rare genetic disorders that are present from birth and characterized by severe neutropenia and increased susceptibility to infections.
- Abnormal neutrophil function can result from defects in the respiratory oxidative burst (as seen in chronic granulomatous disease), abnormal neutrophil motility (as seen in leukocyte adhesion disorder), or defects in interferon gamma and IL-12 pathways. These various disorders cause susceptibility to infections and sometimes immune dysregulation.
- **Chronic granulomatous disease (CGD)**
  - CGD is characterized by inherited defects of neutrophil NAPDH oxidase activity leading to susceptibility to bacterial and fungal infections and granulomatous inflammation.
  - Causes: X-linked recessive (*CYBB* gene, two-thirds of CGD cases in the United States) and autosomal recessive (*CYBA, NCF1, NCF2,* and *NCF4*) modes of inheritance have been identified.
  - Clinical manifestations: Recurrent respiratory tract infections, failure to thrive, skin or organ abscesses, cellulitis, lymphadenitis, and granulomatous inflammations of visceral organs and lymph nodes. Common pathogens include *Staphylococcus aureus, Burkholderia cepacia* complex, *Serratia marcescens, Nocardia* species, *Aspergillus* species, and *Actinomyces* species. Inflammatory conditions, such as IBD and genitourinary tract granulomas, may occur in CGD patients. These patients also tend to develop severe localized reactions to the BCG vaccine.
  - Labs: Impaired neutrophil oxidative burst by dihydrorhodamine (DHR) assay or nitroblue tetrazolium reduction test. If patients have an impaired neutrophil oxidative burst, targeted genetic sequencing of five known responsible genes for CGD should be sent for molecular diagnosis.
  - Treatment: Prophylactic antimicrobials (trimethoprim-sulfamethoxazole and itraconazole), interferon-gamma therapy, and immunosuppressive agents for inflammatory complications. HSCT is the only curative treatment option for CGD.
- **Leukocyte adhesion deficiency (LAD)**
  - LAD is characterized by defects in neutrophil adhesion to the vessel endothelium, an important step required to kill microbes.
  - Causes: There are three different types of LAD. The most common type is LAD 1, which is an autosomal recessive disorder caused by variants in the *ITGB2* gene resulting in defective beta2-integrin (CD18).
  - Clinical manifestations: Recurrent bacterial infections (omphalitis, pneumonia, gingivitis, and peritonitis) with onset in the first weeks of life, poor wound healing, pyoderma gangrenosum, absent pus formation, and delayed umbilical cord separation.
  - Labs: Leukocytosis even in the absence of infection is common. A reduction or absence of CD18 expression by flow cytometry is diagnostic for LAD 1 and absence of CD15a by flow cytometry is diagnostic for type LAD 2.
  - Treatment: HSCT is the definitive treatment for LAD 1. Gene therapy is also available for LAD 1 through clinical trials. In patients with milder phenotypes, prophylactic antibiotics and aggressive treatment of bacterial infections are indicated.

## Complement Deficiencies

- Complement deficiencies are very rare PIs, and patients may present with recurrent bacterial infections and/or systemic lupus erythematosus, depending on the defect.
- Causes: Absent or suboptimal function in any component of the complement system.
- Clinical manifestations: Most early classical and alternative pathway complement defects present with either lupus-like disease or recurrent respiratory tract infections. Deficiencies of terminal components can be associated with increased susceptibility to encapsulated bacteria, especially *Neisseria* species. In addition, abnormalities in complement regulatory proteins can result in atypical hemolytic uremic syndrome.
- Labs: CH50 assay screening for classical pathway defects and AH50 screening for alternative pathway defects. Of note, while mannose binding lectin (MBL) is part of the lectin pathway of the complement system, most individuals with MBL deficiency do not have increased incidence of infections, so serum MBL levels should not be sent routinely.
- Treatment: Antibiotic prophylaxis and immunization against meningococcus and pneumococcus; prompt treatment of acute infections.

## Defects in Intrinsic and Innate Immunity

- The range and type of infections of innate immunity defects depend on the mutated gene and other factors. In additions to the diseases described below, GATA2 deficiency, genetic disorders associated with herpes simplex encephalitis, and disorders with increased risks of chronic mucocutaneous candidiasis are also included in this group of PIs.
- **IL-1 receptor–associated kinase 4 (IRAK-4) and myeloid differentiation primary response 88 (MyD88) deficiencies**
  - IRAK-4 and MyD88 deficiency are rare PIs that are characterized by recurrent invasive infections. The clinical presentation of these two disorders is identical, and they can only be distinguished by genetic testing.
  - Causes: Autosomal recessive mutation in *IRAK4* gene for IRAK4 deficiency and in *MyD88* gene for MyD88 deficiency.
  - Clinical manifestations: Recurrent invasive infections with bacteria (*S. aureus, S. pneumoniae*, and *P. aeruginosa*), and normal workup for defects in antibody production/function, complements, and phagocytes. Patients are usually afebrile with normal inflammatory markers despite severe, acute infections.
  - Labs: Routine screening tests for PIs are usually within normal limits, with the possible exception of vaccine response to pneumococcal polysaccharide antigens. Toll-like receptor (TLR) signaling defects can be screened by measurement of TLR response in vitro. The absence of TLR-induced cytokine production must be followed by targeted genetic sequencing.
  - Treatment: Antibiotic prophylaxis and/or immunoglobulin replacement therapy.
- **Warts, hypogammaglobulinemia, immunodeficiency, and myelokathexis (WHIM) syndrome**
  - WHIM syndrome is a rare PI characterized by increased susceptibility to papilloma viruses, lymphopenia with markedly decreased memory B-cell count, hypogammaglobulinemia, and neutropenia.
  - Causes: Most cases are caused by an autosomal-dominant GOF mutation in CXCR4.

- Clinical manifestations: Widespread recalcitrant wards, condyloma acuminata with risk of malignant transformation, and recurrent bacterial infections in various organs systems.
- Labs: Neutropenia, lymphopenia, low IgG levels, and possibly low IgA levels. Genetic testing is required for a definitive diagnosis.
- Treatment: Immunoglobulin replacement and/or G-CSF therapy. HPV vaccination should be considered. HSCT for WHIM has been rarely reported.

## Diseases of Immune Dysregulation

- This is a group of PIs with autoimmunity as a defining feature; patients may have limited history of infection.
- **Immunodysregulation, polyendocrinopathy, enteropathy, X-linked (IPEX) syndrome**
  - IPEX syndrome is characterized by severe, life-threatening infections due to loss of regulatory T-cell (Treg) differentiation.
  - Causes: X-linked recessive defect in gene encoding FOXP3, a master transcription factor responsible for the development and function of Tregs.
  - Clinical manifestations: Severe infantile-onset enteropathy, insulin-dependent diabetes mellitus, and dermatitis. Other autoimmune features include cytopenias, thyroid disease, renal disease, and hepatitis.
  - Labs: Eosinophilia, hypergammaglobulinemia including elevated IgE levels, and the presence of a variety of autoantibodies.
  - Treatment: Aggressive treatment with immunosuppressive agents is needed in symptomatic patients. HSCT can provide curative immune reconstitution and should be initiated as soon as possible. In spite of these treatments, IPEX syndrome has a high mortality rate.
- **STAT3 gain-of-function (GOF)**
  - STAT3 GOF is characterized by early-onset polyautoimmunity with a wide range of manifestations. Susceptibility to various infections is found in a subset of patients, but this is not always a predominant feature.
  - Causes: Heterozygous GOF variant in *STAT3* gene.
  - Clinical manifestations: Autoimmune cytopenias, lymphoproliferation, enteropathy, autoimmune hepatitis, interstitial lung disease, thyroiditis, arthritis, and growth failure.
  - Labs: Hypogammaglobulinemia and lymphopenia can be seen in some patients.
  - Treatment: Chronic immunosuppression with targeted therapy is required for most symptomatic patients. HSCT has been reported in a small number of patients with life-threatening complications, but the data are limited.
- **Autoimmune polyendocrinopathy-candidiasis-ectodermal dystrophy (APECED)**
  - APECED is characterized by a classic triad of chronic mucocutaneous candidiasis, hypoparathyroidism, and adrenal failure. Other endocrine, skin, and other organ-specific autoimmunity also can occur in APECED patients.
  - Causes: This is an autosomal recessive disorder caused by mutations in the *AIRE* gene.
  - Labs: No specific serologic tests are available for diagnosis of APECED. Genetic testing is required for a definitive diagnosis.
  - Treatment: Life-long antifungal prophylaxis to prevent recurrent candidiasis, replacement therapy for endocrine abnormalities, steroids and steroid-sparing

agents for autoimmunity, and immunoglobulin replacement therapy for antibody deficiency.

- **Autoimmune lymphoproliferative disease (ALPS)**
  - ALPS is characterized by abnormal apoptosis of lymphocytes leading to lymphadenopathy, hepatosplenomegaly, autoimmune cytopenias (often Evans syndrome), autoimmune organ disease, and increased risk of lymphoma.
  - Causes: Both autosomal-dominant (*TNFRSF6, TNFSF6, CASP10,* and *CASP8*) and autosomal recessive (*TNFRSF6,* and *TNFSF6*) inheritance of ALPS-causative genes have been reported. These can be either germline or somatic mutations.
  - Labs: Increased alpha-beta double-negative (DNT) cells in peripheral blood, increased plasma soluble FASL levels, elevated serum levels of IL-10 and/or vitamin B12, and defective FAS-mediated apoptosis on in vitro assay. Genetic sequencing for ALPS-associated genes should be sent to confirm the diagnosis.
  - Treatment: Treatment of ALPS is focused on the management of autoimmune manifestations with immunosuppressive agents. Splenectomy may be indicated for refractory thrombocytopenia/hemolysis. HSCT should be considered in patients with severe manifestations.

## SUMMARY

Clinicians should be concerned for PIs in patients who have recurrent serious infections with common pathogens, serious infections with unusual pathogens, a positive family history of PI, or syndromic features that may be associated with PIs. Certain PIs have immune dysregulation as their primary feature with only a limited history of infection. History taking and focused examination are valuable in guiding initial laboratory evaluation. Genetic diagnosis is essential in many PIs to provide targeted therapy and genetic counseling. Treatment consists of prompt treatment of acute infections, measures to prevent infections, management of complications, immune reconstitution therapy if possible, and psychosocial support.

## SUGGESTED READINGS

Abolhassani H, Azizi G, Sharifi L, et al. Global systematic review of primary immunodeficiency registries. Expert Rev Clin Immunol 2020;16:717–732.

Bonilla FA, Khan DA, Ballas ZK, et al. Practice parameter for the diagnosis and management of primary immunodeficiency. J Allergy Clin Immunol 2015;136:1186–205.e1-78.

Bousfiha A, Jeddane L, Picard C, et al. Human inborn errors of immunity: 2019 update of the IUIS phenotypical classification. J Clin Immunol 2020;40:66–81.

Dorsey MJ, Puck JM. Newborn screening for severe combined immunodeficiency in the United States: lessons learned. Immunol Allergy Clin North Am 2019;39:1–11.

Kitcharoensakkul M, Cooper MA. Rheumatologic and autoimmune manifestations in primary immune deficiency. Curr Opin Allergy Clin Immunol 2019;19:545–552.

Ochs HD, Hagin D, eds. Primary immunodeficiency disorders: general classification, new molecular insights, and practical approach to diagnosis and treatment. Ann Allergy Asthma Immunol 2014;112:489–495.

Perez EE, Ballow M. Diagnosis and management of specific antibody deficiency. Immunol Allergy Clin North Am 2020;40:499–510.

Rezaei N, Aghamohammadi A, Notarangelo LD. Primary Immunodeficiency Diseases: Definition, Diagnosis, and Management. 2nd Ed. Berlin: Springer, 2016.

Rose NR, Mackay IR, eds. The Autoimmune Diseases. 6th Ed. London: Academic Press, 2020.

Smith T, Cunningham-Rundles C. Primary B-cell immunodeficiencies. Hum Immunol 2019;80:351–362.

# Infectious Diseases

Andrew B. Janowski, Carol M. Kao, and Alexis Elward

## COMMON PEDIATRIC INFECTIONS

### Acute Otitis Media

*Epidemiology and Etiology*
- Acute otitis media (AOM) results in fluid accumulation behind the middle ear with subsequent inflammation.
- One of the most common infections for which children are prescribed antibiotics; some estimate 8-12 million prescriptions annually, with the incidence decreasing over the past decade.
- Most commonly seen in conjunction with viral respiratory tract infections, including respiratory syncytial virus (RSV), parainfluenza, influenza, rhinovirus, enterovirus, or adenovirus.
  - Most cases of AOM are viral, without the presence of bacteria.
  - Common bacterial pathogens include *Streptococcus pneumoniae*, *Haemophilus influenzae*, *Moraxella catarrhalis*, group A and B streptococcus, and rarely *Staphylococcus aureus*.

*Clinical Presentation*
- Children present with fever, ear pain, fussiness, and/or impaired hearing.
- Younger infants may present with nonspecific complaints including ear tugging, malaise, vomiting, congestion, cough, fussiness, or fever without localizing symptoms.
- AOM must be differentiated from otitis media with effusion (OME), since OME does not warrant antimicrobial therapy.
  - Otoscopy is essential to the diagnosis. The best and most reproducible finding of AOM is bulging of the tympanic membrane (TM). Other findings that are less specific are retraction, opacification, and decreased mobility of the TM. Presence of purulent-appearing fluid or air bubbles may also be helpful. Erythema may also be present but can be nonspecific and induced by other causes including crying.
  - OME is the presence of a middle ear effusion without signs of inflammation; the TMs are not bulging nor erythematous.

*Treatment*
- Pain control is an essential part of therapy, as NSAIDs or acetaminophen provide symptomatic relief.
- The 2013 American Academy of Pediatrics and the American Academy of Family Physicians produced a guideline of treatment for AOM.
  - Children under the age of 6 months with AOM should be treated with antibiotics. For children 6-23 months with unilateral nonsevere (mild otalgia, otalgia for <48 hours, or temperature below 39°C) AOM, a period of watchful observation may be offered. For children 6-23 months with bilateral AOM, even with mild symptoms, treatment with antibiotics should be prescribed. Watchful waiting can be offered for all situations of AOM in children older than 24 months. Meta-analyses demonstrate

that treatment of AOM with antibiotics only results in modest improvement in symptoms and that many cases are self-resolving and/or caused by viral pathogens.
- If antibiotic therapy is to be initiated, first-line therapy should be amoxicillin 80-90 mg/kg/day in two divided doses. If a child fails to improve, next-line therapy is amoxicillin/clavulanic acid dosed at 90 mg/kg/day (of the amoxicillin component) divided twice a day. The rationale behind this choice is that the pathogens may have beta lactamase resistance to amoxicillin, and the usage of clavulanic acid may restore susceptibility.
- Treatment duration is typically 10 days for children <2 years of age and 5-7 days for children older than 2 years.
- If the infection continues, consider administration of IM ceftriaxone for improved activity against potentially resistant pathogens. ENT referral for tympanocentesis may be indicated.
- If a child has multiple episodes of AOM, at least three episodes in 6 months or four episodes in 1 year, this may be an indication for referral to ENT for myringotomy tube placement. If there is a history of other frequent infections, severe infections requiring hospitalization, or poor weight gain, an underlying immunodeficiency may also be considered.

## Bronchiolitis

*Epidemiology and Etiology*
- One of the most common causes of pediatric hospitalization.
- Typically afflicts children under the age of 2 years, with a peak incidence between 2 and 6 months of age.
- Caused by viral infection, most common agents include RSV, human metapneumovirus, parainfluenza, rhinovirus, influenza, adenoviruses, and coronaviruses. Also associated with *Bordetella pertussis* and *Mycoplasma pneumoniae.*
- Incidence corresponds to peaks in viral activity, predominantly during winter months, although this condition can be seen all times of the year.

*Clinical Presentation*
- Initial symptoms include congestion and nasal discharge. Fever may also be observed:
  - Progression of the disease involves lower airways, leading to cough, tachypnea, and respiratory distress.
- Clinical exam can be quite variable but is typically associated with diffuse crackles or wheezes, associated with signs of respiratory distress including nasal flaring, grunting, and retractions.
  - Hypoxemia is a common indication for hospitalization.
- Clinical course is variable, but younger infants, history of prematurity, immunodeficiency, or chronic lung disease may lead to prolonged duration of illness.

*Laboratory Studies and Imaging*
- Bronchiolitis is a clinical diagnosis; additional testing is not required.
- Blood gases may be helpful in determining which infants may require more intensive respiratory interventions.
- Chest x-ray (CXR) commonly shows atelectasis, hyperexpansion, or diffuse peribronchiolar infiltrates.
- Atelectasis arising from viral bronchiolitis can be confused with lobar consolidation seen with bacterial pneumonia.
- Viral testing is not commonly recommended, although it may be beneficial for infection control and patient cohorting. Testing for influenza allows for identification of infants who would be a candidate for oseltamivir treatment and prophylaxis of close contacts.

*Treatment and Prevention*
- Current recommendations are supportive care, including oxygen as needed, nasal suctioning, and hydration.
  - Bronchodilator therapy, in general, is not of benefit. Other interventions such as nebulized hypertonic saline may lead to potential benefit, but its impact is variable.
  - There is no clear evidence of significant benefit of antivirals or steroids with bronchiolitis, and therefore, these are not recommended.
  - Oseltamivir treatment is recommended for infants with influenza.
  - Severe infections may benefit from interventions like heated humidified high-flow nasal cannula (HFNC), continuous positive airway pressure (CPAP), mechanical ventilation, or rarely extracorporeal membrane oxygenation (ECMO).
- Focal findings on chest auscultation or persistence of symptoms beyond the expected duration of illness should prompt consideration for treatment of bacterial pneumonia.
- Palivizumab (Synagis) is available for prophylaxis of RSV infection in selected infants; see Table 21-1.
- Bronchiolitis is associated with future reactive airway disease (RAD), but it is unclear if this association is due to bronchiolitis increasing the risk of RAD or if infants who have underlying risks for RAD are at increased risk for developing bronchiolitis.

## Pneumonia
*Epidemiology and Etiology*
- One of the leading causes of pediatric death worldwide.
- Increasing data suggest viral pathogens are the most common cause of pneumonia, with up to 80% of community-acquired pneumonia in children under the age of two caused by viruses. Viral pathogens include RSV, parainfluenza, influenza, human metapneumoviruses, adenoviruses, coronaviruses, enteroviruses, and rhinoviruses.
- Common bacterial pathogens include *S. pneumoniae*, *H. influenzae*, *S. aureus*, *M. pneumoniae*, and *B. pertussis*. In newborns, other pathogens must be considered including *group B streptococcus*, enteric gram negatives, *Chlamydia trachomatis*, or *Treponema pallidum*.
  - Depending on the host, immunosuppression, and exposure history, additional infectious agents include *Chlamydophila pneumoniae*, *Chlamydophila psittaci*, *Legionella pneumophila*, *Histoplasma capsulatum*, *Blastomyces dermatitidis*, *Coccidioides immitis*, *Cryptococcus* species, *Francisella tularensis*, cytomegalovirus (CMV), herpes simplex virus (HSV), or *Mycobacterium* sp. (including *M. tuberculosis*).
  - There is a significant incidence of methicillin-resistant *S. aureus* (MRSA) pneumonia that is associated with severe, necrotizing disease.

*Clinical Presentation*
- Children typically present with fever, cough, and tachypnea, less commonly with fatigue, chest pain, or abdominal pain.
- Physical examination typically reveals focal findings of decreased breath sounds, wheezing, crackles, or egophony.
  - Pulse oximetry should be performed in all children with clinical suspicion of pneumonia.

*Laboratory Studies and Imaging*
- Viral testing may aid in the determination to treat with antibiotics or therapy against influenza, but there is a significant false-positive rate for other viruses and cases of coinfection with bacterial superinfection.

| TABLE 21-1 | Palivizumab Prophylaxis for Respiratory Syncytial Virus (Including 2014 Update) |
|---|---|

**Infants eligible for the 1st year of life**

- Any preterm infants born at or before 29 weeks and 0 days of gestation who are younger than 12 months at the start of RSV season
- Preterm infants who have chronic lung disease of prematurity (born prior to 32 weeks and 0 days and required supplemental oxygen above 21% for at least the first 28 days after birth)
- Infants with a hemodynamically significant congenital heart disease, which includes infants receiving medication for heart failure and will require a surgical intervention, or those with moderate to severe pulmonary hypertension[a]
- Infants younger than 12 months of age and requiring medical therapy for congenital heart disease
- Certain infants with neuromuscular disease or congenital abnormalities of the airways

**Infants eligible up through 2nd year of life**

- Preterm infants who have chronic lung disease of prematurity (born prior to 32 weeks and 0 days and required supplemental oxygen above 21% for at least the first 28 days after birth) who continue to require supplemental oxygen, diuretic therapy, or systemic corticosteroid use
- Children under 2 years of age who receive a cardiac transplant during RSV season
- Profound immunosuppression

Start of RSV season depends on location: Southeast Florida, July 1; North Central and Southwest Florida, September 15; most other areas of the United States, November 1.
[a]Discussion with a cardiologist is recommended. Congenital heart disease with hemodynamically insignificant lesions that may not require prophylaxis includes ventricular septal defect, atrial septal defect, aortic stenosis, pulmonic stenosis, patent ductus arteriosus, mild coarctation of the aorta, lesions that have been surgically repaired and do not require medication for congestive heart failure, or mild cardiomyopathy.
Adapted from Committee on Infectious Diseases and Bronchiolitis Guidelines Committee. Updated guidance for palivizumab prophylaxis among infants and young children at increased risk of hospitalization for respiratory syncytial virus infection. Pediatrics 2014;134:415–420; American Academy of Pediatrics; Kimberlin DW, Barnett ED, Lynfield R, et al. Red Book (2021): Report of the Committee on Infectious Diseases. 32nd Ed. Itasca, IL: American Academy of Pediatrics, 2021.

- Additional testing is available for some of the other etiologies of pneumonia, including serology, antigen testing, or polymerase chain reaction (PCR).
- CXR will routinely show lobar consolidation with a typical bacterial pneumonia. With MRSA pneumonia, lung abscess or necrotizing pneumonia may also be seen.
- The American Academy of Pediatrics (AAP), Infectious Diseases Society of America (IDSA), and the Pediatric Infectious Diseases Society (PIDS) do not recommend

routine CXR for patients who that will be managed as an outpatient. Studies have shown CXR findings do not routinely change clinical care in this scenario. CXR should be performed in children being hospitalized or in evaluating children who have not responded to therapy to evaluate for effusion or empyema formation.
- Classically *M. pneumoniae* often appears as a diffuse pneumonia on CXR; however, lobar consolidation can be observed.
- Blood cultures are infrequently positive (1-8.2%).

*Treatment and Prevention*
- In preschool children with mild disease and close follow-up, both IDSA and PIDS recommend against routine antimicrobials as the pneumonia is mostly like of viral etiology and that only supportive care is necessary.
- If a bacterial pneumonia is suspected and antibiotics are to be initiated, the first-line therapy to be used is amoxicillin (90 mg/kg/day divided BID) or ampicillin (150-200 mg/kg/day divided q6h).
  - Azithromycin should be considered if there is a high concern for *Mycoplasma* or *Chlamydophila* pneumonia.
  - Additional therapy with third-generation cephalosporins, clindamycin, or vancomycin may be considered for severe pneumonia or for children who fail to respond to initial therapy.
  - Most treatment regimens are 7-10 days in duration, longer for complicated pneumonia.
- Recurrent pneumonia should be a prompt for an evaluation of immunodeficiency, cystic fibrosis, ciliary dyskinesia, or structural defect.
- Common complications include pleural effusion, empyema, or abscess formation. In children with prolonged fevers or other symptoms despite appropriate antibiotics, imaging is warranted to evaluate for these complications.

## Urinary Tract Infection
*Epidemiology and Etiology*
- Urinary tract infection (UTI) is the most common cause of renal parenchymal damage.
- During the 1st year of life, males are affected more than are females; but after the 1st year, females are more likely to develop a UTI.
- Most common bacterial pathogens include *Escherichia coli*, other gram-negative bacteria (e.g., *Klebsiella* and *Proteus*), enterococci, *Staphylococcus saprophyticus*, and *group B streptococcus.*

*Clinical Presentation*
- Typical symptoms are dysuria, urinary urgency or frequency, suprapubic pain, abdominal pain, and fever.
- Less common symptoms include nausea, vomiting, or fussiness.

*Laboratory Studies and Imaging*
- Diagnosis in immunocompetent patients requires the presence of both: (1) pyuria and (2) isolation of a clinically relevant bacterial pathogen in sufficient quantity. The lack of one of these factors would suggest against a diagnosis of a UTI.
  - Finding pyuria on urinalysis is based on the presence of >5 white blood cells (WBCs)/high-power field (HPF). If urine microscopy is not available, the presence of leukocyte esterase can be substituted.

- Urinary nitrites are seen with only certain pathogens (gram-negative organisms) and if the urine has had sufficient dwell time in the urinary bladder. In younger infants who do not have a long urinary dwell time, nitrites are commonly not detected even when a gram-negative pathogen is present. Positive urinary nitrites have high specificity for UTI.
- Significant urinary culture results depend on the source of sample. Thresholds of >50,000 or >100,000 colony-forming units (CFUs)/mL have been utilized for catheterized or clean catch samples of clinically relevant bacteria.
- Bagged urinary specimens are prone to contamination from perineal organisms, and cultures from bagged specimens should not be used to establish a diagnosis of a UTI. However, a negative bagged specimen does eliminate the possibility of a UTI.
- If a urine sample has a positive culture result, but no evidence of pyuria, this may be reflective of three possibilities: (1) early UTI without a significant inflammatory response, (2) asymptomatic bacteriuria, or (3) contamination of the sample. A repeat sample should be obtained >24 hours later, even if the child is on antibiotics, as presence of pyuria would indicated that the previous sample was indeed consistent with an early UTI. If pyuria remains absent, this would suggest asymptomatic bacteriuria or contamination, and neither condition would require treatment.
- Ultrasound should be considered in febrile infants, children with recurrent UTIs, or children who do not respond to therapy.
- Avoiding cystourethrogram (VCUG) should be considered in children with abnormalities found on ultrasound or in those with recurrent episodes of febrile UTIs. VCUG should not be performed during the acute phase of the UTI.

*Treatment*
- Treatment can be guided toward common urinary pathogens, as antimicrobials such as cephalexin, ceftriaxone, trimethoprim-sulfamethoxazole, and nitrofurantoin all provide excellent empiric coverage as culture results are finalized. Nitrofurantoin should be avoided in cases of suspected pyelonephritis.
  - Based on local susceptibilities at our center, we utilize cephalexin as our first-line antibiotic.
  - Treatment duration is between 3 and 5 days for cystitis, 7 days for pyelonephritis, and 14 days for complicated pyelonephritis.
  - For some children with structural abnormalities or recurrent UTIs, daily prophylaxis can be considered with trimethoprim-sulfamethoxazole, nitrofurantoin, or amoxicillin. The usage of prophylaxis in urinary reflux is controversial, with some evidence demonstrating no benefit and other studies indicating lower incidence of UTI but increased rates of antibiotic resistance among urinary pathogens.
  - Children with structural abnormalities found on ultrasound should be referred to urology.
- At least 1-3% of children develop asymptomatic carriage of bacteria in their urinary tract, which is not associated with future development of UTIs or renal scarring, and should not be routinely treated with antibiotics.

## Approach to the Febrile Infant under 90 Days of Life
- Fever in infants <90 days of life is defined as a temperature ≥38°C.
- Infants with fever present a challenge and deserve special consideration. Infants under 90 days of life lack a well developed immune system, are exposed to a unique group of bacterial pathogens, and often do not localize a source of infection.
- Because of these risk factors, infants are at significant risk for serious bacterial infections (SBIs), including UTI, bacteremia, meningitis, pneumonia, and skin/soft tissue

infection. In one study, up to 13.5% of febrile infants had an identified SBI. UTIs are the most frequently identified infection, accounting for up to 92% of all cases of SBI. Meningitis accounts for around 1% of all febrile cases, with a higher risk for infants under 30 days of life.

• Many studies have evaluated screening tools to identify febrile infants most likely to have an SBI. One approach used by several centers is performing blood, urine, and cerebrospinal fluid (CSF) studies on all infants under 60 days of life, regardless of physical examination and laboratory results. There are cases of infants with normal physical examination and initial laboratory studies who are found to have meningitis. Alternatively, some centers make a clinical decision regarding performing a lumbar puncture (LP) for infants 30-90 days of life. See Table 21-2, which presents one

| **TABLE 21-2** | Approach to the Febrile Neonate |
|---|---|

| Age | Evaluation[a] | Management |
|---|---|---|
| 0-28 days | **1. Detailed history and complete physical examination**<br>**2. Laboratory evaluation for sepsis:**<br>• Blood: CBC with differential and culture<br>• Urine: catheterized urinalysis and culture<br>• CSF: cell count, protein, glucose, and culture<br>• Consider herpes simplex virus, enterovirus, and parechovirus polymerase chain reaction from the CSF<br>• Consider chest radiograph<br>• Consider respiratory viral multiplex | **1. Admit, and consider IV/ IM antibiotics until culture results are available:**<br>**Ampicillin:** Postmenstrual age ≥35 weeks, postnatal age <1 week, 100 mg/kg/dose q8. Age >1 week, 75 mg/kg/dose q6h<br>**Plus**<br>**Ceftazidime:** Postmenstrual age ≥35 weeks, postnatal age <1 week, 50 mg/kg/dose q12h. Age >1 week, 50 mg/kg/dose q8h<br>**Or**<br>**Ceftriaxone:** Postmenstrual age ≥35 weeks, of postnatal age >1 week and no contraindications like hyperbilirubinemia or receiving calcium-containing solutions including parental nutrition, 50 mg/kg/dose q12h<br>**Or**<br>**Gentamicin:** Postmenstrual age ≥35 weeks: 5 mg/kg/day q24h<br>**2. If herpes is suspected, add acyclovir:** 20 mg/kg/dose q8h |

*(Continued)*

**TABLE 21-2** Approach to the Febrile Neonate *(Continued)*

| Age | Evaluation[a] | Management |
|---|---|---|
| 29-60 days | 1. Detailed history and complete physical examination<br><br>2. Laboratory evaluation for sepsis: Same as 0-28 days<br><br>3. Patients who meet all of these criteria may be at lower risk for serious bacterial infection:<br>• Nontoxic appearance<br>• No focus of infection on examination (except otitis media)<br>• No known immunodeficiency<br>• Normal WBC count (5000-15,000 cells/μL)<br>• Band count <1500 cells/μL<br>• Normal urinalysis (<10 WBC/HPF on centrifuged urine)<br>• CSF < 10 WBC/μL, negative Gram stain, normal glucose or protein<br>• Normal chest radiograph (if performed) | 1. If toxic appearing or high risk, hospitalize for IV/IM antibiotics until culture results are available:<br>**Ceftriaxone** 50 mg/kg/dose q12h (meningitis dose)<br>**Plus:**<br>**Vancomycin** 15 mg/kg/dose q8h, if the infant is toxic appearing or high suspicion for bacterial meningitis<br>2. If herpes is suspected, add **acyclovir:** 20 mg/kg/dose q8h<br>3. If low risk, choose option after discussion with attending and/or primary care provider:<br>**Ceftriaxone:** 50 mg/kg IV/IM once and reexamine in 24 and 48 hours (must have LP)<br>**Or**<br>No antibiotics and reexamine in 24 and 48 hours |
| 61-90 days | 1. Detailed history and complete physical examination<br><br>2. Limited laboratory evaluation for sepsis:<br>• Blood: CBC with differential and culture<br>• Urine: catheterized urinalysis and culture<br>• LP if clinical concern for meningitis<br>• Chest radiograph (if indicated)<br>• Stool for heme test and culture (if indicated)<br>• Consider respiratory viral multiplex | 1. If toxic appearing, hospitalize for IV/IM antibiotics until culture results available:<br>**Ceftriaxone** 50 mg/kg/dose q12h<br>**Plus**<br>**Vancomycin** 15 mg/kg/dose q8h, if the infant is toxic appearing or high suspicion for bacterial meningitis<br>2. If nontoxic appearing:<br>No antibiotics and reexamine in 24 and 48 hours |

[a]Evaluation may also include studies for other (e.g., viral) infections as dictated by clinical signs and symptoms and by seasonal and geographic patterns.
CBC, complete blood count; LP, lumbar puncture; WBC, white blood cell; CSF, cerebrospinal fluid.

approach to the febrile infant. Remember that although guidelines and flow charts may be useful in managing certain classes of patients, diagnostic testing and management decisions should always incorporate clinical judgment.

- Although some clinicians would obtain a chest radiograph for all febrile infants, others consider this examination only in infants with signs of respiratory distress including tachypnea, nasal flaring, retractions, grunting, crackles, rhonchi, wheezing, cough, or rhinitis.
- Clinical bronchiolitis or positive testing for RSV or influenza significantly reduces the risk of SBIs. In several medium-sized trials, there have been no cases of meningitis with infants who have bronchiolitis or are positive for RSV or influenza, but there are isolated case reports of meningitis with bronchiolitis. The incidence of UTI and bacteremia is also reduced, but still at significant incidence.
- Indications for HSV testing and empiric acyclovir therapy in neonates with fever
  - There are no published criteria to apply in deciding which febrile neonates should be evaluated and treated empirically for HSV infection. Decisions may be guided by physical findings (e.g., skin lesions), presenting symptoms (e.g., lethargy or seizures), or local practice patterns.
  - Furthermore, there have been case reports of neonates with HSV meningitis who lack a CSF pleocytosis; thus, the lack of CSF pleocytosis cannot be used to rule out the possibility of HSV disease.
- Consultation with an infectious diseases specialist may be warranted.

## Meningitis

*Clinical Presentation*

- Young infants may present only with fever or temperature instability, irritability, somnolence, poor feeding, vomiting, and seizures.
- Older children may experience fever, headache, neck pain or stiffness, nausea and vomiting, photophobia, and irritability.
- The syndrome of inappropriate antidiuretic hormone secretion (SIADH) occurs in 30-60% of children with bacterial meningitis.

*Physical Examination*

- In infants, examination may reveal a bulging fontanelle.
- Common physical findings include lethargy, somnolence, meningismus, rash (including petechiae or purpura), and hemodynamic instability. Kernig and Brudzinski signs may be found in older children, but not typically in infants.
- Seizures can occur in 20-30% of patients within the first 3 days of their meningitis course, usually resulting from inflammation. However, seizures are more common with encephalitis. In many children, fever may persist for 5 days after initiation of antibiotic therapy.

*Laboratory Studies*

- The diagnosis is made on the basis of CSF findings after LP. CSF findings in meningitis are presented in Table 21-3.
- In the event of a traumatic LP, some clinicians use a correction factor to help discern which patients are unlikely to have meningitis and thus do not need to be admitted to the hospital.
  - A recent study found that a CSF WBC to red blood cell (RBC) ratio of ≤1:100 (0.01) and an observed-to-predicted CSF WBC count ratio of ≤0.01 have a high positive predictive value for predicting the absence of meningitis, where CSF predicted WBC count = CSF RBC × (peripheral blood WBC/peripheral blood RBC).
  - However, such ratios must be interpreted in the context of other parameters, including the CSF WBC differential, glucose, and Gram stain, as well as the patient's clinical appearance and whether the patient was pretreated with antibiotics.

| TABLE 21-3 | Cerebrospinal Fluid Parameters in Suspected Meningitis | | | |
|---|---|---|---|---|
| | Leukocytes/ μL | Neutrophils (%) | Glucose (mg/dL) | Protein (mg/dL) |
| Normal children | 0-6 | 0 | 40-80 | 20-30 |
| Normal newborn (under 28 days of life) | 0-18 | 2-3 | 32-121 | 19-149 |
| Bacterial meningitis | >1000 | >50 | <30 | >100 |
| Viral meningitis | 100-500 | <40 | >30 | 50-100 |
| Herpes meningitis | 10-1000 | <50 | >30 | >75 |
| Tuberculous meningitis | 10-500 | Polymorphonuclear neutrophils may predominate early, but typically, there is a lymphocytic predominance. | 20-40 | >400 |

Adapted from Wubbel L, McCracken GH Jr. Management of bacterial meningitis: 1998. Pediatr Rev 1998;19:78–84; Jacobs RF, Starke JR. Mycobacterium tuberculosis. In: Kliegman R, St. Geme J, eds. Nelson Textbook of Pediatrics. 21st Ed. Philadelphia, PA: Elsevier, 2020; Byington CL, Kendrick J, Sheng X. Normative cerebrospinal fluid profiles in febrile infants. J Pediatr 2011;158(1):130–134.

*Treatment*
- Give empiric antibiotic therapy as presented in Table 21-4.
- Duration of therapy varies with etiology, as shown in Table 21-5.
- Corticosteroids have been administered to patients with bacterial meningitis with the purpose of decreasing inflammation and thus decreasing the risk of hearing loss. However, conflicting literature exists regarding the benefit of corticosteroids in improving neurologic sequelae or reducing hearing loss.
  - Current American Academy of Pediatrics (AAP) guidelines state that dexamethasone should be recommended in conjunction with antibiotics for children with *H. influenzae* type b meningitis. The AAP guidelines state that dexamethasone therapy should be considered for infants and children with pneumococcal meningitis who are at least 6 weeks of age.
  - If dexamethasone is used, it should be given prior to or concurrently with the first antibiotic dose.

*Follow-Up*
- Considerations for repeat LP include the following:
  - Meningitis caused by resistant strains of *S. pneumoniae*
  - Meningitis caused by gram-negative bacilli
  - Lack of clinical improvement 24-36 hours after the start of therapy
  - Prolonged (>5 days) or secondary fever

| TABLE 21-4 | Common Etiologies and Empiric Antibiotics for Meningitis | |
|---|---|---|

| Age group | Common organisms | Suggested empiric therapy |
|---|---|---|
| 0-3 months | *Escherichia coli* <br> Group B *Streptococcus* <br> *Listeria monocytogenes* <br> Viruses (HSV, enterovirus, parechovirus) | 0-1 month: ampicillin plus ceftazidime or ceftriaxone or gentamicin; acyclovir if HSV is suspected <br><br> 1-3 months: ceftriaxone and vancomycin; acyclovir if HSV is suspected |
| 3 months to 18 years | *S. pneumoniae* <br> *Neisseria meningitidis* <br> Tuberculosis <br> Viruses (enterovirus, HSV, VZV, WNV, other arboviruses) <br> Tick-borne: *Ehrlichia, Anaplasma, Rickettsia* (Rocky Mountain spotted fever), Lyme disease | Ceftriaxone and vancomycin; acyclovir if HSV encephalitis is suspected |
| Immunocompromised | *S. pneumoniae, N. meningitidis* <br> Fungi (*Aspergillus, Cryptococcus, Blastomycosis, Histoplasmosis*) <br> Viruses <br> *Toxoplasma gondii* <br> Tuberculosis | Antimicrobials tailored to suspected etiology |

*Note: Haemophilus influenzae* is no longer a common pathogen where the Hib conjugate vaccine is routinely administered.
HSV, herpes simplex virus; VZV, varicella-zoster virus; WNV, West Nile virus.

- Recurrent meningitis
- Immunocompromised host
- All children with bacterial meningitis require a hearing evaluation. Sensorineural hearing loss occurs in approximately 30% of children with pneumococcal meningitis and in 5-10% of children with meningococcal and *H. influenzae* meningitis.

## Herpes Simplex Virus Encephalitis

*Clinical Presentation*

- Signs and symptoms include fever, seizures, altered mental status, personality changes, and focal neurologic findings.

| TABLE 21-5 | Duration of Antimicrobial Therapy Based for Children with Meningitis[a] |
|---|---|

| Etiology | Typical length of therapy |
|---|---|
| Enteric gram-negative bacilli | 21 days or longer after documentation of cerebrospinal fluid sterilization |
| Group B *Streptococcus* | 14 days or longer |
| Herpes simplex virus | 21 days |
| *Haemophilus influenzae* | 7 days |
| *Listeria monocytogenes* | 21 days or longer |
| *Neisseria meningitidis* | 5-7 days |
| *Streptococcus pneumoniae* | 10-14 days |

[a]The length of therapy should be considered on an individual basis. Patients with complications such as brain abscess, subdural empyema, delayed cerebrospinal fluid sterilization, or prolonged fever may need extended therapy.

- Onset is acute.
- Untreated disease progresses to coma and death.

*Laboratory Studies*
- CSF reveals elevated WBC (25-1000/µL) with a predominance of lymphocytes.
- HSV-1 or HSV-2 may be detected in CSF by PCR.
- CSF HSV PCR may be negative early in disease.
- Viral cultures are usually negative in patients with encephalitis caused by HSV.

*Diagnostic Studies*
- Electroencephalography may reveal a specific pattern of periodic lateralizing epileptiform discharges (PLEDs).
- Magnetic resonance imaging (MRI) is significantly more sensitive than is computed tomography in HSV encephalitis. Typical MRI findings include abnormal edema or hemorrhagic necrosis involving the white matter of the temporal lobe region (Fig. 21-1), though involvement in children with HSV-1 encephalitis may be more multifocal.

*Treatment*
- IV acyclovir should be given 60 mg/kg/day divided every 8 hours, typically for 21 days.
- Oral suppressive therapy for 6 months following treatment of acute infection has been associated with improved neurodevelopmental outcomes in cases of neonatal HSV encephalitis.

## Infectious Mononucleosis
*Epidemiology and Etiology*
- Infectious mononucleosis is most commonly caused by Epstein-Barr virus (EBV) and is transmitted via close personal contact or sharing of eating and drinking utensils.
- Other causes of infectious mononucleosis-like illness include CMV, toxoplasmosis, human immunodeficiency virus (HIV), rubella, hepatitis A virus (HAV), human herpesvirus 6 (HHV-6), and adenovirus.

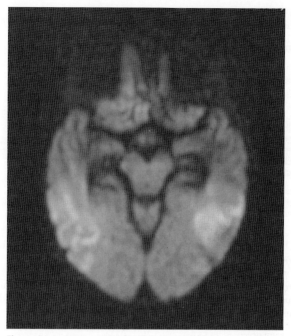

**Figure 21-1.** Temporal lobe white matter changes in a magnetic resonance image of a patient with herpes simplex virus encephalitis.

*Clinical Presentation*

- Signs and symptoms include fever, exudative pharyngitis, headache, generalized lymphadenopathy, malaise, and hepatosplenomegaly. A morbilliform rash may occur in patients with EBV infection who are treated with penicillin antibiotics, especially ampicillin.
- Symptoms typically last 1 week to 1 month in duration, and fatigue may persist for several months.
- Unusual complications include central nervous system (CNS) manifestations (aseptic meningitis, encephalitis, Guillain-Barré syndrome, cranial or peripheral neuropathies), splenic rupture, thrombocytopenia, agranulocytosis, hemolytic anemia, hemophagocytic syndrome, orchitis, and myocarditis.

*Laboratory Studies*

- Although the heterophile antibody test (Monospot) is often negative in children <4 years of age, it can identify 85% of cases in older children and adults.
  - Diagnosis may also be made with EBV antibody tests, including IgM and IgG to the viral capsid antigen (VCA), antibody to the early antigen (EA) complex diffuse component, and antibody to the EBV-associated nuclear antigen (EBNA).
  - All antibody tests may be negative in patients presenting in their first days of illness.
  - EBV DNA can often be detected by PCR in the blood during acute mononucleosis, but this testing is not recommended in the evaluation of routine cases. Viral reactivation during other illnesses is a frequent occurrence.

| TABLE 21-6 | Serum Epstein-Barr Virus (EBV) Antibodies in EBV Infection | | |
|---|---|---|---|
| Infection | VCA IgG | VCA IgM | EBNA |
| No previous infection | – | – | – |
| Acute infection | + | + | – |
| Recent infection | + | ± | ± |
| Past infection | + | – | + |

EBNA, EBV nuclear antigen; Ig, immunoglobulin; VCA, viral capsid antigen (e.g., VCA IgG, IgG class antibody to VCA).

Reprinted from American Academy of Pediatrics. In: Kimberlin DW, Barnett ED, Lynfield R, Sawyer MH, eds. Red Book: 2021 Report of the Committee on Infectious Diseases, 32nd Edition. American Academy of Pediatrics; 2021.

- Table 21-6 presents information about the interpretation of EBV antibodies in infectious mononucleosis.
- Patients with active infection may exhibit elevated serum transaminases.
- A rise in the proportion of atypical lymphocytes in the peripheral smear, often >10%, usually occurs during the 2nd week of illness. However, this finding is less common in young children.

*Treatment*
- Supportive care is appropriate.
- Corticosteroids may be used in patients with marked tonsillar inflammation with impending airway obstruction, massive splenomegaly, myocarditis, hemolytic anemia, aplastic anemia, hemophagocytic syndrome, or neurologic disease.
- Strenuous activity and contact sports should be avoided for at least 21 days after onset of symptoms.
- After 21 days, limited noncontact aerobic activity can be allowed if symptoms have resolved and there is no splenomegaly.
- Clearance to participate in contact sports may be appropriate after 4-7 weeks if the patient's symptoms have resolved and there is no splenomegaly.
- Patients should avoid contact sports until fully recovered and the spleen is no longer palpable.

## CHILDHOOD RASHES

### The Numbered Exanthems
For further information, see Table 21-7.

### Erythema Multiforme
- A benign, self-limited entity consisting of acute, fixed, erythematous macules that develop into papules and target lesions in which the central portion of the lesion becomes dusky or necrotic surrounded by concentric rings of erythema. These target lesions may coalesce to form plaques.

| TABLE 21-7 | The Numbered Exanthems of Childhood | | |
|---|---|---|---|
| Entity | Etiology | Clinical manifestations | Rash |
| First disease: measles (rubeola) | Paramyxovirus | Prodrome: 2-4 days with high fever, cough, coryza, and conjunctivitis | Koplik spots: 1-3 mm elevations may appear on the buccal mucosa; can be white, blue, or gray in color with an erythematous base. About 48 hours later, a maculopapular, erythematous, blanching rash erupts, starting on the head and spreading inferiorly; the rash may become confluent but spares the palms and soles (Fig. 20-2). After 2-3 days, the rash begins to fade and the patient experiences desquamation. |
| Second disease: scarlet fever | *Streptococcus pyogenes* pyrogenic exotoxin A | Sudden onset of fever and sore throat accompanied by malaise, headache, abdominal pain, and nausea and vomiting | Fine, diffuse, blanching red rash, which feels like sandpaper. The rash begins on the face and within 24 hours becomes generalized. The skin folds of the flexor surfaces exhibit intensified erythema, a sign known as "Pastia lines." Desquamation occurs 1 week after the onset of the rash, starting on the face and progressing inferiorly. |
| Third disease: rubella (German measles) | *Rubivirus* | Prodrome: tender lymphadenopathy with mild catarrhal symptoms and fever, eye pain, arthralgia, sore throat, and nausea and vomiting | 1-4 mm erythematous blanching macules begin on the face and spread to the trunk and extremities. The rash then fades to a nonblanching brownish color in the order of its appearance, which is followed by desquamation. |
| Fourth disease: Filatov-Dukes disease | This term is no longer used, but the entity was initially thought to be a "scarlet fever variety" of rubella. More recently, it is thought to be consistent with staphylococcal exotoxin disease (e.g., staphylococcal scalded skin syndrome). | | |

*(Continued)*

| TABLE 21-7 | | The Numbered Exanthems of Childhood *(Continued)* | |
|---|---|---|---|
| Entity | Etiology | Clinical manifestations | Rash |
| Fifth disease: erythema infectiosum | Parvovirus B19 | Prodrome: low-grade fever, headache, malaise, and coryza. These symptoms may be accompanied by pharyngitis, myalgias, arthralgias, arthritis, cough, conjunctivitis, nausea, and diarrhea | Abrupt onset of facial erythema occurring about 7-10 days after initial symptoms, giving the appearance of "slapped cheeks" with circumoral pallor. This is followed by the development of a lacy, erythematous rash on the trunk and extremities. The rash may be exacerbated by hot baths, emotion, sunlight, or exercise. |
| Sixth disease: roseola infantum (exanthem subitum) | HHV-6 and HHV-7 | Intermittent high fevers for 1-8 days accompanied by mild upper respiratory symptoms, adenopathy, and vomiting and diarrhea. Occasionally, the child may have neurologic symptoms including a bulging anterior fontanelle, seizures, or encephalopathy. On physical examination, the child may have pharyngitis or inflamed tympanic membranes | Within 2 days after defervescence, the rash develops, consisting of 2-3 mm rose-colored blanching macules and papules surrounded by a white halo, which begin on the trunk and spread to the face, neck, and extremities. |

HHV, human herpes virus.
*Data from* Wolfrey JD, et al. Pediatric exanthems. Clin Fam Pract 2003;5:557–588; Tanz RR, Shulman ST. Pharyngitis. In: Long SS, Prober CG, Fischer M, eds. Principles and Practice of Pediatric Infectious Diseases. 5th Ed. Philadelphia, PA: Elsevier Saunders, 2018; Weisse ME. The fourth disease, 1900–2000. Lancet 2001;357:299–301.

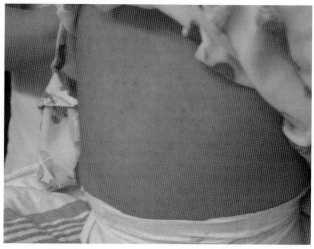

**Figure 21-2. Erythematous rash caused by measles.** (Photo by Stephanie A. Fritz, MD.)

- In many cases, a definite cause is not identified. The most common infectious causes are HSV, *M. pneumoniae*, and group A *Streptococcus*.
- The initial surrounding blanching erythema may resemble hives or insect bites. Lesions in different stages can be seen at the same time. With resolution of the lesions, scaling, desquamation, hyperpigmentation, or hypopigmentation may occur.
- The rash is usually symmetric and involves the hands, mouth, face, palms, soles, and extensor surfaces of the extremities. It may also affect the conjunctiva, genital tract, or upper airway.

## Petechial Eruptions

- Petechial rashes necessitate prompt evaluation to exclude severe, life-threatening illness.
- The most common infectious causes of petechiae are:
  - Meningococcemia (*Neisseria meningitidis*) (Fig. 21-3)
  - Prodrome: cough, headache, sore throat, nausea, and vomiting
  - Acute illness: petechial rash, high spiking fevers, tachypnea, tachycardia, and hypotension
- Other bacterial causes: *Rickettsia rickettsii* (Rocky Mountain spotted fever) (Fig. 21-4), *Rickettsia prowazekii* (endemic typhus), *N. gonorrhoeae*, *Pseudomonas aeruginosa*, *Streptococcus pyogenes*, and *Capnocytophaga canimorsus*.
- Viral causes: *enteroviruses* (*espe*cially coxsackievirus A4, A9, and B2-B5 and e*chovirus 3, 4, 7, 9,* and 18), EBV, CMV, p*arvovirus B19, hepatitis virus B and C, rubeola virus (typical* and *atypical measles), and vir*al hemorrhagic fevers caused by arboviruses and arenaviruses.

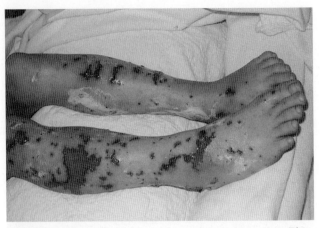

**Figure 21-3. Purpuric lesions in a patient with meningococcemia.** (Photo by David A. Hunstad, MD.)

## CONGENITAL INFECTIONS (SEE TABLE 21-8)

### Toxoplasmosis

*Epidemiology and Etiology*
- Congenital infection occurs when *Toxoplasma gondii* crosses the placenta and invades fetal tissue.
  - The incidence of congenital toxoplasmosis is estimated to be 0.2-1.1/1000 live births in the United States.

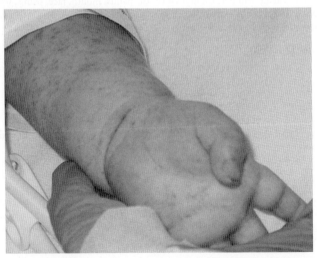

**Figure 21-4. Petechial rash in a patient with Rocky Mountain spotted fever.** (Photo by Celeste Morley, MD, PhD.)

| TABLE 21-8 | Diagnostic Approach to the Newborn with Suspected Congenital Infection |

| Nonspecific tests | Specific tests |
|---|---|
| Complete blood count | CMV PCR from saliva, urine, or blood |
| Lumbar puncture | VZV PCR |
| Long bone radiograph | HIV DNA PCR from blood |
| Head computed tomography | HSV PCR from eyes, mouth, nasopharynx, rectum, blood, and CSF |
| Ophthalmologic evaluation | |
| Audiology evaluation | Serology: |
| | Rubella |
| | *Toxoplasma gondii* |
| | Syphilis |

- The disease severity is worse with a 1st- or 2nd-trimester infection, but the risk of vertical transmission increases as pregnancy advances (15% at 13 weeks, 44% at 26 weeks, 71% at 37 weeks).
- Maternal infection is most commonly acquired by eating cysts in undercooked or raw meat; other sources of infection include receiving blood products, bone marrow, or an organ from a donor with latent infection or inadvertent ingestion of cysts from contaminated cat litter.
- Evaluation of the infant with suspected toxoplasmosis should include ophthalmologic, neurologic, and auditory examinations.

### Clinical Presentation
- Up to 50% of infants are asymptomatic.
- Symptomatic infants may exhibit hepatosplenomegaly, jaundice, lymphadenopathy, thrombocytopenia, rash and meningoencephalitis with hydrocephalus, seizures, calcifications, chorioretinitis, microphthalmia, and microcephaly. Late sequelae include chorioretinitis leading to visual impairment, as well as learning disabilities, intellectual disability, and hearing loss.

### Laboratory Studies and Imaging
- Postnatal diagnosis includes the following:
  - Detection of *Toxoplasma* DNA in blood or CSF by PCR
  - *Toxoplasma*-specific immunoglobulin M (IgM) and IgA
  - *Toxoplasma*-specific IgG persisting beyond 1 year of age
- In cases of suspected toxoplasmosis, head imaging is indicated.

### Treatment and Prevention
- Treatment for symptomatic and asymptomatic infants with congenital disease is pyrimethamine plus sulfadiazine and folinic acid to minimize pyrimethamine toxicity for a prolonged period. Prednisone may be used for severe (vision threatening) chorioretinitis and/or if CSF protein is ≥1 g/dL.
- Pregnant women should wash fruits and vegetables well, avoid undercooked meat, and avoid contact with cat feces and cat litter boxes.

- Spiramycin (<18 weeks) or pyrimethamine, sulfadiazine, and folinic acid (≥18 weeks) may be given to pregnant women with suspected or confirmed primary *Toxoplasma* infection to prevent fetal transmission. Antepartum treatment may reduce the risk of symptomatic congenital toxoplasmosis and may be more effective if initiated within 3 weeks of maternal seroconversion. Consultation with Infectious Diseases and Maternal Fetal Medicine is recommended.

## Rubella
- Congenital infection occurs through maternal viremia with placental seeding leading to fetal infection.
- Infection occurring during the first 8 weeks of gestation carries the worst prognosis.

*Clinical Presentation*
- More than half of all infected infants are asymptomatic at birth but may develop symptoms within the first 5 years of life.
- The most common abnormalities are patent ductus arteriosus or peripheral pulmonary artery stenosis, cataracts, retinopathy, congenital glaucoma, or sensorineural hearing loss, as well as mental retardation, behavioral problems, or meningoencephalitis.
- Other manifestations include radiolucent bone disease, "blueberry muffin" lesions (reflecting extramedullary hematopoiesis), growth retardation, hepatosplenomegaly, and thrombocytopenia.

*Laboratory Studies*
- One of the following:
  - Viral detection in nasopharyngeal secretions, throat, blood, urine, CSF, or stool
  - Persistent or increasing rubella-specific IgG or rubella-specific IgM antibody in the infant

*Treatment and Prevention*
- There is no specific treatment for rubella.
- Prevention involves immunization of all susceptible women before pregnancy, with postpartum immunization of nonimmune women.

## Cytomegalovirus
- CMV is the most common congenital infection, occurring in 1-2% of all live births.
- The virus establishes a chronic infection in the CNS, eyes, cranial nerve VIII, and liver.
- CMV is transmitted transplacentally after maternal primary infection or reactivation of infection. The greatest risk of congenital infection with symptomatic disease occurs after maternal primary infection. CMV can also be transmitted postnatally through contact with cervical secretions or breast milk and occasionally by contact with saliva or urine.

*Clinical Presentation*
- Most infected infants (85-90%) are asymptomatic at birth. Up to 15% of children who are asymptomatic at birth and up to 50% of children symptomatic at birth may develop hearing loss or learning disabilities later in life.
- A minority of infants (5%) are severely affected, with intrauterine growth retardation, jaundice, purpura, hepatosplenomegaly, microcephaly, CNS sequelae, periventricular calcifications, chorioretinitis, and sensorineural hearing loss.

*Laboratory Studies*
- The diagnosis can be made by detection of virus in the infant's urine, saliva, respiratory secretions, blood or CSF obtained within 3 weeks of birth.
- PCR of saliva from newborns obtained within the first 3 weeks of life is >97% sensitive and specific for congenital infection.
- The sensitivity of PCR on dried blood spots is low.

*Treatment*
- Children with symptomatic or asymptomatic infection should have their hearing monitored at regular intervals.
- There is evidence that oral valganciclovir treatment can improve hearing and neurocognitive outcomes at age 2 years in infants with symptomatic CMV disease with or without CNS involvement.
  - Oral valganciclovir (16 mg/kg/dose BID) is equivalent to IV ganciclovir in infants with intact intestinal absorption.
  - Oral valganciclovir may be used for the entire course of treatment.
  - IV ganciclovir is associated with a higher incidence of severe neutropenia in comparison to oral valganciclovir.
  - 6 months of treatment is recommended.
  - Absolute neutrophil counts and serum alanine transaminase concentration should be monitored during treatment.
  - Infants with isolated sensorineural hearing loss without other symptoms and those with mild symptomatic disease should not routinely receive treatment with antivirals as there is a lack of data demonstrating benefit.

## Herpes Simplex Virus Infection

*Epidemiology and Etiology*
- HSV infects 25-60% of exposed infants born vaginally to mothers with primary genital infections acquired near the time of delivery. The risk of transmission to an infant born to a mother with HSV reactivation is much lower (<2%). Over 75% of infants who acquire perinatal HSV are born to women without signs or symptoms of HSV infection before or during pregnancy.
- Postnatal transmission may occur from a caregiver with oral or hand lesions.

*Clinical Presentation*
- Neonatal HSV infections typically present between 5 and 21 days of age, range birth to 6 weeks and they have three types of manifestations.
- Approximately two-thirds of infants with CNS disease or disseminated disease have skin lesions, but lesions may not be visible at symptom onset.
  - Disseminated disease: 25% of all cases
    - Onset at 1-2 weeks of age
    - Involves multiple organs, predominantly the liver and lungs; may include CNS involvement
    - Signs and symptoms: sepsis, liver dysfunction, coagulopathy, and respiratory distress
  - Disease limited to the skin, eye, and mucous membranes (SEMs) (Fig. 21-5): 45% of all cases
    - Onset at 1-2 weeks of age
    - Signs and symptoms: skin or mucosal lesions and keratitis
    - Progresses to more severe disease if not treated

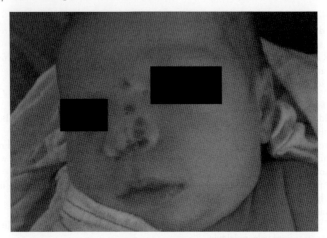

Figure 21-5. **Lesions in a neonate with herpes simplex virus (HSV) skin, eye, and mucous membrane (SEM) disease.** (Photo by Indi Trehan, MD.)

- CNS disease: 30% of all cases
  - Onset at 2-3 weeks of age
  - Signs and symptoms: lethargy, irritability, fever, and seizures

*Laboratory Studies*

HSV DNA can be detected by PCR from CSF, blood, or swabs of skin lesions or mucosal surfaces.

*Treatment*

- IV acyclovir should be given 60 mg/kg/day divided every 8 hours, typically for 14 days (SEM disease) or 21 days (disseminated and CNS disease).
  - Acyclovir can cause neutropenia and renal toxicity.
  - Thus, the WBC count should be monitored 1-2 times per week during course of therapy, and good hydration and monitoring of renal function are required.
- Infants with CNS disease should have an LP repeated near the end of therapy (day 19) to confirm clearance of the virus by PCR, as many providers would extend the course of IV acyclovir until the PCR becomes negative.
- Neonates should be treated with 6 months of suppression with oral acyclovir (300 mg/m$^2$/dose, TID) after completing their initial treatment with IV acyclovir.

*Prevention*

- ACOG recommends that women with recurrent genital herpes be offered suppressive viral therapy at or beyond 36 weeks of gestation and that continuing antiviral therapy until delivery be considered in pregnant women with primary outbreaks occurring in the third trimester.
- Neonates exposed to HSV at delivery should be carefully monitored for evidence of HSV infection. Most experts now recommend further testing and prophylaxis of the infant when the mother has active lesions and delivers vaginally. Any case in which maternal lesions are found at the time of birth should be discussed with an infectious disease specialist.

## Human Immunodeficiency Virus

• See "Human Immunodeficiency Virus" section.

## Syphilis

• Congenital syphilis is primarily transmitted transplacentally and less commonly intrapartum.
• Transmission may occur with maternal primary, secondary, early or late latent disease, but it is greatest with maternal primary and secondary syphilis.

### *Clinical Presentation*

• Syphilis may result in stillbirth, hydrops fetalis, or prematurity.
• Infants symptomatic at birth may present with a rash or mucocutaneous lesions, lymphadenopathy, hepatosplenomegaly, hemolytic anemia, thrombocytopenia, osteochondritis, and rhinitis (snuffles).
• Late manifestations may involve the skin, eyes, ears, teeth, bones, or CNS.

### *Laboratory Studies and Imaging*

• Quantitative nontreponemal test (RPR); confirmation of positive results with a specific treponemal antibody test (e.g., fluorescent treponemal antibody absorption)
• CSF evaluation: cell count, protein, and Venereal Disease Research Laboratory (VDRL) test
• Long bone radiographs for evidence of osteochondritis

### *Treatment and Prevention*

• Administration of aqueous crystalline penicillin G intravenously is effective.
• Prevention is through serologic screening of pregnant women and treatment of infected women during pregnancy with penicillin G. Infected women with a penicillin allergy should be desensitized and given penicillin G, because it is the only documented effective therapy for treating both the mother and the fetus.

## Varicella-Zoster Virus

• Congenital infection of varicella-zoster virus (VZV) occurs via transplacental transmission during maternal viremia.
• Congenital varicella syndrome occurs in 0.4-2.2% of infants born to infected mothers and is most common when the maternal infection occurs in the first 20 weeks of gestation.

### *Clinical Presentation*

• Abnormalities include limb atrophy, scarring of the extremities, CNS, and eye manifestations.
• Neonatal chickenpox develops when maternal infection occurs during the last several weeks of pregnancy.

### *Laboratory Tests*

VZV PCR performed on fluid from the lesion, blood, or CSF

### *Treatment and Prevention*

• Treatment with acyclovir is usually not indicated in healthy children.
• Infants born to mothers who develop clinical varicella infection between 5 days prior to and 2 days after delivery should receive VariZIG or intravenous immune globulin.
  • Susceptible women should be vaccinated before pregnancy.

## Zika Virus

- Congenital infection of Zika virus occurs via transplacental transmission during maternal viremia.
- Transmitted primarily to humans by the *Aedes aegypti* mosquito.
- Humans and nonhuman primates are the main reservoirs of the virus.

*Clinical Presentation*

Microcephaly, brain anomalies, ocular anomalies, clubfoot, arthrogryposis, hypertonia, hypotonia, irritability, tremors, swallowing dysfunction, hearing loss, visual impairment

*Laboratory Tests*

- Testing is recommended for:
  - Infants with possible maternal Zika virus exposure during pregnancy and with clinical findings consistent with Zika virus infection
  - Infants without clinical findings born to women with laboratory evidence of possible infection during pregnancy
- Zika virus RNA RT-PCR from infant serum and urine.
- Zika IgM antibodies from serum.
- RT-PCR and IgM antibodies from CSF (if available, but not necessary for diagnosis).
- Plaque reduction neutralization test (measures virus-specific neutralizing antibodies) can be used to confirm or exclude congenital Zika virus infection at age ≥18 months in infants with clinical findings of Zika infection who were not tested in the newborn period and may also be useful in the newborn period to help identify false-positive results from serology.

*Treatment and Prevention*

- No specific antiviral therapy is available.
- Head ultrasound, ophthalmologic evaluation and follow up, and hearing testing are recommended.
- Referrals to neurology, developmental specialists, and genetics are recommended.
- Pregnant women should postpone travel to areas with ongoing local Zika transmission.

## HEPATITIS

### Hepatitis A Virus

*Epidemiology and Etiology*

- Mode of transmission: fecal-oral
- Common sources of infection:
  - Close personal contact with a person infected with HAV
  - Child care centers
  - International travel
  - Recognized foodborne or waterborne outbreak
  - Male homosexual activity
  - IV drug use

*Clinical Presentation*

- Acute, self-limited illness associated with fever, malaise, jaundice, anorexia, and nausea
- May be asymptomatic in infants
- Can cause fulminant hepatitis in children with underlying liver disease

*Laboratory Studies*
HAV-specific total immunoglobulin and HAV IgM antibody

*Treatment and Prevention*
- Supportive care is appropriate.
- Immune globulin intramuscular (IGIM) may be effective in preventing symptomatic infection if given within 2 weeks of exposure.
- Hepatitis A vaccine is available for all children ≥1 year of age. For infants traveling to hepatitis A endemic regions, the vaccine can be administered to infants 6-11 months of age but will not count toward their routine two-dose series. Preexposure prophylaxis with immunoglobulin should be considered for children <6 months of age or those who cannot receive the vaccine.

## Hepatitis B Virus
*Epidemiology and Etiology*
- Mode of transmission: blood or body fluids.
- Common modes of transmission include percutaneous and permucosal exposure; sharing or using nonsterilized needles, syringes, or glucose monitoring equipment or devices; sexual contact with an infected person; and household exposure to a person with chronic HBV infection.
- Perinatal transmission of HBV is highly efficient particularly in the absence of postexposure prophylaxis.

*Clinical Presentation*
Ranges from a subacute illness with nonspecific symptoms such as anorexia, malaise, and nausea, to clinical hepatitis with jaundice, to fulminant fatal hepatitis.

*Laboratory Studies*
- Serologic antigen and antibody tests are available to diagnose hepatitis B (Table 21-9). In addition, HBV DNA testing has high sensitivity at low levels.
- Recommended screening for hepatitis B infection includes hepatitis B surface antigen (HBsAg) and hepatitis B surface antibody (anti-HBs). If the HBsAg is positive, further serology and antigen testing is recommended.
- Chronic HBV infection is defined as the presence of HBsAg, HBV DNA, or hepatitis B e antigen (HBeAg) in serum for at least 6 months and is likely in the presence of positive testing in a person testing negative for the IgM antibody to hepatitis B core antigen (anti-HBc) (Table 21-9).
- Age at the time of infection is the primary determinant of risk of progression to chronic HBV infection. Up to 90% of perinatal infections lead to chronic HBV, whereas only 5-10% of acutely infected children over age 5 years or adults develop chronic HBV infection.

*Treatment and Prevention*
- No specific treatment is recommended for uncomplicated acute HBV infection.
- Treatment of chronic HBV is recommended if there is evidence of ongoing HBV viral replication and elevated serum ALT concentrations or evidence of chronic hepatitis on liver biopsy.
  - Interferon-α-2b therapy may lead to long-term remission.
  - Tenofovir, entecavir, and telbivudine are antivirals approved for use in children with chronic HBV infection, but require long-term administration.

| TABLE 21-9 | Diagnostic Tests for Hepatitis B Virus (HBV) Antigens and Antibodies | |
|---|---|---|
| Factor to be tested | HBV antigen or antibody | Use |
| Hepatitis B surface antigen (HBsAg) | HBsAg | Detection of acutely or chronically infected people; antigen used in hepatitis B vaccine can rarely be detected up to 3 weeks after vaccination |
| Anti-HBs | Antibody to HBsAg | Identification of people who have resolved infections with HBV; determination of immunity after immunization |
| Hepatitis B early antigen (HBeAg) | HBeAg | Identification of people at increased risk of transmitting HBV |
| Anti-HBe | Antibody to HBeAg | Identification of infected people with lower risk of transmitting HBV |
| Anti-HBc | Antibody to hepatitis B core antigen (HBcAg)[a] | Identification of people with acute, resolved, or chronic HBV infection (not present after immunization) |
| IgM anti-HBc | IgM antibody to HBcAg | Identification of people with acute or recent HBV infections (including HBsAg-negative people during the "window" phase of infection) |

[a]No test is available commercially to measure hepatitis B core antigen (HBcAg).
IgM, immunoglobulin M.
Adapted from American Academy of Pediatrics. In: Kimberlin DW, Barnett ED, Lynfield R, Sawyer MH, eds. Red Book: 2021 Report of the Committee on Infectious Diseases, 32nd Edition. American Academy of Pediatrics; 2021.

- Updated guidance on treatment of HBV can be found at http://aasld.org/publications/practice-guidelines.
- Recombinant HBV vaccine is recommended for all infants. Postexposure prophylaxis is available with hepatitis B immunoglobulin (HBIG).
- Neonates born to hepatitis B–positive mothers should receive HBV vaccine and HBIG within 12 hours after birth to reduce transmission. If mother's HBV status is unknown, mother should be tested for HBsAg, and HBV vaccine should be given to infant within 12 hours of birth. HBIG should be given within 7 days for infant's weighing ≥2 g if mother is confirmed to be positive or within 12 hours for infants <2 g unless mother is confirmed to be negative.
- Breastfeeding of infants by HBsAg-positive mothers poses no additional risk of HBV acquisition.

## Hepatitis C Virus

*Epidemiology and Etiology*
- Mode of transmission: parenteral exposure to blood of hepatitis C virus (HCV)-infected people
- Groups at highest risk
  - IV drug users
  - People who engage in high-risk sexual behaviors
  - Health care professionals because of sporadic percutaneous exposures
- Perinatal transmission
  - Maternal coinfection with HIV has been associated with an increased risk of perinatal transmission of HCV.
  - Approximately 5-6% of children born to women with HCV infection acquire HCV.
  - Method of delivery does not appear to affect vertical transmission rate.
  - Infants born to mothers with HCV infection should be tested for HCV antibody at 18 months of life, and liver enzyme testing can be performed at 6-month intervals. HCV RNA detection can be sent as early as 2 to 6 months of age; however, serologic testing should also be performed at 18 months of age for confirmation.
  - HCV transmission through breastfeeding has not been demonstrated, and thus, HCV-positive mothers may breastfeed. However, mothers should refrain from breastfeeding if the nipples are cracked or bleeding.

*Clinical Presentation*
- Most infections are asymptomatic. Jaundice occurs in <20% of patients.
- Persistent infection with HCV occurs in 80% of infected children.

*Laboratory Studies*
- Anti-HCV Ig can be detected within 15 weeks after exposure and within 5-6 weeks of the onset of hepatitis.
- Reverse transcription-PCR can detect HCV RNA within 1-2 weeks after exposure to the virus.

*Treatment*
A number of regimens are approved for treatment of HCV in children as young as 3 years of age. Referral for treatment and monitoring should be made to a pediatric infectious disease specialist or gastroenterologist. Newer antivirals are available. Updated guidance can be found at https://www.hcvguidelines.org/.

## Hepatitis E Virus

- Transmission is via the fecal-oral route, and outbreaks are often associated with contaminated water.
- Infection with hepatitis E virus (HEV) can be asymptomatic or cause an acute illness with fever, jaundice, anorexia, abdominal pain, malaise, and arthralgia.
- Pregnant women infected with HEV have a high mortality rate.

## HUMAN IMMUNODEFICIENCY VIRUS

### Maternal Infection
- Risk factors for perinatal HIV transmission
  - Maternal viral load is the critical determinant affecting the likelihood of mother to child transmission of HIV.
  - Rupture of membranes >4 hours.

- Breastfeeding.
- Overall, mother-to-child transmission of HIV has been dramatically reduced because of improved ability to rapidly identify HIV-positive mothers, the availability of highly active antiretroviral therapy (HAART) regimens, and the performance of C-section before to labor and before rupture of membranes at 38 weeks of gestation for mothers with viral load ≥1000 copies/mL or with unknown viral load near time of delivery.

*Treatment*
- Intrapartum management
  - Mothers with detectable or unknown viral load near delivery should receive peripartum IV zidovudine (AZT).
  - When possible, invasive procedures (e.g., fetal scalp monitor, artificially rupturing membranes, vacuum, forceps, or episiotomy) should be avoided.
  - A cesarean section is recommended for women with an HIV viral load ≥1000 copies/mL.
  - Because HIV can be transmitted through breast milk, breastfeeding should be avoided where alternative formulas are readily available.
  - Detailed recommendations can be found online at http://clinicalinfo.hiv.gov.
- Management of the HIV-exposed newborn
  - Management of exposed infants is based on the risk of perinatal transmission. For low-risk infants, obtain complete blood count with differential and HIV virologic testing (RNA or DNA PCR) starting at 14-21 days of life. Our local practice is to check HIV PCR at birth.
  - Administer AZT to all newborns as close to birth as possible, preferably within the first 6-12 hours of life and continue as per Table 21-10.

**TABLE 21-10    AZT Dosing in Neonates**

|  | <30 Weeks of gestational age at birth | 30-34 6/7 Weeks of gestational age at birth | ≥35 Weeks of gestational age at birth |
|---|---|---|---|
| 0-2 weeks of age | 2 mg/kg/dose PO q12h | 2 mg/kg/dose PO q12h | 4 mg/kg/dose PO q12h |
|  | OR | OR | OR |
|  | 1.5 mg/kg/dose IV q12h | 1.5 mg/kg/dose IV q12h | 3 mg/kg/dose IV q12h |
| 2-4 weeks of age | 2 mg/kg/dose PO q12h | 3 mg/kg/dose PO q12h |  |
|  | OR | OR |  |
|  | 1.5 mg/kg/dose IV q12h | 2.3 mg/kg/dose IV q12h |  |
| 4-6 weeks of age | 3 mg/kg/dose PO q12h | 3 mg/kg/dose PO q12h |  |
|  | OR | OR |  |
|  | 2.3 mg/kg/dose IV q12h | 2.3 mg/kg/dose IV q12h |  |

Note: Some centers still dose AZT at 2 mg/kg/dose PO q6h.

**TABLE 21-11** Suggested Follow-Up in a Low-Risk[a] HIV-Exposed Infant

| Age of visit | HIV nucleic acid test (NAT) | Complete blood count with differential | Medications |
|---|---|---|---|
| Outpatient 2-3 weeks | RNA or DNA | | AZT (see Table 20-10 for dosing) |
| 6 weeks | RNA or DNA | X | Discontinue AZT at 4 weeks for low-risk infants. TMP/SMX is not needed if infant is low-risk, has normal exam, and negative NAT at 2 weeks and 6-8 weeks. Repeat NAT should be done 2 weeks after prophylaxis ends (i.e., 6 weeks for low-risk who get 4 weeks AZT) |
| 4-6 months | RNA or DNA | | |

[a]Low risk defined as mothers who received ART during pregnancy and had viral suppression near delivery (HIV RNA level <50 copies/mL) and for whom maternal adherence is not of concern.

- Three-drug regimen (AZT + lamivudine + raltegravir or nevirapine) for up to 6 weeks should be considered in high-risk infants. Because of resistance and other factors, the newborn's antiviral regimen should be considered on an individual basis and always discussed with an infectious diseases specialist.
- Suggested follow-up for the uncomplicated HIV-exposed infant is demonstrated in Table 21-11. Two negative virologic tests, one at ≥1 month of age and a repeat ≥4 months of age or two negative HIV antibody tests from separate specimens at age ≥6 months, are required for ruling out infection. HIV ELISA can be checked at age 12-18 months to document loss of maternal HIV antibodies. Our local practice is to check HIV ELISA one time at 2 years of age to document seroreversion to HIV antibody-negative status.
- Complete recommendations can be found at http://clinicalinfo.hiv.gov/en/guidelines/perinatal/whats-new-guidelines.

## Blood-Borne Pathogen Exposure

*Nonoccupational Exposure to HIV*
- HIV is not a hardy virus in the environment, only surviving on the order of hours.
- For direct injection of blood from a known patient with HIV, the risk of transmission of HIV is 0.3%.
- There has never been a documented case of transmission of HIV via accidental injury from a needle found in the community environment.
- A pediatric infectious disease specialist should be contacted for significant exposures in which HIV postexposure prophylaxis may be indicated. Prophylaxis must be started within 72 hours of exposure.

- Postexposure prophylaxis is recommended for 28 days. Given the duration and toxicities, risk/benefit of prophylaxis must be considered.
- Follow-up HIV testing is recommended at the time of exposure, 4-6 weeks, 3 months, and 6 months after exposure.

*Hepatitis B Exposure*
- HBV can survive on environmental surfaces at room temperature for at least 7 days, making it the most likely pathogen found on contaminated items in the environment.
- For children who have completed a full hepatitis B vaccine series, no further intervention is necessary for exposure to a source with unknown HBsAg status or a HBsAg-positive household member; however, a booster dose of hepatitis B vaccine should be given for high-risk situations (percutaneous or mucosal exposure, sexual or needle-sharing contact, sexual assault from a HBsAg-positive source).
- For children who are partially or unimmunized with a significant exposure to a known source of hepatitis B, HBIG should be administered along with the full vaccine series. For additional guidance, see detailed guidelines for specific scenarios.

*Hepatitis C Exposure*
- Hepatitis C can survive in the environment up to a few days.
- No postexposure prophylaxis or vaccination is available.
- Antibody to HCV can be detected 8-11 weeks after exposure and HCV RNA as early as 1-2 weeks after exposure.

## INFECTIONS ASSOCIATED WITH ANIMALS

- Common pathogenic organisms in bite wounds
  - Human: *Streptococcus* species, *S. aureus*, *Eikenella corrodens*, and anaerobes. Between 5% and 15% of bites get infected.
  - Dog or cat: *Pasteurella* species, *S. aureus*, *Moraxella* species, *Streptococcus* species, *Neisseria* species, *Corynebacterium* species, *C. canimorsus* (especially in splenectomized patients), and anaerobes. For cats, up to 50% of bites become infected, whereas 5%-15% of dog bites become infected.
  - Reptile: enteric gram-negative bacteria, anaerobes.
- A 3- to 5-day course of prophylactic antibiotics (e.g., amoxicillin-clavulanate or clindamycin plus trimethoprim-sulfamethoxazole for penicillin-allergic patients) should be considered for "high-risk" injuries such as cat and human bites, bites to the face, genital area, hands, feet, or joints; puncture wounds; wounds >8 hours old; or wounds in immunocompromised and asplenic persons. For infected wounds, antibiotic therapy should be tailored according to culture results.

## Rabies

*Epidemiology*
- Animals most commonly associated with the transmission of rabies infection include bats, skunks, raccoons, and foxes.
- Rabies is rarely or never transmitted by squirrels, chipmunks, rats, mice, guinea pigs, gerbils, hamsters, or rabbits, as these animals commonly die if they are bitten by a larger, rabies-infected animal. However, all wildlife bites should be considered a possible exposure.

*Clinical Presentation*
- Prodromal phase (2-10 days): fever, headache, photophobia, anorexia, sore throat, musculoskeletal pain, itching, pain, and tingling at the site of the bite
- Acute neurologic phase (2-30 days): delirium, paralysis, hydrophobia, coma, and respiratory arrest

*Laboratory Studies*
- The virus may be isolated from the saliva, and viral nucleic acid may be detected in infected tissues.
- Antibody may be detected in the serum or CSF.
- Diagnosis may also be based on fluorescent microscopy of a skin biopsy specimen from the nape of the neck.

*Treatment*
- Scratches or bites should be thoroughly irrigated with soap and water.
- Postexposure prophylaxis should ideally be given as soon as possible.
  - Rabies vaccine is given intramuscularly (1.0 mL) in the deltoid area or anterolateral aspect of the thigh on day 0 and repeated on days 3, 7, and 14.
  - Rabies immune globulin (RIG) should be given concurrently with the first dose of vaccine. The recommended dose is 20 IU/kg; as much of the dose as possible should be used to infiltrate the wound, and the remainder should be given intramuscularly.
  - Rabies vaccine should not be administered in the same part of the body used to administer RIG.
- If a bat is discovered in a room with a sleeping, intoxicated, or very young person, rabies prophylaxis is recommended even if the person does not recall a bite. Likewise, direct contact with a bat that cannot be tested for rabies is another indication for prophylaxis, as bat bites are difficult to find on examination.
- Domesticated dogs and cats that are captured should be observed closely by local animal control officials for 10 days for evidence of rabies. No case of human rabies has been attributed when an animal remained healthy throughout this confinement period. However, animal bites to the face may require immediate prophylaxis, which can be discontinued once rabies testing on the animal is found to be negative.
- Wild animals should be immediately euthanized for examination of the brain by local health officials.

## Catscratch Disease
*Epidemiology and Etiology*
- Cats are the common reservoir for this infection, and children are often infected by kittens through scratches, licks, and bites.
- The causal bacterium is *Bartonella henselae*.
- This is one of the most common identified etiologies in pediatric fever of unknown origin.

*Clinical Presentation*
- Regional lymphadenopathy (usually involving the nodes that drain the site of inoculation) (Fig. 21-6) is accompanied by fever and mild systemic symptoms including malaise, anorexia, and headache.
  - The most commonly affected lymph nodes include the axillary, cervical, epitrochlear, and inguinal lymph nodes.

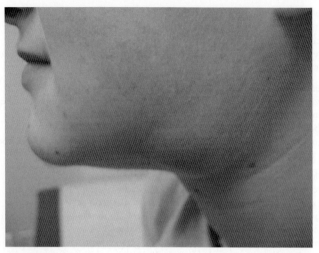

**Figure 21-6. Lymphadenopathy caused by *Bartonella henselae* infection (catscratch disease).** (Photo by David Hunstad, MD.)

- The skin overlying the affected lymph nodes may be normal or may be warm, erythematous, and indurated.
- Other less common manifestations include Parinaud oculoglandular syndrome (inoculation of the conjunctiva results in preauricular or submandibular lymphadenopathy), encephalopathy/encephalitis, aseptic meningitis, granulomatous disease of the liver and spleen, endocarditis, neuroretinitis, osteolytic lesions, hepatitis, pneumonia, thrombocytopenic purpura, and erythema nodosum.

*Laboratory Studies*
Serum antibody assay is available for detection. If a tissue sample is submitted (e.g., lymph node), PCR for *Bartonella* can be performed in some laboratories.

*Treatment*
- Localized adenopathy is usually self-limited, resolving spontaneously in 2-4 months. In immunocompetent individuals, antibiotic therapy is not recommended in most cases. Antibiotics are recommended by some experts for acutely or severely ill immunocompromised patients. Agents with in vitro activity include azithromycin, doxycycline, trimethoprim-sulfamethoxazole, ciprofloxacin, and rifampin.
- Systemic *Bartonella* syndromes should be managed in conjunction with an infectious diseases specialist.

## Q Fever
*Epidemiology and Etiology*
- *Coxiella burnetii* is the causal agent.
- Transmission occurs via inhaled aerosols during the birth of domesticated mammals, including sheep, goats, and cows, by exposure to contaminated materials such as bedding, straw, wool or laundry or unpasteurized dairy products.

*Clinical Presentation*
- Fifty percent of infections are asymptomatic.
- Acute infection follows initial exposure and results in fever, chills, cough, headache, anorexia, pneumonia, diarrhea, vomiting, abdominal pain, rash, and hepatitis. Meningoencephalitis and myocarditis occur rarely. The illness typically lasts 1-4 weeks and resolves gradually. A relapsing illness with fever has been observed in children.
- Chronic infection occurs years after exposure and manifests as fever of unknown origin, chronic relapsing or multifocal osteomyelitis, chronic hepatitis, and endocarditis. There may be a higher risk of persistent localized Q fever in patients with underlying heart disease or prosthetic valves, vascular aneurysms, or vascular grafts and those who are immunocompromised.
- Q fever during pregnancy is associated with miscarriage, premature birth, and low birth weight.

*Laboratory Studies*
- Diagnosis is established by a fourfold change in *C. burnetii* antibody between specimens obtained 2-3 weeks apart by complement fixation, immunofluorescence antibody test, or ELISA or positive immunostaining or PCR for the organism in tissue (e.g., heart valve). PCR may be negative in as many as 66% of patients with endocarditis from Q fever. A biosafety level 3 laboratory is required for culture given the organism is a potential hazard for laboratory workers.
- A single high serum phase II IgG titer ≥1:128 in convalescent serum may be considered evidence of infection.

*Treatment*
- Doxycycline is the drug of choice for acute Q fever. Alternative therapy for patients with allergy to doxycycline is trimethoprim-sulfamethoxazole.
- Chronic Q fever endocarditis in adults is treated with doxycycline and hydroxychloroquine for 18 months. There are limited treatment data in children. Surgical debridement and/or replacement of infected tissue may be needed in some patients.

## Brucellosis
*Epidemiology and Etiology*
- Humans become infected by direct contact with infected animals, their carcasses, or by ingesting unpasteurized milk or milk products. Inoculation may occur through cuts and abrasions in the skin, through inhalation of contaminated aerosols, through contact with conjunctival mucosa, and through oral ingestion.
- Causal agents are *Brucella* species: *Brucella abortus*, *Brucella melitensis*, *Brucella suis*, and *Brucella canis.*

*Clinical Presentation*
- In children, brucellosis is usually a mild, self-limiting disease.
- However, infections with the species *B. melitensis* can be severe and manifest as fever, night sweats, headache, abdominal pain, weakness, malaise, arthralgias, myalgias, anorexia, and weight loss.
- Physical examination findings include lymphadenopathy, hepatosplenomegaly, or arthritis.
- Complications include liver/spleen abscesses, meningitis, endocarditis, and osteomyelitis.

*Laboratory Studies*
- *Brucella* may be grown in culture from blood, bone marrow, or other tissues (cultures should be incubated a minimum of 4 weeks if brucellosis is suspected). Newer BACTEC systems can detect *Brucella* within 7 days making prolonged culture incubation unnecessary.
- The diagnosis may also be made by serologic testing (serum agglutination test) with a fourfold increase in antibody titers collected at least 2 weeks apart.
- Commercially available tests will not detect a serologic response to *B. canis* and *B. abortus* strain RB51.
- Pancytopenia, anemia, or thrombocytopenia can be seen on complete blood cell counts.

*Treatment*
- Combination therapy for 6 weeks with doxycycline and rifampin or with trimethoprim-sulfamethoxazole and rifampin in children <8 years.
- Monotherapy and shorter courses of antibiotics are associated with high rates of relapse.

## Psittacosis
*Epidemiology and Etiology*
- Birds are the major reservoir, and the organism is transmitted by inhaling fecal dust or respiratory secretions.
- The causal agent is *Chlamydia psittaci*.

*Clinical Presentation*
- Signs and symptoms include fever, chills, nonproductive cough, sore throat, headache, and malaise.
- Extensive interstitial pneumonia may develop.
- Rare complications include pericarditis, myocarditis, endocarditis, superficial thrombophlebitis, hepatitis, and encephalopathy.

*Laboratory Studies*
- A fourfold increase in antibody titer by microimmunofluorescence from specimens collected 2-4 weeks apart is consistent with the diagnosis of psittacosis.
- Specialized laboratories offer nucleic acid amplification tests.

*Treatment*
- Doxycycline is the medication of choice, but erythromycin, azithromycin, and clarithromycin are also effective.
- Patients should be treated for 10-14 days after defervescence.

## Rat-Bite Fever
*Epidemiology and Etiology*
- The causal agent, *Streptobacillus moniliformis*, is part of the normal oral flora in rats and can be excreted in rat urine. Of note, the disease is also caused by *Spirillum minus* in Asia.
- Rat-bite fever may also be transmitted by squirrels, mice, gerbils, cats, and weasels; by ingestion of contaminated milk or food; or through contact with an infected animal.

*Clinical Presentation*
- The disease involves the abrupt onset of fever, chills, and macular or petechial rash located predominantly on the extremities (including the palms and soles), myalgias, vomiting, headache, and adenopathy.

- This course may be followed by migratory polyarthritis or arthralgia.
- Complications include relapsing disease, pneumonia, abscess formation, septic arthritis, myocarditis, endocarditis, or meningitis.

*Laboratory Studies*
- *S. moniliformis* can be isolated from blood, material from bite lesions, abscess aspirates, or joint fluid; laboratory personnel should be notified that this organism is suspected since cultures should be held for at least 1 week.
- Giemsa or Wright stain should also be performed on blood specimens.
- 16S ribosomal gene sequencing and MALDI-TOF mass spectrometry may be used as an adjunct to culture.

*Treatment*
- Penicillin G procaine IV for 7-10 days is the drug of choice.
- There is limited experience with ampicillin, cefuroxime, ceftriaxone, and cefotaxime.
- Doxycycline or streptomycin may be used in patients with a penicillin allergy.

## Leptospirosis
*Epidemiology and Etiology*
- The causal organism, *Leptospira*, is excreted by animals in urine, amniotic fluid, or placenta and remains viable in the water or soil for weeks to months. Contact of abraded skin or mucosal surfaces with contaminated water, soil, or animal matter facilitates human infection.
- Outbreaks of disease have been associated with recreational wading, swimming, or boating in contaminated water.

*Clinical Presentation*
- An acute febrile illness may be accompanied by generalized vasculitis.
- The onset of infection is characterized by fever, chills, transient rash, nausea, vomiting, and headache.
- Other notable features include conjunctivitis without discharge and myalgias in the lumbar region and lower leg.
- Severe illness occurs in 5-10% of patients infected, which includes jaundice, renal dysfunction, cardiac arrhythmias, hemorrhagic pneumonitis, or circulatory failure.

*Laboratory Studies*
- The organism may be recovered from blood, urine, or CSF; laboratory personnel should be notified that *Leptospira* infection is suspected.
- Serologic antibody testing, immunohistochemistry, and PCR are available in some laboratories.

*Treatment*
- Patients with severe illness requiring hospitalization should be treated with intravenous Penicillin G. There is evidence from randomized controlled trials that intravenous ceftriaxone and doxycycline have equal efficacy to penicillin G.
- Mild infections may be treated with doxycycline.

## Yersiniosis
*Epidemiology and Etiology*
- The causal pathogen is *Yersinia enterocolitica*.
- The principal reservoir is swine, and thus, infection likely occurs by ingesting contaminated food, including raw or undercooked pork products, unpasteurized milk,

or contaminated water, or contact with animals. Infants may be infected by caregivers who handle raw pork intestines (chitterlings).

*Clinical Presentation*
- The most common finding in young children is enterocolitis with fever and diarrhea in which the stool contains mucus, blood, and leukocytes.
- Older children and young adults may present with a pseudoappendicitis syndrome including fever, right lower quadrant tenderness, and leukocytosis.

*Laboratory Studies*
The organism can be cultured from the stool, throat, mesenteric lymph nodes, peritoneal fluid, and blood during the first 2 weeks of illness.

*Treatment*
- Patients with sepsis, extraintestinal manifestations, neonates, and patients who are immunocompromised should be treated with antibiotics. Isolates are commonly susceptible to third-generation cephalosporins, aminoglycosides, trimethoprim-sulfamethoxazole, fluoroquinolones, and tetracycline or doxycycline.
- The benefit of antibiotic therapy for otherwise healthy patients with enterocolitis, mesenteric adenitis, or pseudoappendicitis syndrome is unclear, but treatment may be considered given that antibiotic therapy decreases intestinal shedding.

## TICK-BORNE INFECTIONS

- Prevention of tick-borne diseases involves the following:
  - Avoid tick-infested areas (woodlands).
  - If entering a tick-infested area, wear light-colored clothing that covers the arms, legs, and other exposed areas.
  - Use tick and insect repellent. The best, all-purpose insect repellent is *N,N*-diethyl-m-toluamide (DEET). In repellents, DEET concentrations between 10% and 30% can be safely used on children's skin. DEET is not recommended for children under 2 months of age.
  - After possible tick exposure, inspect children's clothing and bodies (especially hairy regions of the body, including the head and neck, where ticks often attach).
  - If a tick is found, the tick can be removed with tweezers, with forceful removal of the entire tick with mouth intact. Ticks should never be cut, burned, or removed in pieces.
- For additional details about specific tick-borne diseases and their treatment, see Table 21-12.

## INFECTIOUS DISEASE AND THE INTERNATIONALLY ADOPTED CHILD

- Each year, families in the United States adopt many children from other countries. These children deserve special consideration because many come from countries with limited resources with less than optimal living conditions and may have unknown medical histories.
- Over the past decade, international adoption has dropped, from a peak of 22,991 in 2004 to 2971 in 2019, likely related to shifts in foreign countries' adoption policies toward the United States. The most common countries of origin for adoption in 2019 were China, India, Colombia, and the Ukraine.
- Several screening tests should be performed in internationally adopted children (Table 21-13). In addition, children with serologic evidence of syphilis should undergo radiologic evaluation and LP. Other tests that may be indicated include

**TABLE 21-12** Description and Treatment of Tick-Borne Diseases

| Disease | Organism | Geographic distribution | Reservoir | Common presenting symptoms | Rash | Initial laboratory findings and diagnostic tests | Treatment |
|---------|----------|------------------------|-----------|---------------------------|------|------------------------------------------------|-----------|
| Lyme disease | *Borrelia burgdorferi, Borrelia mayonii* | Northeastern and Midwestern parts of the United States, plus states on the west coast | White-footed mouse | Fever, chills, headache, myalgias, arthralgias Complications: carditis and neurologic manifestations (facial nerve palsy, meningitis) Sequelae of late disease: chronic arthritis, subacute encephalopathy, optic neuritis | Erythema migrans (Fig. 21-7) | Treat based on clinical diagnosis without serologic testing if erythema migrans is present without extracutaneous signs or symptoms, ELISA is negative in the acute infection ELISA or EIA; if positive, confirm by Western blot | Doxycycline[a] or amoxicillin or cefuroxime for erythema migrans; doxycycline for facial nerve palsy; IV ceftriaxone or PO doxycycline for meningitis; amoxicillin or doxycycline for arthritis |
| Tularemia | *Francisella tularensis* | Southern, Southeastern, and Midwestern United States | Rabbits, hares, rodent (muskrats, voles, beavers, prairie dogs), rarely domestic cats | Dependent on route of acquisition Fever, chills, adenopathy, headache, fatigue, cough, pharyngitis, myalgias, vomiting, abdominal pain, diarrhea, skin ulcers, pneumonia | | Normal or slightly elevated white blood cell count and ESR Serology can confirm by 1-2 weeks | Gentamicin, streptomycin, or fluoroquinolones for mild disease |

*(Continued)*

**TABLE 21-12** Description and Treatment of Tick-Borne Diseases *(Continued)*

| Disease | Organism | Geographic distribution | Reservoir | Common presenting symptoms | Rash | Initial laboratory findings and diagnostic tests | Treatment |
|---|---|---|---|---|---|---|---|
| Rocky Mountain spotted fever | *Rickettsia rickettsii* | Southeastern and Midwestern United States | Dogs, cats, rodents, rabbits | Abrupt onset of fever, headache, myalgias, malaise, and vomiting<br><br>Severe disease: heart (myocarditis, arrhythmias, CHF), lungs (pneumonitis, edema, ARDS), central nervous system (meningismus, altered mental status, ataxia, seizures) | Begins as blanching red macules that evolve into petechiae<br><br>Rash starting on wrists and ankles and spreading to extremities and trunk; includes palms and soles (see Fig. 21-4); involves skin necrosis in severe disease | Leukopenia, thrombocytopenia, elevated transaminases, bilirubin, and blood urea nitrogen; hyponatremia<br><br>Possible to make diagnosis with acute and convalescent serology or skin biopsy | Doxycycline[a] |

| Disease | Organism | Geographic distribution | Reservoir | Clinical features | Skin findings | Diagnosis | Treatment |
|---|---|---|---|---|---|---|---|
| Ehrlichiosis | Human monocytic ehrlichiosis (HME): *Ehrlichia chaffeensis*; *Ehrlichia phagocytophilum*. Ehrlichiosis: *Ehrlichia ewingii* | Southern, Southeastern, and Midwestern United States | Dogs, rodents | Fever, chills, myalgias, headache, vomiting, anorexia, hepatosplenomegaly | Petechiae or erythematous maculopapular lesions involving trunk and sparing hands and feet | Leukopenia, thrombocytopenia, anemia, elevated transaminases, cerebrospinal fluid abnormalities (lymphocytic pleocytosis, elevated protein). Wright stain of blood smear: possible morulae. Serology can confirm at 1-2 weeks. Blood PCR | Doxycycline[a] |
| Relapsing fever | *Borrelia recurrentis* (epidemic relapsing fever: louse-borne and tick-borne), *Borrelia hermsii* and *Borrelia turicatae* | Louse-borne: *B. recurrentis*: Africa; Tick-borne: *B. hermsii*: Western mountainous areas; *B. turicatae*: Texas | *B. recurrentis*: no animal reservoir. *B. hermsii* and *B. turicatae*: rodents | Sudden onset of high fever, sweats, chills, headache, arthralgias, myalgias, and weakness. Possible complications: cough, pleuritic pain, pneumonitis, myocarditis, meningitis, hepatosplenomegaly, jaundice, epistaxis, and iridocyclitis | Possible transient maculopapular rash of trunk and petechiae of skin and mucous membranes | Some commercial serologic assays available; antibody tests not standardized. Contact CDC with inquiries about laboratory testing | Penicillin or doxycycline[a] or erythromycin |

*(Continued)*

**TABLE 21-12** Description and Treatment of Tick-Borne Diseases *(Continued)*

| Disease | Organism | Geographic distribution | Reservoir | Common presenting symptoms | Rash | Initial laboratory findings and diagnostic tests | Treatment |
|---|---|---|---|---|---|---|---|
| | (endemic relapsing fever: tick-borne), and other *Borrelia* species | | | Initial febrile episode lasts 3-7 days and is followed by afebrile period lasting days to weeks, which is then followed by one or more relapses | | | |
| Babesiosis | *Babesia microti, Babesia divergens, Babesia bovis* | Coastal areas and islands of Connecticut, Massachusetts, Rhode Island, and New York | Rodents | Malaria-like illness with high fever, weakness, headache, myalgias, nausea, vomiting, arthralgia, weight loss, cough, dyspnea, renal failure

Complications: renal failure, ARDS, CHF, disseminated intravascular coagulation, hypotension and shock, and myocardial infarction | Rash is uncommon | Mild to severe hemolytic anemia; slightly decreased leukocyte count

Diagnosis is usually based on typical blood smear morphology

Giemsa or Wright-stained smear demonstrates intraerythrocytic parasites | Atovaquone plus azithromycin is therapy of choice; clindamycin plus quinine for patients who do not respond to atovaquone and azithromycin |

| Disease | Organism | Location | Host | Symptoms | Additional findings | Diagnosis | Treatment |
|---|---|---|---|---|---|---|---|
| Anaplasmosis | *Anaplasma phagocytophilum* | Northeastern and upper Midwestern states, Northern California, Europe, Asia | | Fever, chills, myalgias, headache, vomiting, anorexia, hepatosplenomegaly | Rash less common than with *Ehrlichia* | PCR on whole blood, occasionally can be seen in Giemsa or Wright-stained peripheral blood smears | Doxycycline |
| Heartland virus | Heartland virus | Midwestern and southern United States | | Fever, fatigue, anorexia, myalgias, headache, nausea, diarrhea, arthralgias | | Heartland virus RNA, IgM and IgG | Supportive care |
| Powassan fever | Powassan virus | Northeast and Great Lakes regions | White-footed mice | Fever, headache, vomiting generalized weakness, encephalitis, meningitis | | Powassan virus IgM from serum and CSF, PCR on serum, CSF, tissue, immunohistochemistry in formalin-fixed tissue | Supportive care |
| Bourbon virus | Bourbon virus | Midwest and Southern United States | | Fever, fatigue, anorexia, nausea, vomiting, maculopapular rash | Thrombocytopenia, leukopenia | Testing available via health department | Supportive care |

[a]Although doxycycline is not generally recommended for children under 8 years of age because of dental staining with older tetracyclines, short courses have been safely used, and it is the agent of choice for *Ehrlichia* and Rickettsial infections in all age groups. Doxycycline is associated with higher relapse rates in treatment of Tularemia. ELISA, enzyme-linked immunosorbent assay; CHF, congestive heart failure; ESR, erythrocyte sedimentation rate; ARDS, acute respiratory distress syndrome; PCR, polymerase chain reaction; CDC, Centers for Disease Control and Prevention.
Adapted from Jacobs RF. Tick exposure and related infections. Pediatr Infect Dis J 1988;7:612–614; Gayle A, Ringdahl E. Tick-borne diseases. Am Fam Physician 2001;64:461–466.
Additional information available at: www.cdc.gov/heartland-virus; www.cdc.gov/powassan; www.cdc.gov/ncezid/dvbd/bourbon

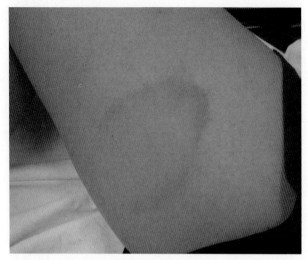

**Figure 21-7. Erythema migrans in a patient with Lyme disease.** (Photo by Indi Trehan, MD.)

| TABLE 21-13 | Screening Tests for Infectious Diseases in Internationally Adopted Children |
|---|---|

Complete blood cell count with red blood cell indices

Consider hepatitis A serological testing, although not routinely recommended

Hepatitis B surface antigen (HBsAg); some experts also include hepatitis B surface antibody (anti-HBs) and hepatitis B core antibody (anti-HBc)

Hepatitis C virus serologic testing (see text)

Syphilis serologic testing
    Nontreponemal test (RPR, VDRL, ART)
    Treponemal test (MHA-TP, FTA-ABS)

Human immunodeficiency virus 1 and 2 serologic testing (repeat 6 months after arrival if initially negative)
    Consider HIV DNA or RNA PCR testing in infants <18 months of age with two samples at least 1 month apart with one sample after 4 months of age

Tuberculin skin test (TST; if under age 2 years)

IGRA preferred in children who are >2 years of age who have received the BCG vaccination

Repeat testing should be performed 3-6 months after arrival if initially negative

Chagas disease serology in children >12 months of age (if immigrating from an endemic country)

Stool examination for ova and parasites (three specimens) or some clinicians will consider presumptive treatment with albendazole

Stool examination for *Giardia lamblia* and *Cryptosporidium* antigen (one specimen)

| TABLE 21-13 | Screening Tests for Infectious Diseases in Internationally Adopted Children (*Continued*) |
| --- | --- |

For children with eosinophilia (absolute eosinophil count >450 cells/µL) and negative stool ova and parasite studies, consider:

Toxocara canis serology and *Schistosoma* serology for children from sub-Saharan African, Southeast Asian, and certain Latin American countries. Strongyloides serology can also be ordered although some clinicians will consider presumptive treatment with ivermectin

Lymphatic filariasis serology in children >2 years (if immigrating from an endemic country)

Urine gonorrhea and chlamydia testing if history of sexual abuse

Urine hCG for all pubertal females

Hemoglobin electrophoresis and G6PD activity in high-risk populations

Lead level

Thyroid-stimulating hormone, free T4 level

RPR, rapid plasma reagin; VDRL, Venereal Disease Research Laboratory; ART, automated reagin test; MHA-TP, microhemagglutination test for *Treponema pallidum*; FTA-ABS, fluorescent treponemal antibody absorption; IGRA, interferon-gamma release assay; BCG, bacillus Calmette-Guérin vaccine.
Reprinted from American Academy of Pediatrics. In: Kimberlin DW, Barnett ED, Lynfield R, Sawyer MH, eds. Red Book: 2021 Report of the Committee on Infectious Diseases, 32nd Edition. American Academy of Pediatrics; 2021.

newborn screening, lead level, urinalysis, thyroid-stimulating hormone and thyroxine, alanine transferase and aspartate transferase, bilirubin, and alkaline phosphatase, as well as vision and hearing screening and developmental testing.
• Common skin infections in international adoptees include impetigo, fungal infections, molluscum contagiosum, and scabies.

### Immunizations

• Many foreign adoptees have deficient immunizations or may have inaccurate or incomplete or missing preadoption immunization records. To address these issues, antibody levels may be measured to verify immunity or the series of immunizations may be repeated.
• The recommended immunization protocol for these children is presented in Table 21-14.

### Intestinal Parasites

• Parasites and other intestinal pathogens are common in children immigrating from or returning from travel to foreign countries.
• Such children who are symptomatic (e.g., signs of gastroenteritis or malnutrition) should have the following testing performed:
  • Three specimens should be tested for ova and parasites.
  • One specimen should be tested specifically for *Giardia lamblia* and *Cryptosporidium parvum* antigens.
• In addition, children with active diarrhea (especially those with bloody stools) should have the stool cultured for *Salmonella*, *Shigella*, *Campylobacter*, and *E. coli* O157:H7. Stool assays for *Shiga* toxins (produced by O157:H7 and other serotypes of diarrheagenic *E. coli*) should be performed.

**TABLE 21-14** Approaches to the Evaluation and Immunization of Internationally Adopted Children

| Vaccine | Recommended approach | Alternative approach |
|---|---|---|
| Diphtheria and tetanus toxoids (DTaP, DT, Td, Tdap) | Immunize with diphtheria and tetanus-containing vaccine as appropriate for age; serologic testing for antitoxoid antibodies 4 weeks after dose 1 if severe local reaction occurs | Children whose records indicate receipt of $\geq 3$ doses: serologic testing for antitoxoid antibody to diphtheria and tetanus toxins before administering additional doses or administer a single booster dose of diphtheria and tetanus-containing vaccine, followed by serologic testing after 1 month for antitoxoid antibody to diphtheria and tetanus toxins with reimmunization as appropriate |
| Haemophilus influenzae type b (Hib) | Age-appropriate immunization | — |
| Hepatitis A | Hepatitis A serology | No vaccination needed if child has positive serology against hepatitis A |
| Hepatitis B | Perform hepatitis B panel | — |
| Influenza | Age-appropriate immunization | — |
| Measles-mumps-rubella (MMR) | Immunize with MMR vaccine or obtain measles antibody, and if positive, give MMR vaccine for mumps and rubella protection | Serologic testing for immunoglobulin G (IgG) antibody to vaccinated viruses indicated by immunization record |
| Pertussis (DTaP, Tdap) | No serologic test routinely available. May use antibodies to diphtheria or tetanus toxoids as a marker of receipt of diphtheria, tetanus, and pertussis-containing vaccine | — |
| Pneumococcal | Age-appropriate immunization | — |

| TABLE 21-14 | Approaches to the Evaluation and Immunization of Internationally Adopted Children *(Continued)* | |
|---|---|---|
| Poliovirus | Immunize with inactivated poliovirus vaccine (IPV) | Serologic testing for neutralizing antibody to poliovirus types 1, 2, and 3 or administer single dose of IPV, followed by serologic testing for neutralizing antibody to poliovirus types 1, 2, and 3 |
| Rotavirus | Age-appropriate immunization | — |
| Varicella | Age-appropriate immunization of children who lack reliable history of previous varicella disease or serologic evidence of protection | — |

Reprinted from American Academy of Pediatrics. In: Kimberlin DW, Barnett ED, Lynfield R, Sawyer MH, eds. Red Book: 2021 Report of the Committee on Infectious Diseases, 32nd Edition. American Academy of Pediatrics; 2021.

- Many intestinal parasites are not considered pathogens. However, their presence suggests that the patient may also be infected with other, pathogenic parasites. Examples of these nonpathogenic parasites include *Trichomonas hominis*, *Endolimax nana*, *Entamoeba coli*, and *Entamoeba dispar*.
- Treatment for pathogenic intestinal parasites is presented in Table 21-15.

## TUBERCULOSIS

### Clinical Presentation

- Although *Mycobacterium tuberculosis* infection (tuberculosis [TB]) is often asymptomatic in children and adolescents, patients may have fever, growth delay or weight loss, night sweats, chills, cough, sputum production, or hemoptysis.
- Extrapulmonary manifestations include meningitis and involvement of the middle ear, mastoid, lymph nodes, bones, joints, and skin.
- Tuberculous infection of the vertebrae (known as Pott disease) manifests as low-grade fever, irritability and restlessness, refusal to walk, and back pain without significant tenderness.
- High-risk populations include immigrants from high-prevalence regions, homeless people, and residents of correctional facilities.

### Laboratory Studies

- Diagnosis is established by acid-fast stain and culture from specimens of gastric aspirates, sputum, bronchial washings, pleural fluid, CSF, urine, or other body fluids or biopsy specimens. The best specimen from young children is three consecutive early morning gastric aspirates.

| TABLE 21-15 | Treatment of Commonly Identified Intestinal Parasites in International Adoptees |
|---|---|
| **Parasite** | **Treatment of choice** |
| *Giardia lamblia* | Tinidazole, nitazoxanide, or metronidazole |
| *Hymenolepis* species (dwarf tapeworm) | Praziquantel, nitazoxanide, or niclosamide |
| *Taenia* species (beef and pork tapeworms) | Praziquantel or niclosamide |
| *Ascaris lumbricoides* (roundworm) | Albendazole, mebendazole, ivermectin, pyrantel pamoate, or nitazoxanide |
| *Trichuris trichiura* (whipworm) | Albendazole or mebendazole, or ivermectin |
| *Strongyloides stercoralis* | Ivermectin or albendazole |
| *Entamoeba histolytica* | Asymptomatic: Iodoquinol, paromomycin, or diloxanide furoate |
| | Intestinal or extraintestinal disease: Metronidazole or tinidazole followed by iodoquinol or paromomycin |
| Hookworm | Albendazole, mebendazole, or pyrantel pamoate |

Reprinted from American Academy of Pediatrics. In: Kimberlin DW, Barnett ED, Lynfield R, Sawyer MH, eds. Red Book: 2021 Report of the Committee on Infectious Diseases, 32nd Edition. American Academy of Pediatrics; 2021.

- The tuberculin skin test (TST) becomes positive within 2-12 weeks of initial infection (Table 21-16). Alternatively, blood-based interferon-gamma release assays (IGRAs) are also available for testing. The TST is preferred for children under age 2, while both tests can be used in children older than age 2. IGRA testing is preferred in children who have received the bacille Calmette-Guérin (BCG) vaccine as it can cause a false-positive TST result. However, the IGRAs can have false-positive and false-negative results, so caution must be taken when interpreting the testing results in light of the patient's history and exposures. Often in complex situations, both TST and IGRA testing are ordered on a child.

### Imaging

A chest radiograph may demonstrate hilar, subcarinal, or mediastinal lymphadenopathy; pleural effusion; segmental lobar atelectasis or infiltrate; cavitary lesion particularly in the upper lung fields; or miliary disease.

### Treatment

- Consultation with infectious diseases or local health officials is recommended as the treatment regimens involve multiple medications and drug resistance is a rising concern.

**TABLE 21-16** Definitions of Positive Tuberculin Skin Test Results in Infants, Children, and Adolescents[a]

**Induration ≥5 mm**

Children in close contact with known or suspected contagious cases of TB

Children suspected to have TB:

- Findings on chest radiograph consistent with active or previously active TB
- Clinical evidence of TB disease[b]

Children receiving immunosuppressive therapy[c] or with immunosuppressive conditions, including HIV infection

**Induration ≥10 mm**

Children at increased risk of disseminated TB:

- Those <4 years of age
- Those with other medical conditions, including Hodgkin disease, lymphoma, diabetes mellitus, chronic renal failure, or malnutrition

Children with increased exposure to TB:

- Those born, or whose parents were born, in high-prevalence regions of the world
- Those with significant travel to high-prevalence regions of the world[d]
- Those frequently exposed to adults who have HIV, experiencing homelessness, incarcerated or institutionalized, people who inject/use drugs, or have an alcohol use disorder

**Induration ≥15 mm**

Children 4 years of age or older without any risk factors for TB

---

[a]These definitions apply regardless of previous bacille Calmette-Guérin (BCG) immunization; erythema at tuberculin skin test (TST) site does not indicate a positive test result. TSTs should be read at 48-72 hours after placement.
[b]Evidence by physical examination or laboratory assessment that would include TB in the working differential diagnosis (e.g., meningitis).
[c]This includes immunosuppressive doses of corticosteroids, tumor necrosis factor-alpha antagonists/blockers, or immunosuppressive drugs used in transplant recipients.
[d]Some experts define significant travel as travel or residence in a country with elevated TB rate for at least 1 month.
TB, tuberculosis.
Reprinted from American Academy of Pediatrics. In: Kimberlin DW, Barnett ED, Lynfield R, Sawyer MH, eds. Red Book: 2021 Report of the Committee on Infectious Diseases, 32nd Edition. American Academy of Pediatrics; 2021.

- Children admitted with TB should be placed in a negative-pressure isolation room, and appropriate particulate respirator masks should be worn by hospital personnel, especially since adult household members (if infected) may be contagious.

## OTHER CHILDHOOD INFECTIONS

Other common childhood infections are described in Table 21-17.

**TABLE 21-17** Other Common Childhood Infections

| Infection | Common etiologies | Initial therapy[a] |
|---|---|---|
| Streptococcal pharyngitis | *Streptococcus pyogenes* | There is no documented beta-lactam antibiotic resistance; use penicillin or amoxicillin; in penicillin allergy, consider cephalexin or clindamycin |
| Acute sinusitis (rare in younger children due to immature sinuses) | Viruses<br>*Streptococcus pneumoniae*<br>*Haemophilus influenzae*<br>*Moraxella catarrhalis* | Amoxicillin (high-dose) or amoxicillin-clavulanate (high-dose); in penicillin allergy consider cefdinir plus clindamycin |
| Skin and soft tissue infection | *Staphylococcus aureus*<br>Group A streptococci | Dependent on local resistance patterns and severity of infection, but might include cephalexin, clindamycin, trimethoprim-sulfamethoxazole, oxacillin, or vancomycin |
| Osteomyelitis | *Staphylococcus aureus*<br>*Kingella kingae* (young children) | Cefazolin<br>If MRSA is likely: Clindamycin<br>If toxic or bacteremic: Vancomycin plus third-generation cephalosporin |
| Infectious arthritis | *S. aureus*<br>*Streptococcus pyogenes*<br>*S. pneumoniae*<br>Gram-negative bacilli<br>*Neisseria gonorrhoeae*<br>*Kingella kingae* (young children) | Cefazolin<br>If MRSA is likely: Clindamycin<br>If toxic or bacteremic: Vancomycin plus third-generation cephalosporin<br>If concern for gram-negative infection or gonorrhea: Ceftriaxone |
| Endocarditis | Viridans streptococci<br>*Streptococcus bovis*<br>Enterococci<br>*S. aureus*<br>Coagulase-negative staphylococci | Treatment dependent on blood culture results and nature of affected valve; refer to the American Heart Association Scientific Statement on Infective Endocarditis for specific treatment regimens |
| Tinea capitis | *Trichophyton tonsurans*<br>*Microsporum canis* | Terbinafine or griseofulvin |

| TABLE 21-17 | Other Common Childhood Infections *(Continued)* | |
|---|---|---|
| **Lymphadenitis** | *Staphylococcus aureus* <br> *Streptococcus pyogenes* | Clindamycin, ampicillin/ sulbactam, cefazolin (if low suspicion of MRSA) |
| **Conjunctivitis** | Ophthalmia neonatorum | None |
| | Onset on day 1 of life: chemical irritation because of silver nitrate prophylaxis | |
| | Onset 2-4 days of age: *N. gonorrhoeae* | Ceftriaxone |
| | Onset 3-7 days of age: *C. trachomatis* | Azithromycin or erythromycin |
| | Onset 2-16 days of age: herpes simplex virus | Consider IV acyclovir |
| | Viral: adenovirus | None |
| | Suppurative conjunctivitis nongonococcal, nonchlamydial: *S. aureus, S. pneumoniae, H. influenzae* | Topical gatifloxacin, levofloxacin, moxifloxacin, or polymyxin B plus trimethoprim solution |

[a]Should be modified when culture results are available.
MRSA, methicillin-resistant *Staphylococcus aureus*; RSV, respiratory syncytial virus.

## SUGGESTED READINGS

American Academy of Pediatrics; Kimberlin DW, Barnett ED, Lynfield R, et al. Red Book (2021): Report of the Committee on Infectious Diseases. 32nd Ed. Itasca, IL: American Academy of Pediatrics, 2021.

American Association for the Study of Liver Diseases and the Infectious Diseases Society for America. HCV Guidance: Recommendations for Testing, Managing, and Treating Hepatitis C-HCV in Children. 2021. Available at www.hcvguidelines.org. Last accessed on 3/16/ 2021.

American College of Obstetricians and Gynecologists. Management of genital herpes in pregnancy. ACOG Practice Bulletin 2020;220:e193–e202.

Avner JR, Baker MD. Management of fever in infants and children. Emerg Med Clin North Am 2002;20:49–67.

Baltimore RS, Gewitz M, Baddour LM, et al. Infective endocarditis in childhood: 2015 update: a scientific statement from the American Heart Association. Circulation 2015;132:1487.

Bradley JS, Byington CL, Shah SS, et al.; Pediatric Infectious Diseases Society and the Infectious Diseases Society of America. The management of community-acquired pneumonia in infants and children older than 3 months of age: clinical practice guidelines by the Pediatric Infectious Diseases Society and the Infectious Diseases Society of America. Clin Infect Dis 2011;53(7):e25–e76.

Brouwer MC, McIntyre P, Prasad K, et al. Corticosteroids for acute bacterial meningitis. Cochrane Database Syst Rev 2015;2015(9):CD004405.

Byington CL, et al. Serious bacterial infections in febrile infants 1–90 days old with and without viral infection. Pediatrics 2004;113:1662–1665.

Byington CL, Kendrick J, Sheng X. Normative cerebrospinal fluid profiles in febrile infants. J Pediatr 2011;158(1):130–134.

Centers for Disease Control and Prevention. CDC Yellow Book 2020: Health Information for International Travel. New York: Oxford University Press, 2017.

Chen LH, Wilson ME. Zika circulation, congenital syndrome, and current guidelines: making sense of it all for the traveler. www.co-infectiousdiseases.com. 2019:381–389.

Gayle A, Ringdahl E. Tick-borne diseases. Am Fam Physician 2001;64:461–466.

Gilbert DN, Chambers HF, Saag MS, et al. The Sanford Guide to Antimicrobial Therapy 2020. Sperryville, VA: Antimicrobial Therapy, Inc., 2020.

Greenhow TL, Hung YY, Herz AM, et al. The changing epidemiology of serious bacterial infections in young infants. Pediatr Infect Dis J 2014;33(6):595–599.

Jain S, Williams DJ, Arnold SR, et al. Community-acquired pneumonia requiring hospitalization among U.S. children. New Engl J Med 2015;371:835–845.

Kimberlin DW, Baley J; Committee on Infectious Diseases; Committee on Fetus and Newborn. Guidance on management of asymptomatic neonates born to women with active genital herpes lesions. Pediatrics 2013;131(2):e635–e646.

Kliegman R, St. Geme J. Nelson Textbook of Pediatrics. 21st Ed. Philadelphia, PA: Elsevier, 2020.

Kuhar DT, Henderson DK, Struble KA, et al. Updated US Public Health Service Guidelines for the management of occupational exposures to human immunodeficiency virus and recommendations for postexposure prophylaxis. Infect Control Hosp Epidemiol 2013; 34(9):875–892.

Lantos PM, Rumbaugh J, Bockenstedt LK, et al. Clinical Practice Guidelines by the Infectious Diseases Society of America, American Academy of Neurology, and American College of Rheumatology: 2020 guidelines for the prevention, diagnosis, and treatment of Lyme disease. Neurology 2021;96:262–273.

Lieberthal AS, Carroll AE, Chonmaitree T, et al. The diagnosis and management of acute otitis media. Pediatrics 2013;131(3):e964–e999.

Litwin CM. Pet-transmitted infections: diagnosis by microbiologic and immunologic methods. Pediatr Infect Dis J 2003;22:768–777.

Long SS, Prober CG, Fischer M. Principles and Practice of Pediatric Infectious Diseases. 5th Ed. Philadelphia, PA: Elsevier Saunders, 2018.

Maldonado YA, Read JS. Diagnosis, treatment, and prevention of congenital toxoplasmosis in the United States. Pediatrics 2017;139:e20163860.

Mazor SS, et al. Interpretation of traumatic lumbar punctures: who can go home? Pediatrics 2003;111:525–528.

McKinnon HD Jr, Howard T. Evaluating the febrile patient with a rash. Am Fam Physician 2000;62:804–816.

National HIV/AIDS Clinician's Consulting Center at 888-448-4911. Available at www.hopkins-hivguide.org

Panel on Treatment of Pregnant women with HIV Infection and Prevention of Perinatal Transmission. Recommendations for Use of Antiretroviral Drugs in Transmission in the United States. Available at http://clinicalinfo.hiv.gov/en/guidelines. Accessed on 3/12/2021.

Parola P, Raoult D. Ticks and tickborne bacterial diseases in humans: an emerging infectious threat. Clin Infect Dis 2001;32(6):897–928.

Ralston SL, Lieberthal AS, Meissner HC, et al. Clinical practice guideline: the diagnosis, management, and prevention of bronchiolitis. Pediatrics 2014;134(5):e1474–e1502.

Ramilo O. Global impact of the HIV/AIDS pandemic. 26th Annual National Pediatric Infectious Disease Seminar, San Francisco, April 20, 2006.

Rawlinson WD, Boppana SB, Fowler KB, et al. Congenital cytomegalovirus infection in pregnancy and the neonate: consensus recommendations for prevention, diagnosis, and therapy. Lancet Infect Dis 2017;17:e177–e188.

Razzaq S, Schutze GE. Rocky Mountain spotted fever: a physician's challenge. Pediatr Rev 2005;26:125–129.

Shulman ST, Bisno AL, Clegg HW, et al. Clinical practice guideline for the diagnosis and management of group A streptococcal pharyngitis: 2012 update by the Infectious Diseases Society of America. Clin Infect Dis 2012;55(10):1279–1282.

Subcommittee on Urinary Tract Infection, Steering Committee on Quality Improvement and Management; Roberts KB. Urinary tract infection: clinical practice guideline for the diagnosis and management of the initial UTI in febrile infants and children 2 to 24 months. Pediatrics 2011;128(3):595–610.

Talan DA, et al. Bacteriologic analysis of infected dog and cat bites. New Engl J Med 1999;340:85–92.

The International Perinatal HIV Group. The mode of delivery and the risk of vertical transmission of human immunodeficiency virus type 1. N Engl J Med 1999;40:977–987.

Tunkel AR, Hartman BJ, Kaplan SL, et al. Practice guidelines for the management of bacterial meningitis. Clin Infect Dis 2004;39(9):1267–1284.

Waggoner-Fountain LA, Grossman LB. Herpes simplex virus. Pediatr Rev 2004;25:86–93.

Weisse ME. The fourth disease, 1900–2000. Lancet 2001;357:299–301.

Wolfrey JD, et al. Pediatric exanthems. Clin Fam Pract 2003;5:557–588.

Wormser GP, Dattwyler RJ, Shapiro ED, et al. The clinical assessment, treatment, and prevention of lyme disease, human granulocytic anaplasmosis, and babesiosis: clinical practice guidelines by the Infectious Diseases Society of America. Clin Infect Dis 2006;43(9):1089–1134.

# 22 Infection Prevention

Patti Kieffer and Patrick J. Reich

## INTRODUCTION

The overarching goals of an Infection Prevention (IP) program are to:

- Maintain health care worker and patient safety during patient care.
- Prevent health care–associated infections (HAIs), including surgical site infections (SSI), central-line associated bloodstream infections (CLABSI), nosocomial viral infections, antibiotic-resistant pathogens, etc.

## STANDARD PRECAUTIONS

Standard Precautions (SP) are work practices required to achieve a basic level of IP to protect patients and health care workers. SP are based on the principle that all blood, body fluids, secretions, excretions (except sweat), nonintact skin, and mucous membranes may contain transmissible infectious agents. SP apply to all patient care encounters regardless of suspected or confirmed diagnosis or presumed infection status and include:

- **Hand Hygiene (HH):** Cleaning your hands is the most basic measure to prevent HAIs.
  - Using an alcohol-based hand sanitizer is generally preferred because it is more effective at killing organisms, is easier to perform during clinical care, and causes less skin irritation and dryness compared to soap and water.
  - Washing with soap and water for at least 15 seconds should be performed when hands are visibly soiled.
  - Performing appropriate technique includes using the right amount of alcohol-based hand sanitizer or soap and ensuring that you cover the entire hands, including the thumbs, fingertips, and areas between fingers.
  - Gloves should be changed if damaged or soiled, and when moving from a contaminated body site (e.g., changing a diaper, assessing a wound) to a clean body site.
  - Historically, there has been a focus on performing HH when entering and leaving a patient's room, but there are multiple opportunities for HH while providing care. The World Health Organization (WHO) 5 Moments of HH (Fig. 22-1) is a summary of critical HH moments.
- **Respiratory Hygiene/Cough Etiquette:**
  - Cover your mouth and nose with a tissue when coughing or sneezing.
  - Perform HH after having contact with any respiratory secretions or contaminated objects.
- **Personal Protective Equipment (PPE):**
  - Wear a gown and gloves if there is risk of contact with blood or other bodily fluids.
  - Wear an isolation mask and eye protection if there is risk of respiratory droplet exposure, splashes, or other bodily fluid exposure.

# Your 5 moments for
## HAND HYGIENE

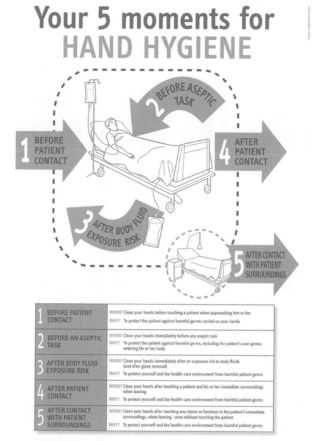

| | | |
|---|---|---|
| **1** BEFORE PATIENT CONTACT | WHEN? | Clean your hands before touching a patient when approaching him or her |
| | WHY? | To protect the patient against harmful germs carried on your hands |
| **2** BEFORE AN ASEPTIC TASK | WHEN? | Clean your hands immediately before any aseptic task |
| | WHY? | To protect the patient against harmful germs, including the patient's own germs, entering his or her body |
| **3** AFTER BODY FLUID EXPOSURE RISK | WHEN? | Clean your hands immediately after an exposure risk to body fluids (and after glove removal) |
| | WHY? | To protect yourself and the health-care environment from harmful patient germs |
| **4** AFTER PATIENT CONTACT | WHEN? | Clean your hands after touching a patient and his or her immediate surroundings when leaving |
| | WHY? | To protect yourself and the health-care environment from harmful patient germs |
| **5** AFTER CONTACT WITH PATIENT SURROUNDINGS | WHEN? | Clean your hands after touching any object or furniture in the patient's immediate surroundings, when leaving - even without touching the patient |
| | WHY? | To protect yourself and the health-care environment from harmful patient germs |

**Figure 22-1. The World Health Organization 5 moments for hand hygiene.** (Reprinted from World Health Organization. Your 5 Moments for Hand Hygiene. October 2006. Available at https://www.who.int/gpsc/tools/5momentsHandHygiene_A3.pdf?ua=1)

- Proper cleaning and disinfecting patient care equipment, instruments/devices, and high touch surfaces per manufacturer's recommendations.
- **Safe use and disposal of needles and other sharps,** follow safe injection practices.

## TRANSMISSION-BASED PRECAUTIONS

**Transmission-Based Precautions** are the second tier of basic IP and are to be used in conjunction with SP for patients who may be infected or colonized with certain infectious agents. A detailed list of specific pathogens and corresponding isolation precautions is found in Appendix A of the SLCH Isolation Table, a summary of the most common pathogens is found in Table 22-1.

**TABLE 22-1** Common Pathogens and Isolation Recommendations

| Disease | Category | Single room? | PPE |
|---|---|---|---|
| Respiratory viral infections (e.g., influenza, adenovirus, seasonal coronaviruses, parainfluenza, rhinovirus/enterovirus, metapneumovirus, etc.) | Contact + Droplet | Preferred | Gowns, gloves, isolation mask, eye protection |
| Active MRSA infection | Contact | Preferred | Gowns, gloves |
| MDR—multidrug-resistant gram-negatives (e.g., ESBL—extended spectrum beta-lactamase producing gram-negatives, CRE—carbapenem-resistant gram-negatives) | Contact | Preferred | Gowns, gloves |
| *C. difficile* | Contact | Preferred | Gowns, gloves |
| Pulmonary tuberculosis | Airborne with N95 (or equivalent) | Required, must be negative pressure | N95 or equivalent |
| Measles | Contact + airborne with N95 (or equivalent) | Required, must be negative pressure | Gowns, gloves, N95 or equivalent, eye protection |
| Varicella (chickenpox) | Contact + airborne without N95 | Required, must be negative pressure | Gowns, gloves **Only immune HCWs should enter the room** |

- **Contact Precautions** should be used for patients with known or suspected infections that are transmitted by direct contact with patients or contaminated environmental surfaces. Gowns and gloves are required. The patient should have a dedicated stethoscope.
- **Droplet Precautions** are intended to prevent transmission of pathogens spread through close respiratory or mucous membrane contact with respiratory secretions. Close contact (within 3-6 feet) is usually required for transmission. An isolation mask and eye protection should be worn upon room entry. Special air handling and ventilation are not required to prevent droplet transmission.
- **Airborne Precautions** are indicated to prevent transmission of infectious agents that remain infectious over long distances when suspended in the air (TB, measles, varicella, etc.). A properly fitted N95 respirator (or equivalent) is required when entering the room. All persons wearing N95 respirators must be fit tested. Patients should be admitted to a private, negative pressure ventilation (NPV) room. The doors should remain closed and in and out traffic limited.
- Room air pressure relationships range from NPV to neutral to positive pressure ventilation (PPV). Generally:
  - NPV rooms are indicated for patients with airborne-transmitted infections (e.g., TB, measles, varicella, COVID-19 undergoing aerosol-generating procedures, etc.).
  - PPV rooms are used in the operating room to decrease SSI risk and for severely immunocompromised patients (e.g., BMT, AML patients) to minimize general exposure risk.

## MANAGEMENT OF OUTBREAKS, CLUSTERS, AND EMERGING PATHOGENS

- Disease outbreaks can occur at the local, national, and global levels. Surveillance programs and emergency preparedness measures are necessary to detect, contain, and ideally prevent these outbreaks.
  - The 2003 severe acute respiratory syndrome (SARS) outbreak, West African Ebola outbreaks beginning in 2013, and 2019 novel Coronavirus (COVID-19) pandemic are examples of local outbreaks that developed into regional and ultimately global epidemics.
- Contact tracing and exposure investigation are important components of outbreak investigation and control. Based on the transmission characteristics of the specific disease, quarantine of exposed individuals and postexposure prophylaxis may be indicated.

## UNIQUE ASPECTS IN PEDIATRIC INFECTION PREVENTION

- Infants and young children pose unique challenges to IP. The health care worker plays an important role in providing a safe and infection-free environment in the pediatric setting. It is vital that IP programs that serve pediatric patients be tailored to meet the needs of this specialized population, taking into account age-related factors that create challenges for the health care worker as well prevent the child from adhering to IP standards. The IP processes established must meet the growth and development needs of the child.
- Infants, particularly premature infants, pose unique IP challenges given their small size and immature skin, lung development, gut integrity, and immune system func-

tion. Standard prevention measures used in adult patients (e.g., weekly changing of central line dressings, daily chlorhexidine bathing, etc.) may not be easily adapted in this population.

- Parents and other caregivers provide essential components of patient care and emotional support, and so their presence at the bedside should be encouraged and accommodated whenever possible.
  - This includes situations when visitation for adult patients may not be recommended (e.g., patient with a communicable disease such as COVID-19).

## FREQUENTLY ASKED INFECTION PREVENTION QUESTIONS AND ANSWERS

- *When can my patient come off transmission-based precautions for MRSA, adenovirus, norovirus, Clostridium difficile, etc.?*
  Each case is unique and the criteria for removal of isolation varies based on organism and patient-level factors (e.g., isolation precautions are often extended in immunocompromised compared to immunocompetent patients). Specific information on removal of isolation precautions are found in Appendix A of the SLCH Isolation Table.
- *I have a fever, cough, diarrhea, or other symptoms. Should I come to work today?*
  It is imperative that employees do not come to work when symptoms of viral infections or other contagious conditions are present (e.g., fever, diarrhea, pink eye, etc.). Occupational Health is available to help answer questions regarding when to stay home and when to return to work.
- *I was exposed to a patient with pertussis. Do I need postexposure prophylaxis?*
  There are specific indications for postexposure antibiotic prophylaxis after a pertussis exposure, including direct contact with respiratory, oral, or nasal secretions from a symptomatic patient. If you think you have been exposed to pertussis, please contact Occupational Health for further guidance.
- *What criteria are used to decide whether it is appropriate to cohort two patients in a semiprivate room?*
  Cohorting guidelines are very specific. Generally, cohorting patients with the same illness (e.g., influenza A with influenza A, RSV with RSV, etc.) is acceptable, but many factors are considered when making these decisions. It is best to discuss cohorting options with the charge nurse of the floor and the administrative supervisors who can help make the best possible decisions around cohorting.

## SUGGESTED READINGS

Kimberlin DW, Barnett ED, Lynfield R, Sawyer MH, eds. *Red Book: 2021 Report of the Committee on Infectious Diseases*. Itaska, IL: American Academy of Pediatrics: 2021.

Centers for Disease Control and Prevention. Available at https://www.cdc.gov/handhygiene/science/index.html

Centers for Disease Control and Prevention. Available at https://www.cdc.gov/infectioncontrol/basics/standard-precautions.html

Centers for Disease Control and Prevention. Available at https://www.cdc.gov/infectioncontrol/basics/transmission-based-precautions.html

Centers for Disease Control and Prevention. Available at https://www.cdc.gov/csels/dsepd/ss1978/lesson6/index.html

Centers for Disease Control and Prevention. Available at https://www.cdc.gov/infectioncontrol/pdf/guidelines/isolation-guidelines-H.pdf

Solutions for Patient Safety Prevention Bundles. Available at https://www.solutionsforpatient-safety.org/wp-content/uploads/SPS-Prevention-Bundles_FEB-2021.pdf

St. Louis Children's Hospital Isolation Table Appendix A. Available at https://www.stlouis-childrens.org/sites/default/files/pdfs/Copy%20of%20SLCH_Appendix.A.IsolationTable.final.1.2019.pdf

The Society for Healthcare Epidemiology of America. The Society for Healthcare Epidemiology of America Compendium of Strategies to Prevent Healthcare-Associated Infections in Acute Care Hospitals. Available at https://shea-online.org/index.php/practice-resources/priority-top-ics/compendium-of-strategies-to-prevent-hais

World Health Organization. World Health Organization 5 Moments of Hand Hygiene. Available at https://www.who.int/docs/default-source/save-lives---clean-your-hands/5may-advo-cacy-toolkit.pdf?sfvrsn=8301e563_2

# 23 Night Curriculum for Cross Coverage

Amanda Reis Dube and Chrissy Hrach

## ON CALL PROBLEMS

This chapter outlines common medical problems encountered at night on the general pediatric wards, with suggestions for rapid diagnosis and treatment. Clinical situations and institutional guidelines may vary and treatment should be modified based on these factors.

## RESPIRATORY DISTRESS

- Immediate questions
  - What are the vital signs of the patient and are they appropriate for age?
  - What is the degree of respiratory distress?
  - Does the patient need escalation of care that you cannot provide on the inpatient general pediatric unit?
- Key content
  - Targeted examination: Include a rapid assessment and a quick determination of the severity of the respiratory condition including A, B, C's—Airway, Breathing and Circulation
    - ○ Airway—is it clear and maintainable?
      - – Does the patient require support or a jaw thrust?
      - – Does the patient require suctioning or repositioning?
    - ○ Breathing—rate, effort and mechanics, grunting, nasal flaring
      - – Air entry—is there stridor or wheeze?
  - Identify children at high risk for respiratory failure:
    - ○ Increased respiratory rate or effort or diminished breath sounds
    - ○ Decreased level of consciousness
    - ○ Poor muscle tone
    - ○ Cyanosis
  - Scoring: Utilize the CAB (Children's Asthma/Bronchiolitis) score, for example, as part of the assessment (Table 23-1). This score is a way to report an objective measurement of examination findings and compare changes over time and in response to treatment. Please note that this score is not yet validated.
    - ○ There are other bronchiolitis scoring tools published such as the WARM tool, as well as other asthma scoring tools such as pediatric asthma severity score (PASS) and pediatric respiratory assessment measure (PRAM). No single tool has been universally adopted.
  - Initial management
    - ○ Allow child to assume position of comfort.
    - ○ Consider placing child on pulse oximetry and ECG monitor.
    - ○ Administer oxygen as needed and as tolerated.

| TABLE 23-1 | Children's Asthma/Bronchiolitis (CAB) Score |

| | Respiratory rate | | | | | |
|---|---|---|---|---|---|---|
| Score | 1-12 months | 1-5 years | 6-11 years | ≥12 years | Wheezing | Accessory Muscle Use |
| 0 | ≤50 | ≤40 | ≤30 | ≤20 | None | No apparent activity |
| 1 | 51-60 | 41-50 | 31-40 | 21-25 | Terminal expiration with good aeration | Mild increase (subcostal retractions) |
| 2 | 61-75 | 51-60 | 41-45 | 26-30 | Entire expiration | Moderate increase (subcostal and intercostal retractions) |
| 3 | >75 | >60 | >45 | >30 | Inspiration and expiration OR absent wheezing due to poor aeration | Maximal increase (subcostal, intercostals, and supraclavicular retractions) |

Courtesy of Anne E. Borgmeyer, DNP, RN, CPNP-PC, AE-C.

- Determine whether patient merits escalation to a higher level of care, such as an ICU, taking into account local policies and degree of respiratory support needed.
- Initial studies
  - Consider obtaining a chest plain radiographs in patients with a focal lung examination or sudden change or to look for pneumonia, effusion, pneumothorax, cardiomegaly, or evidence of a foreign body aspiration.
  - Consider blood gas and/or blood glucose, and/or urine toxicology if patient has altered mental status.
  - In general, stabilize patient first, then obtain labs and imaging.
- Differential diagnosis
  - Upper airway obstruction—symptoms are more apparent during inspiration than expiration
    - With a partial obstruction may have stridor, choking, gagging
    - With a complete obstruction—no audible speech, cry, or cough
  - Lower airway obstruction—symptoms are more apparent during expiration than inspiration
  - Parenchymal lung disease—hypoxemia, tachypnea, increased work of breathing
  - Disordered control of breathing—apnea or abnormal rhythm
- Uncommon but important not to miss
  - Tension pneumothorax
  - Pulmonary embolism
  - Heart failure

- Empiric therapy
  - Upper airway obstruction—common examples include croup and anaphylaxis
    - Croup treatment: nebulized racemic epinephrine and corticosteroids. Common practice is dexamethasone either IM or PO depending on the degree of respiratory distress.
    - Anaphylaxis: first step is to remove the offending agent if known. Then IM epinephrine, inhaled bronchodilator if wheezing is present, and treat hypotension if present. Can consider H1 and H2 blockers once patient is stabilized, if desired.
  - Lower airway obstruction—common examples are bronchiolitis and asthma
    - Bronchiolitis: suctioning, oxygen as needed
      - High-flow nasal cannula (HFNC) therapy: this intervention is commonly used for patients with bronchiolitis and can also be useful for patients with other etiologies of respiratory distress. HFNC delivers humidified, warmed oxygen at adjustable rates.
    - Asthma: oral corticosteroids, inhaled bronchodilators, consider magnesium sulfate, and oxygen
  - Parenchymal lung disease: main treatment is oxygen delivery. May additionally benefit from positive pressure (e.g., HFNC, CPAP, or BiPAP), antibiotics for pneumonia, and diuretics in the case of volume overload.
  - Disordered control of breathing: determine the underlying etiology such as altered level of consciousness, or neuromuscular disease. Support oxygenation and ventilation.

## VOLUME STATUS/SHOCK

- Immediate questions
  - What is the fluid status of the patient?
  - What are the most recent set of vital signs?
- Key content
  - What is shock?
    - When perfusion of the vital organs is inadequate to meet organ tissue demands
      - This can lead to accumulation of lactic acid and irreversible cellular damage.
  - Major categories of shock
    - Hypovolemic shock: inadequate intravascular volume relative to the vascular space. This is the most common type of shock in pediatric patients, often related to dehydration or hemorrhage.
    - Cardiogenic shock: myocardial dysfunction. Inadequate myocardial function limits stroke volume and cardiac output. Large heart size on chest plain radiographs in a child with evidence of shock and poor cardiac output is the hallmark.
    - Distributive shock: inappropriate distribution of blood flow. This type of shock is seen in cases of anaphylaxis and sepsis, due to peripheral vasodilation.
    - Obstructive shock: outflow from left or right side of heart is physically impaired. This could be seen from a large pulmonary embolism, tension pneumothorax, or pericardial effusion.
    - Neurogenic shock: children usually present with hypotension, bradycardia, and sometimes hypothermia.
  - Compensated versus hypotensive shock
    - Compensated shock: systolic blood pressure is within the normal range for age.
    - Hypotensive (decompensated) = systolic blood pressure <5th percentile for age

- Assessment for shock
  - Heart rate: Sinus tachycardia is commonly seen as an initial sign of shock in children. Improvement in heart rate in response to interventions is an important indication of success, while worsening of heart rate is a concerning indication of deterioration.
  - Blood pressure: In a patient with possible shock, both the systolic and diastolic blood pressures should be frequently assessed. Hypotension is a late and often sudden sign of cardiovascular decompensation. Thus, even mild hypotension should be treated urgently. Hypotension is present if the systolic blood pressure is **<70 mm Hg + (2 × age in years)** for children 1-10 years of age.
  - Systemic perfusion: Assessing these indicators of blood flow and systemic vascular resistance are very important in determining the type and severity of shock.
    - Pulse location: Can you palpate pulses centrally and peripherally? If peripheral pulses are weak or absent, then the patient is in decompensated shock.
    - Pulse volume: Are the pulses are thready or bounding. Thready pulses indicate peripheral vasoconstriction, as is often seen in hypovolemic shock, while bounding peripheral pulses indicate peripheral vasodilation, as is often seen in distributive shock.
    - Skin temperature: Note color and capillary refill.
    - CNS function: Evaluation for altered mental status is critical. For younger children who might not respond to standard questions at baseline, evaluate the response to environment. One option for categorizing levels of consciousness in young children is the AVPU scale:
      - **A**lert
      - Responsive to **V**oice
      - Responsive to **P**ain
      - **U**nresponsive
    - Urine output—monitoring urine output directly reflects renal blood flow and glomerular filtration rate. Normal urine output averages 1-2 mL/kg/hr in children.
- Initial management of shock
  - Rapid cardiopulmonary assessment: This is covered by the basic PALS algorithms and includes assessment of airway, breathing, and circulation. After initial assessment, you can categorize the patient as stable, in respiratory distress, in respiratory failure, in shock (compensated or uncompensated), or in cardiopulmonary failure.
  - Overall goal is to normalize blood pressure and tissue perfusion.
  - Targets for physiologic indicators
    - Blood pressure: normal
    - Skin perfusion: warm, with capillary refill 1-2 seconds
    - Mental status: normal, or "awake" on the AVPU scale
    - Urine output: at least 1 mL/kg/hr
  - Once shock has been identified, prompt action is required for optimal patient outcomes
    - First 15 minutes
      - Recognize decreased mental status and perfusion.
      - Establish IV access.
      - Maintain airway based on PALS guidelines.
      - Administer 20 mL/kg isotonic saline or colloid boluses via push-pull bolus up to and over 60 mL/kg.

- If concern for cardiogenic shock, it may be reasonable to start with only 10 mL/kg. For any patient, reassessment after each bolus is imperative to assess for improvement versus deterioration due to volume overload.
  - Assess for and correct hypoglycemia and hypocalcemia.
  - After giving fluids, it is important to determine if the patient is fluid responsive; that is, if fluid administration has been sufficient to stabilize the patient.
    - Fluid responsive shock: Continue current management.
    - Fluid refractory shock: Begin pressor therapy, establish central venous access, and transfer to ICU.
- Remember to ask for help early when you have a patient in shock. Early reversal of shock is associated with a decrease in mortality and morbidity regardless of underlying etiology.

## FEVER

- Initial questions
  - Is this a new fever?
  - How old is the patient?
  - Is the patient immunocompromised?
  - Does the patient have any implanted hardware?
  - On examination, does the patient have normal perfusion and mental status?
- Key content
  - How do we define fever?
    - ≥ 38.0 for infants <6 months, and the immunocompromised
    - ≥ 38.5 for other patients
    - Severity of illness does not correspond with the degree of fever
  - What are the major categories of illnesses that can cause fevers?
    - Infectious
      - Systemic bacterial infections, such as bacteremia, sepsis, meningitis, or endocarditis
      - Systemic viral infections, such as Epstein-Barr Virus (EBV), Cytomegalovirus (CMV), or disseminated Herpes Simplex Virus (HSV)
      - Respiratory infections, such as Upper Respiratory Tract Infection (URI), acute otitis media, pharyngitis, pneumonia, or bronchiolitis
      - Skin and soft tissue infections, such as cellulitis or abscess
      - Abdominal/pelvic infections, such as appendicitis, abscess, pyelonephritis, or Urinary Tract Infection (UTI)
      - Bone/joint infections, such as septic arthritis or osteomyelitis
      - Hardware infections, such as central line or urinary catheter associated
    - Inflammatory: for example, Kawasaki, Juvenile Idiopathic Arthritis (JIA), lupus, Inflammatory Bowel Disease (IBD) or Henoch-Schonlein Purpura (HSP)
    - Malignancy: for example, leukemia, lymphoma, neuroblastoma, or Wilms tumor
    - Other: consider drug fevers or Central Nervous System (CNS) dysfunction
  - Key considerations in assessment of the child with a fever
    - Vital signs
    - Physical examination, including general appearance, mental status, perfusion, respiratory effort, lines and hardware, wounds
    - Repeated examinations and assessments over time are key
  - Laboratory evaluation: Not every patient will need labs drawn, but some may.
    - Infants <2 months of age: consider Complete Blood Count (CBC) with differential, blood culture, urinalysis/urine culture, and lumbar puncture (consult AAP Guidelines

2021 [see Pantell et al., 2021 suggested reading], REVISE guidelines [see Biondi et al., 2019 suggested reading], or your institutional guidelines for particular situation)

- ○ Patients with hardware: CBC, blood culture; consider urinalysis if indwelling or intermittent catheter; consider lumbar puncture if patient has a ventriculoperitoneal shunt
- ○ Other high-risk patients: consider CBC, blood culture, urinalysis
- ○ Other labs to consider: Erythrocyte Sedimentation Rate (ESR), C-Reactive Protein (CRP) chest plain radiographs, respiratory viral panel, and abdominal or other imaging, depending on clinical situation
- Antipyretics
  - ○ Fevers themselves are not dangerous, but there may be some situations in which giving antipyretics can be advantageous.
    - – More accurate mental status examination: If a young child seems irritable and has a fever, reassessing after antipyretic therapy can help distinguish the expected discomfort of a fever from pathologic irritability.
    - – Decreased insensible water loss: Treatment with antipyretics may reduce insensible water losses, which can be of benefit in children who have, or are at risk for developing, dehydration.
    - – Improved ability to hydrate: Children with fevers may feel uncomfortable, and thus less likely to willingly take PO fluids. Antipyretics may improve their ability to keep themselves hydrated.
    - – Known history of febrile seizures: Giving antipyretics to children with a history of febrile seizures does not prevent febrile seizures during future fever episodes although there is some evidence that they may help prevent recurrent febrile seizures during the same fever episode.
- Empiric therapy
  - ○ High-risk patient populations who may merit empiric antibiotics include the following:
    - – Patients with a central line
    - – Infants <2 months old
    - – Neutropenic patients
    - – Some immunocompromised/immunosuppressed patients

## ACUTE SEIZURE MANAGEMENT

- Key questions
  - • Does the patient have a history of seizures?
  - • When did the current episode start?
  - • What medications is the patient taking? Any missed doses or overdoses?
  - • Any known lab abnormalities or risk factors for lab abnormalities? (especially glucose and sodium)
- Key content
  - • Initial steps in management of a seizing patient:
    - ○ If not in a safe place, position in hospital bed, laying down, and remove sharp/hard objects from vicinity.
    - ○ Put on monitors; specifically, apply a sensor to measure $SpO_2$, and, ideally, leads for a CR monitor and a blood pressure cuff.
    - ○ Start a timer to time seizure.
    - ○ Check a finger stick blood glucose, and administer glucose if low.
    - ○ Call for additional help (nursing support, rapid response, respiratory therapy).

○ Consider potential causes of seizure.
  – Differential may include febrile seizure, toxic ingestion, hypoglycemia, hypo- or hypernatremia, medication or medication withdrawal, CNS infection, head trauma, hypoxia, or stroke.
○ Seizure management: In general, benzodiazepines should be administered starting at 3-5 minutes if the seizure has not self-resolved. If the patient has an IV, intravenous lorazepam is the preferred starting medication. If the patient does not have an IV, intramuscular or intranasal midazolam or rectal diazepam are reasonable alternatives. If benzodiazepines do not successfully terminate the seizure after two doses at 5 minute intervals, loading with an antiepileptic medicine is generally the preferred second-line treatment.
○ Status epilepticus: Generally defined as a seizure lasting longer than 30 minutes, or back-to-back seizures without return to mental status baseline lasting longer than 30 minutes. Status epilepticus has high morbidity/mortality.
○ Continued vital sign monitoring is critical, especially as benzodiazepines and antiepileptic medications may result in respiratory depression. If hypoxia develops, consider repositioning the patient's head to a "sniffing" position, administration of oxygen via nasal cannula or nonbreather, and intubation if necessary.
○ Once patient is stable, initiate workup
  – Initial workup may include CBC, CMP, calcium, magnesium, and urine drug screen. Neuroimaging, lumbar puncture, and specific drug levels (e.g., to check for appropriate blood levels of antiepileptic drugs in patients with known epilepsy) should be considered depending on the particular patient and situation.
• Febrile seizure
  ○ Age range: 6 months through 5 years
  ○ Fever: ≥100.4°F or 38°C; may occur before or after the seizure
  ○ Prevalence: 2-5% of children will experience a febrile seizure. Approximately 30% of children who experience one simple febrile seizure will have another
  ○ Simple versus complex
    – Simple: generalized, last <15 minutes, no recurrence within 24 hours
    – Complex: focal, last longer than 15 minutes, or recur within 24 hours
  ○ Management: for febrile seizures lasting longer than five minutes, acute management is the same as for other seizure types (see above)
  ○ Workup
    – Simple febrile seizure: If patient is otherwise healthy, returns to baseline spontaneously, and has no concern for serious bacterial infection, no workup is needed.
    – The approach to a patient with a complex febrile seizure depends on the patient's particular circumstances. Consider CBC, CMP, LP, neuroimaging, and/or EEG.
    – If meningeal signs/symptoms present, obtain LP.
    – If patient is <12 months old and underimmunized, consider obtaining LP.

## POSITIVE BLOOD CULTURES

• Immediate questions
  • Was sterile technique done when obtaining blood culture?
  • What is the organism that is growing?
  • Is that organism real or contaminant?
  • Is the patient stable?

- What is the time to positivity of the blood culture?
- Does the patient need to be started on antibiotics or change the current antibiotic regimen?
- Key content
  - Collection technique
    - Blood cultures should be obtained prior to starting antibiotic therapy.
    - Two sets of blood cultures obtained from separate venipuncture sites are preferred. Often in pediatrics, only one set of blood cultures is obtained due to smaller blood volumes and fewer options for venipuncture sites.
    - To decrease the chances of contamination, blood cultures should be obtained via venipuncture rather than via an existing IV site.
  - Volume: Volume of blood is a key factor in maximizing the yield of true pathogens.
    - In pediatrics, volumes of blood to be collected are guided by body weight and range from 2 mL for premature infants to 20-30 mL for adolescents.
    - A blood culture set is often one aerobic bottle and one anaerobic bottle; however, for otherwise healthy pediatric patients without indwelling hardware, inoculating two aerobic bottles is often advisable as anaerobic bacteria are a far less common true source of infection.
  - Timing of collection
    - Commonly, blood cultures are obtained when fever is detected. However, studies have shown that the timing of blood cultures relative to fever is not predictive of true positivity.
  - Interpretation of results
    - There are multiple considerations where determining the clinical significance of a positive blood culture, including the number of positive cultures out of the total number obtained; which organism was recovered; time to positivity; the site of the culture collection (peripheral IV vs. central line vs. venipuncture); and the likelihood of bacteremia based on the patient's overall clinical picture.
      - Organisms that are usually true pathogens: *Staphylococcus aureus*; *Streptococcus pneumonia*; group A Streptococcus; Enterobacteriaceae; *Haemophilus influenzae*; *Pseudomonas aeruginosa*; Bacteroidaceae; *Candida* species
      - Organisms that are more commonly contaminants: coagulase negative staphylococci; *Corynebacterium* species; *C.* (formerly *Propionibacterium*) *acnes*; *Bacillus* species; *Micrococcus* species
    - Time to positivity
      - According to a large, multicenter study by Biondi et al. in 2014, 91% of true positive blood cultures are positive by 24 hours. The yield increases to 96% and 99% by 36 and 48 hours, respectively. This, combined with data from Lefebvre et al. in 2017, who found that mean time to positivity was 14.4 hours for true pathogens and 23.1 hours or contaminants, has led many institutions to shorten the required observation period after blood cultures to 24-36 hours for some patient populations.
  - Hospital blood culture systems: Most modern clinical microbiology laboratories utilize an automated continuous monitoring blood culture system for detecting bacteremia.
    - Most systems will include a 5-day incubation period.
    - Clinically significant bacteremia are usually detected within 48 hours.
  - Empiric therapy: If it is determined that the patient has a clinically significant positive blood culture result and is not yet on antibiotics, antibiotics should be initiated promptly. The patient's age and clinical picture, as well as your local antibiograms, can be used to determine the most appropriate empiric antibiotic choice.

## SODIUM ABNORMALITIES

- Key questions
  - How was the sample drawn?
  - What underlying medical problems does the patient have?
  - What medications is the patient on?
  - What is the patient's volume status?
  - What is the patient's mental status?
- Key content
  - Hypernatremia: serum sodium concentration >145 mEq/L
    - ○ Causes
      - – Hypernatremia should be thought of as a deficiency of water rather than an excess of sodium.
      - – Decreased fluid intake
        - - Fluid restriction, ineffective/insufficient feeding of infant
      - – Water loss
        - - Renal: diabetes insipidus (central or nephrogenic), diuretics, hyperglycemia, tubular impairment
        - - GI: gastroenteritis, osmotic diarrhea, ostomy, malabsorption
      - – Excessive sodium intake
        - - Administration of normal saline, hypertonic saline, or blood products; inappropriate formula mixing for infant
    - ○ Importance: Hypernatremia can lead to shrinkage of cerebral neurons, which can lead to intracranial or intracerebral hemorrhage secondary to bridging vein damage. Hypernatremia can also predispose to venous sinus thrombosis. Rapid correction of hypernatremia can lead to cerebral edema.
    - ○ Investigation
      - – A thorough history to identify possible risk factors is the most important means of investigation.
      - – Physical examination should focus on assessing for signs of altered mental status, which often initially manifests as agitation and irritability, progressing to lethargy. Tone may also initially increase, and seizures can be seen.
      - – Ensure that, if the blood sample was drawn through an IV, sufficient blood was wasted as to prevent contamination from IV fluids.
    - ○ Management: Interventions focus on administration additional fluids, the exact type of which may depend on the specific cause of hypernatremia.
      - – An estimate of the total free water deficit can be made with the following calculation: 4 mL × body weight × desired change in sodium. How this relates to the total volume of fluid to administer depends on the type of fluid chosen. For example, 0.45% sodium chloride is about 50% free water.
      - – Be sure to also account for maintenance fluid needs and ongoing fluid losses.
      - – Goal rate of correction is 0.5 mEq/L/h.
      - – Transfer to an ICU for closer monitoring is often appropriate.
  - Hyponatremia: serum sodium concentration <135 mEq/L
    - ○ Causes
      - – Hyponatremia should be thought of as an excess of water rather than a deficiency of sodium.
      - – Excessive intake of water +/− decreased ability to secrete free water.
    - ○ Importance: Hyponatremia can lead to cerebral edema and ultimately herniation if not appropriately managed. Rapid correction of hyponatremia can result in central pontine myelinolysis.

○ Investigation
  – Detailed history, including of fluid balance, changes in weight, medications (e.g., diuretics), and other medical disorders
  – Physical examination, focusing on mental/neurologic status—early symptoms of hyponatremic encephalopathy can include headache, nausea/vomiting, and weakness, which may progress to behavioral changes, latency to respond to verbal/tactile stimuli, and ultimately seizures, pupillary changes, and posturing
  – Assessment of serum and urine osmolality
    - Serum osmolality: serum osm > 280 suggests pseudohyponatremia, for example, from hyperglycemia or mannitol
    - Urine osmolality: urine osm < 100 indicates excessive water intake, such as from psychogenic polydipsia or water intoxication
    - If urine osm > 100 and patient is normovolemic, hyponatremia could be due to hypothyroidism, postoperative hyponatremia, glucocorticoid insufficiency, or SIADH
    - If urine osm > 100 and patient is hypovolemic, causes of hyponatremia include edema, hypoalbuminemia, mineralocorticoid deficiency, or cerebral salt wasting
    - Urine electrolytes may also be helpful in some situations
○ Treatment
  – Asymptomatic hyponatremia
    - Treatment depends on cause, but in many cases can begin with fluid restriction and/or addressing underlying risk factors.
  – Symptomatic hyponatremia
    - Administration of 3% hypertonic saline is the mainstay of treatment.
    - Seizures: Goal is to increase serum sodium enough to stop the seizure, by a maximum of 4-8 mEq/L in the 1st hour. 1 mL/kg of 3% hypertonic saline is often a good starting rate.
    - If not seizing or once seizure stops, goal is increase in plasma sodium concentration by 0.5-1 mEq/L per hour until mental status changes resolve, not exceeding 12 mEq/L per 24 hours.
    - Transfer to an ICU for closer monitoring is often appropriate.

## POTASSIUM ABNORMALITIES

• Immediate questions
  • How was the level collected?
  • What other underlying disease processes does the patient have, if any?
  • Is the patient getting any supplemental potassium?
  • What medications is the patient getting?
  • Are there EKG changes?
• Key content
  • Potassium is important in maintaining the resting membrane potential in neurons, muscle cells, and cardiac cells.
    ○ Hypo- or hyperkalemia increases the risk of arrhythmias. Acute changes are more dangerous than chronic depletion or excess.
    ○ At baseline, approximately 98% of total body potassium is located intracellularly. Potassium can be shunted toward the intracellular or extracellular environment, so serum potassium concentration is not always reflective of total body potassium.
    ○ Serum potassium level is primarily regulated via exchange with sodium using a NA/K ATPase pump.

- Hypokalemia: definition: <3.5 mEq/L. Severe hypokalemia <2.5 mEq/L
  ○ Common causes: due to decreased intake, increased excretion, or intracellular shifting
    – Decreased intake: rare cause; potassium is present in a variety of food groups, and healthy kidneys are efficient at reabsorbing potassium.
    – Causes of increased potassium excretion: diarrhea, vomiting, osmotic diuresis, potassium-wasting diuretics (e.g., furosemide, dialysis, low magnesium, corticosteroids, Cushing syndrome, diabetic ketoacidosis).
    – Causes of shift to intracellular potassium shifts: metabolic alkalosis, B-adrenergic agonists (e.g., insulin, albuterol, epinephrine), hyperthyroidism.
    – Pseudohypokalemia: can happen with delayed handling of blood specimen.
  ○ Manifestations
    – Weakness, muscle achiness, and muscle cramps, which can progress to hyporeflexia, flaccid paralysis, and respiratory depression
    – EKG changes: increased P wave amplitude, prolonged PR interval, ST depression, QT prolongation, reduced T wave amplitude, T wave inversion, and U waves
  ○ Management
    – For symptomatic hypokalemia, adding potassium-rich foods to a patient's diet is unlikely to be sufficient to replete their potassium.
    – Oral potassium chloride can be administered to patients with mild to moderate symptoms.
    – Intravenous potassium chloride should be used in patients with severe symptoms and/or EKG changes.
    – Many patients with hypokalemia have concurrent hypomagnesemia—this is important to assess for and should be corrected if present, as continued hypomagnesemia will interfere with potassium repletion.
- Hyperkalemia: >5.5 mEq/L for children and adults; >6.0 mEq/L in newborns; severe hyperkalemia (>7 mEq/L) can be life threatening
  ○ Common causes
    – Increased potassium load can occur any time there is substantial cell lysis. Some examples include burns, trauma, hemolysis, rhabdomyolysis, tumor lysis syndrome, tissue necrosis, blood transfusion, GI hemorrhage.
    – Causes of decreased excretion: renal failure (acute or chronic), aldosterone deficiency, or mineralocorticoid deficiency (e.g., Addison disease), type IV renal tubular acidosis, potassium-sparing diuretics (e.g., spironolactone), ACE inhibitors, NSAIDs, trimethoprim.
    – Causes of shift to extracellular space: metabolic acidosis, catecholamines, beta agonists, hyperglycemia.
    – Pseudohyperkalemia: Falsely elevated serum potassium measurements are commonly caused by cellular lysis, which releases intracellular potassium into the serum. This is particularly common for samples drawn through small IVs, obtained via heel stick, or obtained with use of a tourniquet. If there is concern for pseudohyperkalemia, make sure to get a free-flowing venous sample prior to making management decisions.
  ○ Manifestations: weakness, confusion, and EKG changes
    – EKG changes: peaked T waves, decreased R wave amplitude, widened QRS, prolonged PR interval. Can progress to complete heart block, ventricular arrhythmias, and cardiac arrest.
    – Treatment is generally merited when potassium level is > 6-6.5 mEq/L, or anytime EKG changes are present.

- ○ Management
  - – Decrease/eliminate oral (food, supplements) and parenteral (IV fluids, TPN) sources of potassium.
  - – Assess medication list to see if patient is on any drugs that would be expected to increase potassium levels—if so, remove/decrease drug.
  - – Administer calcium to stabilize cardiac myocytes if EKG changes are present.
  - – Use medications (e.g., insulin + glucose, sodium bicarbonate, albuterol) to temporarily shift potassium intracellularly.
  - – Use exchange resins (slow), diuretics (medium), or dialysis (fast) to decrease total body potassium.
- • Populations at high risk
  - ○ Diabetic ketoacidosis (DKA): Patients in DKA often present with high serum potassium due to extracellular shifts but have low total body potassium due to osmotic diuresis. Manage by monitoring closely and adding potassium to IV fluids once serum K levels drop below 5.5 mmol/L.
  - ○ HUS: Both hemolysis and acute renal failure put these patients at high risk of hyperkalemia. Manage by keeping potassium out of IV fluids and initiating dialysis if necessary.
  - ○ Malnourished patients undergoing refeeding: These patients may be at particularly high risk as insufficient caloric intake or starvation are often associated with decreased potassium intake, and refeeding leads to an influx of glucose and insulin, which can shift potassium intracellularly.

## PAIN

- • Key questions
  - • How is the pain level being assessed, or how can it be assessed?
  - • What is the likely underlying cause of the patient's pain?
  - • What pharmacologic and nonpharmacologic methods are already being employed for pain control?
  - • When was the patient's last dose of any pain medication?
- • Key content
  - • Assessment of pain
    - ○ Infants, toddlers, and children with neurocognitive delays: Behavioral scales, such as the *Face, Legs, Activity, Cry, Consolability* (FLACC) scale, the *Premature Infant Pain Profile* (PIPP), or the *Crying, Requires O₂, Increased vital signs, Expression, Sleepless* (CRIES) score, can provide a visual assessment of pain and distress by quantifying assessment of facial expression, motor responses/tone, vital signs, and verbal responses.
    - ○ Preschool to young school age: For children approximately ages 3-7 years old, a faces scale (drawings or photos of faces showing increasing degrees of distress) or color intensity scales can be used.
    - ○ School age: 1-10 scales are generally appropriate for children over 8 years.
  - • Nonpharmacologic options
    - ○ Physical therapy (PT) and occupational therapy (OT) have been shown to be very beneficial for patients with chronic pain.
    - ○ Art therapy, music therapy, and/or play therapy may provide benefit under some circumstances.
    - ○ Distraction or guided imagery: can be helpful for acute/procedural pain and anxiety. Child life therapists, where/when available, can assist with these and a variety of other nonpharmacologic pain management techniques.

- Heat or cold therapy: Heat can be a useful adjunctive technique for abdominal pain, particularly when crampy in nature. Heat or cold may be useful for decreasing pain from musculoskeletal injuries.
- For infants, swaddling, offering a pacifier, and giving an oral sucrose solution can decrease distress in response to painful procedures.
- Nonopioid pain medications
  - Ibuprofen: most commonly used nonsteroidal anti-inflammatory drug (NSAID) analgesic
    - Particularly helpful for cases that involve tissue inflammation
    - Precautions
      - Only FDA approved for patients ≥6 months of age
      - Avoid in situations of increased bleeding risk, such as post-tonsillectomy
      - Avoid in patients with gastric ulcers or serious GI bleeding
      - Often not appropriate for chronic abdominal pain, gastritis, or reflux, because NSAIDs promote gastric irritation
  - Ketorolac: NSAID which, unlike ibuprofen, comes in IV form
    - Useful for moderate to severe pain, such as postsurgical, severe migraine, kidney stone, or vasoocclusive episode in a patient with sickle cell disease.
    - Up to 5 days of scheduled use is considered safe in children who do not have other contraindications to NSAIDs.
  - Acetaminophen
    - Useful in children who have contraindications or relative contraindications to NSAIDs
      - Can be administered rectally for children who are NPO or otherwise unable/unwilling to take PO medications.
      - An IV form is available in some hospitals.
    - Precautions: liver failure, use with hepatotoxic medications
  - Tricyclic antidepressants and selective norepinephrine reuptake inhibitors: consider for neuropathic pain
  - Gabapentin: useful for some instances of neuropathic or chronic pain; can cause sedation and lightheadedness. Use must be titrated; not appropriate as a PRN medication
  - Lidocaine: use for local anesthesia prior to procedures (e.g., LP, suturing, I&D). Can also use topical formulation (e.g., EMLA or LMX) on intact skin to reduce pain of needle stick, such as during IV placement or lab draws
- Opioids
  - Some appropriate situations for opiate use in children include: postoperative pain, acute trauma, preprocedural analgesia, appendicitis, vasoocclusive episodes for children with sickle cell disease, cancer pain, and air hunger at end-of-life
  - Consider coadministration with an NSAID to decrease the amount of opiate needed
  - Ensure appropriate monitoring (e.g., continuous pulse ox, along with regular assessments of blood pressure and level of consciousness)
  - Advantages and disadvantages of specific opiates
    - Morphine: often a first-line IV medication for trauma or acute surgical abdominal pain. Can cause itching; consider coadministering nalbuphine if patient reports this side effect. Avoid morphine in patients with chronic kidney disease (delayed clearance due to renal clearance).
    - Oxycodone: oral option for some patients postoperatively or post-trauma.

– Fentanyl: 100 times more potent than morphine but with short half-life; can be used for brief procedural analgesia.
– Tramadol: moderate/weak opiate with a lower risk of serious side effects (less sedation, respiratory depression, and dependence risk compared to stronger opiates). Can still cause itching, nausea, and constipation. Avoid in patients with seizure history of recent traumatic brain injury.
– Patient-controlled analgesia (PCA) with a combination of continuous and bolus-dose narcotics may be the most effective way to provide pain control for patients with sickle cell disease, some postoperative patients, and some patients with cancer pain. This strategy is generally successful only in older children, often age 7 and up, although can be considered in children as young as 5.
  ○ Side effects
    – Respiratory depression: All children receiving opiates should be monitored via continuous pulse oximetry, and careful attention should be paid to using the lowest effective dose. In the case of overdose, give naloxone to reverse opiate effect.
    – Constipation: Consider initiating a bowel regimen simultaneously with initiating opiates to prevent narcotic-induced constipation.
• Special circumstances
  ○ Migraines: A combination of NSAIDs (e.g., ibuprofen or ketorolac) + antiemetics (e.g., compazine or ondansetron) + fluid bolus +/− diphenhydramine can be used as a "cocktail" for the initial management of severe migraine.
  ○ Functional abdominal pain: heat packs, diphenhydramine, fluid boluses, acetaminophen, and distraction can be considered acutely. PT/OT and psychology should be involved for medium- to long-term management. If your institution has a Pain Team, consulting this team may be helpful for complex pain patients.
  ○ Procedural pain (e.g., LP): injected 1% buffered lidocaine at the site of needle insertion. Also consider oral sucrose solution + non-nutritive sucking in infants.

## BEHAVIOR

• Immediate questions
  • What is the cause of escalation in this patient?
  • What underlying factors may be contributing?
  • What steps can I take to facilitate de-escalation in this agitated patient?
  • Is this patient a danger to themselves or others?
• Key content
  • Suicide assessment
    ○ Suicide is the second leading cause of death among high school-aged youths 14-18 years of age after unintentional injuries in 2019 according to US Department of Health and Human Services/Centers for Disease Control and Prevention.
    ○ Multiple assessments exist for suicidality screening:
      – Suicidal Ideation Questionnaire: This 30-question assessment serves as a valuable component of adolescent mental health. It is appropriate for teens in grades 10-12.
      – The Ask-Suicide Screening Questions (ASQ): For situations in which a 30-question assessment is not feasible, the ASQ, which consists of only four items, has been shown to have acceptable sensitivity in the ED (Table 23-2).

| TABLE 23-2 | ASQ Screening Questions |
|---|---|

The Ask-Suicide Screening Questions (ASQ)

1. In the past few weeks, have you ever felt that your family would be better off if you were dead?

2. In the past few weeks, have you wished you were dead?

3. In the past week, have you been having thoughts about killing yourself?

4. Have you ever tried to kill yourself?

Adapted from Horowitz LM, Bridge JA, Teach SJ, et al. Ask suicide-screening questions (ASQ): a brief instrument for the pediatric emergency department. Arch Pediatr Adolesc Med 2012;166(12):1170–1176.

- The Columbia-Suicide Severity Rating Scale (C-SSRS) (COLUMBIA-SUICIDE SEVERITY RATING SCALE (C-SSRS) Posner, Brent, Lucas, Gould, Stanley, Brown, Fisher, Zelazny, Burke, Oquendo, & Mann © 2008 The Research Foundation for Mental Hygiene, Inc.) is a questionnaire used for suicide assessment developed by multiple institutions, including Columbia University and NIMH support. This scale is evidence supported and is a part of a national and international public health initiative. The risk assessment is three pages long and is intended to help establish a person's immediate risk of suicide and is used in acute care settings.
    - Other screening tools include the Patient Health Questionnaire for Adolescents (PHQ-A), the Beck Depression Inventory-Primary Care Version (BDI-PC), the Mood and Feelings Questionnaire, the Center for Epidemiologic Studies Depression Scale for Children, and the PRIME MD-PHQ2.
  ○ Key topics to address during suicidality screening:
    - Presence and frequency of suicide thoughts
    - Reasons for ideation
    - Intensity, duration, and controllability or these thoughts
    - Deterrents against suicide
    - Accessibility of means for suicide
  ○ Assess for risk factors at different levels such as individual, family, social, and system.
  ○ Assess for psychological factors such as hopelessness, black/white thinking, negative thinking bias, poor social problem solving, impaired decision-making, feeling deflated, and feeling burdensome to others.
- Inpatient suicide precautions: These guidelines are intended both to keep the patient safe and provide distance from the stressors of their usual environment.
  ○ Room set up: Remove all sharp objects, telephone and unnecessary cables, cords, shoe laces, and equipment. Limit linen. No personal belongings except for quality of life items such as glasses.
  ○ 1:1 sitter at all times. Constant visual observation.
  ○ No access to personal phone or electronics.
  ○ Visitor belongings should be kept outside room in locker, nothing at the bedside.
- De-escalation techniques—Pediatric hospitals utilize various de-escalation strategies. Some examples include Safe Training and Responsible Restraints (STARR) response or Crisis Prevention Institute (CPI) training. CPI training has been selected to utilize at our hospital. It has an increased attention on prevention

through a focus on trauma, de-escalation, and an understanding of how behaviors (ours) influence behaviors (others).

- ○ Your safety is primary: Do not let the patient get between you and the exit. Never turn your back on the patient. Stand near the door, but not blocking it.
- Management of agitation
  - ○ Agitation is a symptom.
  - ○ It is ideal to identify the cause of the agitation to help with mitigation.
  - ○ Agitation can be verbal or physical.
    - − As a first step, ask family what has worked in the past for the patient—for example, specific pharmacologic or behavioral interventions.
    - − Agitation is a psychiatric emergency: There should be one person in charge, just one person talking, and that person should lower the volume of their voice in order to help calm the room. Limit staff in room, with just enough for safety.
    - − Maintain a supportive stance and a safe location.
    - − Give safe choices to the patient. Examples include food or distractions such as a preferred activity.
      - - Give clear messages.
    - − Why do patients get agitated?
      - - Fear, anger, helplessness, and inability to control their environment are common triggers.
      - - Strange people, places or words; feelings of being ill or vulnerable, and parents who are scared or utilize inconsistent parenting can also be triggers.
      - - Violence becomes a defense against an overwhelming sense of fragility and helplessness.
    - − De-escalation key points: According to a consensus statement by Richmond et al., there are 10 domains of de-escalation:
      - - Respect personal space
      - - Do not be provocative
      - - Establish verbal contact
      - - Be concise
      - - Identify wants and feelings
      - - Listen closely to what the patient is saying
      - - Agree or agree to disagree
      - - Lay down the law and set clear limits
      - - Offer choices and optimism
      - - Debrief the patient and the staff
    - − The Modified Overt Aggression Scale (MOAS) is a widely used rating scale made up of four categories: verbal aggression, aggression against objects, aggression against self, and aggression against others. Responses in each category can be used as an objective measure to track the patient's behavior over time.
    - − Pharmacologic management of agitation
      - - Should be a stepwise approach.
      - - Redirection is always first line.
      - - Utilize first what has worked well in the past. Past response predicts future response.
      - - Can consider an additional dose of a standing medication.
      - - Try to limit the number of agents.
      - - Ideal to offer oral medications first.
      - - Remember that PRN medications need some time to work.
      - - Attempt to use a "trauma informed" approach.

## SUGGESTED READINGS

American Heart Association, Subcommittee on Pediatric Resuscitation. Pediatric Advanced Life Support Provider Manual. 2016.

American Heart Association, Subcommittee on Pediatric Resuscitation. Pediatric Advanced Life Support Provider Manual. 2016.

Aquino J. Abnormal Sodium National Pediatric Nighttime Curriculum. Floating Hospital for Children at Tufts Medical Center.

Bandstra NF, Skinner L, LeBlanc C, et al. The role of child life in pediatric pain management: a survey of child life specialists. J Pain 2008;9(4):320–329. https://doi.org/10.1016/j.jpain.2007.11.004

Barbance O, De Bels D, Honoré PM, et al. Potassium disorders in pediatric emergency department: clinical spectrum and management. Arch Pediatr 2020;27(3):146–151. https://doi.org/10.1016/j.arcped.2019.12.003

Berde CB, Sethna NF. Analgesics for the treatment of pain in children. N Engl J Med 2002;347(14):1094–1103. https://doi.org/10.1056/nejmra012626

Biondi EA, McCulloh R, Staggs VS, et al. Reducing variability in the infant sepsis evaluation (revise): A national quality initiative. Pediatrics 2019;144(3):e20182201. https://doi.org/10.1542/peds.2018-2201

Biondi EA, Mischler M, Jerardi KE, et al. Blood culture time to positivity in febrile infants with bacteremia. JAMA Pediatr 2014;168(9):844–849. doi:10.1001/jamapediatrics.2014.895

Byrnes MC, Stangenes J. Refeeding in the ICU: an adult and pediatric problem. Curr Opin Clin Nutr Metab Care 2011;14(2):186–192. https://doi.org/10.1097/MCO.0b013e328341ed93

Campbell L. Respiratory Distress National Pediatric Nighttime Curriculum. Lucile Packard Children's Hospital, Stanford University.

Carcillo JA, Fields AI. Clinical practice parameters for hemodynamic support of pediatric and neonatal patients in septic shock. Crit Care Med 2002;30:1365.

Chow A, Robinson JL. Fever of unknown origin in children: a systematic review. World J Pediatr 2011;7(1):5–10. https://doi.org/10.1007/s12519-011-0240-5

Daly K, Farrington E. Hypokalemia and hyperkalemia in infants and children: pathophysiology and treatment. J Pediatr Health Care 2013;27(6):486–496. https://doi.org/10.1016/j.pedhc.2013.08.003

Debbie S. Fever. National Pediatric Nighttime Curriculum. Lucille Packard Children's Hospital.

Duffner PK, Berman PH, Baumann RJ, et al. Clinical practice guideline—neurodiagnostic evaluation of the child with a simple febrile seizure. Pediatrics 2011;127(2):389–394. https://doi.org/10.1542/peds.2010-3318

Farrell C, Del Rio M. Hyponatremia. Pediatr Rev 2007;28(11):426–428. https://doi.org/10.1542/pir.28-11-426

Fein JA, Zempsky WT, Cravero JP, et al. Relief of pain and anxiety in pediatric patients in emergency medical systems. Pediatrics 2012;130(5):e1391–e1405. https://doi.org/10.1542/peds.2012-2536

Gabhart JM. Pediatric Shock. National Pediatric Nighttime curriculum. Lucille Packard Children's Hospital at Stanford.

Gary D. Detection of Bacteremia: Blood Cultures and Other Diagnostic Tests. Up to Date. 2020. Available at https://www.uptodate.com/contents/detection-of-bacteremia-blood-cultures-and-other-diagnostic-tests. Last accessed on 4/12/2021.

Gershel J, Rauch D, eds. Caring for the Hospitalized Child: A Handbook of Inpatient Pediatrics. 2nd Ed. 2018.

Hampers LC, Spina LA. Evaluation and management of pediatric febrile seizures in the emergency department. Emerg Med Clin North Am 2011;29(1):83–93. https://doi.org/10.1016/j.emc.2010.08.008

Horowitz LM, Bridge JA, Teach SJ, et al. Ask suicide-screening questions (ASQ): a brief instrument for the pediatric emergency department. Arch Pediatr Adolesc Med 2012;166(12), 1170–1176. https://doi.org/10.1001/archpediatrics.2012.1276

Howard RF. Current status of pain management in children. JAMA 2003;290(18):2464–2469. https://doi.org/10.1001/JAMA.290.18.2464

Ivey-Stephenson AZ, Demissie Z, Crosby AE, et al. Suicidal ideation and behaviors among high school students—youth risk behavior survey, United States, 2019. MMWR Suppl 2020;69(1):47–55. https://doi.org/10.15585/mmwr.su6901a6

Jackson JM, Williams DM. Chasing fevers: an interactive exercise for pediatrics residents on triaging and assessing in patients with fever. MedEdPORTAL 2020;16:10907. https://doi.org/10.15766/mep_2374-8265.10907

Jannuzzi RG. Nalbuphine for treatment of opioid-induced pruritus. Clin J Pain 2016;32(1): 87–93. https://doi.org/10.1097/AJP.0000000000000211

Kazl C, LaJoie J. Emergency seizure management. Curr Probl Pediatr Adolesc Health Care 2020;50(11):100892. https://doi.org/10.1016/j.cppeds.2020.100892

Kee PPL, Chinnappan M, Nair A, et al. Diagnostic yield of timing blood culture collection relative to fever. Pediatr Infect Dis J 2016;35(8):846–850.

Kraemer FW, Rose JB. Pharmacologic management of acute pediatric pain. Anesthesiol Clin 2009;27(2):241–268. https://doi.org/10.1016/j.anclin.2009.07.002

Laino D, Mencaroni E, Esposito S. Management of pediatric febrile seizures. Int J Environ Res Public Health 2018;15(10):2232. https://doi.org/10.3390/ijerph15102232

Lefebvre CE, Renaud C, Chartrand C. Time to positivity of blood cultures in infants 0 to 90 days old presenting to the emergency department: is 36 hours enough? J Pediatric Infect Dis Soc 2017;6(1):28–32. https://doi.org/10.1093/jpids/piv078

Maslow GR, Dunlap K, Chung RJ. Depression and suicide in children and adolescents. Pediatr Rev 2015;36(7):299–310. https://doi.org/10.1542/pir.36-7-299

McClain BC, Ennevor S. The use of gabapentin in pediatric patients with neuropathic pain. Semin Anesth 2000;19(2):83–87. https://doi.org/10.1053/sa.2000.6788

Michael C. Intravascular Non-Hemodialysis Catheter-Related Infection: Clinical Manifestations and Diagnosis. Up to Date. 2021. Available at https://www.uptodate.com/contents/intravascular-non-hemodialysis-catheter-related-infection-clinical-manifestations-and-diagnosis. Last accessed on 4/12/2021.

Moritz ML, Ayus JC. Disorders of water metabolism in children: hyponatremia and hypernatremia. Pediatr Rev 2002;23(11):371–380. https://doi.org/10.1542/pir.23-11-371

Murata S, Okasora K, Tanabe T, et al. Acetaminophen and febrile seizure recurrences during the same fever episode. Pediatrics 2018;142(5):e20181009. https://doi.org/10.1542/peds.2018-1009

Pantell RH, Roberts KB, Adams WG, et al. Evaluation and management of well-appearing febrile infants 8 to 60 days old. Pediatrics 2021;148(2):e2021052228. doi:10.1542/peds.2021-052228

Rabin J, Brown M, Alexander S. Update in the treatment of chronic pain within pediatric patients. Curr Probl Pediatr Adolesc Health Care 2017;47(7):167–172. https://doi.org/10.1016/j.cppeds.2017.06.006

Richmond JS, Berlin JS, Fishkind AB, et al. Verbal de-escalation of the agitated patient: Consensus statement of the American Association for emergency psychiatry project BETA De-escalation workgroup. West J Emerg Med 2012;13(1):17–25. https://doi.org/10.5811/westjem.2011.9.6864

Rosenbloom E, Finkelstein Y, Adams-Webber T, et al. Do antipyretics prevent the recurrence of febrile seizures in children? A systematic review of randomized controlled trials and meta-analysis. Eur J Paediatr Neurol 2013;17(6):585–588. https://doi.org/10.1016/j.ejpn.2013.04.008

Section on Clinical Pharmacology, Committee on Drugs, Sullivan JE, Farrar HC. Fever and antipyretic use in children. Pediatrics 2011;127(3):580–587. https://doi.org/10.1542/peds.2010-3852

Shastri N. Intravenous acetaminophen use in pediatrics. Pediatr Emerg Care 2015;31(6): 444–448. https://doi.org/10.1097/PEC.0000000000000463

Sherman JM, Sood SK. Current challenges in the diagnosis and management of fever. Curr Opin Pediatr 2012;24(3):400–406. https://doi.org/10.1097/MOP.0b013e32835333e3

Short S, Pace G, Birnbaum C. Nonpharmacologic techniques to assist in pediatric pain management. Clin Pediatr Emerg Med 2017;18(4):256–260. https://doi.org/10.1016/j.cpem.2017.09.006

Singh RK, Gaillard WD. Status epilepticus in children. Curr Neurol Neurosci Rep 2009;9(2):137–144. https://doi.org/10.1007/s11910-009-0022-9

# 24 Neurology

Cameron Crockett, Sarah Dixon, Cristina M. Gaudioso, and Jennifer L. Griffith

## NEUROLOGIC EXAMINATION

### Head Circumference

- Always document the occipital frontal circumference (OFC) in children <2 years of age and in those you are seeing for the first time. The "rule of 3s and 9s" (birth: 35 cm; 3 months: 40 cm; 9 months: 45 cm; 3 years: 50 cm; 9 years to adult: 55 cm) is helpful to remember the approximate OFC appropriate for age.
- Document parental OFCs if there is a concern for macrocephaly or microcephaly; benign familial macrocephaly is a leading cause of macrocephaly.
- Posterior fontanelle closes 1-3 months postnatally. Anterior fontanelle closes 7-19 months postnatally in most children. Fontanelles may be enlarged or have delayed closure in trisomy 21, hypothyroidism, and achondroplasia.

### General Examination

Be sure to assess the following: vital signs, including respiratory pattern; dysmorphic features, including ambiguous genitalia and sacral anomalies; the pulmonary, cardiac, and gastrointestinal systems; cutaneous manifestations (look for such features such as café au lait macules, neurofibromas, ash leaf spots, hypomelanotic macules, whorled lines); spine; and extremities.

### Mental Status

- Level of consciousness and response to stimulus (e.g., awake, asleep, opens eyes to voice, grimace to sternal rub, unresponsive).
- In infants, assess visual fixation/tracking, and if irritable, whether consolable with pacifier, swaddling, etc.
- Language: assess expressive language (fluency), receptive language (following commands), and ability to repeat.
- Orientation to person, place, time (year, month, day), situation.
- Assessment of higher cognitive functions must be tailored to patient's developmental level.
  - Registration and recall of three words (chair, candle, dog)
  - Ability to name colors, animals
  - Counting or basic calculations, reading

### Cranial Nerves

- Olfactory (CN I): not routinely tested, but in cases of facial trauma, evaluate using non-noxious stimuli, such as coffee or vanilla
- Optic nerve (CN II)
  - Pupillary examination: Document pupil size, symmetry, and reactivity to light.
  - Funduscopic examination—evaluate for the following:
    - Papilledema (may take 24 hours or longer to develop following acute increase in intracranial pressure [ICP])

- ○ Hemorrhage (most sensitive clinical indicator of subarachnoid hemorrhage, easier to demonstrate with pupillary dilation)
- ○ Venous pulsations (present when ICP is below 180 mm $H_2O$; note that approximately 20% of normal people do not have venous pulsations)
- Visual fields, visual acuity: This helps differentiate between optic neuritis and papilledema because there is little change in fields or acuity with papilledema. Red desaturation often occurs in optic neuritis and can be tested by comparing the intensity of a red object between two eyes, or using Ishihara color plates. Bitemporal hemianopsia indicates chiasmatic lesion; homonymous hemianopsia or quadrantanopsia indicates lesion of optic radiations or occipital cortex.
- Relative afferent pupillary defect: This is brought out by the swinging flashlight test, which documents abnormality in afferent arc of pupillary light response proximal to dorsal midbrain (i.e., lesion in the macula, retina, optic nerve or tract, brainstem).
- Red reflex: Hold the ophthalmoscope at arm's length in a darkened room and examine for equivalence in color, intensity, clarity, and absence of opacities or white spots. In an infant with retinoblastoma, red reflex will be absent. If abnormal, examine dilated pupils or refer to ophthalmology.
- Oculomotor, Trochlear, and Abducens Nerves (CNs III, IV, and VI)
  - Extraocular movements: Use H-shaped path to isolate muscles. CN VI (lateral rectus) or CN III palsies (affecting the pupil) are often early signs of increased ICP. Evaluate for nystagmus (end-gaze nystagmus that extinguishes is normal, most often indicative of myopia).
  - Conjugate gaze: Examine whether light reflects identically from each iris; does alternating cover test uncover a latent esophoria (inward deviation) or exophoria (outward)? CN IV palsy causes hypertropia (elevation) and excyclotorsion of the affected eye, and the patient may tilt the head away from the affected eye to compensate.
- Facial nerve (CN VII): Assess symmetry of upper and lower facial movements. If the whole face is weak, then lesion is of lower motor neuron (LMN), but if only the lower face is weak, then it is upper motor neuron (UMN) because of bilateral cortical input to the forehead.
- Vestibulocochlear nerve (CN VIII): Head impulse test, Dix-Hallpike maneuver indicate peripheral lesion if positive, can help to exclude a central lesion. Hearing: Test with Weber and Rinne (512-Hz tuning fork) to distinguish conductive and sensorineural hearing loss.
- Glossopharyngeal and vagus nerves (CNs IX and X): Ask about any changes in voice, and evaluate symmetry of palate elevation. In unresponsive person, check gag reflex.
- Accessory nerve (CN XI): Test strength of shoulder shrug and head rotation.
- Hypoglossal nerve (CN XII): Check tongue movements and look for atrophy or fasciculations.

## Motor Examination

- Assess muscle bulk, tone (appendicular and axial), and strength graded on the Medical Research Council (MRC) scale (0—no contraction, 1—flicker or trace of contraction, 2—movement across joint with gravity eliminated, 3—movement against gravity, 4—movement against gravity and resistance, 5—normal strength). In infants, hold under the arms and in ventral suspension to assess axial tone.
- Observe for adventitious movements (e.g., tics, chorea, dystonia).

## Sensory Examination

Check four modalities (light tactile, temperature/pinprick, vibration, joint position sense) and assess for hemisensory neglect with bilateral, simultaneous stimulation. Romberg maneuver tests for sensory ataxia.

## Deep Tendon Reflexes

- Check reflexes in biceps, triceps, at patella, and ankle. Testing of the planter reflex may reveal Babinski sign (upgoing big toe when the sole of the foot is stroked) in patients with UMN lesions. However, Babinski sign in an infant is considered normal.
- Grading scale: 0—no reflex (loss of reflexes occurs faster in neuropathy compared with myopathy); 1+—trace reflex; 2+—normal reflex; 3+—very brisk; 4+—hyperreflexia with clonus.
- Perform special reflexes (jaw jerk, trapezius, pectoralis, abdominal, cremasteric) as needed.

## Primitive Reflexes

- Palmar grasp: present from birth to 2-4 months
- Plantar grasp: present from birth until 8 months
- Moro: birth until 4-6 months
- Tonic neck: birth until able to roll over (3-6 months)
- Galant (ipsilateral trunk curvature with stroking along spine): birth until 2-3 months

## Coordination

- Young children may not cooperate with commands, so look for velocity and accuracy on reaching for objects as a surrogate.
- Use eye saccades (may overshoot or undershoot), fast tapping of fingers or toes, finger-nose-finger movements, and heel-knee-shin movements.

## Gait

- Observe stance, leg swing, and arm swing for evidence of hemiplegic or diplegic gait.
- Walking on heels and tiptoes, running, and tandem gait can help bring out subtle weakness or other gait abnormalities that are less apparent during normal gait.

## Coma Examination

- Critical in all patients with an altered level of consciousness. Localize pathology to the bihemispheric, bithalamic, or reticular activating system (brainstem).
- Mental status: Document level of alertness, response to commands, regard, and speech.
- Respiratory pattern: If intubated, determine whether the patient is breathing at a rate above that set by the ventilator and if breathing pattern is regular or irregular.
- Pupillary reactivity
  - Document size, symmetry, and reactivity.
  - Response is resistant to metabolic disturbance with the following exceptions:
    - Opiates: pinpoint
    - Anticholinergics and sympathomimetics: fixed and dilated
    - Cholinergics: pinpoint
    - Hypoxia or hypothermia: midpoint and fixed

- Extraocular movements
  - Cold water calorics (20 mL in each ear) to activate the vestibulo-ocular reflex. Be sure there is no wax in the ears and that the tympanic membrane is intact. The doll's eye (oculocephalic reflex) examination may be used if the cervical spine is stable.
- Corneal reflex: tests afferent CN V and efferent CN VII
- Facial grimace to noxious stimuli: nail bed pressure, nostril swab, or mandibular pull are preferable to sternal rub
- Cough/gag reflex
- Response to pain
  - Check for purposeful withdrawal, triple flexion (stereotyped response), decerebrate (extensor) or decorticate (flexor) posturing, or no response.
  - Asymmetry or gradient between upper and lower extremities will help localization.
- Note tremor, myoclonus, or other involuntary movements
- Reflexes
  - Hyperreflexia often indicates CNS lesion, whereas hyporeflexia often indicates metabolic or spinal cord injury (acutely). However, uremia, hypo/hyperglycemia, and hepatic coma may give focal signs with hyperreflexia.

## Localizing the Lesion

Patterns of motor, sensory, and reflex abnormalities can indicate which part of the nervous system is affected by the lesion or disease process and can, therefore, guide testing. See Table 24-1.

## STROKE

### General Principles

While rarer than in adult patients, stroke should be considered as an etiology for any acute neurologic change in pediatric patients. Stroke in pediatric patients is often underrecognized.

*Ischemic Stroke*
- In pediatric population may present as focal deficits (weakness, speech abnormality, visual disturbance, ataxia) or generalized symptoms (headache, AMS, vomiting)
- More likely to present with seizure or headache than adult population

*Hemorrhagic Stroke*
Can present similarly to ischemic stroke, best differentiated by imaging (see below)

*Cerebral Venous Sinus Thrombosis (CVST)*
- Variable presentation, which may be acute, subacute, or chronic in nature.
- Headache is most frequent symptom and may be accompanied by vomiting, papilledema, visual symptoms, focal or generalized neurologic deficits.

### History and Examination

- Initial evaluation should be focused on differentiating between stroke and stroke mimics, and determining if candidate for hyperacute intervention (i.e., tPA or thrombectomy).
- The most common presentation involves motor weakness, but a stroke can include loss of any other neurologic function, including sensory abilities, language, or vision.
- There is typically a loss of function, not a gain. However, up to 1/3 of pediatric strokes present with seizures and over half may experience headache at stroke onset.

**TABLE 24-1  Localizing the Lesion**

| | Brain | Spinal cord | Motor neuron | Peripheral nerve | Neuromuscular junction | Muscle |
|---|---|---|---|---|---|---|
| Pattern of motor impairment | Pyramidal (UE extensors, LE flexors), usually asymmetric, multiple CN | Often bilateral, pyramidal | Proximal > distal | Distal > proximal | Ptosis, ophthalmoplegia, proximal > distal | Proximal > distal, symmetric |
| Sensory changes | All modalities, CN affected | Sensory level | None (cramps) | Usually, distal > proximal | None | None (myalgias) |
| Reflexes | Increased | Increased (may be decreased early) | Decreased | Decreased/absent | Normal until severe weakness | Normal until severe weakness |
| Other features | Aphasia, altered mental status, field cut | Bowel/ bladder, decreased rectal tone | Fasciculations, atrophy | Autonomic symptoms, pes cavus, hammer toes | Fatiguability, improves with ice (MG) | Myotonia, myokymia, pseudohypertrophy |

## Differential Diagnosis

- Stroke mimics: Seizure with postictal (Todd's) paralysis, migraine, Bell palsy, PRES, ADEM, and others.
- Stroke etiologies: trauma, arteriopathies, vasospasm, vasculitis, systemic vascular disease, hematologic disorders including neoplasia, prothrombotic states (acquired and congenital), metabolic disorders, and congenital and acquired heart disease.
- Caution: Up to 15% of children with known congenital cardiac defects and stroke also have other definable risk factors such as a prothrombotic state.

## Evaluation

- MRI with diffusion sequences and magnetic resonance angiography to evaluate for dissection, vasculopathy, or large vessel occlusion.
- Consider MR venography with contrast if signs of elevated ICP, risk factors for hypercoagulability; MR spectroscopy if there is suspicion for mitochondrial disorder.

## Treatment

- Hyperacute interventions for ischemic stroke including intravenous tissue plasminogen activator (tPA) and endovascular mechanical thrombectomy. IV tPA can be given in adolescents who present within 4 hours of time last known well.
- Mechanical thrombectomy can be considered in patients with evidence of large vessel occlusion on vascular imaging. Thrombectomy may be performed in patients who are not candidates for IV tPA due to exclusion criteria, or in whom symptoms do not rapidly improve after IV tPA given.
- Consider admission to an intensive care unit (ICU), permissive hypertension that allows blood pressure to be moderately elevated early after acute stroke, prevention of hypoglycemia, aggressive treatment of fevers, use of isotonic fluids (to prevent worsening of cerebral edema), and close monitoring. Lay head of the bed flat unless there is a concern for increased ICP.
- There are no randomized controlled trials in children regarding anticoagulation or antiplatelet therapy. However, neonates with stroke have low risk of recurrence; hence, aspirin is not routinely recommended. Older children have a recurrence risk of 7-20%, so aspirin should be considered.
- In sickle cell patients with stroke, consult hematology for urgent exchange transfusion.
- Patients with evidence of CVST should be started on immediate anticoagulation, with usual initial management with continuous heparin infusion.
- Patients with intracranial hemorrhage should have neurosurgical consultation.

## SEIZURES

### Definition and Classification

- Seizure occurs with abnormal excessive or synchronous electrical discharge of cerebral neurons, manifested as transient impairment of function of the region(s) that are involved—motor, sensory, cognitive (language), visual, and/or auditory.
- Many disorders can mimic seizures (see Nonepileptic Paroxysmal Events section). A detailed history of early clinical features/aura, any focal features, level of awareness during the event, and postictal course should be obtained from observers.

- Per the International League Against Epilepsy 2017 revised seizure classification, a seizure is classified primarily by its location of onset:
  - Focal seizure may be further classified by awareness (intact or impaired), or motor (clonic, hyperkinetic, or automatisms), or nonmotor (behavior arrest, sensory, emotional) symptoms at onset.
  - Generalized seizure is classified as motor (clonic, tonic-clonic, myoclonic, atonic) or nonmotor (absence).

## Etiology

- Seizures may be acute symptomatic (occur in close temporal association with CNS or systemic stress/illness) or unprovoked (no clear precipitating factor).
- Epilepsy is defined as 2 or more unprovoked seizures occurring >24 hours apart or one unprovoked seizure with high likelihood of further seizures based on EEG, MRI, or other testing.
- Epilepsy etiologies include genetic, structural, metabolic, immune, infectious, and unknown.
- Birth, developmental, and family histories are important to obtain, as well.
- In a patient with known epilepsy, breakthrough seizures may occur due to missed doses of antiseizure medication, concurrent illness, sleep deprivation, or an unknown factor.

## Management of First-Time Unprovoked Seizure

- Complete physical and neurologic examination, particularly looking for any focal neurologic abnormalities.
- Evaluate for possible provoking factors: Fever/illness, head trauma, CNS infection, tumor, ingestion/intoxication, and electrolyte disturbance.
- Clinical laboratory studies: Glucose, electrolytes, CBC, UDS, and EKG. Consider evaluation for infection based on history. Consider screening metabolic labs if there is clinical concern for inborn error of metabolism (global developmental delay, regression, organomegaly, altered mental status, vomiting, or multiorgan dysfunction).
- EEG: May identify focal background abnormality, epileptiform discharges, subtle seizures, or other abnormalities consistent with a known epilepsy syndrome. Note that a normal EEG does not rule out seizures or epilepsy.
- Urgent imaging (CT or MRI) should be obtained for any patient where there is concern for stroke, CNS infection, hemorrhage, or tumor.
- Brain MRI should be considered for most new-onset seizures but may not be necessary in a typically developing child with generalized epilepsy syndrome (e.g., childhood absence epilepsy).
- If the seizure is brief and self-resolves, await EEG, MRI, and laboratory studies before determining treatment. If no cause is found, most first-time seizures are not treated with antiseizure medication.
- Consider rescue medication such as rectal diazepam (for children >6 months) or intranasal midazolam (for children <6 months or >12 years) for home use for any child with history of status epilepticus.
- Seizure safety precautions: Close observation in water (encourage showers over baths, requires 1:1 supervision when swimming), no activities involving heights or open fires, and no driving until seizure free for at least 6 months (this varies state to state).

## STATUS EPILEPTICUS

### General Principles

- Although defined as any seizure (or group of seizures without recovery to baseline) lasting >30 minutes, pharmacologic treatment of seizures is typically required for any seizure >5 minutes in duration.
- Status epilepticus is an emergency. All medications are more effective when used early. Order the next anticipated medication immediately after giving the first.
- Prognosis is generally related to underlying medical diagnosis. Overall mortality is 1-3%.

### Treatment

- First 5 minutes
  - Airway, breathing, circulation (ABCs), turn to side, do not place anything in the mouth, and time seizure.
  - Establish IV access.
  - Check POC glucose, electrolytes, CBC, UDS, and antiepileptic drug levels (if necessary).
  - Administer IV lorazepam (0.1 mg/kg; maximum dose 4 mg) over 2-4 minutes.
  - If no IV access, give rectal diazepam (age 6 months-5 years: 0.5 mg/kg; 6-11 years: 0.3 mg/kg; 12+ years: 0.2 mg/kg, max 20 mg). May also use intranasal midazolam, 0.2 mg/kg (max 10 mg), particularly for age <6 months.
- 6-10 minutes
  - Reassess ABCs and address any problems. Call for additional help and assign team roles.
  - Five minutes after first dose, give second dose of IV lorazepam 0.1 mg/kg (max 4 mg), OR rectal diazepam, OR intranasal midazolam 0.2 mg/kg (max 10 mg).
  - If 2 benzodiazepine doses given in the last 6 hours, may go to 11-20 minutes treatment.
- 11-20 minutes
  - Reassess ABCs and address any problems. Call for additional help and assign team roles.
  - Administer long-acting antiseizure medication (fosphenytoin 20 mg/kg over 7-10 minutes or phenobarbital 20 mg/kg over 20 minutes).
  - Reexamine patient, monitor for respiratory depression and hypotension.
- 21+ minutes
  - If seizure continues after completing long-acting antiepileptic drug load, give medication in 11-20 minute stage that was not already used.
  - If seizure has clinically stopped, consider possibility of nonconvulsive status epilepticus if the patient is not waking or arousable.
- After 30 minutes
  - Plan on admission to ICU.
  - Consider intubation and central lines.
  - Give additional fosphenytoin 10 mg/kg or phenobarbital 10 mg/kg.
  - Consider treatment with midazolam infusion or other agent to induce pharmacologic coma.
- Special considerations
  - If the patient has Dravet syndrome or juvenile myoclonic epilepsy (JME), do not give fosphenytoin. Consider IV valproate 40 mg/kg after initial benzodiazepine for

these patients. Avoid valproate in children <2 and if there is suspicion for mitochondrial disorder. May also use IV levetiracetam 60 mg/kg for status epilepticus.
• Refractory status epilepticus typically has an underlying etiology that needs to be addressed: look for abnormal electrolytes, infection, hemorrhage, stroke, genetic, or metabolic syndrome.

## FEBRILE SEIZURES

### Definition
• Febrile seizures are seizures occurring in children 6 months to 60 months of age and are associated with febrile illness (T ≥ 100.4°F) not caused by an infection of the CNS. Seizures must not meet criteria for other acute symptomatic seizures and patients must not have history of previous unprovoked seizures.
• Simple febrile seizures are generalized in onset, last <15 minutes, *and* do not recur within 24 hours. They constitute 85% of all febrile seizures.
• Complex febrile seizures are focal in nature, last >15 minutes, or recur within 24 hours.
• Febrile status epilepticus is defined as seizure lasting 30 minutes or longer.

### Epidemiology
• The most common age for febrile seizures is 6 months to 3 years; they are rare after 6 years of age.
• Overall risk in children is 2-5%; if parent or sibling has had febrile seizures, the risk is 10-20%.
• The seizures may occur early in illness as a temperature rises or even before a fever/illness is recognized.
• Risk of febrile seizure recurrence is 25-30%. Risk factors for recurrence:
  • First febrile seizure before 1 year
  • Febrile seizures following low-grade fevers
  • Family history of febrile seizures
  • Epilepsy in first-degree relatives, complex febrile seizures, or neurodevelopmental abnormalities
• Risk of epilepsy later in life after febrile seizure is about 2-4% overall. Risk factors for eventual epilepsy:
  • Complex febrile seizures (raise recurrence risk twofold)
  • Neurodevelopmental abnormalities, including abnormal examination
  • Afebrile seizures in first-degree relatives
  • Recurrent febrile seizures

### Evaluation
• If seizure lasts >5 minutes, treat as status epilepticus.
• Routine labs may be performed in evaluation of underlying infection.
• Recommend LP for all infants <6 months of age. Strongly consider LP for infants <12 months if unvaccinated or pretreated with antibiotics and for any child with meningeal signs.
• Consider urgent imaging (CT or MRI) if there are focal features or if seizure is prolonged.
• EEG is recommended for patients with more than 1 complex feature to febrile seizure or if the patient has abnormal development.

## Treatment

- Prophylactic treatment is not typically recommended because most febrile seizures are self-limited.
- Rectal diazepam for seizure longer than 5 minutes should be prescribed for children with history of prolonged or multiple seizures.

## INFANTILE SPASMS

### Definition and Classification

- Infantile spasms (West syndrome) is an epileptic encephalopathy of infancy with peak incidence at 3-7 months. It is defined by epileptic spasms, hypsarrhythmia on EEG, and developmental arrest/regression.
- Clinical epileptic spasms consist of brief, symmetric, synchronous contractions of the head, neck, trunk, and/or extension of the arms/legs. They tend to cluster and occur most commonly around sleep-wake transitions.
- Etiologies include symptomatic (brain injury associated with prematurity or infection, hypoxic-ischemic injury, cortical malformation, tuberous sclerosis, trisomy 21, other genetic conditions), or cryptogenic (no identified etiology).

### Evaluation/Treatment

- Inpatient admission to expedite diagnostic workup and initiate treatment may be considered. Earlier identification and treatment of infantile spasms is associated with improved outcome.
- Physical examination should include detailed skin examination with Wood lamp to evaluate for ash leaf spots associated with tuberous sclerosis.
- Evaluation includes EEG capturing awake and asleep states, epilepsy protocol brain MRI, metabolic and genetic studies.
- First-line treatment for patients with infantile spasms due to tuberous sclerosis is vigabatrin.
- For all other patients, first-line treatment is ACTH or high-dose oral steroids.
- Patients with rapid initiation of treatment, normal development prior to onset of spasms, and no identified underlying cause may have better outcome.
- Many patients will develop other seizure types and may progress to Lennox-Gastaut syndrome.

## NONEPILEPTIC PAROXYSMAL EVENTS

### Common Seizure Mimics

History is the most important diagnostic tool to distinguish seizure from nonepileptic event. Having observers obtain a video of events can also be very helpful. Several seizure mimics exist and tend to occur at various developmental stages.

*Common Seizure Mimics in Infancy*

- Benign sleep myoclonus: Quick jerking movement of limb or face lasting seconds that only occurs in sleep in an otherwise healthy infant.
- Jitteriness: Affects one or more limbs, often switching sides from one event to another. Increases with unbundling, stimulation, startle, and crying but is suppressible with tactile stimulation.
- Hyperekplexia: Excessive startle that occurs with noise or touch. Can be elicited by gently tapping the glabella, triggering excessive startle which doesn't habituate with repeated taps.

- Benign myoclonus of infancy: Quick jerking movement of limbs without altered awareness, occur during sleep and wakefulness, and are suppressible.
- Shuddering attacks: Brief stiffening and shivering movements with preserved awareness. Often occur in late infancy and provoked by excitement or frustration.
- Sandifer syndrome: Back arching, stiffening of extremities, and head turning/tilting, which occurs due to reflux. Often provoked by feeding or lying flat.

*Common Seizure Mimics in Early Childhood*
- Breath-holding spells: Typically triggered by crying, pain, or strong emotion causing child to cry, hold their breath at end of exhalation, and become briefly tonic. Associated with cyanotic or pallid color change. Important to check ferritin in these patients as breath-holding spells are associated with iron-deficiency anemia and can improve with iron supplementation.
- Stereotypies: Simple (body rocking, head banging) or complex (wrist flapping, head shaking) mannerisms that are interruptible by tactile or verbal stimulation. More commonly seen in those with autism or intellectual disability but can also occur in neurotypical kids.
- Daydreaming: Staring off may mimic absence seizure but can be interrupted with verbal or tactile stimulation. Often occurs when engaged in quiet activities.
- Parasomnias: Night terrors, confusional arousals, and sleepwalking occur in first few hours of sleep and typically last longer than 3-5 minutes. May be confused for nocturnal frontal lobe seizures, which are typically brief (<2 minutes) and occur several times per night.

*Common Seizure Mimics in Adolescence*
- Vasovagal syncope: Loss of tone may be followed by postsyncopal convulsions. Prodromal symptoms precede syncope (light-headedness, blurred vision, tinnitus, pallor, diaphoresis). Often provoked by prolonged standing, dehydration, orthostatic changes, heat exposure, or strong emotion. Have rapid return to baseline after event.
- Cardiac syncope: Sudden loss of consciousness without warning, may occur with exertion.
- Periodic limb movements in sleep: Repetitive jerking movements of lower extremities that only occur in sleep.
- Panic attack: Sudden onset of intense fear, palpitations, dyspnea, diaphoresis, chest pain, paresthesia, light-headedness, and trembling with preserved awareness, which can last 10-30 minutes. There is no postictal confusion.
- Narcolepsy/cataplexy: Sudden brief loss of voluntary muscle tone in response to strong emotion. Occurs due to intrusive REM sleep during daytime.
- Functional neurologic disorder/nonepileptic spells: Common semiologies include altered mental status with or without motor phenomena. Features that favor nonepileptic spells include irregular, nonrhythmic jerking or thrashing movements, side to side head shaking, and eyes closed during the event.

## MOVEMENT DISORDERS

### General Principles
- Hyperkinetic movements are unwanted, excess movements and include dystonia, chorea, athetosis, myoclonus, tremor, tics, and stereotypies.
- These may be distinguished from one another based on rhythmicity, posture, whether movement is stereotyped, and/or suppressible (Table 24-2).

### Status Dystonicus
- A neurologic emergency characterized by increasingly severe/frequent episodes of generalized dystonia.

| TABLE 24-2 | Classification of Abnormal Movements | |
|---|---|---|

| Movement | Description | Example |
|---|---|---|
| Dystonia | Involuntary muscle contractions causing abnormal posturing. Posturing can be sustained or brief and may be triggered by specific voluntary movement/ position | Dystonic reaction from medication, focal hand dystonia (writer's cramp), or generalized dystonia due to neurodegenerative condition such as PKAN (pantothenate kinase–associated neurodegeneration) |
| Chorea | Continuous, random-appearing involuntary movements | Sydenham chorea as sequelae of infection with group A streptococcus |
| Athetosis | Slow, continuous writhing movements preventing ability to maintain stable posture | Can co-occur with chorea forming choreoathetosis, a sequela of basal ganglia injury from kernicterus |
| Myoclonus | Brief, shock-like jerking movement. Can be repeated but often nonrhythmic | Myoclonic jerks, seen in patients with juvenile myoclonic epilepsy, classically occur early in the morning. Can also see postanoxic myoclonus following cardiac arrest |
| Tremor | Rhythmic, oscillating involuntary movements with symmetric velocity in all directions | Intention tremor occurs when tremor worsens upon approaching a target (localizes to cerebellum). Other potential causes: essential tremor, hyperthyroidism, Wilson disease, medications (valproic acid), psychogenic, or enhanced physiologic tremor |
| Tics | Intermittent, rapid, recurrent, nonrhythmic, stereotyped movements, which are at least briefly suppressible, and preceded by premonitory urge | Simple motor tic: eye blinking, shoulder shrug, facial grimace<br><br>Complex motor tic: series of movements involving multiple muscle groups<br><br>Phonic tics: humming, throat clearing, sniffing, grunting, coprolalia |
| Stereotypies | Repetitive, often rhythmic movements that can be voluntarily suppressed, but lack premonitory urge. Tend to occur when excited, stressed, distracted, or heavily engaged in activity | Hand-flapping, hand-wringing, and body rocking |

- Differential diagnosis includes status epilepticus, neuroleptic malignant syndrome, or serotonin syndrome.
- Treatment includes dystonia specific medications (benzodiazepine, sedative infusions, baclofen, trihexyphenidyl), address precipitating factors (pain, infection, distress), supportive care (IV fluids), and cardiorespiratory monitoring likely in ICU setting.

## Tics

- Tics are intermittent, recurrent, nonrhythmic, stereotyped movements, which are at least briefly suppressible, and preceded by premonitory urge.
- Tics are present in up to 5% of population.
- Typical age of onset is 4-15 years old (median 7 years), with peak severity 9-11 years.
- Individual tics can wax and wane over months to years, typically worsen with physical or emotional stress.
- Rarely a sign of structural CNS pathology. If accompanied by other movement/neurologic abnormalities, consider basal ganglia pathology.
- Generally do not treat unless tics are bothersome to the child, causing harm, or interfering with school/daily activities.
- First-line treatment options include habit reversal therapy, α2-adrenergic agonists (clonidine, guanfacine), and atypical antipsychotics (risperidone, ziprasidone).

### Provisional Tic Disorder

Diagnostic criteria: Onset <18 years, one or more motor or vocal tic present for <1 year.

### Chronic Motor or Vocal Tic Disorder

Diagnostic criteria: Onset <18 years, one or more motor or vocal tic but NOT both lasting more than 1 year.

### Tourette Syndrome

- Diagnostic criteria: Onset <18 years, two or more motor tics AND one or motor vocal tics for at least 1 year.
- Affects 1-3% of children in the United States. Boys more commonly affected than girls.
- High comorbidity of attention deficit disorder, anxiety, and obsessive-compulsive disorder.
- Overall good prognosis: Majority have improvement in tics by late adolescence/early adulthood. Comorbid conditions may be longer lasting.

## POSTERIOR REVERSIBLE ENCEPHALOPATHY SYNDROME (PRES)

### General Principles

Clinical radiographic syndrome characterized by altered consciousness, headache, visual symptoms, and/or seizures as well as MRI findings of vasogenic edema, predominantly in the posterior cerebral hemispheres. Risk factors include hypertension, renal disease, immunosuppressive therapy, and autoimmune disorders.

### History and Examination

Rapid onset (hours to days) of altered consciousness, headache, visual symptoms, and/or seizures (typically generalized tonic-clonic). Often associated with hypertension.

### Differential Diagnosis

Acute altered mental status has a broad differential. See Table 24-3.

| TABLE 24-3 | Evaluation of Altered Mental Status | |
|---|---|---|
| **Category of disease** | **Examples** | **Diagnostic testing** |
| Ingestion/toxic | Illicit drugs, prescription drug overdose, serotonin syndrome, neuroleptic malignant syndrome, baclofen pump malfunction | Urine and serum drug screen |
| Metabolic | Hypo- and hyperglycemia, hypo- and hypernatremia, hypercalcemia, hyperthermia/hypothermia, mitochondrial, urea cycle defects, aminoacidopathies | Serum glucose, electrolytes, lactate/pyruvate, serum/csf amino acids, urine organic acids, ammonia, acylcarnitine profile |
| Endocrine | Thyroid storm, diabetic ketoacidosis | TSH, free T4, blood gas, urinalysis |
| Vascular | Hypoxic-ischemic brain injury (postarrest), bithalamic infarct/venous sinus thrombosis, vasculitis | Brain MRI, consider MR angiography and/or venography with contrast |
| Seizure | Subclinical status epilepticus, postictal state | EEG |
| Infection | Sepsis, meningitis, encephalitis | CSF culture, PCR for HSV-1,2, EMV, CMV, VZV; HIV; arbovirus/rickettsial titers |
| Autoimmune/ postinfectious | ADEM, NMDAR encephalitis, Hashimoto encephalopathy | MRI, LP, paraneoplastic antibodies, antithyroid antibodies |
| Malignancy | Lymphoma, paraneoplastic syndrome, mass lesion, thromboembolism | Brain MRI w/wo contrast, CSF cytology and flow cytometry, paraneoplastic Ab, PET scan |
| Trauma | Cerebral edema, diffuse axonal injury, subarachnoid hemorrhage, epidural or subdural hematoma | Head CT, MRI Caution with LP in setting of possible increased ICP |
| Hydrocephalus | VP shunt malfunction, mass lesion, posttraumatic | Head CT, shunt series, MRI brain |
| Psychiatric | Conversion disorder, nonepileptic seizure/dissociative spell, catatonia | Video EEG |

## Evaluation

• Noncontrast MRI brain is essential in all patients with suspected PRES. Characteristic MRI findings include symmetric vasogenic edema within the occipital and parietal lobes. The edema may, however, involve nonposterior regions (mainly in watershed areas).

- In addition to imaging, labs including CBC, CMP, and toxicology screen should be obtained. A lumbar puncture should be done in patients for whom meningitis or encephalitis is on the differential. EEG should be strongly considered given high risk for seizures.

### Treatment

Treatment of hypertension and discontinuation of immunosuppressive agents, when applicable, are the mainstay of treatment. Discontinuation of immunosuppression should be discussed with the prescribing physician. Individuals with seizures should be treated with an appropriate antiseizure medication.

## ACUTE CEREBELLAR ATAXIA

### Definition

Syndrome of acute-onset cerebellar dysfunction that occurs in previously healthy children, usually younger than 6 years. Often associated with a prodromal illness.

### History

Rapid onset (hours to days) of cerebellar dysfunction. Abnormal gait is the most common presenting symptom, although children may also present with nystagmus, speech problems, fine motor problems, and/or irritability.

### Examination

A complete neurologic examination should be performed with particular attention to cerebellar signs. Findings include ataxic gait (wide-based and unsteady), ataxic speech (scanning with fluctuations in rhythm/tone/volume), dysmetria (as seen on finger-nose testing), dysdiadochokinesia (as seen on rapid-alternating movement testing), action tremor, and nystagmus.

### Differential Diagnosis

See Table 24-4.

### Workup

Obtain routine screening labs (CBC, CMP, Mg, Phos) and a toxicology screen. Acute neuroimaging is not typically warranted, unless another neurologic process is suspected. May consider MRI brain with and without contrast.

### Treatment

Treatment is supportive only. PT evaluation prior to discharge may be beneficial. Symptoms will resolve gradually over 2-3 weeks.

## DEMYELINATING DISORDERS

### Categories

- Optic Neuritis
- Optic neuritis is an inflammatory, demyelinating condition of the optic nerve that results in acute vision loss. It is highly associated with multiple sclerosis (MS) but may also occur in other autoimmune disorders such as neuromyelitis optica spectrum disorder (NMOSD), myelin oligodendrocyte glycoprotein (MOG) antibody disease (MOGAD), and acute disseminated encephalomyelitis (ADEM).

**TABLE 24-4** Differential Diagnosis of Ataxia

| Category of disease | Examples | Diagnostic testing |
|---|---|---|
| Ingestion/toxic | Antiepileptic medications, sedatives | Urine and serum drug screen |
| Migraine variants | Benign paroxysmal vertigo, basilar migraine | History, normal MRI |
| Postinfectious | Acute cerebellar ataxia, acute cerebellitis, acute demyelinating encephalomyelitis (ADEM) | MRI, LP |
| Infectious | Meningitis, encephalitis, labyrinthitis | CSF culture, PCR for HSV-1,2, EMV, CMV, VZV; HIV |
| Demyelinating/ autoimmune | MS, Sjögren's, Behcet's, neuromyelitis optica (NMO), celiac | MRI brain, CSF oligoclonal bands, NMO Ab, ANA/ENA |
| Paraneoplastic | Opsoclonus-mycoclonus, NMDA-receptor encephalitis, GAD-65 encephalitis | Paraneoplastic Ab, urine HVA+VMA, CT abdomen, testicular U/S, PET scan |
| Malignancy | Posterior fossa tumors | Brain MRI with/without contrast |
| Vascular | Posterior circulation stroke, vertebral or basilar artery dissection, vasculitis | Brain MRI, MR angiography |
| Episodic ataxia | EA1: last minutes, myokymia, carbamazepine responsive<br><br>EA2: hours-days, headache, acetazolamide responsive<br><br>EA3-7: variable medication response | Acetazolamide or carbamazepine trial, genetic testing |
| Peripheral nerve (sensory ataxia) | Acute inflammatory demyelinating polyradiculoneuropathy (AIDP), Miller-Fisher syndrome | EMG/NCS, LP for albuminocytologic dissociation |
| Metabolic | Mitochondrial, urea cycle disorders, aminoacidopathies (MSUD), GLUT-1 deficiency, pyruvate dehydrogenase deficiency | Lactate/pyruvate, CSF glucose, serum/CSF amino acids, urine organic acids, ammonia, acylcarnitine profile |
| Inner ear | Benign paroxysmal positional vertigo (BPPV), Ménière's, vestibular Schwannoma | Electronystagmography, MRI |
| Psychogenic | Conversion disorder | Astasia-abasia gait |
| Epilepsy | Postictal state | EEG |

- Vision loss typically develops over hours to days. It is usually monocular but may be binocular. Most patients report eye pain that worsens with eye movements.

*Transverse Myelitis*

Acute transverse myelitis (TM) is an immune-mediated condition of the spinal cord that presents with rapid-onset weakness, sensory deficits, bowel/bladder dysfunction, and/or autonomic dysfunction. TM may be idiopathic (usually a postinfectious process) or may be caused by an underlying demyelinating autoimmune disorder such as MS, NMOSD, MOGAD, ADEM, and MS.

*Acute Disseminating Encephalomyelitis (ADEM)*

- ADEM is a demyelinating condition of the central nervous system characterized by encephalopathy.
- Acute-onset encephalopathy is the hallmark (and a required) feature of pediatric ADEM. It is usually accompanied by neurologic deficits, such as cranial neuropathies, hemiparesis, myelopathy, and/or ataxia. It is often associated with seizures. Most children will report a viral/febrile illness within 2 weeks of onset of neurologic symptoms and many have fever, vomiting, and meningismus at time of presentation.

## Examination

- Perform a complete neurologic examination in any patient with suspected demyelinating disease.
- Optic neuritis: fundoscopic examination (to assess for disc swelling and/or venous distension), visual acuity and color vision (loss of color vision > loss of visual acuity is indicative of optic nerve disease), visual fields (to assess for field defect, especially central scotoma), and pupillary reaction (to assess for afferent pupillary defect). A formal eye examination should be completed by ophthalmology.
- Transverse myelitis: include sensory level, strength and tone, deep tendon reflexes, cremasteric reflex (in males), and digital rectal examination.
- ADEM: detailed mental status examination, cranial nerve examination (including fundoscopic examination, visual acuity and color vision), sensory (including sensory level), motor examination, deep tendon reflexes, gait, and coordination.

## Evaluation

- Imaging
  - For optic neuritis, MRI brain and orbits with and without contrast (imaging shows increased T2 signal of the optic nerves, often with gadolinium enhancement), and consider MRI cervical spine with and without contrast.
  - For TM and ADEM: MRI brain and total spine with and without contrast. Patients with TM will have T2 hyperintense lesions (+/− gadolinium enhancement) extending one or more spinal cord segments, while patients with ADEM have brain, brainstem, or spinal cord lesions that are typically bilateral, asymmetric, and poorly marginated).
- CSF: cell count and differential, protein, glucose, IgG index (with serum), oligoclonal bands (with serum), culture and viral studies (based on season).
- Serum: MOG antibody, NMO antibody, CBC, CMP, vitamin D level. Consider ANA, ENA, ANCA, and dsDNA.

## Treatment

- High-dose IV steroids (methylprednisolone) for 3-5 days, which have been shown to improve outcomes and shorten time to recovery.
- In patients with severe neurological deficits or symptoms refractory to steroids, treatment with IVIG or plasmapheresis can be considered.

## HEADACHE

### Definition

- The International Classification of Headache Disorders, 3rd edition (ICHD-3) classifies headaches as either primary or secondary.
  - Primary headaches include migraine, tension-type headache, and trigeminal autonomic cephalgias. Migraine and tension-type headaches are the most common in children.
  - Secondary headaches are those caused by an underlying condition such as trauma, infection, intracranial mass, or idiopathic intracranial hypertension (IIH) and should always be considered in individuals presenting with new or atypical headache.
- Diagnostic criteria for pediatric migraine without aura:
  - Five or more headaches lasting 1-72 hours
  - Have at least two of the following four features: either bilateral or unilateral location, pulsatile quality, moderate to severe intensity, aggravated by routine physical activity
  - Accompanied by nausea/vomiting and/or photophobia and phonophobia (which may be inferred from behavior)

### History

- Document the onset, duration, location, quality, and severity of pain, alleviating/aggravating factors, any associated features, and personal/family history of headaches. Any history of aura (visual, sensory, brainstem type, etc.) should also be noted.
- Headache red flags include pain worse when lying down, pain that awakens patient from sleep, associated early morning vomiting, associated fever, recent head trauma, "worst headache of my life," history of malignancy, or any alteration of mental status or focal deficit.

### Examination

Complete neurologic examination with special attention to fundoscopic examination (to look for papilledema, optic pallor, retinal hemorrhages), extraocular movements (to look for ocular palsies), visual fields (to look for a field cut), gait, and coordination (to look for ataxia).

### Evaluation

- For individuals with a history of migraine headaches and absence of red flags on history and examination, further workup with labs and neuroimaging is not necessary.
- For individuals with signs of elevated ICP, focal neurologic deficits, or concern of hypercoagulable state, evaluation for acute stroke or CVST is warranted. See Stroke section.
- A lumbar puncture with opening pressure should be performed in individuals with suspected IIH (symptoms of elevated ICP, papilledema, CN VI palsy, MRI brain that is normal or with abnormalities suggestive of IIH [flattening of the posterior sclera, partially empty sella, bilateral venous sinus stenosis]). An LP should also be performed in those with suspected CNS infection.

### Treatment

- First-line abortive treatments for pediatric migraine include nonsteroidal anti-inflammatory drugs (NSAIDs) and triptans.

- In the emergency department, we recommend treatment with IV fluids, IV NSAIDs (ketorolac), and IV prochlorperazine. Dystonic reactions secondary to prochlorperazine may be prevented or treated with diphenhydramine. If this therapy regimen fails, IV magnesium or IV valproate should be considered (if there are no contraindications).
- If ER treatment is ultimately unsuccessful, the patient may be admitted for ongoing IV therapy with the above medications, dihydroergotamine (DHE), or steroids.
- Individuals with frequent migraines (>2 episodes per week) or with migraine episodes that significantly reduce quality of life may benefit from a daily medication for headache prevention. Common first-line choices for migraine prevention in children include β blockers (e.g., propranolol), anticonvulsants (e.g., topiramate), and tricyclic antidepressants (e.g., amitriptyline or nortriptyline).

## NEONATAL ENCEPHALOPATHY

### Definition
- Syndrome of abnormal neurologic function in a newborn infant ≥35 weeks estimated gestational age, as evidenced by altered level of consciousness, seizures, abnormal vital signs, and abnormal tone and deep tendon reflexes.
- Neonatal encephalopathy is a broad term encompassing many etiologies, while hypoxic-ischemic encephalopathy (HIE) refers to neonatal encephalopathy attributable to asphyxia at birth.

*History and examination*
- Review of birth history for a "sentinel event"—events in the peripartum period, which may explain the infant's presentation—should be coupled with rapid clinical evaluation.
- Severity of encephalopathy can be scored using the following criteria: level of consciousness, degree of spontaneous activity, muscle tone, posture, suck, Moro reflex, pupil size/reactivity, heart rate, and respiratory pattern.

### Differential Diagnosis
May include sepsis, hypoglycemia (especially in infants of diabetic mothers), inborn errors of metabolism, genetic disorders affecting brain development, and maternal medications

### Evaluation
- Cord blood analysis for pH and base deficit.
- Placental pathology to evaluate for potential contributors to presentation.
- Lumbar puncture if concerned for infection.
- Consider evaluation for metabolic and/or genetic etiologies pending clinical course.

### Treatment
- Therapeutic hypothermia has been the only proven neuroprotective intervention available for treatment of neonatal encephalopathy. Hypothermia should be initiated within first 6 hours or life and continued for 72 hours. Morphine or dexmedetomidine infusions should be used to limit shivering.
- Head ultrasound on first day of life, followed by brain MRI at day of life 4 and 10.
- EEG monitoring, particularly during the first 24 hours, and longer if seizures identified.

## APPROACH TO THE HYPOTONIC INFANT

- Tone is the resistance of muscle to passive movement and includes appendicular (extremities) and axial (muscles of neck, back and trunk).
- Tone can be decreased (hypotonia) or increased (hypertonia). Spasticity is defined as velocity-dependent increased tone.
- Tone is state dependent: An agitated infant is likely to have increased tone and a sleeping infant will have decreased tone. Serial examinations are essential.

### History and Examination
- Document prenatal history, including maternal assessment of fetal movement.
- Use pull-to-sit maneuver, scarf sign, vertical, and ventral suspension tests to assess axial tone and passive movement of extremities to assess appendicular tone. Mental status, strength, and deep tendon reflexes should be assessed carefully.
- A term baby should be able to hold the head in the plane of the body for a few seconds and head lag should be absent by 2 months.
- Examining the parents can often provide useful clues to congenital or genetic conditions (myotonia, fatigable weakness).

### Differential Diagnosis
- Specific findings can help localize the underlying process. See Localizing the Lesion section and Table 24-1.
- Other diagnoses such as congenital heart disease or sepsis may present with a hypotonic infant.

### Evaluation
- Labs: CK, TSH, electrolytes, ionized calcium, magnesium, ammonia, and newborn state screening. Additional testing based on examination findings and history
- Imaging: MRI of the brain without contrast

## SPINAL MUSCULAR ATROPHY (SMA)

- Characterized by progressive muscle weakness and atrophy due to degeneration of the anterior horn cells in the spinal cord and lower brainstem.
- Autosomal recessive condition due to mutations in the *SMN1* gene, which produces the survival motor neuron (SMN) protein important for the health of anterior horn cells.
- A modifying gene called *SMN2* creates a truncated, partially functional version of the protein; the number of SMN2 copies affects clinical trajectory.

### History and Examination
- The more SMN protein there is, the later the symptoms begin and the milder the disease. In the most severe type, an infant will present with severe weakness and hypotonia with absent reflexes, with intact mental status.
- Hallmark symptom is weakness of the voluntary muscles, with proximal muscles most affected, and lower extremities affected more than upper. Tongue fasciculations and bulbar symptoms (weak cry, poor suck or feeding, and impaired secretion clearance) are often present. Deep tendon reflexes are significantly decreased or absent.

## Differential Diagnosis

Will vary based on age of presentation, but consider myotonic dystrophy, congenital myasthenic syndromes, congenital myopathies, infantile botulism, Prader-Willi syndrome, and metabolic or mitochondrial diseases.

## Evaluation

- SMA testing is now included on standard newborn screening in a majority of states.
- Genetic testing remains the gold standard and should be performed in any infant with unexplained hypotonia and hyporeflexia, even with previous normal newborn state screening.

## Treatment

- Previously supportive only, including pulmonary (due to respiratory muscle weakness), nutritional (due to bulbar muscle weakness), and orthopedic (due to progressive scoliosis).
- New disease-modifying therapies are now available, which have shown significant benefit for patients with SMA.

## DUCHENNE MUSCULAR DYSTROPHY (DMD)

### Definition

- One of the dystrophinopathies, a group of diseases characterized by progressive muscle degeneration due to the alterations of the dystrophin protein.
- Inheritance is X linked and, therefore, primarily affects boys, but girls who carry mutation can rarely have symptoms.

### History and Examination

- Symptom onset is usually in early childhood, around age 2-3 years.
- Weakness first starts in proximal muscles and later affects distal limb muscles, with lower extremities affected first. Children are noted to have difficulty running, jumping, or walking. They may also have waddling gait and be noted to have calf hypertrophy. On examination, they may show the Gower maneuver: to go from sitting to standing, the child will get into prone position, with hands and feet underneath them, then use hands to "climb" thighs to standing position.
- Later the heart and respiratory muscles are affected as well.

### Differential Diagnosis

Becker muscular dystrophy (a milder form of dystrophinopathy arising from mutations leading to semifunctional dystrophin rather than near-total loss as with DMD), limb girdle muscular dystrophy, mild SMA (SMA type III), Pompe disease, and dermatomyositis

### Evaluation

- Early in the diagnosis, the creatine kinase level is significantly elevated, climbing to 10-20 times the upper limit of normal by age 2 years, then falls as muscle tissue is replaced by fat.
- Genetic testing for mutation in *DMD* gene is confirmatory.

## Treatment

- Mainstay of treatment is corticosteroids, which have been shown to be effective at improving strength and slowing progression.
- Newer gene therapies can be used in patients with select mutations to convert DMD phenotypes to BMD phenotypes.
- Other treatment is supportive and includes physical therapy, braces or mobility devices (walkers, wheelchairs), monitoring of cardiac and respiratory function, and management of scoliosis. Some patients with DMD will have cognitive challenges.

## GUILLAIN-BARRÉ SYNDROME

### Definition

- Also called acute inflammatory demyelinating polyradiculoneuropathy.
- An antecedent viral infection (*Campylobacter jejuni*, cytomegalovirus [CMV], Epstein-Barr virus [EBV], and *Mycoplasma pneumoniae*) occurs in 60-70% of cases.

### History and Examination

- Initial symptoms are typically sensory (numbness and paresthesia) with progression to hallmark features of ascending weakness and areflexia.
- Symmetric weakness reaches its nadir by 2 weeks in 50% of patients. Progression for over 8 weeks suggests alternative diagnosis of chronic inflammatory demyelinating polyneuropathy (CIDP).
- Autonomic dysfunction is common, including tachycardia, postural hypotension, and hypertension.
- Back and extremity pain, extreme enough to mimic encephalopathy, can be a significant part of the presentation in young children.

### Evaluation

- Cerebrospinal fluid (CSF) albuminocytologic dissociation (elevated protein with normal cell count) is present in over 80% of patients by 2 weeks. CSF protein can be normal in 1/3 of patients within the first week of symptoms.
- Nerve conduction studies may demonstrate either axonal or demyelinating neuropathy, although these changes may take between 1 and 2 weeks to develop. Axonal form has a worse prognosis for recovery.
- Laboratory evaluation may include serum for EBV and CMV antibodies, stool culture (especially for *C. jejuni*), and serum for peripheral neuropathy antibody panel (before giving intravenous immune globulin [IVIG]).

### Treatment

- Treatment is recommended for patients too weak to ambulate independently, and ideally should begin within the first 7-10 days of symptoms.
- Treatment of choice: IVIG
  - Pretreat with acetaminophen and diphenhydramine.
  - IVIG may cause anaphylaxis in individuals with immunoglobulin A (IgA) deficiency. Consider sending IgA level before treatment.
  - Plasma exchange is also effective.
- Steroids have not been shown to be beneficial, and some patients may actually decline with steroid treatment.

- Follow respiratory function closely with forced vital capacity (FVC) and negative inspiratory function (NIF), particularly during the first few days of illness when weakness progresses most rapidly. Intubation may be necessary if FVC falls to 50% of normal or if NIF is low.
- Monitor for vasomotor instability (i.e., labile blood pressures), but treat cautiously.

## SUGGESTED READINGS

Amlie-Lefond C. Evaluation and acute management of ischemic stroke in infants and children. Continuum (Minneap Minn) 2018;24(1, Child Neurology):150–170.

Bodesteiner JB. The evaluation of the hypotonic infant. Semin Pediatr Neurol 2008;15(1):10–20.

Fine A, Wirrell EC. Seizures in children. Pediatr Rev 2020;41(7):321–347.

Fisher RS, et al. Operational classification of seizure types by the International League Against Epilepsy: Position Paper of the ILAE Commission for Classification and Terminology. Epilepsia 2017;58(4):522–530.

Friedman DI, Liu GT, Digre KB. Revised diagnostic criteria for the pseudotumor cerebri syndrome in adults and children. Neurology 2013;81(13):1159–1165.

Glauser T, Shinnar S, Gloss D, et al. Evidence-based guideline: treatment of convulsive status epilepticus in children and adults: report of the guideline committee of the American Epilepsy Society. Epilepsy Curr 2016;16(1):48–61.

Hulbert ML, et al. Exchange blood transfusion compared with simple transfusion for first overt stroke is associated with a lower risk of subsequent stroke: a retrospective cohort study of 137 children with sickle cell anemia. J Pediatr 2006;149:710–712.

Jacobs SE, et al. Cooling for newborns with hypoxic ischaemic encephalopathy. Cochrane Database Syst Rev 2013;(1):CD003311.

Oskoui M, et al. Practice guideline update summary: pharmacologic treatment for pediatric migraine prevention. Neurology 2019;93(11):500–509.

Patel AD, Vidaurre J. Complex febrile seizures: a practical guide to evaluation and treatment. J Child Neurol 2013;28(6):762–767.

Pringsheim T, et al. Practice guideline recommendations summary: treatment of tics in people with Tourette syndrome and chronic tic disorders. Neurology 2019;92(19):896–906.

Sanger TD, Chen D, Fehlings DL, et al. Definition and classification of hyperkinetic movements in childhood. Mov Disord 2010;25(11):1538–1549.

Sheridan DC, Spiro DM, Meckler GD. Pediatric migraine: abortive management in the emergency department. Headache 2014;54(2):235–245.

Subcommittee on Febrile Seizures; American Academy of Pediatrics. Neurodiagnostic evaluation of the child with a simple febrile seizure. Pediatrics 2011;127(2):389–394.

# 25 Nephrology

Brian R. Stotter and Vikas R. Dharnidharka

## INTRODUCTION

The first part of this chapter serves as a quick reference for fluid, electrolyte, and acid-base disorders in children, focusing on definitions, differential diagnosis, common presentations, and basic approach to management. The second part focuses on history and presentation of common kidney diseases in children, assessment of kidney function, and interpretation of laboratory studies.

## FLUIDS, ELECTROLYTES, AND ACID-BASE DISORDERS

### MAINTENANCE FLUIDS

- Maintenance fluid requirements are determined by sensible (measured) and insensible (unmeasured) fluid losses:
  - Sensible losses: Urine, stool, bleeding, drains, vomiting/gastric suction
  - Insensible losses: Skin, respiratory tract
- Maintenance intravenous fluids (IVFs) are provided when patients are unable to take fluid orally. They are not a substitute for fluids already lost; repletion fluids should be provided in addition to maintenance fluids for this purpose. The clinician should also consider ongoing fluid losses when providing supplemental IVF.
  - Calculation of maintenance IVF (in mL/hr):

$$(\text{Body Surface Area (BSA)} \times 1500 \text{ mL}) \div 24 \text{ hr}$$

$$\text{BSA m}^2 \text{ (Mosteller formula)} = \sqrt{[(\text{Height})(\text{cm}) \times \text{Weight (kg)} \div 3600]}$$

- Previous practice was to give dextrose-containing maintenance fluids with 77 mEq/L of sodium chloride (NaCl), which is 0.45% NaCl or half normal saline (½ NS). However, this approach has been associated with a high incidence of hyponatremia in hospitalized children. For children 28 days to 18 years old, dextrose-containing maintenance fluids with isotonic fluid (e.g., 0.9% NaCl, lactated Ringer's solution) is advised.
  - This excludes neonates <28 days old or adolescents over 18 years of age and patients with neurosurgical disorders, heart disease, liver disease, kidney dysfunction, cancer, diabetes insipidus, voluminous diarrhea, or severe burns.

### DEHYDRATION AND HYPOVOLEMIA

- Dehydration is common in children, and is most commonly due to gastroenteritis, with fluid losses in excess of fluid intake.
- Dehydration may be classified as isotonic (equal loss of water and electrolytes), hypotonic (water loss is lower compared to electrolyte loss), and hypertonic (water loss is

higher compared to electrolyte loss). History will suggest the etiology. The following section discusses isotonic dehydration.

- Assessment of dehydration:

  Percent dehydration = (pre-illness weight − current weight)/pre-illness weight

- Pre-illness weight is often not accurately known. Table 25-1 gives physical examination findings that allow estimation of the degree of dehydration.
- Management
  - Mild dehydration (3-5%):
    - Oral rehydration therapy (ORT): 50 mL/kg plus replacement of ongoing losses with oral rehydration solution (ORS) over 4 hours
    - If vomiting, give small amounts (5-10 mL) every 1-2 minutes to give total volume of ORS calculated over 4 hours.

| TABLE 25-1 | Symptoms Associated with Dehydration | | |
|---|---|---|---|
| Symptom | Minimal or no dehydration (<3% loss of body weight) | Mild-to-moderate dehydration (3-9% loss of body weight) | Severe dehydration (≥10% loss of body weight) |
| Mental status | Well; alert | Normal, fatigued or restless, irritable | Apathetic, lethargic, unconscious |
| Thirst | Drinks normally; might refuse liquids | Thirsty; eager to drink | Drinks poorly; unable to drink |
| Heart rate | Normal | Normal to increased | Tachycardia, with bradycardia in most severe cases |
| Quality of pulses | Normal | Normal to decreased | Weak, thread, or impalpable |
| Breathing | Normal | Normal; fast | Deep |
| Eyes | Normal | Slightly sunken | Deeply sunken |
| Tears | Present | Decreased | Absent |
| Mouth and tongue | Moist | Dry | Parched |
| Skin fold | Instant recoil | Recoil in <2 sec | Recoil in >2 sec |
| Capillary refill | Normal | Prolonged | Prolonged; minimal |
| Extremities | Warm | Cool | Cold; mottled; cyanotic |
| Urine output | Normal to decreased | Decreased | Minimal |

Source: Adapted from Duggan C, Santosham M, Glass RI. The management of acute diarrhea in children: oral rehydration, maintenance, and nutritional therapy. Morb Mortal Wkly Rep 1992;41(RR-16):1–20; World Health Organization. The Treatment of Diarrhea: A Manual for Physicians and Other Senior Health Workers. Geneva, Switzerland: World Health Organization, 1995. Available at http://www.who.int/child-adolescent-health/New_Publications/CHILD_HEALTH/WHO.CDR.95.3.htm

○ Reassess hydration status and ongoing losses every 2 hours.
○ Serum electrolyte measurement is not necessary for mild and moderate dehydration when isotonic dehydration is suspected.
• Moderate dehydration (6-9%):
  • Attempt ORT with 100 mL/kg plus replacement of ongoing losses with ORS over 4 hours.
  • If ORT fails, then begin intravenous (IV) rehydration with NS, with a goal of replacing the fluid deficit over 4 hours.
• Severe dehydration (≥10%):
  • Severe dehydration is a medical emergency and can result in shock.
  • Obtain serum electrolytes and glucose.
  • Treat hypoglycemia (glucose < 60 mg/dL) and electrolyte abnormalities.
  • Give a rapid IV bolus of 20 mL/kg NS and repeat as necessary to improve perfusion.
  • Once pulse, perfusion, and mental status return to normal, ORT can begin, with a goal of replacing the remaining deficit over 2-4 hours.
• Replacement of ongoing losses
  • Consider the patient's underlying source(s) of fluid loss when choosing the composition of replacement fluids. For example, fecal losses contain more water than sodium (35-60 mEq Na/L), so ½ NS would be an appropriate replacement fluid.
• Indications for inpatient management: intolerance of ORS (intractable vomiting, refusal, or inadequate intake), inability to provide adequate care at home, acute bloody diarrhea, concern for complicating illnesses, severe dehydration, lack of follow-up, progressive symptoms, young age, or diagnostic uncertainty.
• See Table 25-2 for the composition of common oral fluids compared with the WHO recommendations for the composition of ORS.

## ELECTROLYTE ABNORMALITIES

### Hypernatremia

*Definition*
• Hypernatremia is defined as a serum or plasma sodium >150 mEq/L.

*Etiology*
• Etiology of hypernatremia can be divided into two categories:
  • Dehydrated states (hypernatremic dehydration).
    ○ Water deficit, for example, due to increased fluid losses (fever, tachypnea, prematurity, diabetes insipidus) or inadequate oral water intake (adipsia, child abuse/neglect, ineffective breastfeeding).
    ○ Water and sodium deficit, for example, due to emesis, diarrhea, burns, or urinary losses, as seen in diabetes mellitus (DM) and certain causes of chronic kidney disease (CKD).
    ○ Hypernatremic dehydration is always hypertonic.
• Excess sodium intake, for example, from incorrectly prepared formula, salt ingestion, and iatrogenic causes such as sodium bicarbonate or hypertonic (3%) saline.

*Clinical Presentation*
• Hypernatremia most commonly presents in the setting of dehydration. Central nervous system (CNS) symptoms such as irritability, restlessness, weakness, lethargy, and hyperreflexia predominate. Nausea and thirst are also typically present.

**TABLE 25-2  Composition of ORS Compared with Common Oral Fluids**

| ORS | Carbohydrate (mmol/L) | Sodium (mmol/L) | Potassium (mmol/L) | Chloride (mmol/L) | Osmolarity (mOsm/L) |
|---|---|---|---|---|---|
| WHO recommendations | Should equal Na, but not >110 | 60-90 | 15-25 | 50-80 | 200-310 |
| WHO ORS (2002, reduced osmolarity) | 75 | 75 | 20 | 65 | 245 |
| WHO ORS (1975) | 111 | 90 | 20 | 80 | 311 |
| Pedialyte | 139 | 45 | 20 | 35 | 250 |
| Apple juice | 667 | 0.4 | 44 | 45 | 730 |
| Gatorade | 323 | 20 | 3.2 | 11 | 299 |
| Soda | 622 | 1.6 | N/A | N/A | 650 |

Adapted from King CK, Glass R, Bresee JS, et al. Managing acute gastroenteritis among children: oral rehydration, maintenance, and nutritional therapy. MMWR Recomm Rep 2003;52(RR-16):1–16.

- Cerebral hemorrhage is possible due to water shifts out of cells to the hypernatremic intravascular space. This leads to decreased brain volume and shearing and rupture of bridging veins. Seizure and coma may result.
- Water movement from the intracellular to the extracellular space helps preserve the intravascular volume. Patients often do not appear dehydrated until it is severe.

*Treatment*
- If dehydrated, first restore intravascular volume with isotonic fluid boluses of 20 mL/kg NS.
  - Next, calculate the free water deficit to determine replacement needs:

$$\text{Freewater deficit (L)} = [0.6 \times \text{weight (kg)}] \times [(\text{current Na}/140 - 1)]$$

where

$$(0.6 \times \text{weight}) = \text{total body water (TBW)}$$

- Replace free water enterally or intravenously. Enteral replacement is preferred but may be contraindicated due to the patient's condition.
  - IV free water replacement can be done with one of several IVF, each with varying sodium ($Na^+$) concentrations. The decision to use D5W, ¼ NS (38.5 mEq/L), ½ NS (77 mEq/L), or lactated Ringer's solution (130 mEq/L), each with glucose and potassium, depends on the degree and duration of hypernatremia.
  - If delivered at the same rate, the IVF with lower sodium concentration will correct serum sodium faster than an IVF with a higher sodium content.
  - Chronic hypernatremia should be corrected slowly, whereas acute hypernatremia can be treated more rapidly.
  - The volume (in liters) of chosen infusate to be delivered can be calculated as follows:

$$(\text{Serum Na} - \text{desired Na})/(\text{Change in Na/L of fluid delivered})$$

where

$$\text{Change in Na/L} = (\text{Infusate Na (mEq/L)} - \text{Serum Na})/[(0.6 \times \text{weight}) + 1]$$

- The goal is to reduce serum sodium by no more than 10-12 mEq/L in 24 hours. This equates to a fall in sodium by no more than 0.5 mEq/L/hr.
  - Infusion rate is calculated by dividing the volume to be given by the goal correction time.
  - In practice, typically 1.25-1.5 × maintenance infusion rate is appropriate.
- Correct hypernatremia with caution. Monitor serum sodium concentration every 4-6 hours (more frequently if severe) and adjust infusion rate as needed.
  - As hypernatremia develops, brain cells generate idiogenic osmoles to retain water within the intracellular space. Rapid correction of hypernatremia can create an osmotic gradient that encourages further water movement into cells, producing cerebral edema. Seizures, brain herniation, and death can result.
- Treat the underlying cause of the hypernatremia.

## Hyponatremia
*Definition*
Hyponatremia is defined as a serum or plasma sodium <135 mEq/L.

*Etiology*
- Etiology of hyponatremia can be divided into categories:

- Dehydrated states, for example, gastroenteritis and runner's hyponatremia.
  - Hypovolemia stimulates vasopressin release, reducing free water excretion by the kidneys; oral fluid replacement is often hypotonic relative to the fluid lost in these conditions.
- Reduced effective circulating volume, for example, congestive heart failure (CHF) and nephrotic syndrome.
  - Like true hypovolemia, reduced effective circulating plasma volume results in vasopressin release and subsequent hyponatremia.
- Excess water intake (water intoxication), for example, primary polydipsia or excessive caregiver water administration.
- Decreased free water excretion, for example, syndrome of inappropriate antidiuretic hormone (SIADH) secretion from adrenal insufficiency, hypothyroidism, infection, or medication side effect. Advanced CKD is associated with hyponatremia due to impaired water excretion, but vasopressin is typically suppressed.
- Excess sodium loss, for example, cerebral salt wasting (CSW), salt-losing nephropathies (e.g., renal dysplasia and obstructive uropathy), primary renal tubulopathies (e.g., Bartter and Gitelman syndromes), and acute or chronic interstitial nephritis.
  - CSW is believed to be caused by increased atrial natriuretic peptide release, resulting in high output of sodium-rich urine and hyponatremia.
  - Sodium loss also results in hypovolemia and vasopressin release.
- Pseudohyponatremia (e.g., hypertriglyceridemia and hyperproteinemia).
  - Hypertonic hyponatremia (e.g., hyperglycemia, azotemia, use of mannitol).
    – Caused by the presence of another osmotically active substance.
    – Measured serum sodium decreases 1.6 mEq/L for every 100 mg/dL and the serum glucose concentration is above normal (over 100 mg/dL by convention).

*Clinical Presentation*
- An acute osmotic gradient between the intracellular and extracellular space results in cellular swelling that primarily affects the brain, causing nausea, headache, lethargy, confusion, agitation, and hyporeflexia. If severe, seizures, coma, and/or death may ensue.
- Chronic hyponatremia presents with nausea, fatigue, dizziness, confusion, cramps, and gait disturbances.
- Low body temperature despite warm environment may also be seen.

*Treatment*
- If dehydrated, first restore intravascular volume with 20 mL/kg isotonic fluid boluses.
- Hyponatremia causing cerebral dysfunction is an emergency and requires immediate attention. Water restriction and hypertonic (3%) saline are critical therapies. Only enough 3% saline to improve mental status should be given (usually to increase serum sodium by 5 mEq/L).
- Outside of the acute setting, IV sodium replacement can be done with one of several IVF, each with varying sodium concentrations. Normal saline (154 mEq/L) or 3% saline (513 mEq/L) are typically used.
- First, calculate the sodium deficit (NaD):

$$\text{NaD (in mEq / L)} = (\text{Desired Na} - \text{Patient's Na}) / 2$$

(Divide by 2 because it is convention to replace half of the sodium deficit.)

- Next, calculate the total body sodium deficit (TBNaD):

$$\text{TBNaD (in mEq / L)} = \text{NaD} \times (0.6 \times \text{weight})$$

(pre-illness weight should be used)

- The volume (in liters) of chosen infusate to be delivered can be calculated as follows:

TBNaD/(Infusate Na (mEq/L))

- The goal is to increase serum sodium by 0.5 mEq/L/hr.
- Infusion rate is calculated by dividing the volume to be given by the goal correction time.
- Additional management of hyponatremia depends on the underlying etiology. Rehydrate if dehydrated, restrict water intake in cases of excess water intake or decreased water excretion, and replace sodium if there is excess sodium loss.
- Osmotic demyelination syndrome (previously known as central pontine myelinolysis) occurs from rapid correction of chronic hyponatremia. While the mechanism is unclear, brain adaptation to chronic hyponatremia involves extrusion of intracellular ions that cannot be replaced quickly during hyponatremia treatment, resulting in demyelination and potentially irreversible brain damage. Hyponatremia that develops over hours is much less likely to result in this complication.

## Hyperkalemia

*Definition*
- Hyperkalemia is defined as a serum potassium >5.5 mEq/L in children, or >6 mEq/L in neonates and young infants.
  - Higher normal range of potassium in neonates due to reduced urinary potassium excretion and relative aldosterone insensitivity.

*Etiology*
- Etiology of hyperkalemia can be divided into categories:
  - Pseudohyperkalemia (measured serum potassium is not reflective of the patient's true serum potassium level), such as from a hemolyzed blood specimen
  - Increased potassium intake, for example, from massive blood transfusion, total parenteral nutrition, or intravenous medications with high potassium content
  - Transcellular potassium shift, for example, from cellular breakdown (e.g., tumor lysis syndrome, rhabdomyolysis, extreme exercise), metabolic acidosis, insulin deficiency, or hyperkalemic periodic paralysis
  - Decreased potassium excretion, for example, in acute kidney injury (AKI) or CKD, type IV renal tubular acidosis (RTA), adrenal insufficiency, hypoaldosteronism, and medications (e.g., potassium-sparing diuretics, angiotensin-converting enzyme inhibitors [ACEI], nonsteroidal anti-inflammatory drugs [NSAIDs], or trimethoprim)

*Clinical Presentation*
- Patients with mild or moderate hyperkalemia (between 6 and 7 mEq/L) are often asymptomatic. At higher levels, symptoms may include muscle weakness, paralysis, palpitations, or syncope.
- Hyperkalemia promotes depolarization of the resting cell membrane. Cardiac depolarization is the most concerning due to the risk of arrhythmias and cardiac arrest.
- Electrocardiogram (EKG) changes worsen with rising potassium levels.
  - 5.5-6.5 mEq/L: Peaked T waves and shortened QT interval.
  - 6.5-8 mEq/L: Peaked T waves, prolonged PR interval, decreasing or disappearing P wave, widened QRS, amplified R wave.
  - >8 mEq/L: Absent P wave, bundle branch blocks, progressively widened QRS that merges with the T wave to form a sinusoidal pattern resulting in ventricular fibrillation or asystole.

- Not all children with hyperkalemia have EKG changes, and absence of EKG changes does not preclude the need for therapy. EKG changes that occur in children >7 mEq/L with chronic hyperkalemia may occur at lower levels in children with acute hyperkalemia.

*Treatment*
- Repeat the test to ensure value is not falsely elevated due to a hemolyzed specimen. Obtain a free-flowing venous sample rather than a heel stick, which is more prone to hemolysis.
- Stop potassium-containing IVF and oral supplements.
- Obtain an EKG and monitor with telemetry.
- Calcium gluconate stabilizes the myocardium by antagonizing hyperkalemia-induced depolarization. It should only be given when there are EKG abnormalities (beyond peaked T waves) or if potassium is >7 mEq/L. Note that calcium gluconate is cardioprotective but does not lower the serum potassium level.
- Loop diuretics enhance urinary potassium excretion, and exchange cation resins (e.g., sodium polystyrene sulfonate) reduce gastrointestinal potassium absorption. These are the only medications that reduce total body potassium.
- Albuterol and insulin (given with glucose to prevent hypoglycemia) promote intracellular potassium shift. Though controversial, sodium bicarbonate is believed to work similarly.
- Consider dialysis if hyperkalemia is life-threatening and/or refractory to medical therapy.

## Hypokalemia
*Definition*
Hypokalemia is defined as a serum potassium <3.5 mEq/L.

*Etiology*
- Etiology of hypokalemia can be divided into categories:
  - Decreased potassium intake, for example, from malnutrition or anorexia nervosa (decreased intake is unlikely to cause hypokalemia in otherwise healthy children).
  - Intracellular potassium uptake, for example, in alkalosis, use of insulin or β-adrenergic agents, or hypokalemic periodic paralysis.
  - Increased gastrointestinal losses, for example, from emesis or nasogastric suctioning, diarrhea, or laxative use.
    ○ This is the most common cause of hypokalemia in children.
  - Increased urinary losses, for example, from diuretics, type I or II RTA, tubulointerstitial injury (e.g., interstitial nephritis, as well as cisplatin, amphotericin B, and other medications that cause tubular injury), genetic tubulopathies (e.g., Bartter syndrome or Gitelman syndrome), and increased mineralocorticoid activity (hyperaldosteronism).
  - Volume depletion is the most common cause of increased mineralocorticoid activity in children.

*Clinical Presentation*
- Patients with serum potassium >2.5 mEq/L are frequently asymptomatic.
- Symptoms start to manifest once the serum potassium drops below 2.5 mEq/L and include muscle weakness, cramps, fasciculations, constipation or ileus, urinary retention, and ascending paralysis. Severe hypokalemia can trigger a spontaneous rhabdomyolysis.
- Hypokalemia can affect urinary concentrating ability and present as polyuria, with or without polydipsia.

*Treatment*
- Potassium supplementation can be provided enterally or parenterally. Enteral preparations are preferred due to the slower uptake and decreased risk of hyperkalemia.
- If there is symptomatic hypokalemia (e.g., severe muscle weakness or paralysis, arrhythmias), rapid IV potassium administration can be provided. Potassium chloride is most commonly used and should be given at a rate no higher than 0.5-1 mEq/kg/hr.
  - IV potassium can cause peripheral vein pain and phlebitis, thus administration through a central line is preferred when available.
- Correct hypomagnesemia if present, as hypomagnesemia promotes potassium wasting in the distal nephron and may blunt the response to potassium repletion.
- Treat the underlying cause.

## Hypercalcemia
*Definition*
- Normal calcium levels vary with age and the laboratory.
- Serum calcium >10.5 mg/dL and ionized calcium >5.0 mg/dL are typically considered to be elevated levels.

*Etiology*
Causes of hypercalcemia include primary hyperparathyroidism (e.g., parathyroid adenoma, neonatal severe hyperparathyroidism, transient neonatal hyperparathyroidism, or multiple endocrine neoplasia type 1 or 2A syndromes), malignancy (e.g., lymphoma, leukemia, dysgerminoma, rhabdomyosarcoma, neuroblastoma, or congenital mesoblastic nephroma), familial hypocalciuric hypercalcemia, granulomatous diseases, Williams syndrome, milk-alkali syndrome, subcutaneous fat necrosis, adrenal insufficiency, hypervitaminosis D, thiazide diuretic use, or prolonged immobilization.

*Clinical Presentation*
- Symptoms of hypercalcemia include muscle weakness, fatigue, headache, anorexia, nausea, vomiting, constipation, abdominal pain, polyuria, polydipsia, weight loss, mental status changes, and lethargy.
- Examination may demonstrate bradycardia, proximal muscle weakness, hyperreflexia, abnormal mental status, and signs of the underlying condition.

*Diagnostic Evaluation*
- Laboratory testing includes total serum and ionized calcium, albumin, parathyroid hormone (PTH), phosphorus, alkaline phosphatase, electrolytes, creatinine, magnesium, vitamin D levels, urine calcium, urine phosphorus, and urine creatinine.
  - Measurement of PTH is important for differentiating PTH-dependent causes of hypercalcemia (e.g., primary or tertiary hyperparathyroidism, genetic syndromes with hyperparathyroidism) from PTH-independent causes (e.g., granulomatous diseases, hypervitaminosis D, malignancy).
- Other evaluation depending on suspected cause of hypercalcemia might include radiographs, EKG, renal ultrasound, karyotype, thyroid function, or evaluation for malignancy (e.g., PTH-related peptide).

*Treatment*
- If asymptomatic, treatment may be delayed until there is diagnosis of the underlying cause.

- If symptomatic or serum calcium >12 mg/dL:
  - IV hydration with normal saline is the mainstay of treatment.
  - Loop diuretics may be used to increase urinary calcium excretion once the patient is adequately hydrated.
- Bisphosphonates and calcitonin may be used for refractory hypercalcemia.
- Glucocorticoids may be used to decrease calcium absorption from the intestine, by way of decreasing production of 1,25-dihydroxyvitamin D, to treat hypercalcemia resulting from granulomatous disease.
- For severe hypercalcemia refractory to medical therapies, dialysis may be necessary.

## Hypocalcemia

*Definition*
- Normal values for calcium levels vary with age and the laboratory.
- Serum calcium <8.5 mg/dL and ionized calcium <4.0 mg/dL are typically considered low levels.
- The total calcium level should be corrected for serum albumin level using the formula:

$$\text{Corrected calcium} = 0.8 \times (4 - \text{serum albumin}) + \text{serum calcium}$$

  - Ionized calcium is the active form. With normal ionized calcium, a low total calcium due to hypoalbuminemia will not cause hypocalcemic symptoms.

*Etiology*
Causes of hypocalcemia include hypoparathyroidism (e.g., DiGeorge syndrome, Kearns-Sayre syndrome, postthyroidectomy, autoimmune parathyroiditis, or secondary to elevated maternal calcium), pseudohypoparathyroidism, transient neonatal hypocalcemia, vitamin D deficiency, iatrogenic causes (e.g., aminoglycosides, loop diuretics, or short bowel syndrome), hypomagnesemia, Wilson disease, or sequestration (e.g., pancreatitis, hyperphosphatemia, receiving citrated products, or hungry bone syndrome).

*Clinical Presentation*
- Symptoms of hypocalcemia include paresthesias (particularly the perioral area, hands, and feet), muscle pain, cramps, irritability, mental status changes, seizures, muscle weakness/spasm, and respiratory distress. Hypotension is commonly seen in the setting of acute hypocalcemia.
- Patients may exhibit tetany (increased peripheral neuromuscular excitability), elicited on examination as Chvostek sign (tapping the facial nerve anterior to the ear causes contraction of ipsilateral facial muscle) or Trousseau sign (placing a blood pressure cuff on the arm and inflating above systolic blood pressure for 3-5 minutes causes wrist flexion).
- EKG demonstrates arrhythmias or prolonged QTc.

*Diagnostic Evaluation*
- Laboratory evaluation includes total and ionized calcium, albumin, electrolytes, creatinine, alkaline phosphatase, phosphorus, magnesium, PTH, vitamin D levels, urine calcium, urine creatinine, and urine phosphorus.
- Other testing to determine the etiology may be necessary, as well as an EKG to evaluate for QTc abnormalities and arrhythmias.

*Treatment*
- Correct the underlying cause if possible.
- If the patient is asymptomatic, oral calcium and vitamin D supplements may be sufficient.

- If symptomatic, treat with IV calcium gluconate (preferred to calcium chloride due to lower risk of subcutaneous tissue necrosis from extravasation).
- Correct hypomagnesemia and vitamin D deficiency.

## Hyperphosphatemia

*Definition*
- Hyperphosphatemia is defined as an elevated serum phosphorus level, which varies by age. Note that different laboratories may have slight variations in their reference intervals:
  - Infants <12 months old: Phosphorus >7 mg/dL.
  - Children 1-5 years old: Phosphorus >6.5 mg/dL.
  - Children 6-12 years old: Phosphorus >5.8 mg/dL.
  - Adolescents and adults: Phosphorus >4.5 mg/dL.

*Etiology*
- Etiology of hyperphosphatemia can be divided into categories:
  - Spurious hyperphosphatemia, for example, from a hemolyzed blood specimen, hyperglobulinemia, or hyperlipidemia. Sample contamination with heparin or tissue plasminogen activator (tPA) can cause spurious hyperphosphatemia as well.
  - Acute phosphate load, for example, exogenous phosphate (phosphate-containing enemas, parenteral nutrition).
  - Acute or chronic kidney disease (due to phosphate retention).
  - Increased tubular phosphate reabsorption, for example, in hypoparathyroidism, hypervitaminosis D, acromegaly, use of bisphosphonates, and familial tumoral calcinosis.
  - Transcellular phosphate shift, for example, from cellular breakdown (tumor lysis syndrome, rhabdomyolysis), certain causes of metabolic acidosis (lactic acidosis, diabetic ketoacidosis).

*Clinical Presentation*
Patients are typically asymptomatic. Patients have symptoms from the underlying condition or may have signs and symptoms of hypocalcemia.

*Treatment*
- Treat the underlying cause.
- For acute hyperphosphatemia, provide volume expansion with IVF.
- Chronic hyperphosphatemia requires treatment with a low-phosphate diet and use of phosphate binders (e.g., calcium carbonate, sevelamer carbonate) to limit intestinal phosphate absorption.
- Consider dialysis in medically refractory causes, particularly if associated with symptomatic hypocalcemia.

## Hypophosphatemia

*Definition*
- Hypophosphatemia is defined as a low serum phosphorus, which varies by age. Note that different references and laboratories may have slight variations in their reference intervals:
  - Neonates and infants <12 months old: Phosphorus <5 mg/dL
  - Children 1-2 years old: Phosphorus <3.8 mg/dL
  - Children 2-5 years old: Phosphorus <3.5 mg/dL
  - Children >5 years old and adolescents: Phosphorus <2.5 mg/dL

*Etiology*
Causes of hypophosphatemia include diuretics, hypoparathyroidism, diabetic ketoacidosis (with administration of insulin), Fanconi syndrome, refeeding syndrome, inadequate dietary intake, and aluminum toxicity.

*Clinical Presentation*
- Phosphorus is required for producing adenosine triphosphate (ATP), which provides energy for numerous metabolic processes. Symptoms of hypophosphatemia include lethargy, ileus, myalgias, and weakness.
- Chronic hypophosphatemia can lead to short stature and rickets.
  - Clinical signs of rickets include craniotabes, frontal bossing, widening of the wrist and ankle joints, rachitic rosary along the costochondral junctions, and bowing of legs.

*Treatment*
- For acute treatment, give oral or IV phosphorus repletion.
- Treat the underlying cause.

## ACID-BASE DISORDERS

- Normal blood pH is 7.35-7.45. The lungs and kidneys work to maintain normal acid-base balance through exhalation of carbon dioxide ($CO_2$) and excretion of the daily acid load, respectively.
- Simplified Henderson-Hasselbalch equation:

$$pH \propto [HCO_3^-]/[pCO_2]$$

$$HCO_3^- = \text{bicarbonate concentration}$$

$$pCO_2 = \text{partial pressure of dissolved carbon dioxide}$$

- In a primary acid-base disorder, compensation occurs to minimize large changes in pH.
  - In respiratory disorders, the kidneys compensate by modifying $HCO_3^-$.
  - In metabolic disorders, the lungs compensate by modifying $pCO_2$.
  - Example: In metabolic acidosis, the primary disturbance is a decrease in $HCO_3^-$ that lowers pH. To compensate, there is increased expiration of $CO_2$ (i.e., tachypnea) to bring the pH back close to normal range.
  - See Table 25-3 for more details on the compensatory response for each primary acid-base disorder. Lack of appropriate compensation suggests the presence of more than one acid-base disorder.

### Metabolic Acidosis
- Metabolic acidosis is defined as an acid-base disorder leading to a low serum $HCO_3^-$ and an arterial blood pH < 7.35.
- Caused by increased acid production or intake, extracellular shift of hydrogen ions, or decreased acid excretion from the kidneys.
- Metabolic acidosis can be described as high anion gap (indicating the presence of unmeasured anions) or normal anion gap:
- Serum anion gap = $[Na^+] - ([Cl^-] + [HCO_3^-])$. Normal anion gap is usually 4-12 mEq/L, but exact range is dependent on the laboratory analyzer. If serum potassium is included in the anion gap calculation (preferred when serum potassium is elevated), then the normal anion gap is 8-16.

| TABLE 25-3 | Primary Acid-Base Disorders and Expected Compensatory Response | | |
|---|---|---|---|
| Acid-base disorder | Primary disturbance | Compensation | Expected compensatory response |
| Metabolic acidosis | $\downarrow HCO_3^-$ | $\downarrow pCO_2$ | Winter's formula: $pCO_2 = 1.5 \times [HCO_3^-] + 8 \pm 2$ |
| Metabolic alkalosis | $\uparrow HCO_3^-$ | $\uparrow pCO_2$ | $\Delta pCO_2 = 0.7 \times \Delta [HCO_3^-]$ |
| Respiratory acidosis | $\uparrow pCO_2$ | $\uparrow HCO_3^-$ | Acute: $\Delta [HCO_3^-] = 0.1 \times \Delta pCO_2$ <br> Chronic: $\Delta [HCO_3^-] = 0.4 \times \Delta pCO_2$ |
| Respiratory alkalosis | $\downarrow pCO_2$ | $\downarrow HCO_3^-$ | Acute: $\Delta [HCO_3^-] = 0.2 \times \Delta pCO_2$ <br> Chronic: $\Delta [HCO_3^-] = 0.4 \times \Delta pCO_2$ |

Chronic respiratory acidosis and respiratory alkalosis take 3-5 days for renal compensation.

- Examples of causes of high anion gap metabolic acidosis: diabetic ketoacidosis, lactic acidosis, uremia, ingestion of salicylates, and toxic alcohols (ethylene glycol, methanol).
- Examples of causes of normal anion gap metabolic acidosis: GI bicarbonate losses (diarrhea, intestinal/pancreatic fistulas, ostomies), NS infusion (due to elevated chloride load), and RTA.

### Metabolic Alkalosis

- Metabolic alkalosis is defined as an acid-base disorder leading to a high serum $HCO_3^-$ and an arterial blood pH > 7.45.
- Caused by GI or renal losses of hydrogen ions, intracellular shift of hydrogen ions, excess bicarbonate intake, or volume contraction in the setting of a fixed amount of extracellular bicarbonate (contraction alkalosis).
- Can differentiate by response to IV hydration (chloride-responsive vs. chloride-resistant):
  - Chloride-responsive metabolic alkalosis is associated with low urine chloride (<20 mEq/L) and volume depletion (e.g., vomiting, nasogastric suctioning, remote diuretic therapy). Volume repletion corrects the metabolic alkalosis.
  - Chloride-resistant metabolic alkalosis is associated with high urine chloride (>20 mEq/L) and does not correct with volume repletion.
    ○ Normal blood pressure (BP): Bartter syndrome, Gitelman syndrome, alkali loading, active diuretic therapy, hypomagnesemia
    ○ Elevated BP: Hyperaldosteronism or increased mineralocorticoid-like effect (e.g., renal artery stenosis, Liddle syndrome, syndrome of apparent mineralocorticoid excess, licorice ingestion)

### Respiratory Acidosis

- Respiratory acidosis is defined as an acid-base disorder leading to a high $pCO_2$ (hypercapnia) and an arterial blood pH < 7.35.

- Caused by reduction in minute ventilation. Increased endogenous $CO_2$ production is uncommon.
- Can occur as a result of respiratory tract obstruction (e.g., adenotonsillar hypertrophy, status asthmaticus), decreased thoracic excursion (e.g., obesity, progressive scoliosis, thoracic trauma, pneumonia, spinal cord injury, myopathy), or CNS depression (head trauma, CNS infection or tumor, sedatives, anesthetics).

### Respiratory Alkalosis

- Respiratory alkalosis is defined as an acid-base disorder leading to a low $pCO_2$ and an arterial blood pH $> 7.45$.
- Excessive alveolar ventilation can provoke neuromuscular irritability (e.g., paresthesias), decrease cerebral blood flow, and lower myocardial contractility.
- Can occur as a result of CNS disorders (e.g., hyperventilation from stress/anxiety, traumatic brain injury, stroke, tumors), respiratory disorders (e.g., pneumonia, status asthmaticus, excessive noninvasive or mechanical ventilation), or medication toxicity (e.g., salicylates, caffeine).

## KIDNEY DISEASES

### KIDNEY FUNCTION AND URINE STUDIES

- The kidneys perform several essential homeostatic functions:
  - Maintain fluid, electrolyte, and acid-base balance.
  - Remove waste products (e.g., uremic toxins), drugs, and metabolites through glomerular filtration and tubular secretion.
  - Regulate BP, through secretion of renin and adjustment of sodium/potassium balance.
  - Produce erythropoietin, important for stimulating red blood cell (RBC) production.
  - Convert inactive vitamin D to the active form (1,25-dihydroxyvitamin D), important for bone and mineral metabolism.

### History

- Frequently asymptomatic, may not experience symptoms until kidney disease is advanced.
- General: fatigue, malaise, anorexia, growth failure, swelling (from fluid retention).
- Cardiopulmonary: chest pain, palpitations, cough, shortness of breath.
- Gastrointestinal: feeding difficulties, nausea/vomiting, abdominal pain.
- Genitourinary: flank pain, dysuria, hematuria, polyuria or oliguria.
- Neurologic: altered mental status, headache, visual changes, muscle weakness, seizures.
- Neonatal history.
  - Prenatal diagnosis of abnormal kidneys (e.g., small or enlarged kidneys, increased echogenicity, cysts, dysplasia), urinary tract dilatation (e.g., hydronephrosis, hydroureter), abnormal bladder appearance, presence of oligo- or anhydramnios.
  - Fetal urine production is the source of amniotic fluid after the 1st trimester of pregnancy and important for fetal lung development.

- Intrauterine growth restriction (IUGR), preterm birth, and low birth weight (LBW) associated with increased risk of hypertension (HTN) and CKD later in life due to decreased nephron endowment (Brenner hypothesis).
- Maternal history: Use of certain medications (e.g., NSAIDs, ACE inhibitors) during pregnancy can negatively affect fetal kidney development; perinatal asphyxia can cause neonatal AKI in addition to other organ dysfunction.
- Family history.
  - Hereditary kidney diseases, such as polycystic kidney disease, Alport syndrome or thin basement membrane disease, and nephrotic syndrome (some cases are associated with single gene mutations within families). Inquire about any family members who have received dialysis or a kidney transplant.
- Past medical history.
  - Recurrent gross hematuria, UTIs, kidney stones, unexplained swelling, elevated BP, medication exposures, daytime urinary incontinence or nocturnal enuresis.
- Dietary history.

## Physical Examination

- Growth and nutrition.
- BP.
  - Use an appropriately-sized cuff and correct techniques, confirm elevated measurements from oscillometric devices with manual auscultation.
  - Upper and lower extremity BPs if hypertensive (to screen for aortic coarctation).
- Volume status.
  - Tachycardia, hypotension, delayed capillary refill, sunken eyes, dry mucous membranes, and decreased skin turgor suggest hypovolemia.
  - HTN, shortness of breath and rales (pulmonary edema), ascites, and peripheral edema are signs of hypervolemia.
- Abdomen.
  - Auscultate for renal bruits (suggestive of renal artery stenosis).
  - Palpate for enlarged kidneys (can be seen with ureteropelvic junction obstruction, multicystic dysplastic kidney, renal vein thrombosis, and kidney masses) and bladder (lower urinary tract obstruction, neurogenic bladder).
- Maintain a broad assessment, especially in newborns, as many kidney diseases are associated with other congenital anomalies (vertebral defects, anal atresia, cardiac defects, tracheo-esophageal fistula, renal anomalies, and limb abnormalities (VACTERL) association).

## Urinary Assessment

- Abnormal urine volume
  - Anuria: no urine output
  - Oliguria: insufficient urine output for homeostasis (after the immediate neonatal period, this is defined as <500 mL/24 hr/1.73 m$^2$)
  - Polyuria: high urine output, no strict definition in children
    ○ Important to distinguish polyuria from urinary frequency, in which small urine volumes are produced frequently over a 24-hour period
- Visual appearance
- Color
  - Dark yellow/amber urine suggests dehydration.

- Red or reddish-brown urine is seen with hematuria.
  - Confirmed by urinalysis with the presence of RBCs.
  - Pseudohematuria refers to urine discoloration with heme positivity on urinalysis (see below) but no RBCs on urine microscopy (e.g., myoglobinuria).
- Clarity (cloudy urine is suggestive of infection or crystalluria).
- Urinalysis.
  - Urine pH: Measure of acidification in the urine. Depending on systemic acid-base balance, the urine pH can range from 4.5 to 8 (lower in the setting of an acid load, higher in the setting of impaired urinary acidification such as RTA).
  - Specific gravity: Indirect way to assess urine osmolality, but determined by number AND size of particles (e.g., urea, sodium, potassium) in urine.
    - Maximally diluted urine has a specific gravity <1.005 (e.g., diabetes insipidus).
    - Maximally concentrated urine has a specific gravity of 1.030 but can be higher if large molecules (e.g., glucose, protein, radiocontrast) are in the urine.
    - Specific gravity 1.008-1.012 is considered isosthenuria, in which urine is neither more dilute or more concentrated than protein-free plasma.
  - Blood: Tests for heme moiety (hemoglobin and myoglobin). If positive, it is necessary to confirm RBC morphology by microscopic examination.
  - Protein: Semiquantitative assessment of albumin in the urine. Insensitive for non-albumin proteinuria (e.g., immunoglobulin light chains, low molecular weight [LMW] proteins).
  - Glucose: A modern urine dipstick detects glucose only; to test for other sugars, urine reducing substances should be ordered.
  - Leukocyte esterase: Marker for the presence of white blood cells (WBCs), as this enzyme is released by lysed neutrophils and macrophages.
  - Nitrite: 90% of common urinary pathogens are nitrite-forming bacteria.
  - Bilirubin: Elevated in any disease that causes increased conjugated bilirubin in the bloodstream (negative in hemolytic disease).
  - Urobilinogen: Increased in conditions that increase production of bilirubin or decrease the liver's ability to remove reabsorbed urobilinogen from the portal circulation (positive in both liver disease and hemolytic disease).
- Microscopy
  - In healthy children, having 1-5 RBCs/high-power field (HPF) or 1-2 WBCs/HPF is normal.
  - Casts: Tube-shaped particles in the urine sediment that can contain cells (RBCs, WBCs, tubular epithelial cells), fat, protein, or other debris
    - Hyaline casts: Suggestive of low renal blood flow (e.g., dehydration)
    - RBC casts: Hematuria of glomerular origin, suggestive of glomerulonephritis (GN)
    - "Muddy brown" casts: Consist of tubular epithelial cells, pathognomonic for acute tubular necrosis (ATN)
    - Fatty casts: Commonly seen in nephrotic syndrome
    - Waxy casts: Associated with advanced kidney disease
- Crystals
  - Calcium oxalate: Hypercalciuria (envelope or dumbbell shape of crystals)
  - Uric acid crystals: Hyperuricosuria (appear as rhombic plates or rosettes)
  - Hexagonal (benzene ring structure) cystine crystals: Cystinuria
  - Struvite (ammonium magnesium phosphate) crystals: Only form in alkaline pH; seen with urease-splitting organisms (coffin-lid appearance of crystals)
  - Fine, needle-like crystals: Tyrosinemia

## Glomerular Filtration Rate Estimation

- Bedside Schwartz formula: Used in children to estimate glomerular filtration rate (GFR) from serum creatinine (SCr) measurement. eGFR (mL/min/1.73 m$^2$) = 0.413 [height (cm)/SCr (mg/dL)]
- Blood urea nitrogen (BUN), in isolation, is not an accurate marker of kidney function.
  - Factors that increase BUN: GI hemorrhage, dehydration, increased protein intake, and increased protein catabolism (sepsis, burns, glucocorticoid therapy, early phase of starvation).
  - Factors that decrease BUN: high fluid intake, decreased protein intake, advanced starvation, and liver disease.
- Serum cystatin C (CysC): Endogenous protein produced constitutively by all nucleated cells that has been studied as another marker of kidney function. Useful in children with low or high muscle mass, which may influence SCr measurement.
  - Several equations have been derived that use CysC with/without SCr for GFR estimation (calculators can be found at https://ckid-gfrcalculator.shinyapps.io/eGFR/ and https://www.kidney.org/professionals/kdoqi/gfr_calculatorped).
- Estimation of GFR using 24-hour creatinine clearance (U × V/P)
  - To standardize: creatinine clearance

$$(mL/min/1.73m^2) = \frac{U_{Cr}(mg/dL) \times V(mL) \times 1.73}{P_{Cr}(mg/dL) \times 1440 \times SA(m^2)}$$

  - $U_{Cr}$ = urinary concentration of creatinine
  - V = urine volume in 24 hours
  - $P_{Cr}$ = plasma concentration of creatinine
  - SA = body surface area
  - If a child >3 years of age has <15 mg/kg/day of creatinine in a 24-hour urine collection, it probably means that the collection did not actually occur over 24 hours or that not all the urine has been collected.
- For normal values of GFR by age, see Table 25-4.

| TABLE 25-4 | Normal Glomerular Filtration Rate (GFR) by Age |
| --- | --- |
| **Age** | **GFR (mL/min/1.73 m$^2$)** |
| Birth | 20.8 |
| 1 week | 46.6 |
| 3-5 weeks | 60.1 |
| 6-9 weeks | 67.5 |
| 3-6 months | 73.8 |
| 6 months-1 year | 93.7 |
| 1-2 years | 99.1 |
| 2-5 years | 126.5 |
| 5-15 years | 116.7 |

| TABLE 25-5 | Summary of Diagnostic Evaluation by Kidney Function | |
|---|---|---|

| Glomerular function | Tubular function | Hormonal function |
|---|---|---|
| Blood urea nitrogen | Water metabolism<br>• Urine specific gravity<br>• Urine osmolality<br>• Maximal urine concentrating ability | Erythropoietin<br>• Hematocrit<br>• Reticulocyte count |
| Serum creatinine | Acid-base metabolism<br>• Urine pH | Vitamin D<br>• Serum 1,25-dihydroxyvitamin D concentration |
| Iothalamate or iohexol GFR scan | • FE of bicarbonate at normal serum bicarbonate level<br>• Urine ammonium excretion<br>• Urine-blood pCO$_2$ | • Serum calcium concentration<br>25-hydroxyvitamin D |

GFR, glomerular filtration rate; FE, fractional excretion.

- While kidney function frequently implies glomerular filtration, the different functions of the kidneys can be categorized as glomerular, tubular, or hormonal in nature (Table 25-5).

## ACUTE KIDNEY INJURY

- Defined as an abrupt loss of kidney function, resulting in decreased GFR, retention of waste products, and fluid and electrolyte derangements.
  - Acute rise in SCr with or without decreased urine output.
- Kidney Disease Improving Global Outcomes (KDIGO) criteria for AKI:
  - Increase in SCr by ≥0.3 mg/dL from baseline within 48 hours, OR
  - Increase in SCr to ≥1.5 times baseline within the prior 7 days, OR
  - Urine volume ≤0.5 mL/kg/hr for 6 hours

### Etiology
- Traditionally, the etiologies of AKI have been divided into prerenal, intrinsic, and postrenal causes (Table 25-6).
  - Prerenal AKI: injury related to decreased kidney perfusion.
  - Intrinsic AKI: direct damage to the kidney tissue.
  - Postrenal AKI: injury related to obstruction of urine flow.
- In many cases, there can be several contributing factors to a single AKI event and overlap of etiologies (e.g., hypotension and nephrotoxic antibiotic exposure in a child with septic shock).

| TABLE 25-6 | Etiologies of Acute Kidney Injury (AKI) | |
|---|---|---|
| **Prerenal** | **Intrinsic** | **Postrenal** |
| Hypovolemia | Glomerular<br>• Postinfectious GN<br>• IgA nephropathy<br>• C3 glomerulopathy<br>• Lupus nephritis<br>• ANCA vasculitis | Nephrolithiasis |
| Hypoxia | Vascular<br>• Vasculitis (IgA, ANCA)<br>• TMA (e.g., HUS)<br>• Renal vein thrombosis | Tumors and masses |
| Hypotension | Tubular/interstitial<br>• Acute tubular necrosis<br>• Acute interstitial nephritis<br>• Pyelonephritis | Congenital anomalies<br>• Posterior urethral valves<br>• UPJ and UVJ obstruction |
| Hepatorenal syndrome | | |
| Cardiac dysfunction | | |
| Sepsis | | |
| Third spacing (e.g., hypoalbuminemia) | | |
| Renovascular disease (e.g., renal artery stenosis) | | |
| Medications (e.g., NSAIDs) | | |

NSAIDs, nonsteroidal anti-inflammatory drugs; GN, glomerulonephritis; ANCA, antineutrophil cytoplasmic antibody; TMA, thrombotic microangiopathy; HUS, hemolytic uremic syndrome; UPJ, ureteropelvic junction; UVJ, ureterovesical junction.

## Laboratory Studies

• Urinalysis/microscopy.
  • Prerenal AKI: May have specific gravity >1.020 or hyaline casts on urine sediment, but otherwise normal urinalysis and microscopy.
  • Intrinsic AKI: Isosthenuria is common (from impaired urinary concentration capacity with direct tubular damage), as well as proteinuria and/or hematuria. Various types of urinary casts and cellular elements on urine microscopy depending on underlying cause (e.g., muddy brown and renal tubular epithelial cell casts in ATN, RBCs, and RBC casts in acute GN, WBCs in acute interstitial nephritis).
• Urinary indices may be helpful in differentiating prerenal from intrinsic AKI (Table 25-7).

**TABLE 25-7** Urinary Indices in AKI

| Test | Prenatal[a] | Intrinsic[a] |
|------|-------------|--------------|
| Specific gravity | >1.020 (>1.015) | <1.010 (<1.010) |
| Urine osmolality (mOsmol/kg) | >500 (>400) | <350 (<400) |
| Urine/plasma osmolality | >1.3 (>2.0) | <1.3 (<1.0) |
| Urine sodium (mEq/L) | <20 (<30) | >40 (>70) |
| $FE_{Na}$ | <1 (<2.5) | >3 (>10) |
| Urine/plasma urea | >8 (>30) | <3 (<6) |
| $FE_{Urea}$ | <30 | >70 |
| Urine/plasma creatinine | >40 (>30) | <20 (<10) |
| $FE\beta_{2\text{-microglobulin}}$ | <0.4 | >0.5 |

[a]Indices for neonates who are >32 weeks are given in parentheses.
FE, fractional excretion.

## RENAL TUBULAR ACIDOSIS

- Type I (distal RTA): Defective urinary acidification in the distal nephron
- Type II (proximal RTA): Defective $HCO_3^-$ reabsorption in the proximal tubule
- Type IV (hyperkalemic RTA): Defective urinary acidification in the cortical collecting duct due to hypoaldosteronism or aldosterone resistance (impaired $Na^+$ reabsorption and $K^+$ secretion)
  - Tests for diagnosis of RTA (Table 25-8)
- Urine anion gap (UAG)
  - Used to determine whether urinary $NH_4^+$, a carrier of acid ($H^+$), is increased or decreased when normal anion gap metabolic acidosis is present
  - UAG = urine $[Na^+] + [K^+] - [Cl^-]$
  - Negative UAG implies high amount of unmeasured $NH_4^+$ and therefore normal urinary acidification (e.g., diarrhea, type II RTA).
  - Positive UAG implies low or absent $NH_4^+$ and thus impaired urinary acidification (e.g., type I and type IV RTA).

## PROTEINURIA

### Definitions

- Normal protein excretion: <4 mg/m²/hr or 150 mg/1.73 m²/day.
  - Due to the difficulty of obtaining 24-hour urine collections in children, especially if not toilet trained, a spot urine sample may be used (preferably from a first morning void).
  - Normal urine protein-to-creatinine (UPC) ratios:
    ○ <0.5 mg/mg in children 6-24 months of age
    ○ <0.2 mg/mg in children >24 months of age
- Proteinuria: >4 mg/m²/hr or > 150 mg/1.73 m²/day (>300 mg/1.73 m²/day if <6 months old).
  - Usually implies glomerular proteinuria or albuminuria.

**TABLE 25-8  Types of Renal Tubular Acidosis (RTA)**

| | Type I (distal) | Type II (proximal) | Type IV (hyperkalemic) |
|---|---|---|---|
| Urine anion gap | Positive | Negative | Positive |
| Urine ammonia | Low | Appropriately high | Low |
| Serum potassium | Low | Low | High |
| Urine pH | >5.5 | <5.5 | <5.5 |
| Defect | Impaired distal H+ excretion | Impaired HCO₃⁻ reabsorption | Hypoaldosteronism or aldosterone resistance |
| | | Can be part of more global proximal tubular dysfunction (Fanconi syndrome) with hypophosphaturia, glycosuria, and aminoaciduria | |
| Treatment | Alkali therapy (potassium citrate) | Alkali therapy (usually needs higher dosing than for type I RTA) | Remove offending agent, treat underlying cause |
| | Remove offending agent, treat underlying cause | Remove offending agent, treat underlying cause | Alleviate urinary obstruction if present |
| | | | May need fludrocortisone and alkali therapy |
| Example causes | Hereditary, drugs (amphotericin), autoimmune diseases (SLE, Sjögren syndrome), hypercalciuria (nephrocalcinosis) | Hereditary (cystinosis), drugs (ifosfamide), heavy metal poisoning, hyperparathyroidism | Adrenal insufficiency, urinary tract obstruction, pyelonephritis, drugs (NSAIDs, CNIs, amiloride, spironolactone), pseudohypoaldosteronism |

SLE, systemic lupus erythematosus; NSAIDs, nonsteroidal anti-inflammatory drugs; CNIs, calcineurin inhibitors.

- Transient proteinuria is of no renal consequence, persistent proteinuria suggests kidney disease.
- Nephrotic range (heavy) proteinuria: $>40$ mg/m$^2$/hr or $>3$ g/1.73 m$^2$/day.
  - UPC $> 2$ mg/mg.
- Microalbuminuria: Early marker of kidney disease in patients with DM and sickle cell disease that precedes overt proteinuria.
  - Albumin-to-creatinine (ACR) ratio: 30-300 mg/g.
- LMW proteinuria: Increased excretion of tubular protein (freely filtered by the glomerulus, but typically reabsorbed by the renal tubules). Examples of LMW proteins include $\beta_2$-microglobulin and retinol-binding protein.
  - Typically elevated in hereditary or acquired causes of tubular dysfunction.
  - Qualitative urine protein detection on urinalysis is selective for albumin, thus, if LMW proteinuria is suspected it needs to be measured directly.
- Both glomerular and tubular protein excretion is higher in neonates and infants (lack of renal maturation).

## History

- History of present illness
  - Symptoms associated with GN (edema, concurrent hematuria), CKD (poor growth/short stature, polyuria, nocturia), and HTN
  - Urologic symptoms (burning micturition, red or brown colored urine, urinary urgency or hesitancy, incontinence, enuresis)
  - Recent illnesses
  - New and chronic medication exposures (e.g., NSAIDs)
  - Extrarenal symptoms that may suggest a secondary glomerulopathy (e.g., recurrent fevers, weight loss, arthritis, photosensitivity, malar rash, purpura)
- Past medical history
  - Prenatal ultrasound of the kidneys and urinary tract, presence of amniotic fluid
  - Gestational age, birth weight
  - Recurrent febrile UTIs or unexplained febrile illnesses in infancy
  - VUR
  - HTN
  - History of AKI
  - History of hepatitis B, hepatitis C, or HIV in high-risk patients
- Family history:
  - Hearing loss, deafness (suggestive of hereditary nephritis)
  - Nephrotic syndrome
  - Polycystic kidney disease
  - CKD, need for dialysis, or kidney transplantation
  - HTN
  - Kidney stones

## Physical Examination

- Weight, height, head circumference
- BP and heart rate
- Ear pits and tags, low-set/malformed ears, branchial cleft cysts, brachydactyly, single umbilical artery, midline posterior sacral lesions: may suggest an underlying congenital anomaly of the kidneys and urinary tract
- Generalized and pitting edema, ascites, pleural effusion, scrotal/labial edema: fluid overload from nephrotic syndrome, GN, or CKD

- Palpable kidneys: obstructive uropathy, cystic kidney disease
- Large palpable bladder: neurogenic bladder, bladder outlet obstruction
- Ambiguous genitalia: Denys-Drash syndrome, WAGR syndrome
- Hypoplastic nails and patellae: Nail-patella syndrome

## Laboratory Studies

- Urinalysis on first morning void (rule out orthostatic proteinuria)
  - Qualitative protein measurement
    - False-positive result: concentrated urine, alkaline urine, and contamination with mucus/blood/pus/semen/vaginal secretions
    - False-negative result: dilute urine, acidic urine, nonalbumin proteinuria (LMW proteins, globulins)
  - Microscopic examination: look for signs of concurrent hematuria (dysmorphic or eumorphic RBCs, RBC casts), other cellular casts, crystals, bacteria, lipid bodies
  - Quantitative protein measurement: timed 24-hour urine collection or spot urine protein-to-creatinine measurement
  - 24-hour urinary protein measurement includes both albumin and nonalbumin protein
  - Limitations in spot urine testing for children with severe malnutrition and significant GFR reduction (lower urine creatinine overestimates true protein excretion)
- Complete blood count (CBC), basic metabolic panel (BMP), serum albumin
- C3/C4 complement
- Other laboratory tests, depending on differential diagnosis

## Imaging

- Kidney and bladder ultrasound to rule out anatomical abnormalities
- Consider voiding cystourethrogram (VCUG) if the patient has a history of recurrent UTIs.
- Consider dimercaptosuccinic acid (DMSA) renal scan if renal scarring is suspected, even if not seen on kidney and bladder ultrasound (low sensitivity for scars).

## Differential Diagnosis

- First step in evaluation is to differentiate transient proteinuria from persistent proteinuria.
  - Prevalence of proteinuria on a single urine sample ranges from 1.2% to 15% based on large school screening programs. Prevalence of persistent proteinuria is much lower.
  - Orthostatic proteinuria, or elevated protein excretion in the upright position with normal protein excretion when supine, is the most common cause of isolated proteinuria in children.
- Important to exclude nephrotic syndrome or an acute GN, as these require urgent evaluation and management.
- Causes of proteinuria can be found in Table 25-9.

## Treatment

- Treat the underlying cause if known.
- For significant albuminuria, ACE inhibitors and ARBs may decrease urine protein excretion and delay progression of kidney disease.

## Indications for Kidney Biopsy

- Persistent significant proteinuria (>1 g/1.73 m$^2$/day or UPC > 0.5 mg/mg)

| TABLE 25-9 | Differential Diagnosis of Proteinuria in Children | |
|---|---|---|
| | **Persistent proteinuria** | |
| **Intermittent proteinuria** | **Glomerular** | **Tubular** |
| Orthostatic (postural) | Primary glomerulopathies | Hereditary |
| Fever | • Minimal change disease | • Cystinosis |
| Exercise | • Congenital nephrotic syndrome | • Dent disease |
| Seizures | • FSGS | • Lowe syndrome |
| Hypovolemia | • IgA nephropathy | • Wilson disease |
| | • C3 glomerulopathy | • Galactosemia |
| | • Membranous nephropathy | • Tyrosinemia |
| | • Alport syndrome | • Mitochondrial disorders |
| | Secondary glomerulopathies | • Polycystic kidney disease |
| | • Postinfectious GN | Acquired |
| | • Lupus nephritis | • ATN |
| | • ANCA vasculitis | • AIN |
| | • IgA vasculitis (formerly Henoch-Schönlein purpura nephritis) | • Pyelonephritis |
| | • Chronic infection (hepatitis B, hepatitis C, HIV) | • Obstructive uropathy |
| | Hemolytic uremic syndrome | • Analgesic nephropathy |
| | Diabetic nephropathy | • Medications (e.g., penicillamine) |
| | Sickle cell disease | |
| | Hypertension | • Heavy metal poisoning |
| | Hyperfiltration injury (e.g., following nephron loss) | |
| | Overflow proteinuria (e.g., after albumin infusion) | |

GN, glomerulonephritis; FSGS, focal segmental glomerulosclerosis; ANCA, antineutrophil cytoplasmic antibody; HIV, human immunodeficiency virus; ATN, acute tubular necrosis; AIN, acute interstitial nephritis.

• Most common scenario is steroid-resistant nephrotic syndrome
• Proteinuria with concurrent microscopic hematuria
• Decreased GFR
• Persistently low C3 after 3 months
  • Postinfectious GN is associated with low C3, but it is expected to normalize after 8-12 weeks. Persistently low C3 may be concerning for C3 glomerulopathy.
  • Clinical or serologic evidence of vasculitis (lupus nephritis [LN], ANCA vasculitis, IgA vasculitis [formerly Henoch-Schönlein purpura nephritis])

## NEPHROTIC SYNDROME

### Definition

- Nephrotic syndrome is a clinical state characterized by:
  - Nephrotic range proteinuria (>40 mg/m$^2$/hr or UPC > 2 mg/mg)
  - Hypoalbuminemia (albumin ≤2.5 g/dL)
  - Edema
  - Hyperlipidemia

### Classification

- Congenital and infantile nephrotic syndrome: Finnish type, diffuse mesangial sclerosis, or secondary to congenital infection.
  - Onset in children <12 months of age.
  - As high as 85% of cases have a genetic basis, associated with poor outcomes.
- Primary nephrotic syndrome: no identifiable underlying disease present.
  - Most common form of childhood nephrotic syndrome (>90% of cases in children under 10).
  - Most common histologic lesion is minimal change disease. Other pathologic lesions seen in primary nephrotic syndrome include focal segmental glomerulosclerosis (FSGS), membranous nephropathy, C3 glomerulopathy, and IgA nephropathy.
- Secondary nephrotic syndrome: Nephrotic syndrome in the presence of an underlying disease.
  - Examples include LN, chronic hepatitis B infection, secondary FSGS (e.g., from HIV infection), postinfectious GN, and vasculitides (e.g., IgA vasculitis).

### Treatment

- The majority of children with primary nephrotic syndrome will have underlying minimal change disease, which typically responds to steroids.
- Prednisone 60 mg/m$^2$/day or 2 mg/kg/day for 4-6 weeks, followed by 40 mg/m$^2$/day or 1.5 mg/kg every other day for 4-6 weeks. Subsequent taper over 2-5 months.
- Relapse: defined as ≥3+ on urine dipstick or UPC > 2 mg/mg for 3 consecutive days.
  - Typically treated with prednisone 60 mg/m$^2$/day until proteinuria is in remission (trace or negative for protein on dipstick for 3 consecutive days), followed by tapering. Some patients may respond to lower steroid dosing.
- For frequently relapsing nephrotic syndrome (4+ relapses/year or 2+ relapses within 6 months) and steroid-dependent nephrotic syndrome (relapses during steroid therapy or within 2 weeks of discontinuing steroids after a taper), consider steroid-sparing agents such as mycophenolate mofetil, calcineurin inhibitors (e.g., tacrolimus), rituximab, or alkylating agents (e.g., cyclophosphamide).
- If unable to achieve remission of proteinuria after 4 weeks of full prednisone dosing, the child is considered steroid-resistant.
- Additional considerations
  - Fluid and sodium restriction during relapses to mitigate worsening edema.
  - May require IV albumin and furosemide for forced diuresis.
  - Adequate protein in diet for endogenous synthesis of albumin.
  - Monitor for decreased growth velocity and other complications of chronic steroid therapy.

- Infection control, including vaccination with the 23-valent polysaccharide (PPSV23) pneumococcal vaccine.
  ○ Live vaccines should be avoided while on steroid therapy.

## Complications (Table 25-10)

### Indications for Kidney Biopsy
- Steroid-resistant nephrotic syndrome
- Low C3 complement at presentation
- Patient presentation <1 year of age
- Evidence of CKD
- Suspicion for secondary nephrotic syndrome (e.g., membranous LN), including cooccurrence of gross hematuria, HTN, or increased serum creatinine
- Frequently relapsing or steroid-dependent nephrotic syndrome, before considering steroid-sparing agents

## HEMATURIA

### Definitions and Epidemiology
- Defined as >5 RBCs/HPF in a centrifuged urine specimen.
  - Macroscopic (gross) hematuria: Hematuria visible to the naked eye.
  - Microscopic hematuria: Hematuria detected only on urinalysis.
- Prevalence: Most children with gross or microscopic hematuria have transient hematuria. 0.5-1% of children are estimated to have persistent microscopic hematuria.

| TABLE 25-10 | Complications of Nephrotic Syndrome |
|---|---|
| **Complications** | **Cause** |
| Infection: peritonitis (e.g., *Streptococcus pneumoniae*) | Edema |
| | Low serum IgG |
| | Low factor B |
| | Decreased mesenteric blood flow |
| Deep vein thrombosis | Loss of antithrombin III in urine |
| | High fibrinogen |
| | High blood viscosity |
| | Decreased renal blood flow |
| Hyperlipidemia | Increased very low-density lipoproteins produced by liver |
| | Urinary loss of high-density lipoprotein and lipoproteins |
| Hypocalcemia | Artifactual hypocalcemia secondary to hypoalbuminemia and true hypocalcemia from urinary loss of vitamin D |
| Copper, zinc, and iron deficiencies | Loss of carrier proteins |
| Hypothyroidism | Loss of thyroxine-binding globulin |

## Etiology (Table 25-11)

- The differential diagnosis can be approached by determining the source of bleeding.
  - Glomerular: Urine can be red, but usually described as cola-colored or smoky brown.
    - Proteinuria may be present, no clots.
    - RBCs appear dysmorphic on urine microscopy, RBC casts may be present.
  - Nonglomerular: Urine is red or pink-tinged.
    - Proteinuria usually absent or minimal. Clots may be present.
    - RBCs appear normal or eumorphic on urine microscopy, RBC casts are absent.

## History

- Characteristics of hematuria: timing, onset, and duration
- History of recent exercise, trauma, passage of kidney stones
- History of recent skin or respiratory infections
- Medication use (e.g., calcium or vitamin D)
- Associated signs and symptoms: fever, nasal congestion/coryza, sore throat, cough, hemoptysis, abdominal pain, hematochezia, flank pain, dysuria, urinary urgency/frequency, joint pain, rash
- Past medical history: cystic kidney disease, sickle cell disease/trait, lupus, malignancy
- Family history: hematuria, hearing loss/deafness, polycystic kidney disease, nephrolithiasis, CKD, need for dialysis or kidney transplantation, sickle cell disease/trait, autoimmune diseases, coagulopathy

**TABLE 25-11** | **Example Causes of Hematuria in Children**

| Glomerular | Nonglomerular |
| --- | --- |
| Acute or chronic GN | UTI |
| • Postinfectious GN | Hypercalciuria |
| • C3 glomerulopathy | Nephrolithiasis |
| • Membranous nephropathy | Interstitial nephritis |
| • IgA nephropathy/vasculitis | Cystic kidney disease |
| • Lupus nephritis | Sickle cell disease |
| • IgA vasculitis | Viral or chemical cystitis |
| • ANCA vasculitis | Renal trauma |
| Familial hematuria | Renal vein thrombosis |
| • Alport syndrome | Exercise-induced |
| • Thin basement membrane disease | Vascular malformations |
| | Coagulopathy |
| Hemolytic uremic syndrome | Nutcracker syndrome |
| | Malignancy |
| | • Wilms tumor |
| | • Bladder rhabdomyosarcoma |
| | Menarche |

GN, glomerulonephritis; ANCA, antineutrophil cytoplasmic antibody; UTI, urinary tract infection.

## Physical Examination

- Hearing loss: Alport syndrome
- Abdominal mass: polycystic kidney disease, Wilms tumor, bladder rhabdomyosarcoma
- Flank pain/tenderness: UTI, nephrolithiasis, sickle cell disease/trait, loin pain hematuria syndrome
- Edema: acute GN of various causes
- Rash, joint pain: LN, ANCA vasculitis, IgA vasculitis
- Genitourinary trauma

## Laboratory Studies and Imaging

- Confirm the presence of hematuria with urine microscopy.
- Many conditions can cause red or cola-colored colored urine and have no RBCs on urine microscopy ("pseudohematuria").
  - Heme-positive: Hemoglobinuria, myoglobinuria, porphyria.
  - Heme-negative: Rifampin, phenazopyridine, certain foods (beets, blackberries, rhubarb).
- If dipstick is positive for heme, this must be followed with a microscopic examination to determine presence of true hematuria.
- An evaluation for persistent hematuria is necessary if microscopic hematuria persists on 3 consecutive urine samples, obtained at least 7 days apart.
- Urinalysis can provide a hint to the location of the bleeding (e.g., presence of dysmorphic RBCs or RBC casts suggests glomerular bleeding).
  - Urine culture in any child presenting with gross hematuria.
  - Urine protein should be quantified (i.e., UPC) if dipstick is positive for protein, as this may suggest more serious kidney disease.
- CBC, BMP, and serum albumin.
- Kidney/bladder ultrasound.
- Additional studies depending on differential diagnosis:
  - C3/C4 complement
  - Serologies: Antinuclear antibody (ANA), antistreptolysin O (ASO), ANCA
  - Urine calcium measurement (screen for hypercalciuria)
    - Urine calcium-to-creatinine ratio >0.2 mg/mg creatinine for children 2 years of age and older, or urine calcium >4 mg/kg/day on a 24-hour urine collection
  - Hemoglobinopathy screen
  - CT abdomen/pelvis
  - Cystoscopy

## Treatment

- Therapy depends on the underlying cause.
- For acute GN (postinfectious or otherwise), use sodium and fluid restriction, as well as diuretics as needed to mitigate edema and HTN. Monitor closely for AKI.
- Autoimmune GNs (e.g., LN, ANCA vasculitis) should be treated with corticosteroids and other immunosuppressants.
- For Alport syndrome, start ACE inhibitor/ARB at the onset of microalbuminuria or overt proteinuria. Perform hearing and vision screening. Provide anticipatory guidance on CKD progression and end-stage kidney disease (ESKD).
- For hypercalciuria, increase oral hydration, encourage low sodium diet, and consider thiazide therapy for lowering urinary calcium excretion (dietary calcium restriction not needed). Consider sodium or potassium citrate for concurrent hypocitraturia (citrate inhibits kidney stone formation) and magnesium oxide for concurrent hypomagnesuria (magnesium also inhibits calcium stone formation).

- If there is isolated hematuria (i.e., no concurrent proteinuria, HTN, or kidney dysfunction) and no serious pathologic cause is identified, follow-up evaluation every 6-12 months without additional workup is acceptable. Follow growth curves, BP, and urinalysis. See "Glomerulonephritis" section.

## GLOMERULONEPHRITIS

- A group of disorders resulting in inflammation and damage of the glomerular tuft. Presents clinically with hematuria, proteinuria, edema, oliguria, azotemia, and HTN.
- Example causes of GN are presented in Table 25-12.

### Diagnosis
- CBC, BMP, and serum albumin
- Urinalysis with microscopy
- C3/C4 complement
- Serologies:
  - ANA and antidouble stranded DNA (dsDNA): lupus nephritis
  - ANCA, antiproteinase 3 (PR3), antimyeloperoxidase (MPO): ANCA vasculitis
  - Antiglomerular basement membrane (GBM) antibody: anti-GBM disease
  - Serum IgA level is not helpful in the diagnosis of IgA nephropathy/vasculitis
- Kidney biopsy
  - Not all patients presenting with acute GN require a diagnostic biopsy
  - Indications for kidney biopsy:
    - AKI or rapidly progressive GN
    - Persistent hypocomplementemia (low C3/C4)
    - Progressive proteinuria
    - Concurrent nephrotic syndrome
    - New diagnosis of lupus with clinical/laboratory evidence of kidney involvement

### Treatment
- Supportive care: antihypertensive therapy as needed, fluid/sodium restriction and diuretics for oliguria and edema
- Immunosuppressive therapy: depending on the cause of GN and its severity
- For associated AKI, dialysis may be required if refractory to medical management

## HYPERTENSION

### Definitions
- Definitions for normal BP, elevated BP (previously "prehypertension"), and HTN are determined by normative BP data for a child's age, sex, and height (see Appendix F).
- Children ages 1-13:
  - Normal BP: <90th percentile
  - Elevated BP: ≥90th percentile to <95th percentile, or 120/80 to <95th percentile (whichever is lower)
  - Stage 1 HTN: ≥95th percentile to <95th percentile + 12 mm Hg, or 130/80 to 139/89 (whichever is lower)
  - Stage 2 HTN: ≥95th percentile + 12 mm Hg or ≥140/90 (whichever is lower)
- Children ≥13 years:

**TABLE 25-12  Example Causes of Glomerulonephritis**

| Glomerular disease | Serologic findings | Biopsy findings | Management |
|---|---|---|---|
| Postinfectious GN | Low C3 Normal C4 | LM: Endocapillary proliferative GN<br>IF: Granular C3/IgG deposits<br>EM: Subepithelial "humps" | Conservative management; treat hypertension and edema with fluid/sodium restriction and diuretics |
| IgA nephropathy | Normal C3/C4 | LM: Mesangial hypercellularity and increased mesangial matrix<br>IF and EM: Mesangial IgA-dominant deposits | Subnephrotic range proteinuria: ACEI/ARB<br>NS or RPGN: Corticosteroids, other immunosuppressants |
| IgA vasculitis | Normal C3/C4 | Similar to IgA nephropathy, may have more endocapillary and extracapillary inflammation | Similar to IgA nephropathy<br>Pain control for extrarenal symptoms |
| C3 glomerulopathy (C3GN and DDD) | Low C3 +/– C4 | LM: Variable (classic "membranoproliferative" pattern occurs in up to 55% of biopsies). Can have mesangial or endocapillary proliferative GN.<br>IF: C3-dominant capillary loop and mesangial deposits, typically without immunoglobulin.<br>EM: Mesangial, subendothelial, and occasional subepithelial deposits (C3GN), ribbon-like "osmophilic" GBM deposits (DDD) | Immunosuppressive therapy based on biopsy findings |

| | | | |
|---|---|---|---|
| Lupus nephritis | Low C3/C4<br>ANA positive<br>Anti-dsDNA positive | LM: Variable depending on ISN/RPS class and acuity/chronicity, with mesangioproliferative GN (class II), endocapillary proliferative GN (class III/IV), and/or membranous (class V) features<br><br>IF: "Full-house" immunostaining for IgG, IgM, C3, and C1q<br><br>EM: Subendothelial, mesangial, subepithelial deposits, can have diffuse foot process effacement (lupus podocytopathy) or tubuloreticular inclusions | Immunosuppressive therapy based on biopsy findings<br>Induction: Corticosteroids with CYC or MMF, consider RTX in severe disease<br>Maintenance: MMF or AZA |
| ANCA vasculitis | Normal C3/C4<br>ANCA positive<br>Anti-MPO and/or anti-PR3 positive | LM: Crescentic GN with necrotic lesions, may have granulomas<br><br>IF/EM: Pauci-immune pattern (few or no electron dense deposits) | Induction: Corticosteroids with CYC or RTX, consider PLEX in severe disease<br>Maintenance: MMF or AZA |

GN, glomerulonephritis; LM, light microscopy; IF, immunofluorescence microscopy; EM, electron microscopy; ACEI, angiotensin-converting enzyme inhibitor; ARB, angiotensin receptor blocker; NS, nephrotic syndrome; C3GN, C3 glomerulonephritis; DDD, dense deposit disease; GBM, glomerular basement membrane; ANA, antinuclear antibody; ISN/RPS, International Society of Nephrology/Renal Pathology Society; ANCA, antineutrophil cytoplasmic antibody; MPO, myeloperoxidase; PR3, proteinase 3; CYC, cyclophosphamide; RTX, rituximab; PLEX, plasma exchange; MMF, mycophenolate mofetil; AZA, azathioprine.

- Normal BP: <120/80
- Elevated BP: 120-129/<80
- Stage 1 HTN: 130-139/80-89
- Stage 2 HTN: ≥140/90

## Epidemiology

- Prevalence: persistent elevated BP estimated at 2.2-3.5%, HTN 3.5% in children.
  - Higher among children with overweight/obesity.
- Elevated BP and HTN are not diagnosed until multiple BPs obtained, due to BP variability and accommodation effect (patient acclimates to BP measurement).
- Screening: Annual BP measurement should be performed starting at 3 years of age, or at every office visit if at risk for developing HTN (e.g., obesity, CKD, aortic arch obstruction, DM, use of medications known to elevate BP).
  - BP screening should start younger in certain children (e.g., prematurity and/or low birth weight, congenital heart disease, congenital anomalies of the kidneys and urinary tract, malignancy, bone marrow or solid organ transplant, use of medications known to elevate BP).

## Etiology

- HTN can be divided into primary (essential) and secondary HTN.
  - Primary HTN: No identifiable underlying cause, most common cause of pediatric HTN
    - More common in older children (≥6 years), overweight/obesity, or with positive family history of HTN
    - Isolated systolic HTN more predictive of primary HTN, diastolic HTN more predictive of secondary HTN
    - No difference in severity of BP elevation between primary and secondary HTN
  - Secondary HTN: A specific identifiable disorder is present
    - Kidney disease and renovascular disease are the most common causes in children.
    - Other important causes include coarctation of the aorta, endocrine disorders, medication/toxin exposures, and monogenic disorders (Table 25-13).

## History

- Birth history: Pregnancy complications (known as prenatal congenital renal/urologic anomalies, IUGR, low birth weight, prematurity), NICU course (bronchopulmonary dysplasia, umbilical artery catheterization, AKI)
- History of febrile UTIs or undifferentiated febrile illnesses: HTN related to renal scarring
- Abdominal/flank pain, dysuria, hematuria, frequency, nocturia, or enuresis: Underlying kidney or urologic disease
- Weight gain: Overweight/obesity, acute or chronic GN, Cushing syndrome
- Weight loss, skin flushing, palpitations: Hyperthyroidism, pheochromocytoma
- Muscle weakness, constipation: Hypokalemic hypertensive disorders (e.g., hyperaldosteronism, certain monogenic causes of HTN)
- Claudication: Vascular disorders (e.g., large vessel vasculitis, midaortic syndrome)
- Symptoms of severe HTN: Fatigue, headache, visual disturbance, tinnitus, epistaxis, chest pain, palpitations, shortness of breath, nausea/vomiting, and seizures
- Medication use: Corticosteroids, calcineurin inhibitors, oral contraceptives, stimulant medications, caffeine, tobacco, and other illicit substances

**TABLE 25-13** Example Causes of Secondary Hypertension

| Kidney disease | Vascular | Endocrine | Medications/toxins |
|---|---|---|---|
| Primary and secondary glomerular disorders | Renal artery stenosis | Hyperthyroidism | Corticosteroids |
| CAKUT | Aortic coarctation | Cushing syndrome | Calcineurin inhibitors |
| Hemolytic uremic syndrome | PDA | Congenital adrenal hypoplasia | Sympathomimetics |
| Polycystic kidney disease | Large vessel vasculitis (e.g., Takayasu arteritis) | Hyperaldosteronism | Stimulants |
| Renal trauma | Midaortic syndrome | Pheochromocytoma | Oral contraceptives |
| Renal masses | Renal vein thrombosis | Hypercalcemia | Cocaine |
| | | | Anabolic steroids |
| | | | Nicotine |
| | | | Caffeine |
| | | | Licorice |

| Monogenic HTN | Genetic syndromes | Neurologic | Other |
|---|---|---|---|
| Gordon syndrome (PHA2) | Neurofibromatosis | Increased ICP | Pain |
| Liddle syndrome | Tuberous sclerosis | Guillain-Barré syndrome | Stress/anxiety |
| GRA | Turner syndrome | | Collagen vascular disorders |
| AME | Down syndrome | | Bronchopulmonary dysplasia |
| | | | Heavy metal poisoning |

CAKUT, congenital anomalies of the kidneys and urinary tract; PDA, patent ductus arteriosus; PHA2, pseudohypoaldosteronism type 2; GRA, glucocorticoid-remediable aldosteronism; AME, apparent mineralocorticoid excess; ICP, intracranial pressure.

- Dietary and activity history: Salt and sugar intake, amount of physical activity
- Family history: HTN, stroke, cardiovascular disease, CKD, diabetes mellitus

## Physical Examination

- General
  - Examine the skin for pallor, flushing, increased sweating, and pale mucous membranes.
  - Note edema, Cushingoid features, dysmorphic features (Turner or Williams syndrome), thyroid enlargement, and birthmarks, such as café au lait spots or neurofibromas.
- Cardiovascular
  - Note femoral pulses if absent or delayed or if there is a discrepancy between upper and lower extremity pulses. Obtain four extremity blood pressures.
  - Examine heart rate, rhythm, murmurs, work of breathing, hepatomegaly, and bruits over major vessels.
- Abdomen
  - Palpate for masses (unilateral or bilateral), auscultate for abdominal bruits.
- Neurologic
- Examine fundi and note neurologic deficits.

## Evaluation

- Confirm elevated BPs by manual auscultation (oscillometric devices tend to overestimate), using the correct BP cuff size and measurement technique.
- 24-hour ambulatory blood pressure monitoring (ABPM) should be performed if available to confirm office BP readings and rule out white coat HTN.
- Screening laboratory studies for all patients: BMP, urinalysis with microscopy, lipid panel, kidney/bladder ultrasound (in children <6 years old, or older children with abnormal urinalysis or kidney function)
- In obese children, screen for comorbidities: Hemoglobin A1c (diabetes), AST/ALT (fatty liver disease), and fasting lipid panel (dyslipidemia)
- Additional studies, depending on differential diagnosis: CBC, thyroid-stimulating hormone, plasma renin and aldosterone activity, plasma metanephrines, drug screen, sleep study, DMSA renal scan, abdominal CT or MR angiography
- Echocardiography: Assess for end-organ damage (left ventricular hypertrophy)

## Treatment

- Goals for HTN management should be reduction in BP to <90th percentile for age, sex, and height, or <130/80 for adolescents ≥13 years old.
- Nonpharmacologic therapy: Dietary modification (e.g., low-sodium, plant-based diet), weight loss, increased physical activity (exercise 3-5 times per week, 30-60 minutes per session), and smoking cessation.
- Pharmacologic therapy: For children who remain hypertensive despite a trial of nonpharmacologic therapy, HTN associated with CKD or diabetes mellitus, or stage 2 HTN without a modifiable factor such as overweight/obesity.
- Most common first-line agents include calcium channel blockers, ACEI/ARBs, and thiazide diuretics.
- β-Blockers are not recommended for initial treatment.
- ACEI/ARBs are contraindicated in pregnancy and in children with bilateral renal artery stenosis due to risk of AKI.

- A stepwise approach is useful. Begin one medication at a low dose and increase until BP is controlled, the maximum dose is reached, or side effects occur. Failing adequate control, add a second agent and proceed as above.
- Severe HTN (hypertensive crisis)
  - Traditionally categorized as hypertensive emergency (with evidence of life-threatening symptoms of HTN or acute end-organ injury) and hypertensive urgency (without symptoms or acute end-organ injury), though this is arbitrary.
  - Acute, severe HTN most commonly manifests as altered mental status, coma, or seizures (hypertensive encephalopathy). Can also have end-organ injury to the eyes (papilledema, retinal hemorrhage), heart (heart failure), or kidneys (AKI).
  - Children should be immediately referred to the emergency department for any of the following:
    - Stage 2 HTN with serious symptoms.
    - BP > 30 mm Hg above the 95th percentile for children under age 13.
    - BP > 180/120 in an adolescent.
  - Initial management involves stabilization of airway, breathing, and circulation (due to risk of rapidly developing altered mental status, seizures, or heart failure), confirmation of BP elevation, and assessment for end-organ injury.
  - Hypertensive emergency: Goal is to lower BP to a value that causes symptoms to stop and prevents further end-organ damage: typically systolic BP < 95th percentile for age, sex, and height in children under age 13 or <130/80 in adolescents.
  - Treatment should be in a controlled fashion, using IV bolus and continuous IV infusion medications.
    - Nicardipine and labetalol are preferred to hydralazine (less predictable response to IV bolus dosing) or nitroprusside (may increase ICP, risk of cyanide toxicity with prolonged use or with kidney injury).
    - **BP should be lowered by no more than 25% of anticipated total systolic BP reduction in the first 8 hours** (e.g., if starting systolic BP is 210 mm Hg and goal is 130 mm Hg, the systolic BP should be no lower than 190 mm Hg after 8 hours).
    - Rapid lowering of BP is associated with irreversible end-organ damage, including permanent neurologic injury, myocardial ischemia, and AKI.
  - Hypertensive urgency: Goal BP is the same as for any hypertensive child (<90th percentile for age, sex, and height if under age 13, or <130/80 in adolescents).
    - For children with acute HTN, IV boluses of labetalol or hydralazine, or a continuous IV nicardipine infusion, can be used.
    - For children with chronic HTN, BP should be lowered more slowly using oral medications.

## SUGGESTED READINGS

Adrogué HJ, Madias NE. Hypernatremia. N Engl J Med 2000;342(20):1493–1499.

Adrogué HJ, Madias NE. Hyponatremia. N Engl J Med 2000;342(21):1581–1589.

Feld LG, Kaskel FJ, eds. Fluid and Electrolytes in Pediatrics: A Comprehensive Handbook. New York: Springer, 2010.

Feld LG, Neuspiel DR, Foster BA, et al. Clinical practice guideline: Maintenance intravenous fluids in children. Pediatrics 2018;142(6):e20183083.

Flynn JT, Kaelber DC, Baker-Smith CM, et al. Clinical practice guideline for screening and management of high blood pressure in children and adolescents. Pediatrics 2017;140(3):e20171904.

Geary DF, Schaefer F, eds. Pediatric Kidney Disease. 2nd Ed. Berlin: Springer-Verlag, 2016.

King CK, Glass R, Bresee JS, et al. Managing acute gastroenteritis among children: Oral rehydration, maintenance, and nutritional therapy. MMWR Recomm Rep 2003;52(RR-16):1–16.

Leung J, Crook M. Disorders of phosphate metabolism. J Clin Pathol 2019;72(11):741–747.

Lietman SA, Germain-Lee EL, Levine MA. Hypercalcemia in children and adolescents. Curr Opin Pediatr 2010;22(4):508–515.

Nadar R, Shaw N. Investigation and management of hypocalcaemia. Arch Dis Child 2020;105(4):399–405.

Rose BD, Post TW, eds. Clinical Physiology of Acid–base and Electrolyte Disorders. 5th Ed. New York: McGraw-Hill, 2001.

Viera AJ, Wouk N. Potassium disorders: Hypokalemia and hyperkalemia. Am Fam Physician 2015;92(6):487–495.

Viteri B, Reid-Adam J. Hematuria and proteinuria in children. Pediatr Rev 2018;39(12):573–587.

Wang CS, Greenbaum LA. Nephrotic syndrome. Pediatr Clin North Am 2019;66(1):73–85.

Wenderfer SE, Gaut JP. Glomerular diseases in children. Adv Chronic Kidney Dis 2017;24(6):364–371.

# **Palliative Care**

Will Johansen and Joan L. Rosenbaum

"You matter because you are you. You matter to the last moment of your life, and we will do all we can, not only to help you die peacefully, but also to live until you die."

—Dame Cicely Saunders

Palliative care has a growing evidence base and requires clinicians to draw on a distinct set of communication skills. Patients with advanced and often incurable diseases are dealing with the emotional impact of a life-limiting illness, treatment decisions that are complex and frequently involve consideration of clinical trials, and the challenges of sustaining hope while also having realistic goals. Patients feel emotionally supported when their doctor shows care for them as a person, by spending enough time with them, allowing them to ask questions, and listening to their concerns. Providers can show emotional support by using specific language that expresses empathy, which is simply acknowledging the presence of a patient's emotion concerns. Providers can show emotional support by listening and using specific language, as outlined below.

## NURSE STATEMENTS (SEE TABLE 26-1)

- Use this mnemonic to respond to a patient/family's emotional statement.
- The goal is to validate the emotion, not to fix/quiet the emotion.
- Be ready to expect more emotion after using a NURSE statement.
- This is not a mnemonic that has to be followed in chronological order. You choose which statements you want to use as they fit your style.
- Examples of emotional statements:
  - "I'm just so nervous about what the scans may show."
  - "This headache is killing me!"
  - "It's tearing me apart that I can't feed my baby."
  - "You have absolutely no idea what I'm going through!"
- **N**—Name the emotion. Make sure you are not telling the patient what emotion they are showing.
  - "It sounds like you are very anxious about these scans."
  - "It sounds like this headache has been very frustrating."
  - "It sounds like not being able to feed your baby is very sad."
  - "It sounds like this has all been very difficult."
- **U**—Understand. This shows the patient/family you are trying to comprehend what they're going through.
  - "I imagine this must be very scary to be waiting for those scans."
  - "I bet it's so hard to be in pain like that."
  - "I can't imagine how frustrating it is to not be able to feed your baby."
- **R**—Respect. This is a way to praise the patient/family

| TABLE 26-1 | NURSE Statements for Responding to Emotions | |
|---|---|---|
| | Examples | Notes |
| Naming | "It sounds like you are frustrated" | In general, turn down the intensity a notch when you name the emotion |
| Understanding | "This helps me understand what you are thinking" | Think of this as another kind of acknowledgment but stop short of suggesting you understand everything (you don't) |
| Respecting | "I can see have really been trying to follow our instructions" | Remember that praise also fits in here, e.g., "I think you have done a great job with this" |
| Supporting | "I will do my best to make sure you have what you need" | Making this kind of commitment is a powerful statement |
| Exploring | "Could you say more about what you mean when you say that…" | Asking a focused question prevents this from seeming too obvious |

From VitalTalk. NURSE statements for articulating empathy. Available at http://williamwolff.org/wp-content/uploads/2018/08/nurse-statements.pdf and vitaltalk.org. Accessed August 24, 2021. Copyright © 2021 Vital Talk. All rights reserved.

- "You are really brave for being able to go through this."
- "I'm really impressed with your ability to deal with these headaches for so long."
- "Thank you for being so involved with your child's care. It's obvious you care a great deal for (patient's name)."
- "It takes a lot of strength and love to be the parent of a child who is sick."
- **S**—Support. This shows that you are willing support and follow-up with the patient/family and that they won't be abandoned.
  - "I'll come back once the scans are done to discuss what our next steps will be."
  - "I'll be back in the morning to check in on you and your child."
  - "I'll stop by once (an intervention) is done to see how (patient's name) is doing."
- E—Explore. This allows the patient/family to further explain their thoughts/concerns/worries.
  - "Tell me more."
- There are also best practice recommendations that are helpful to clinicians in giving bad news. The SPIKES protocol provides a stepwise framework for difficult discussions. These can be practiced and successfully taught in a safe setting for learners.

## SPIKES

- Use this mnemonic when you need structure in delivering bad news. It works best when followed in chronologic order.
  - **S**—Setup/Start

- ○ This is done BEFORE you meet the patient/family.
- ○ Review medical chart to have an idea of medically what has happened, what is currently happening, and what tentative plans are happening in the future.
- ○ Create a suitable environment for the conversation. The more quiet, more private and less distractions the better.
- ○ Determine who should be present. Ex: a member of your team, a member of a consultant team (if appropriate), bedside nurse, chaplain, social worker, etc.
- ○ Review the goals of the meeting w/ your team and then again once the family is present. This provides structure to the discussion and prepares your team and the family for what to expect.
  - – "We are meeting today because we wanted to discuss the results of CJ's most recent imaging."
- **P**—Perception
- ○ Assess the family's medical education level so you know best to communicate information to them.
- ○ Assess what the patient/family knows about the current medical situation and be aware of possible patient/parent misinterpretations of previous information which will need to be corrected prior to delivering bad news.
  - – "Let's make sure we are all on the same page. What have you been told thus far?"
- **I**—Invitation
- ○ Start w/a "warning shot" so the family can prepare themselves BEFORE you break the bad news.
- ○ Asking permission BEFORE you break the bad news givens the family a sense of control of a situation that otherwise is relatively uncontrollable to them.
  - – "I do have some serious news to discuss w/ you. Would that be alright?"
- **K**—Knowledge
- ○ When you deliver the bad news, do so in a "headline" format, meaning it should be direct, concise, and w/o medical jargon. Make sure you allow time/space for family to process and ask if they have any questions.
  - – "CJ's head imaging has raised concern for a mass in his brain."
  - – "You've just received some very heavy information. What questions can I answer?"
- **E**—Emotion
- ○ You should expect an emotional response after you deliver bad news.
- ○ Use your "NURSE" statements to respond/validate that emotion.
- ○ Make sure you respond to the emotion in the room BEFORE trying to move on and provide more medical information/plans.
- **S**—Summarize
- ○ This is the wrap up where you summarize the meeting.
- ○ Recommend a plan moving forward. This again gives structure to the discussion and give the patient/family something to expect/look forward to.
- ○ Continue to ask if there are any questions and let patient/family know that you will be there to support them.
  - – "To summarize, CJ's most recent head imaging is concerning for a mass in his brain. Moving forward, we will have our Neurosurgery and Oncology teams come speak with you and we will continue to closely watch CJ here in the hospital and keep him safe and comfortable."

## PAIN

Pain is one of the most common symptoms experienced by children receiving palliative care and a cause of distress for parents and loved ones. A child's pain may represent a complex mix of physical, psychological, social, and spiritual factors, which must all be considered in order to manage effectively. Pain management plans should be developed with patient and family goals of care in mind.

- Definition—unpleasant sensory and/or emotional experience associated w/ actual or potential tissue damage or described in terms of such damage.
- There are several different assessment tools for pain based on patient age, comorbid conditions, etc. The following mnemonic is useful when asking about a pain history in a patient.
  - "PQRST"
    - P—Palliative/provocative factors
    - Q—Quality (stabbing, burning, dull, etc.)
    - R—Region/radiation
    - S—Severity/scale (1-10).
    - T—Temporal factors
  - Nociceptive
    - Somatic
      - Typically associated w/ well-localized/focal pain
      - Examples—postoperative incision, tumor invasion into soft tissue, arthritis, bed sore, etc.
      - Descriptors—sharping, aching, throbbing, stabbing, or squeezing
    - Visceral
      - Typically associated with some type of noxious stimuli regarding a hollow organ
      - This pain is typically NOT well localized/focal in nature
      - Examples—constipation causing abdominal pain, a tumor pressing on the small intestine, bowel ischemia
      - Descriptors—cramping, gnawing, squeezing, or pressure
    - Management
      - Typically start with acetaminophen and NSAIDs before moving on to opiates and/or muscle relaxers.
      - Muscle relaxer
        - Methocarbamol
          - MOA—not fully understood; however, may inhibit acetylcholinesterase
          - Side effects—drowsiness, dizziness, respiratory depression
          - Dose = (15 mg/kg), IV/PO, q8h. Max dose = 1000 mg/day and do NOT use >3 days if in IV formulation
        - Tizanidine
          - MOA—alpha-2 agonist which will increase the inhibition on presynaptic neurons resulting in less spasticity
          - Side effects—dizziness, drowsy, weakness, nausea, dry mouth
          - Dose = (2-4 mg), PO, tid
        - Diazepam
          - MOA—potentiates GABA
          - Side effects—drowsiness, dizziness, confusion, respiratory depression

- Dose = (0.1 mg/kg), PO, PRN q4-6h. Max = 10 mg/dose
  – Opiates—most will have the same MOA of agonizing the Mu-receptor agonism, which inhibits presynaptic calcium channel peptides resulting in less release of excitatory neurotransmitters which deliver the message of pain to the cerebral cortex
    - Most will also have a similar side effect profile consisting of constipation, urinary retention, respiratory depression, itchiness, nausea, vomiting, and confusion.
    - Morphine
      - PO = 0.2-0.5 mg/kg, PRN q4-6h
      - IV = 0.1 mg/kg, PRN q4-6h (max 2-4 mg)
    - Hydromorphone
      - PO = 0.03-0.08 mg/kg, PRN q4-6h
      - IV = 0.01 mg/kg, PRN q4-6h
    - Oxycodone
      - PO = 0.05-0.2 mg/kg, PRN q4-6h
- Neuropathic
  ○ Central
    – Typically due to repeated or extremely intense stimulation of the CNS pain pathway
    – Examples—multiple sclerosis, phantom limb pain, chronic pain syndromes, etc.
  ○ Peripheral
    – Usually due to some irritant (i.e., toxin, trauma, ischemia, etc.) of the peripheral nervous system.
    – Examples—chemotherapy-induced polyneuropathy, diabetic neuropathy, postherpetic neuralgia, HIV, etc.
  ○ Descriptors—tingling, shock/electric-like, paresthesia, allodynia, hyperalgesia, etc.
    – Allodynia—pain from a nonnoxious stimulus (i.e., light touch).
    – Hyperalgesia—pain response that is out of proportion to a painful stimulus.
  ○ Management
    – Gabapentin
      - MOA—mimics GABA; however, it will cause inhibition of voltage-gated calcium channels to modulate pain messages.
      - Side effects—dizziness, sleepiness, nausea, vomiting, and abnormal vision.
      - Dose = 10-15 mg/kg, PO, tid. Typically start at daily and titrate upward to tid. Max = 3600 mg/day.
    – Pregabalin
      - MOA—mimics GABA; however, it will cause inhibition of voltage-gated calcium channels to modulate pain messages.
      - Side effects—headache, sleepiness, dizziness
      - Dose = 50 mg, PO, tid
    – TCAs (amitriptyline)
      - MOA—blocks the reuptake of serotonin and norepinephrine neurotransmitters
      - Side effects—nausea, vomiting, drowsiness, constipation, prolonged QTC, vision problems
      - Dose = 0.1 mg/kg, PO, nightly. Max = 1 mg/kg

- Total pain
  - The psychological, social, emotional, spiritual, and physical experience of pain; each domain contributing in a specific way to the individual pain experience.
  - Sometimes coined as "existential suffering." Note that this type of suffering is resistant to pharmacologic analgesia alone.
- Nausea and vomiting
  - The vomiting center (VC) of the brain is the relay station for nausea and vomiting. There are several pathways that lead to the VC, and it is key to determine which one(s) are at work to best create an antiemesis treatment plan.
    - Note that the VC lies at the base of the 4th ventricle OUTSIDE of the blood brain barrier.
  - It is useful to know which chemoreceptors are present in each of the nausea and vomiting pathways to understand why certain medications are used to target them.
    - VC chemoreceptors: H-1, Ach, and 5HT-2.
  - Cortical
    - Anxiety can cause anticipatory nausea prior to a medical intervention/medication administration. Pretreat w/ therapy and/or PRN benzodiazepine.
      – Lorazepam (0.5-1 mg), PO, PRN q4h
    - CNS tumors increased intra-cranial pressure, and/or meningeal irritation can cause nausea and vomiting alongside of other neurological findings.
    - Chemoreceptors: stimulation from CTZ and VC.
  - Vestibular/middle ear
    - Vestibular disease can present as vertigo or nausea and vomiting which is exacerbated w/ movement of the head. Treat w/ Meclizine.
      – Meclizine (25-50 mg), PO, PRN daily
    - Motion sickness can be a cause of N/V and is typically treated w/a Scopolamine patch.
      – Scopolamine patch (1 mg), q72h
    - Chemoreceptors: NK-1, H-1, and Ach.
  - Chemoreceptor Trigger Zone (CTZ)
    - Medications (i.e., chemotherapy, opiates, antibiotics, etc.) can cause this, and down-titration/rotation of each (if possible) should be attempted before adding more medications on to control nausea and vomiting.
    - Metabolic derangements (i.e., uremia, azotemia, hypo-Na, hyper-Ca, etc.) can result in nausea and vomiting.
    - Chemoreceptors: 5HT-3 and D-2.
      – Tx—Haloperidol (0.5-1 mg), PO, PRN q4h
      – Tx—Olanzapine (2.5-5 mg), PO, daily/bid
  - GI Tract
    - Mechanoreceptors play a large role in this pathway as they respond to GI irritation (i.e., ulcers, bleeding, gastritis, etc.) and/or visceral stretch/compression (i.e., obstruction from stool burden, tumor burden, etc.).
    - Chemoreceptors: vagus nerve, H-1 and 5HT-3
      – Tx—Ondansetron (0.15 mg/kg), PO, PRN q6h. Max = 8 mg

## END OF LIFE (FIG. 26-1)

Relief of suffering is a core principle of pediatric palliative and is a primary responsibility of the entire interdisciplinary palliative care team as end-of-life approaches.

This requires recognition of the signs that end of life is near and expertise in pain and symptom management.

## Symptoms/Physical Examination

- The time frame(s) over which death is occurring have different physical examination findings associated with each.
  - *Acutely dying* means ≥48 hours prior to death.
  - *Actively dying* meant <48 hours prior to death.
- Pulmonary
  - Diagnosis
    - Dyspnea—this is a subjective feeling of breathlessness. NOT the same as hypoxia (an objective measurement) or tachypnea.
    - The rate can be variable (fast, slow, both) and eventually absent.
      - Apnea—typically ≥10 seconds of not breathing.
    - The sound:
      - Agonal—gasping/labored breathing
      - Noisy breathing—moaning/groaning sound with some "wet" sounds. Likely due to secretion buildup and weakening of the upper respiratory musculature
  - Management
    - Opiates are the primary medication to use for EOL pulmonary symptoms, primarily dyspnea. Note that typically these medications will NOT drastically change the rate or sound(s) of the pulmonary system as it shuts down.
      - MOA—decrease chemoreceptor response to hypercapnia effectively altering the patient's perception of dyspnea. May also cause vasodilation causing reduction in cardiac preload and decreasing pulmonary congestion
      - Side effects—nausea, vomiting, sedation, constipation
      - Morphine (0.05 mg/kg), IV/PO, q4h w/ PRN q1h
    - Benzodiazepines can assist with anxiety management which can exacerbate dyspnea.
      - MOA—potentiates GABA receptors in the CNS to decrease nervous excitation
      - Side effects—sedation, paradoxical reaction
      - Ativan (0.05 mg/kg), IV/PO, q4h w/ PRN q1h. Maximum of 2 mg/dose
    - Anti-cholinergic medications can assist with secretion management by drying them up.
      - MOA—blocks acetylcholine at parasympathetic sites at several sites (including salivary glands) resulting in decreased rate of saliva production.
      - Side effects—urinary retention, constipation, delirium (excluding glycopyrrolate, which does not cross the blood/brain barrier).
      - Glycopyrrolate (0.2-0.4 mg), SQ/IV, PRN q3h.
      - Atropine 1% ophthalmic solution, 1-4 drops sublingually, q4h.
    - Fans to assist with J-receptors modulation can be beneficial.
- Cardiovascular
  - Diagnosis
    - Color change typically occurs distally before it occurs proximally.
    - Variable pattern of color change; however, a common one is mottled → cyanotic → grey.
    - Rate variability. A common pattern is tachycardia → bradycardic → pulseless.
- Gastrointestinal

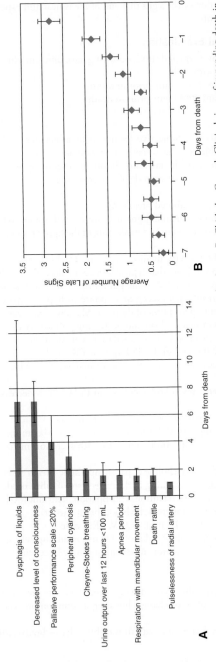

**Figure 26-1. A and B.** Timeline of end-of-life symptoms. (Reprinted from Hui D, dos Santos R, Chisholm G, et al. Clinical signs of impending death in cancer patients. Oncologist 2014;19(6):681–687, by permission of Oxford University Press.)

○ Diagnosis
  – Look for signs of decreasing muscle mass and adiposity, especially around the temporal region of the face.
  – Overall slowing of GI transit; however, even without PO intake, there still can be stool from sloughing of the intestinal lining.
  – The body's demand for nutrition/hydration diminishes progressively as death approaches.
○ Management
  – Tapering down/discontinuing nutrition (typically TPN).
  – Allow patient to eat for comfort if they so choose. This will unlikely be the case they approach closer to death.

• Neurologic
○ Progressive decline in level of alertness/awareness. Sleepy → Lethargic → Obtunded.
○ Delirium, hallucinations, myoclonus, seizures, etc. may all occur. This can be dependent on the underlying disease(s) that are currently ongoing w/ the patient (i.e., CNS lesions, electrolyte imbalances, etc.).
○ Pain is assumed to be a part of the dying process, even without a focal source.
○ Management (primarily for terminal delirium)
  – Anti-dopaminergic medications are the main stay of treatment. It is very important to determine route(s) you have available to you with which to administer these drugs.
    - MOA—antagonism of D2-receptors in the CNS
    - Side effects—sleepiness, urinary retention, rigidity, prolonged QTC, tardive dyskinesia, neuroleptic malignant syndrome
    - Haldol (0.05-0.15 mg/kg), IV/IM, PRN q1h (max dose of 5 mg)
    - Zyprexa (2.5-5 mg), PO, daily-bid

• Dermatology
○ Color change to be expected (see Cardiology section).
○ Skin breakdown not uncommon as the body shuts down and enters the dying process.
○ Providing hydration to dry skin/chapped lips can be very therapeutic for both the patient as well as the care giver(s).

## HOSPICE AND PALLIATIVE CARE

Hospice care is similar to palliative care. Both are meant to bring comfort and relief from pain, but they differ in some important ways. As a general pediatrician caring for children with complex medical illness, it is important have a good idea of what each service offers.

• Palliative care is:
  • a philosophy and an organized method which improves quality of life of children and families facing life-threatening illness
  • Accomplished through prevention and relief of suffering by:
    ○ early identification of care issues
    ○ care coordination
    ○ treatment of pain and other problems
    ○ attention to psychological/emotional, social, *educational*, and spiritual issues
• Hospice is for someone:

- whose goal for treatments is to enhance comfort and quality of remaining life, not to cure
- whose prognosis is <6 months based on the clinical judgment of their attending physician and a hospice medical director
- Covered benefit includes:
  - care from nurses, physicians, home health aides, social workers, bereavement and spiritual counselors, volunteers, and therapists
  - equipment related to hospice diagnosis and needed to provide comfort: (hospital bed, oxygen, wheelchair, pads/air mattresses, nebulizers)
  - medications related to hospice diagnosis (primary and secondary) needed to provide comfort
- What are the types of hospice care levels?
  - Routine home care
    - Routine care provided in the patient's home/residence.
    - Ex: A baby diagnosed w/ holoprosencephaly who is clinically stable gets a home nursing visit once per week from a hospice nurse and hospice social worker to provide support and complete a clinical assessment.
  - General inpatient care
    - Used primarily for control of an acute symptom exacerbation (such as pain) or to support the active phase of dying.
    - This typically is done at a hospice inpatient facility, hospital or nursing home.
    - Ex: A young girl w/ DIPG is transferred to the hospital when she had progressively declining levels of consciousness, likely due to disease progression/dying. Her family previously had said that it would be "too much" for them for her to pass away at home.
  - Continuous home care
    - Intended for extended periods of crisis management of acute symptoms w/ the goal of keeping patients in the home setting.
    - This is NOT 24-hour nursing care.
    - Ex: A teenage girl w/ progressive gliosarcoma appears to be in the active phase of dying but has been having more episodes of pain/agitation, so a hospice nurse is called out to the home to assess and likely make some changes to the patient's PCA. After discussion w/ the hospice physician on call, they determine the need for intense symptom management, which will require her to be the bedside for an extended period of time.
  - Respite care
    - This level of care allows for the caregivers of a patient (whose symptoms are currently well-controlled) enrolled on hospice to have some relief.
    - Typically covers a brief (no more than 5 consecutive days) admission to a hospital, in patient unit, or nursing home.
    - Ex: A young man w/ adrenoleukodystrophy (whose symptoms are at his normal baseline) is admitted to the hospital so his mother can attend the graduation of her oldest child in another state.
- Documentation:
  - Medicare hospice has two initial 90-day certification periods with potentially unlimited additional 60-day certification periods thereafter if patient continues to meet hospice eligibility criteria.
  - Face-to-face visit.
  - Private insurance and medicaid hospice can vary.
  - Patients are discussed in Interdisciplinary Team meetings at least every 2 weeks, and plan of care is adjusted as needed and communicated to attending physician.

## SUGGESTED READINGS

Acquaviva KD. LGBTQ-Inclusive Hospice and Palliative Care: a Practical Guide to Transforming Professional Practice. Harrington Park Press, 2017.

Back A, et al. Mastering Communication with Seriously Ill Patients: Balancing Honesty with Empathy and Hope. Cambridge University Press, 2010.

CCHMC PACT. Palliative Service Medication Dosing Guide. Publisher is CCHMC (Cincinnati Children's Medical Center). Updated 2017.

Friebert SE. Pediatric Hospice and Palliative Care America. NHPCO, 2015.

Friebert SE, et al. Palliative Care for Infants, Children, and Adolescents: A Practical Handbook. Johns Hopkins University Press, 2011.

Hauer JM. Caring for Children Who Have Severe Neurological Impairment: A Life with Grace. The Johns Hopkins University Press, 2013:48–80.

Heneghan C, et al. Pediatric Palliative Care Approach to Pain and Symptom Management (Dana Farber Cancer Institute/Boston Children's Hospital). 2020.

McPherson MLM. Demystifying Opioid Conversion Calculations: A Guide for Effective Dosing. American Society of Health-System Pharmacists, 2019.

Shega JW, Paniagua MA. Essential Practices in Hospice and Palliative Medicine. AAHPM, 2017.

Twycross A, et al. Managing Pain in Children: A Clinical Guide for Nurses and Healthcare Professionals. Wiley-Blackwell, 2014.

Wolfe J, et al. Textbook of Interdisciplinary Pediatric Palliative Care. Elsevier/Saunders, 2011.

# Pulmonary Diseases

Cadence Kuklinski and Katherine Rivera-Spoljaric

## CROUP (VIRAL LARYNGOTRACHEOBRONCHITIS)

### Definition and Epidemiology

- Croup, or viral laryngotracheobronchitis, is an acute inflammation of the entire airway, mainly in the glottic and subglottic areas, resulting in airway narrowing, obstruction, and voice loss. Therefore, it has generally been described as a triad of hoarse voice, harsh barking cough, and inspiratory stridor.
- Typically, the condition affects younger children (6-36 months), with a peak incidence at 2 years of age and uncommon >6 years of age. It is the most common cause of acute upper airway obstruction in young children.
- Seasonal outbreaks occur in the fall and winter, although may occur year-round in some areas.
- Males are more commonly affected than females and are more likely to be hospitalized.

### Etiology and Pathophysiology

- Viral infection is the predominant etiology; parainfluenza virus (types 1 [most common], 2, and 3) (more severe) is the most common agent. Other viral agents associated with the development of croup are coronavirus respiratory syncytial virus (RSV), adenovirus, influenza virus, rhinovirus, and enterovirus.
- *Mycoplasma pneumoniae* is one of the few bacterial microorganisms that has been reported as an etiologic agent.
- In children, the larynx is narrow and is composed by the rigid ring of the cricoid cartilage; a viral infection causing inflammation of this area leads to airway edema and subsequent obstruction. This obstruction results in the classic symptoms of stridor and cough.

### Clinical Presentation

- Croup usually presents initially with a coryzal prodrome (1-4 days).
- Common symptoms include clear rhinorrhea, low-grade temperature, and mild tachypnea followed by barking cough, hoarseness, and stridor.
- Obstructive symptoms occur most commonly at night.
- Severity of airway narrowing may be determined by the presence of stridor at rest, tachypnea, retractions, tracheal tug, cyanosis, and pallor as well as decreased breath sounds, which indicate critical narrowing.

### Diagnosis

- The diagnosis is clinical.
- Radiography of the neck is not necessary but may show the typical "steeple sign" or subglottic narrowing. Radiographic appearance does not correlate with disease severity.

- Radiographs should be obtained if there is concern about the diagnosis, and they may distinguish croup from other causes of upper airway obstruction such as epiglottitis or foreign body.
- Oxygen saturations should be obtained, and obtain blood gas measurement if there is evidence of significant hypoxemia or signs of restlessness, altered mental status, and/or cyanosis.
- The differential diagnosis includes epiglottitis (but the patient is usually toxic appearing), spasmodic croup (no viral prodrome and mostly in atopic children), bacterial tracheitis, laryngitis, foreign body, and laryngospasm.

## Treatment

- A few clinical scoring systems that guide assessment and management have been described in the literature. The most commonly used is the Westley score system, which is described below:
  - Scores are given based on the presence of stridor (none 0, when agitated 1, at rest 2), retractions (none 0, mild 1, moderate 2, severe 3), level of air entry (normal 0, decreased 1, markedly decreased 2), cyanosis in room air (none 0, with agitation 4, at rest 5), and level of consciousness (normal 0, disoriented 5).
  - Mild croup is described as scores 1-2, moderate croup as scores 3-8, and severe croup as scores >8, with consideration of pharmacologic therapy and hospitalization in moderate and severe cases. And score >12 is consistent with impending respiratory failure.
- In general, patients without signs of severe airway narrowing or stridor at rest may be managed on an outpatient basis after appropriate observation. Parents should be reassured and instructed about signs of worsening respiratory distress.
- General supportive measures such as increased fluid intake, decreased handling, and careful observation are usually recommended.
- Management strategies may include use of cool mist vaporizer, cold air exposure when riding in a motor vehicle, and use of steam inhalation, although these methods are anecdotal and have not proved beneficial in reducing symptom scores during several studies.
- For children with evidence of stridor at rest and/or signs of moderate to severe airway compromise, pharmacologic therapy is indicated.
  - Patients with hypoxemia should be treated with humidified supplemental oxygen. There has not been an established benefit of high-flow oxygen over traditional nasal cannula.
  - Nebulized racemic epinephrine acts by reducing vascular permeability of the airway epithelium, therefore diminishing airway edema and improving airway caliber by decreasing resistance to airflow.
  - It should be administered at doses of 0.25-0.5 mL along with humidified oxygen as needed. If no response is elicited after the first treatment, the dose may be repeated.
  - The patient may return to pretreatment state 30-60 minutes after a dose, and therefore, he or she should be observed for at least 2-3 hours after administration due to "rebound phenomenon."
- Systemic corticosteroids are effective in reducing symptoms within 6 hours and for at least 12 hours after initial treatment.
  - Dexamethasone 0.6 mg/kg/dose IM, IV, PO single dose is the glucocorticoid most commonly used, but prednisolone 1-2 mg/kg/dose PO for 3 days is an alternative.
  - Studies have shown that high-dose nebulized budesonide (2 mg) is superior to placebo and as effective as dexamethasone in reducing symptom scores, but the cost-benefit ratio limits its use.

# EPIGLOTTITIS

## Definition and Epidemiology

- Epiglottitis represents a true pediatric emergency with acute infectious supraglottic obstruction that may rapidly lead to life-threatening airway obstruction.
- It affects children of all ages, with a peak around 3-6 years of age, although its incidence has declined significantly since *Haemophilus influenzae* type B immunization was introduced in 1998.

## Etiology and Pathophysiology

- *H. influenzae* type B is the most common cause in children, although its prevalence has markedly decreased in the postvaccine era. Other agents include group A *Streptococcus, H. influenzae* (types A, F, and nontypeable), *Staphylococcus aureus, Candida albicans,* and *Streptococcus pneumoniae.*
- Direct invasion by the inciting agent causes inflammation of the epiglottis, aryepiglottic folds, ventricular bands, and arytenoids. Subsequently, there is accumulation of inflammatory cells and edema fluid where the stratified squamous epithelium is loosely adherent to the anterior surface and the superior third of the posterior portion of the epiglottis.
- Diffuse infiltration with polymorphonuclear leukocytes, hemorrhage, edema, and fibrin deposition occurs. Microabscesses may form. As the edema increases, the epiglottis curls posteriorly and inferiorly. This causes airway obstruction.
- Inspiration tends to draw the inflamed supraglottic ring into the laryngeal inlet.

## Clinical Presentation

- Epiglottitis is a rapidly progressing illness, even in previously healthy individuals. Patients are usually anxious and toxic appearing and assume the classic "tripod position" (forward-leaning posture with bracing arms and extension of the neck that allows for maximal air entry).
- Other symptoms typically present are high fever, muffled or absent voice ("hot potato"), sore throat, drooling, inspiratory stridor, dysphagia, protruded jaw, and extended neck.

## Diagnosis

- Presumptive diagnosis should be made on clinical grounds.
- If patient is in little distress, and the diagnosis is unclear, a lateral neck radiograph may be obtained, which shows the classical thumbprint sign that represents a swollen epiglottis and aryepiglottic folds. Radiographs can be normal in 20% of the patients.
- The definitive diagnosis requires direct visualization of a red swollen epiglottis under laryngoscopy, but this examination should be attempted only in a controlled setting in collaboration with an anesthesiologist and an otolaryngologist.
- The differential diagnosis includes foreign body aspiration, anaphylactic reaction, angioedema, caustic ingestion, thermal injury, inhalation injury, and laryngotracheobronchial and retropharyngeal infection.

## Treatment

- Airway stabilization and maintenance must be performed quickly and early in the course.
- Oxygen should be administered at the onset of minimal sign of distress.

- Stimulation and patient disturbance should be minimized to avoid complete obstruction.
- An artificial airway should be available next to the patient, and it should always be ready for use.
- After appropriate management of the airway has been established, empiric intravenous (IV) antibiotic therapy against β-lactamase–producing pathogens should be initiated promptly. For severely ill patients, consider combination therapy with an antistaphylococcal agent active against MRSA.
- The use of IV glucocorticosteroids is controversial and not shown to be beneficial in the initial management; however, doses are frequently administered for the management of airway inflammation especially on patients that have had difficulty with extubation.

## BACTERIAL TRACHEITIS

### Definition and Epidemiology

- This acute bacterial infection of the trachea often also involves the larynx and bronchi. It has been called bacterial laryngotracheobronchitis and pseudomembranous croup.
- A cause of acute airway obstruction, this condition may potentially be life threatening.
- Most patients are <6 years of age, although older children may be affected. There is a slight male predominance.
- There seems to be no seasonal preference.

### Etiology and Pathophysiology

- The most common cause is *Staphylococcus aureus*, but other encountered agents are *Streptococcus pneumoniae*, *Streptococcus pyogenes*, *Moraxella catarrhalis*, and *H. influenzae*. Anaerobic organisms have also been reported.
- Invasion of opportunistic bacterial organisms, often following an upper airway viral infection, causes subglottic edema with ulcerations, copious and purulent secretions, and pseudomembrane formation.

### Clinical Presentation

- The typical presentation involves a history of an upper respiratory infection (URI) for approximately 3 days characterized by a low-grade fever and a "brassy" cough. The illness then evolves rapidly with high fever and signs of airway obstruction, including stridor, cough, drooling, and supine positioning (preference to lie flat).
- Patients generally appear toxic.
- There is also evidence of purulent airway secretions.

### Diagnosis

- Diagnosis is clinical. Direct visualization of the trachea via laryngoscopy demonstrates thick, abundant, and purulent secretions.
- The differential diagnosis includes epiglottitis (although no dysphagia, and patient may lie flat), croup (although voice is normal and there is a lack of a barky cough), and laryngeal and retropharyngeal abscess.

## Treatment

- Management of the airway is critical with intubation.
- There is no proven role for bronchodilators or corticosteroids.
- Antimicrobial therapy should be immediately instituted. Choice of therapy includes broad-spectrum antibiotics with antistaphylococcal activity.
- Management and treatment of tracheitis in patients with an existing tracheostomy may be different. Intubation is rarely needed, as patients can typically be supported via their tracheostomy with invasive ventilation. A tracheal aspirate may be obtained for cell count and culture. A tracheal aspirate with abundant polymorphonuclear lymphocytes (PMNs) may help to differentiate between active bacterial infection and colonization. If an active infection is determined to be present, antibacterial coverage should be guided by historical and current culture results.

## FOREIGN BODY ASPIRATION

### Definition and Epidemiology

- This occurs when an object is accidentally inhaled into the airway. It occurs more commonly in children <5 years of age but has been described at any age.
- Younger children are typically at higher risk because of oral exploration and immaturity of their swallowing functions.
- This situation may be life threatening; it is the leading cause of accidental death by ingestion in younger children.

### Etiology and Pathophysiology

- Ingested food and toy parts are aspirated into the airways.
  - A foreign body can be localized in the larynx, trachea, or bronchi.
  - Impaction of the larynx is particularly dangerous, although most particles travel well into the airways and lodge in the intrathoracic area.
- The foreign particle provokes localized airway inflammation with mucosal edema, inflammation, and over time can lead to the development of granulation tissue. Atelectasis of the area involved and empyema may occur.

### Clinical Presentation

- In general, following a witnessed aspiration or choking episode, patients develop a loud persistent cough along with gagging and stridor. However, the symptoms manifested are largely dependent on the localization of the particle, its size, and its composition.
- Foreign bodies in the larynx may cause hoarseness, aphonia, croupy cough, odynophagia, wheezing, and difficulty breathing, depending on the degree of obstruction.
- Foreign bodies in the trachea can cause what has been described as an audible slap, a palpable thud, and wheezing.
- Foreign bodies in the bronchus usually are manifested by coughing and wheezing.
- Regardless of the position of the foreign body, if the event is unwitnessed and the particle remains lodged in the airway for a prolonged period of time, the patient usually develops a chronic cough, with or without wheeze that is often mistakenly treated as asthma.
- Hemoptysis may be a sign of airway injury.
- There is no fever associated such as in acute infectious airway obstruction.

- Position of the patient has no effect on the degree of airway obstruction, as in epiglottitis.
- Asymmetric findings on chest auscultation may provide a diagnostic clue but should not serve as an exclusion criterion.

## Diagnosis

- A history of the choking event sometimes can be elicited from parents. The diagnosis should also be entertained when a child exhibits unexplained symptoms that fail to respond to standard medical treatment, such as treatment for asthma or antibiotic therapy for suspected pneumonia.
- Radiography of the upper airway and the chest can be useful to confirm aspiration of a radiopaque particle, but if negative, should not exclude the possibility of foreign body aspiration.
- Inspiratory and expiratory chest films as well as a lateral decubitus view may show a "ball-valve" effect or persistent hyperinflation of the area suspected to be lodging the particle. Other radiographic findings may include persistent unilateral infiltrates or atelectasis.
- If suspicion is high, referral for laryngoscopy and rigid bronchoscopy is often the only method of visualizing (and removing) the foreign body.
- The differential diagnosis includes epiglottitis, viral laryngotracheobronchitis, bacterial tracheitis, asthma, pneumonia, airway malacia, and psychogenic cough.

## Treatment

- Management usually involves removal of the foreign body via bronchoscopy (typically rigid) for appropriate control of the airway.
- There is no established role for antibiotic or corticosteroid use.
- If the particle remains in the airway for a prolonged period of time, potential complications may arise, including bronchial stenosis, distal bronchiectasis, tracheoesophageal fistula, abscess formation, and airway lacerations or perforation.

# BRONCHIOLITIS

## Definition and Epidemiology

- Bronchiolitis is an acute infectious disease of the lower respiratory tract, specifically the small passages in the lungs (bronchioles), usually caused by a viral infection.
- It is usually most prominent during winter and early spring, with annual epidemics in temperate climates. However, sporadic infections can occur year-round.
- It occurs in the first 2 years of life (0-24 months), and it peaks at 6 months of age (2-8 months). It is more common in male infants (1.5:1), bottle-fed infants, infants living in crowded conditions, and infants with cigarette-smoking mothers.

## Etiology

- Etiology is predominantly viral. The most common source of the virus is a family member with a URI.
- The most common viral agents is RSV, followed by rhinovirus. Other causative agents include human metapneumovirus, parainfluenza, adenovirus, coronavirus, rhinovirus, and less frequently influenza.
  - RSV is spread primarily by direct contact of <6 feet distance with an infected person. Large droplets can survive up to 6 hours on surfaces and up to 30 minutes

in the hands. Therefore, frequent hand washing is essential for infection control. Virus shedding occurs for approximately 3-8 days, but in young infants, shedding may last 3-4 weeks.

- This infection is the leading cause of infant hospitalization and the leading cause of lower respiratory tract infection in infants and small children, with two-thirds of the infants infected in their 1st year and universal infection by 2 years of age. The mortality rate from RSV infection may be as high as 5% in high-risk patients.
- Reinfection is common because infection does not provide long-lasting immunity.
- Human metapneumovirus
- Infection occurs via aerosol or direct contact. Peaks in March and April.
- Parainfluenza virus
  - This virus is unstable in the environment, and spread occurs from respiratory secretions.
- Adenovirus
  - Survival outside of the body is prolonged, and transmission can occur via direct contact, the fecal-oral route, and occasionally water. Shedding can occur for months or years.
  - Infection is endemic in all seasons.
- Coronavirus
  - Can be spread through direct contact or aerosols. Most serotypes are fairly unstable in the environment.
  - Endemic throughout all seasons.
- Rhinovirus
  - Transmission is by aerosol or direct contact. Most cases are mild and self-limited, but shedding may last up to 3-4 weeks (peak, 2-7 days).
- The infection is endemic in all seasons.
- Influenza
  - Chiefly transmitted in the fall, winter, and early spring

## Pathophysiology

- Disease occurs by invasion of the smaller bronchioles by the viral particles followed by viral colonization and replication. Necrosis and sloughing of ciliated cells and proliferation of nonciliated cells follows, which leads to impaired clearance of secretions, submucosal edema, and congestion. The resulting plugging of bronchioles from mucus and debris and peripheral airway narrowing from edema causes small airway (bronchiole) obstruction and increased respiratory effort.
- The resulting changes to respiratory mechanics are characterized by increased functional residual capacity, decreased compliance, increased airway resistance, and increased physiologic dead space with increased shunt. Therefore, a ventilation-perfusion mismatch with impaired gas exchange occurs, resulting in hypoxia and $CO_2$ retention.
- Infants are particularly more susceptible to severe disease. Their airways are easily plugged by mucus or inflammatory debris because of their smaller diameter, relative increased number of mucous glands, and greater collapsibility in response to pressure changes. Additionally, their collateral pathways of ventilation (pores of Cohn and Lambert) are less well developed, increasing the risk of atelectasis.

## Clinical Presentation

- Usually, there is a history of exposure to URI within 1 week of onset of illness.
- First symptoms are usually a mild URI (1-4 days), decreased oral intake, and fever with gradual development of respiratory distress. If RSV is the etiology, symptoms usually peak at approximately the 5th day of illness.

- Patients develop a paroxysmal wheezy cough and dyspnea. In mild cases, symptoms last for approximately 1-3 days. Severe cases have a protracted course.
- Pertinent physical examination findings include tachypnea (60-80 breaths per minute), hyperexpanded chest, nasal flaring, use of accessory muscles, widespread fine crackles, prolonged expiration, diffuse wheezes, and decreased breath sounds.
- Risk factors for severe disease include prematurity, age <12 weeks, chronic pulmonary disease, congenital airway anomalies, congenital heart disease, immunodeficiency, neurologic diseases, and history of poor feeding.
- Infants born prematurely and those younger than 2 months may be at risk for apnea, which may be unrelated to respiratory distress.

## Diagnosis

- Diagnosis is based on clinical presentation.
- Aids to confirm diagnosis and predict the course of the illness include nasopharyngeal swab for viral diagnostics (enzyme-linked immunosorbent assay, direct fluorescent antibody, or PCR-based tests). Other less-timely approaches include viral culture and serology for viral antibodies.
- Routine radiographs are not recommended but may be helpful if there is suspicion of bacterial pneumonia.
  - Radiographic findings may include hyperinflation, increased anteroposterior chest diameter, peribronchial thickening, diffuse interstitial infiltrates, and atelectasis.
  - There is no correlation between radiographic findings and severity of illness. Ten percent of chest radiographs are normal.
- Complete blood counts and electrolytes are nonspecific and therefore not routinely recommended unless there is suspicion of sepsis or dehydration.
- Pulse oximetry is recommended to assess the degree of hypoxia and response to oxygen.
- Arterial oxygen saturation while feeding has been described as the single best objective predictor of severe disease in the literature. Blood gas sampling is recommended in severe respiratory disease to assess possible impending respiratory failure.
- The differential diagnosis includes asthma, cystic fibrosis (CF), myocarditis, congestive heart failure, foreign body or aspiration, pertussis, organophosphate poisoning, bacterial bronchopneumonia, *Mycoplasma* or *Chlamydia* infection, and anatomic abnormality.

## Treatment

- In general, the most important foundation for treatment is supportive care, careful monitoring, and minimal handling.
- Consider admission to the hospital if there is apnea, resting respiratory rate >70 breaths per minute, decreased arterial oxygen saturation (<95%), atelectasis on chest radiograph, or ill appearance. Hospitalization may also be appropriate for those at high risk of severe disease.
  - About 2-7% of infants with severe disease progress to respiratory failure and require intubation. Indications for intubation include severe respiratory distress, apnea, hypoxia or hypercapnia, lethargy, poor perfusion, and metabolic acidosis.
- Nonpharmacologic methods
  - Positioning. Usually, it is recommended that the patient be positioned at a sitting angle of 30-40 degrees, with slight head and chest elevation.
  - Assessment of hydration and fluid administration as needed.

- Saline nasal drops and mechanical aspiration of nares on a regular basis has shown effectiveness (decreased hospital stay).
- Cool, humidified oxygen supplementation as needed via nasal prongs or face mask to maintain oxygen saturation >90%.
- Chest physiotherapy has no role in the treatment of bronchiolitis.
- Pharmacologic methods
  - Bronchodilators (albuterol, levalbuterol, racemic epinephrine, ipratropium bromide)
    ○ Their use is controversial. Although some studies have shown improvement in clinical scores such as decreased respiratory rate and increased arterial oxygen saturation, there has been no significant decrease in hospitalization rate with the use of bronchodilator therapy.
  - Glucocorticoids
    ○ Use is also controversial. Dexamethasone has shown no beneficial effect when used as monotherapy in various studies.
  - Antibiotics
    ○ Secondary bacterial infection is uncommon; therefore, routine use of antibiotics is rarely indicated.
    ○ Use should be considered in persistently febrile young children given reports in the literature of bacteremia, UTI, and bacterial otitis media in children with bronchiolitis.
    ○ The use of azithromycin is being studied as an adjunct therapy to prevent the progression to recurrent wheezing and asthma in patients with RSV bronchiolitis early in life. However, this is not standard of care in the treatment of bronchiolitis.
  - Antivirals
    ○ Use is controversial. Consider inhaled ribavirin in high-risk infants. Ribavirin has virostatic activity; it interferes with messenger RNA and prevents replication of the virus. The American Academy of Pediatrics recommends its use based on an individual basis in patients with specific conditions such as complicated congenital heart disease, CF, chronic lung disease (CLD), underlying immunosuppression, and severe illness as well as in patients <6 weeks of age.
  - Nebulized hypertonic saline has been suggested as an agent to reduce airway edema and mucus plugs with some studies suggesting that this treatment can reduce length of stay and need for hospitalization; however, these findings have not been consistently replicated and therefore, its use remains controversial at this time.

### Prevention

- Most important method of prevention: frequent hand washing, along with hospital control measures (isolation), and patient education
- Pharmacologic methods
  - Palivizumab RSV prophylaxis
    ○ The American Academy of Pediatrics (2014) recommends its use for:
      - Infants born at ≤29 weeks of gestational age and <12 months at the start of RSV season
      - Infants ≤12 months of age with hemodynamically significant congenital heart disease
      - Infants and children <12 months of age with CLD of prematurity and <24 months of age with CLD of prematurity necessitating medical therapy (e.g., supplemental oxygen, bronchodilator, diuretic, or chronic steroid therapy) within 6 months prior to the beginning of RSV season

○ It also recommends to consider prophylaxis for:
  – Infants <12 months of age with congenital airway anomalies or neuromuscular disorder that decreases the ability to manage airway secretions
  – Infants <12 months of age with CF with clinical evidence of CLD and/or nutritional compromise
  – Children <24 months with CF with severe lung disease (previous hospitalization for pulmonary exacerbation in the 1st year of life or anomalies on chest radiography or chest computed tomography that persist when stable) or weight for length less than the 10th percentile
  – Infants and children <24 months who are profoundly immunocompromised
  – Infants and children <24 months undergoing cardiac transplantation during RSV season
○ Prophylaxis should be initiated before the onset of the RSV season (beginning of November), and it should be terminated at the end of RSV season (beginning of March). Health care practitioners should individualize the season according to their area.
○ Palivizumab does not interfere with responses to vaccines.

## CYSTIC FIBROSIS

### Epidemiology

- CF is the most common life-shortening genetic disorder in the Caucasian population, with an estimated incidence of 1:2000-1:3000 live births in the United States and an estimated mean survival age of 36.8 years in the United States.
- CF occurs more often in northern Europeans and Ashkenazi Jews, but it is also present with less frequency in African Americans (1:15,000), Hispanics (1:9200), Native Americans (1:10,900), and Asians (1:30,000).

### Pathophysiology

- CF is an autosomal recessive disorder caused by mutations of both alleles of the CF gene (chromosome 7), resulting in abnormalities in the production of gene product CF transmembrane conductance regulator (CFTR).
- The most common mutation is a three-base pair deletion that encodes for phenylalanine at position 508 of the CF gene, or F508del, and at least one copy of this mutation is found in approximately 90% of patients with CF.
- CFTR allows chloride to be transported out of the cell to the epithelial surface and determine hydration of the mucous gel. Inadequate hydration of the gel is believed to cause inspissated secretions and organ damage. It affects the lungs, sinuses, liver, pancreas, and genitourinary tract. In the lungs, it impairs ciliary clearance, promoting bacterial infection, which accounts for most of the morbidity and mortality of the disease.
- There are five classes of CFTR mutations, which are disease causing. Class I and II generally cause more severe disease, with Class IV and V leading to more mild phenotypes. However,
  ○ Class I results in defective protein production. Premature termination of the mRNA results in a complete absence of CFTR protein. Common examples include G542X, W1282X, R553X, 621+G>T, and 1717-1G>A. A Class I mutation occurs in about 20% of patients with CF.
  ○ Class II leads to defective protein processing and prevents the CFTR protein from trafficking to the correct cellular location. The most common is F508del,

with approximately 50% of patients with CF being homozygous for that mutation, and about 90% of patients with CF having at least one copy.

- ○ Class III causes defective regulation and are also known as gating mutations and lead to the channel having a diminished response to ATP. The response can be variable and depends on the region of the gene that is altered. G551D is the most common Class III mutation in White populations.
- ○ Class IV results in defective conduction, meaning that although the protein is made and trafficked correctly, the rate of ion flow and duration of channel opening is reduced as compared to normal CFTR. R117H is the most common Class IV in White populations.
- ○ Class V results in a reduced amount of functional CFTR protein and can include mutations that alter the stability of the mRNA and those that reduce the stability of mature CFTR protein. A455E has been placed in Class V.
- ○ Class I, II, and III generally cause more severe disease, with Class IV and V leading to more mild phenotypes. However, there can be a wide variety of phenotypes even within the same genotype in CF, possibly because of the influence of gene modifiers. The correlation of genotype and phenotype is stronger for pancreatic function than it is for pulmonary disease.
- The major colonizing microorganisms are *Staphylococcus aureus*, *H. influenzae*, and *Escherichia coli* early in the disease; then *Pseudomonas aeruginosa*, *Stenotrophomonas maltophilia*, and *Achromobacter xylosoxidans*; and finally *Burkholderia cepacia* complex later in the disease. In this later complex, *Burkholderia cenocepacia* (genomovar III) accounts for increased morbidity and mortality in the CF population.

## Clinical Presentation

- The most common clinical manifestations involve the gastrointestinal and respiratory tract.
  - Gastrointestinal manifestations usually are evident early in life, with meconium ileus occurring in 20% of the neonates. Other common gastrointestinal manifestations include failure to thrive, steatorrhea, obstructive jaundice, rectal prolapse, and hypoproteinemia.
  - Respiratory manifestations become evident during the 1st years of life with recurrent respiratory tract infections (pneumonia, chronic sinusitis), cough, and wheezing that may be misinterpreted as asthma.
- Other clinical signs and symptoms that should prompt evaluation for CF include delayed passage of meconium (>24-48 hours after birth), meconium plug syndrome, prolonged cholestasis, distal intestinal obstruction, recurrent or chronic pancreatitis, nasal polyps, chronic sinusitis, allergic bronchopulmonary aspergillosis (ABPA), *Pseudomonas* bronchitis, spontaneous pneumothorax, hyponatremic dehydration, hypochloremic metabolic alkalosis, obstructive azoospermia (congenital bilateral absence of the vas deferens), hypertrophic osteoarthropathy, and digital clubbing.
- A CF pulmonary exacerbation is defined inconsistently in the literature, but in general, it is characterized by all or some of the following: increased cough, fever, changes in spirometry (change in $FEV_1 > 10\%$), change in activity level, decreased appetite, weight loss, new findings on chest radiograph (increased mucous plugging or new infiltrates), new adventitious sounds on auscultation (new rales), change in respiratory rate, exercise intolerance, school or work absenteeism, increased sputum production, and hemoptysis.

## Diagnosis

- Most cases of CF are now diagnosed by newborn screening, which is conducted in all 50 states. All states test for a chemical made by the pancreas, called immunoreactive trypsinogen (IRT), which is found normally in the body, but tends to found at elevated levels in people with CF.
  - IRT can also be elevated with prematurity, stressful delivery, or other GI conditions. Some states follow up an elevated IRT with DNA tests, looking for the most common CF-causing genes.
- The gold standard for diagnosing CF continues to be two positive sweat chloride tests using pilocarpine iontophoresis (60 mmol/L) along with classic clinical findings and a history of CF in an immediate family member.
  - False-positive sweat test results are uncommon but may occur in the presence of adrenal insufficiency, nephrogenic diabetes insipidus, type I glycogen storage disease, hypothyroidism, hypoparathyroidism, familial cholestasis, and malnutrition.
- Almost all patients with CF undergo genotyping for CFTR mutations (two mutations confirm the diagnosis), as the presence of certain mutations can help to guide treatment.
  - Additional testing in the workup of CF includes a computed tomography scan of sinuses demonstrating pansinusitis, 24-hour fecal fat measurement looking for signs of pancreatic insufficiency, and ultrasound to assess absence of the vas deferens in males.
- CFTR-related disease include diseases that are associated with CFTR mutations but do not meet diagnostic criteria for CF including chronic pancreatitis, ABPA, idiopathic bronchiectasis, chronic sinusitis, and congenital bilateral absence of the vas deference.
- CFTR-related metabolic syndrome includes infants with abnormal newborn screening that subsequently show (1) intermediate sweat chloride level with one CF-causing mutation or (2) normal sweat chloride level with two CFTR mutations (one CF causing and one non-CF causing).

## Treatment

- Treatment goals include delaying or preventing lung disease, promoting good nutrition and growth, and treating complications.
- Maintenance treatment for patients with classic CF
  - Airway clearance. Daily airway clearance is one of the most important methods of prevention of respiratory tract infections.
    - There are many different methods, including manual chest physiotherapy, postural drainage, autogenic drainage, high-frequency chest oscillation vests, and manual percussion therapy.
    - Adjunctive therapies include the flutter valve and Acapella device.
    - The use of a specific method is mostly dependent on patient preferences; no studies demonstrate superiority of one method over another.
    - Dornase alfa promotes airway clearance by cleaving DNA released by degenerating neutrophils, thus decreasing mucus viscosity. Its use has been shown to improve pulmonary function. It should be considered in children 6 years and older as a daily inhalation (2.5 mg).
    - Hypertonic saline (7%) promotes airway clearance by hydrating inspissated airway mucus. It has shown to reduce frequency of pulmonary exacerbations. It should be considered in children 6 years and older.

- Optimization of nutrition. Nutritional failure has been proven to be closely related to increased morbidity and frequency of pulmonary exacerbations. Therefore, it is important to maintain adequate nutrition via encouragement of a high-calorie and high-protein diet.
  - For patients who are not able to achieve appropriate oral caloric intake, a feeding gastrostomy tube may be an option.
- Pancreatic enzyme supplementation. Patients with the pancreatic-insufficient form of CF manifest signs of malabsorption. Pancreatic enzyme supplementation is essential for these patients.
  - Usual dose ranges from 1500 to 2500 units of lipase per kilogram of patient's weight per meal.
  - Dosing is usually started at the lowest level and titrated up as needed, and it should not exceed 2500 lipase units/kg/meal because high doses have been associated with chronic intestinal strictures.
- Lipid-soluble vitamin supplementation (vitamins A, D, E, and K). Lipid-soluble vitamins are not well absorbed in patients with pancreatic insufficiency.
- Antimicrobials. Chronic antimicrobial therapy is frequently used in patients with increased morbidity from colonizing microorganisms to attempt prevention of pulmonary exacerbation. These are commonly used against methicillin-resistant *Staphylococcus aureus*, methicillin-sensitive *Staphylococcus aureus* (Panton-Valentine leukocidin positive), *Pseudomonas*, and *Aspergillus*. In addition, chronic azithromycin therapy has proven beneficial in terms of its immunomodulatory effects; it interferes with *Pseudomonas* biofilm formation in the CF airways.
- Anti-inflammatory agents
  - Oral glucocorticoid therapy and nonsteroidal anti-inflammatory drugs such as high-dose ibuprofen have proven benefits for some patients; however, the side effects of long-term therapy should be weighed against the benefits.
  - Azithromycin has been shown to improve respiratory function and reduce frequency of exacerbation, and its use is recommended for children 6 years and older. Its mechanism of action remains unclear.
- CFTR modulators
  - Ivacaftor monotherapy has shown to be effective at potentiating chloride channel function in cells with expressing one of 97 mutations, the most common being G551D and R117H. Its use is recommended with patients who carry an approved mutation and are 4 months and older.
  - Lumacaftor/ivacaftor is approved for people with two copies of the F508del mutation. Lumacaftor helps the resulting protein form the right shape, get to the cell surface, and stay there longer, and is ivacaftor helps to improve opening of the resulting channel. It is approved for ages 2 and older.
  - Tezacaftor/ivacaftor is another combination med which works similarly to lumacaftor/ivacaftor and has been shown to have fewer side effects and fewer drug interactions. It is approved for people ages 6 and older with two copies of F508del or with a single copy of 1 of 154 other mutations.
  - Elexacaftor/tezacaftor/ivacaftor is known as the triple combination therapy. Elexacaftor is a next-generation corrector and helps additional F508del-CFTR protein to form the correct shape and traffic to the cell surface. The addition of elexacaftor helps the CFTR protein perform better and makes this drug effective for a greater number of people with CF. It is approved for ages 12 and over in those who have at least one copy of 177 specified mutations.

- Therapy for a pulmonary exacerbation
  - This should always include intensive chest physiotherapy 3-4 times a day along with good nutritional support. Outpatient antibiotic therapy should always be attempted first if there are no signs of respiratory distress or decompensation. Choice of therapy should be based on previous sputum cultures.
  - The duration of therapy depends on clinical improvement but is generally between 2 and 3 weeks.
    - If there is failure to improve clinically while on outpatient therapy, the patient should be admitted to initiate IV antibiotic therapy for a total of 2-4 weeks.
    - All patients should be hospitalized in separate rooms with strict isolation measures as needed for resistant organisms.
    - The duration of admission depends on the severity of the patient's illness and clinical judgment (clinical improvement, improvement in spirometry, easiness of completing IV treatment at home).
- Special considerations
  - Allergic bronchopulmonary aspergillosis (ABPA)
    - ABPA is an exaggerated immunologic response in the lungs against *Aspergillus* that results in signs of airway obstruction. It occurs in 2-9% of patients with CF.
    - Criteria for diagnosis include positive skin prick testing against *Aspergillus*, along with detection of specific *Aspergillus* anti-IgG and anti-IgE in serum. Radiographic evidence of central bronchiectasis is suggestive of the diagnosis.
    - Treatment includes oral corticosteroids and antifungals such as itraconazole.
  - Cystic fibrosis–related diabetes mellitus (CFRD)
    - CFRD is caused by destruction of pancreatic islet cells and resultant insulin deficiency. Patients with CF should undergo frequent (annual) oral glucose tolerance tests to screen for evidence of CFRD.
    - Treatment is generally managed by a pediatric endocrinologist. It frequently involves administration of insulin and carbohydrate counting without compromising lipid intake and high caloric necessities.
  - Lung transplantation
    - The most common cause of death related to CF is advanced lung disease, and for these patients, lung transplantation may be the only alternative to prolong survival.
    - Referral for lung transplantation should be considered when $FEV_1 < 30\%$ of predicted (<50% for early referral), hypercarbia (>50 mm Hg), hypoxemia (<55 mm Hg), young age, female gender, and nutritional failure.

## SUGGESTED READINGS

Baird SM, Marsh PA, Padiglione A, et al. Review of epiglottitis in the post *Haemophilus influenzae* type-b vaccine era. ANZ J Surg 2018;88(11):1135–1140. doi: 10.1111/ans.14787.

Burton LV, Silberman M. Bacterial tracheitis. In: *StatPearls* [Internet]. Treasure Island, FL: StatPearls Publishing, 2021.

Casazza G, Graham ME, Nelson D, et al. Pediatric bacterial tracheitis—a variable entity: case series with literature review. Otolaryngol Head Neck Surg 2019;160(3):546–549. doi: 10.1177/0194599818808774.

Dowdy RAE, Cornelius BW. Medical management of epiglottitis. Anesth Prog 2020;67(2): 90–97. doi: 10.2344/anpr-66-04-08.

Epps QJ, Epps KL, Young DC, et al. State of the art in cystic fibrosis pharmacology—optimization of antimicrobials in the treatment of cystic fibrosis pulmonary exacerbations: I. Anti-methicillin-resistant *Staphylococcus aureus* (MRSA) antibiotics. Pediatr Pulmonol 2020;55(1):33–57. doi: 10.1002/ppul.24537.

Gates A, Gates M, Vandermeer B, et al. Glucocorticoids for croup in children. Cochrane Database Syst Rev 2018;8(8):CD001955. doi: 10.1002/14651858.CD001955.pub4.

Gates A, Johnson DW, Klassen TP. Glucocorticoids for croup in children. JAMA Pediatr 2019;173(6):595–596. doi: 10.1001/jamapediatrics.2019.0834.

Johnson DW. Croup. BMJ Clin Evid 2014;2014:0321.

Kirolos A, Manti S, Blacow R, et al.; RESCEU Investigators. A systematic review of clinical practice guidelines for the diagnosis and management of bronchiolitis. J Infect Dis 2020;222(Suppl 7):S672–S679. doi: 10.1093/infdis/jiz240. Erratum in: J Infect Dis 2020;221(7):1204.

Ren CL, Morgan RL, Oermann C, et al. Cystic Fibrosis Foundation Pulmonary Guidelines. Use of cystic fibrosis transmembrane conductance regulator modulator therapy in patients with cystic fibrosis. Ann Am Thorac Soc 2018;15(3):271–280. doi: 10.1513/AnnalsATS.201707-539OT.

VanDevanter DR, Kahle JS, O'Sullivan AK, et al. Cystic fibrosis in young children: a review of disease manifestation, progression, and response to early treatment. J Cyst Fibros 2016;15(2):147–157. doi: 10.1016/j.jcf.2015.09.008.

Yalamanchi S, Saiman L, Zachariah P. Decision-making around positive tracheal aspirate cultures: the role of neutrophil semiquantification in antibiotic prescribing. Pediatr Crit Care Med 2019;20(8):e380–e385. doi: 10.1097/PCC.0000000000002014.

# Patient Safety and Quality Improvement

Kevin O'Bryan and Chrissy Hrach

## INTRODUCTION

Upholding patient safety is critically important in providing effective care to patients. Reducing adverse medical events and associated harm is essential for all health care providers. Constant vigilance to prevent medical errors requires the cooperation of the entire health care team. To reduce errors and provide safe care to patients, health care systems must be designed with highly reliable processes incorporated to the system. Quality improvement describes the efforts to augment the quality of health care delivery and to make safe, effective patient care become possible.

Much of the recent work on patient safety has focused on the creation of safety culture and high reliability systems. A workplace culture is the values and personality of a workplace. The culture focus of an organization could be on a variety of topics such as efficiency, customer satisfaction, or financial growth. Organizations typically ascribe to values that they focus on to set their local culture. Culture can be influenced by these organizational values but equally impactful is how management and employees interact and what elements are areas of focus in the day-to-day work. A culture of safety is one where the elements of patient safety are set as organization values as well as focuses of day-to-day work. High reliability systems are workflows or processes that rely less on well educated people to do things well and are structure in a way to ensure success.

To develop a culture of safety, and to incorporate high-reliability practices, teaching hospitals must integrate physicians into all phases of quality improvement efforts. Medical students and resident physicians deliver a substantial percentage of direct patient care in these institutions and directly impact patient care outcomes through their knowledge, skills, and attitudes. Furthermore, residents' active participation in all phases of health care makes them a powerful force for changing hospital culture. Efforts focused on improved communication during handoffs and transfers of care, serve as educational experiences for the entire health care team, as well as provide opportunities to reduce preventable errors. Incorporating trainee physicians into quality improvement activities not only improves their knowledge and confidence but also engages these key stakeholders in promoting the principles of safety and quality.

## HANDOFFS AND SIGN-OUTS

With the advent of duty hour restrictions and the transition of medical care to more shift-based care models, patient care responsibility is frequently handed off from provider to provider throughout an inpatient visit. It is well recognized that these transitions in care are high risk and frequently implicated in medical errors that reach patients. To address this, it is recommended that all providers complete handoffs in a standardized fashion to ensure that required information is transmitted successfully. There are a number of ways to do so including using the I-PASS pneumonic for standardized sign-out. I-PASS stands for: **I**llness severity, **P**atient summary, **A**ction list, **S**ituational awareness with contingency planning, and **S**ynthesis by receiver.

- Regardless of what system is used, there are a number of components that are essential:
  - Minimization of distractions: Accurate sign-out between care services is critical to providing safe care. This should happen in a quiet environment with the minimum of distractions. This may mean working with nursing staff and peers to establish a quiet "no interruptions" time and/or a separated area dedicated especially for this activity.
  - Handoffs should follow a standardized process: The handoff should be performed according to a standard workflow that applies to all patients. By following a standardized approach, both the giver and receiver of information know what to expect next and can hold each other accountable to providing full, accurate information in the correct order.
  - Closed loop communication: The person receiving the sign-out repeats back his or her understanding of the patient to the person giving sign-out to ensure that critical information is understood. Not all the data need to be repeated back, but critical elements should be restated such that the giver can assess the receiver's understanding of the handoff and ensure its accuracy. There are other handoffs that occur on a less frequent basis throughout care delivery including transitions in care provider teams. This can be when a patient is transferred in or out of an ICU or goes to the operating room. This can also be when a patient is admitted or discharged from the hospital and transitions between outpatient and inpatient providers. During these transitions, a modified verbal handoff should occur similar to the model described above. Because these occur between different structures, such as a pediatric clinic and a hospital unit, regrettably, these interactions are more difficult to structure and standardize but still benefit from efforts to do so.

## WRITTEN COMMUNICATION

Written communication is another important component of providing safe care to patients. To supplement the verbal handoffs during these transitions in care, written confirmation is required. This can be a transfer note, an off service note, or a discharge summary depending on the situation. Timeliness is essential for this written supplement to be effective. Documents of this nature should be completed as soon as possible and ideally before the receiving caregiver provides care. This can be difficult to accomplish when a patient is transferred to the ICU but should definitely be accomplished when patients are discharged or transferred back to outpatient providers. A discharge summary or letter should be available to any care provider in time for their follow-up visit. A good rule of thumb is that a discharge letter should be completed prior to the first outpatient appointment.

Written communication should also be accurate and easily interpretable. Ideally, notes are concise and accurate, and provide the reader with all the necessary information to continue care. Many electronic notes are prone to "note bloat" from unnecessary use of copy and paste behaviors where extraneous or inaccurate information is copied from previous notes. These practices should be avoided, and, when used, should be done in a fashion where copied information is carefully reviewed and edited to ensure accuracy. Copy and paste ideally should only be used as a tool to ensure information is not lost between encounters and not a tool for documentation efficiency.

| TABLE 28-1 | Official "Do Not Use" List[a] | |
| --- | --- | --- |
| **Do not use** | **Potential problem** | **Use instead** |
| U, u (unit) | Mistaken for "0" (zero), the number "4" (four) or "cc" | Write "unit" |
| IU (International Unit) | Mistaken for IV (intravenous) or the number 10 (ten) | Write "International Unit" |
| Q.D., QD, q.d., qd (daily) | Mistaken for each other | Write "daily" |
| Q.O.D., QOD, q.o.d, qod (every other day) | Period after the Q mistaken for "I" and the "O" mistaken for "I" | Write "every other day" |
| Trailing zero (X.0 mg)[b] | Decimal point is missed | Write X mg |
| Lack of leading zero (.X mg) | | Write 0.X mg |
| MS | Can mean morphine sulfate or magnesium sulfate | Write "morphine sulfate" |
| MSO4 and MgSO4 | Confused for one another | Write "magnesium sulfate" |

[a]Applies to all orders and all medication-related documentation that is handwritten (including free-text computer entry) or on preprinted forms.
[b]Exception: A "trailing zero" may be used only where required to demonstrate the level of precision of the value being reported, such as for laboratory results, imaging studies that report size of lesions, or catheter/tube sizes. It may not be used in medication orders or other medication-related documentation.

Another component of ensuring safe practices as well as making notes readable is the appropriate use of abbreviations. Users of abbreviations are susceptible to error because their meaning may differ between institutions and individuals. Your organization should have a list of approved and prohibited abbreviations, and if you intend to use abbreviations, you should be familiar with these rules. Listed in Table 28-1 is the JAHCO "do not use" list of terms for medication ordering.

## RESIDENT PHYSICIAN ROLE IN PATIENT SAFETY

Residency is a busy and stressful time in a physician's education. There is a constant tension between gaining independence and providing safe and effective care. It is important that trainees experience independence in a graduated fashion while still insuring appropriate care of their patients. Increases in autonomy can be associated with a greater risk for medical errors. Efforts should be taken to minimize the risk of injury. To reduce preventable harm, strategies you should employ include:

• Double-check your work and the work of those around you. Important items should be promptly reviewed, and high-risk situations, such as ordering a new drug or treatment, must be double-checked. You should always be confident in the orders you place and not rely on the safety checks of others to correct your mistakes. Many hospitals have a pharmacist who double checks inpatient orders prior to releasing medications for administration. This added layer of safety can be effective in preventing errors but trainees should be careful to not be overly reliant on these safety measures as they are not present in all care settings.

- Maintain a questioning attitude toward plans and diagnoses. Keep your differential diagnoses broad and try to avoid "diagnostic inertia," the concept of maintaining a particular diagnosis or assessment provided by a previous care provider. Diagnostic inertia prevents you from considering alternative diagnoses and recognizing errors in the initial evaluation.
- Seek help when you need it, and escalate that assistance as appropriate. First consider consulting the literature or reference materials, followed by discussion with a peer, consultation with an ancillary professional such as a pharmacist, as well as seeking help from your supervising physician and/or consultative assistance from another specialty or a critical care physician when indicated. Attentiveness to all of avenues of support is critical to practicing physicians, as well as skill in using them in the appropriate setting.

Unfortunately, all physicians make mistakes and trainees are especially prone. Errors can be of various magnitudes and may occur regardless of a physician's experience. It is important that one recognizes when an error occurs, report it, and then try to mitigate the damages. You should understand and follow your local institution's policies for managing medical errors. Here is a generic approach to managing a medical error:

- Recognize the error: Patients may have negative outcomes with or without the occurrence of an error, and errors that occur may or may not have impact on a patient. It is important to be vigilant for errors and report them when they occur regardless of their impact.
- Report the error: All hospitals have a mechanism for reporting medical errors. These should be reported factually and avoid emotional or blaming language. The relevant facts should simply be stated without judgment.
- Disclosing errors: Research has shown that disclosure of errors at, or close to, the time of occurrence has reduced medical liability. Doing so also helps to salvage the therapeutic relationship with the patient and family. This should be done carefully and in accordance with your institution's approach. Your supervising physician should always be aware of the disclosure plan and will usually participate. When disclosing, it is important not to blame other members of the care team but to take responsibility as the care team as a whole. Using the term "we" and explaining the circumstances fully can be helpful. After the disclosure has occurred, the discussion should be fully documented in the medical record. Again your institution should have guidelines for accomplishing this.
- Care team after care: Medical errors affect not only the patient but also the care team. Care team function can be diminished if there is associated blame; further, individuals may experience significant guilt after being involved in such an event. Depending on the impact of the situation, it may be important to debrief the event as a care team and seek and provide support to affected team members. Be aware that the impact to a care provider is not necessarily correlated to the severity of error itself.
- Follow up the event: Entry of the event into a safety event reporting system will usually trigger some type of monitoring or follow-up. Depending on local practice and error severity, this may result in an investigation and/or a root cause analysis. A root cause analysis is a process when a group of frontline providers get together to identify

where the safety mechanisms in the system broke down and how future events can be prevented. If you get the opportunity to participate in one of these sessions, it can be an invaluable learning opportunity.

## QUALITY IMPROVEMENT

Skills in quality improvement are becoming essential for all physicians. Trainees as well as practicing physicians are now being required to participate in quality improvement as part of their certification and maintenance of certification. Most residency programs require trainees to complete a quality improvement project as part of their training. There are numerous methodologies for quality improvement and extensive literature available addressing health care quality improvement opportunities and methodologies. Factors to consider in successfully accomplishing a quality improvement project should include the following:

- Pick a project that interests you—your organization may have projects available for you to choose from, or you may be asked to develop your own project. You will enjoy the project and learn more if you are engaged and interested.
- Find a mentor who is interested in the project and has some competency in quality improvement methodology. If your project is large, you may want to recruit peers to participate in the project to spread the workload.
- Define the scope of your project and focus! Remember that you only have a finite period of time to complete this work and you will be very busy throughout residency. Work with your mentor to find a small enough piece that you can accomplish. Certain projects may be more successful if they rely on process measures rather than outcome measures. For example, it may be preferable to measure the percentage of providers using a new safety checklist in a 1-week period of well child encounters rather than trying to measure if ER visits for preventable accidents are decreased after implementation of this same checklist.
- You should create a SMART aim statement for your project. SMART = Specific, Measurable, Achievable, Realistic, and Timely. A specific aim statement will help describe clear and specific plans for the improvement ahead.
- Engage with the relevant key stakeholders. You need to work with the people that will be impacted by the change you are making. You should engage with these individuals to get their impressions, suggestions, and buy in. You cannot simply ask them to change their workflow without their input. Be mindful to include a multidisciplinary group so that you can include multiple viewpoints. Work within the quality improvement structure in your institution, but tools such as key driver diagrams and fishbone diagrams are very effective for improving engagement and planning.
- Write up your project as you go. Writing down your plan and interventions keeps you accountable to your plan and helps your mentor keep you on track and avoids the problem of the scope of your project growing as you engage with other stakeholders.

A common process used for implementing quality improvement projects is the PDSA cycle. The PDSA cycle is an iterative method used to continually improve a process and involves four steps that repeat until you achieve success: Plan, Do, See, and Act. To illustrate this process, here is an example of a PDSA cycle to improve hand washing in a clinic.

- **Plan**: The first step is to **plan** an intervention to improve the process you are interested in. This means measuring the process you want to change and then using those measurements or observations to create a directed intervention to improve the process. For a hand-washing example, you would want to first know how well you are currently doing with hand washing. Therefore, you might measure for an hour each day what percentage of the time people wash their hands when leaving a patient's room. After collecting these data, create a plan to improve the rates of hand washing in the clinic. This might be to add hand sanitizer dispensers to the doorways of all clinic rooms, for example. It is very important that you plan your intervention based on your measurements. If the percentage before the intervention is 100%, there is not much point in targeting this process.

- **Do**: The **do** portion of the cycle is to implement your plan or in the example, install hand sanitizer dispensers.
- **See**: In the see, or **study**, portion of the cycle, observe and measure changes after the intervention. In this example, measure the percent compliance of hand washing. Also you will want to observe and possibly survey for other changes related to the intervention. For example, you might find that in room 6, hand washing has decreased because that room has a different layout and the hand sanitizer is not visible when leaving that room.
- **Act**: The final step is to act, which is to decide to keep or reject the change you made and decide if you have achieved adequate success. In the hand-washing story, we might find that we have achieved success except in room 6 and we need to do another PDSA cycle to change the hand sanitizer location in room 6 and again assess for improvement.

In conclusion, health care providers must follow other industries in establishing highly reliable processes to reduce preventable harm. The incorporation of patient safety and quality improvement activities into medical training programs will ultimately help to achieve these outcomes and reduce the risk of adverse medical events.

## SUGGESTED READINGS

Berwick DM, Nolan TW, Whittington J. The triple aim: care, health and cost. Health Aff 2008;27(3):759–769.

Resar R, Griffin FA, Haraden C, et al. Using Care Bundles to Improve Health Care Quality. Cambridge, MA: IHI Innovation Series white paper, Institute for Healthcare Improvement, 2012. Available at www.IHI.org

Starmer AJ, Spector ND, Srivastava R, et al. Changes in medical errors after implementation of a handoff program. NEJM 2014;371(19):1803–1812.

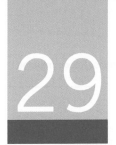

# Radiology

Ting Y. Tao and William McAlister

## ORDERING A RADIOLOGY EXAMINATION

- Imaging procedures may be requested depending on the clinical condition of the patient. Recommendations for imaging may represent either optimal selection (based on availability) or complementary examinations that build on each other.
- The radiologist may customize the examination or even suggest a different one to answer the specific clinical question. Key information should be provided:
  - Radiologic procedure requested
  - Specific clinical question or clinical situation
    - Gastrointestinal (GI)/abdominopelvic conditions (see Table 29-1)
    - Head and neck conditions (see Table 29-2)
    - Selected other conditions (see Table 29-3)
  - Relevant clinical history, diagnoses, and surgeries
    - Cancer patients: last chemotherapy or radiation therapy
  - Prior imaging studies and reports (especially if studies were performed elsewhere)
  - Allergy to iodinated or gadolinium intravenous (IV) contrast
  - Renal function (serum creatinine) if IV contrast is to be used
  - IV access (location and gauge)
  - Patient factors: stability (examination at bedside or in radiology department), nothing by mouth (NPO) status, mechanical ventilation, cooperativeness, and need for sedation

### Safety Considerations

- Monitored conscious sedation with agents such as IV pentobarbital, midazolam, or propofol is appropriate for young patients who cannot stay still, for uncooperative patients, and for potentially painful procedures.
- Make patients NPO when ordering any sedated examination, computed tomography (CT) that involves IV contrast, MRI with IV contrast, or a GI fluoroscopic examination.

### Radiation Considerations

- Radiography, fluoroscopy, and CT expose the patient to ionizing radiation, whereas ultrasound and magnetic resonance imaging (MRI) do not.
- At children's hospitals and imaging centers, radiation doses can be, and often are, significantly reduced by modification of imaging technique.

### Gastrointestinal Contrast Considerations

- Barium and water-soluble contrast agents.
  - Barium is usually the GI contrast of choice but should not be used if a leak is suspected because it can cause peritonitis or mediastinitis or if surgery is imminent. In addition, barium can limit future abdominal CT imaging because of scatter artifact from retained material.

| TABLE 29-1 | Gastrointestinal/Abdominopelvic Conditions: Recommended Imaging |
|---|---|

| Condition | Imaging used |
|---|---|
| Abdominal trauma | CT with IV contrast is the study of choice. |
| Appendicitis | Abdominal radiographs are often nonspecific, although occasionally appendicoliths may be seen (15%). US is imaging study of choice in young, thin children. Computed tomography (CT) is study of choice in older children with moderate body fat. Typically, intravenous contrast is used. MRI can be used to diagnose appendicitis. |
| Ascites | US can diagnose and localize for drainage. |
| Biliary atresia | US is useful to assess for presence of the gallbladder and its size (often <1.5 cm) as well as to exclude biliary obstruction from choledochal cysts. "Triangular cord sign," which is tubular echogenic cord of fibrous tissue at porta hepatis. HIDA scan is useful in diagnosing obstruction. |
| Bowel perforation | Obstructive series may show free air. Erect and decubitus radiographs are needed. CT may be useful in demonstrating small amounts of free air and suggesting a cause. |
| Duodenal atresia | Abdominal radiographs are diagnostic. "Double-bubble" sign is due to a distended stomach and proximal duodenum with an otherwise gasless abdomen. |
| Esophageal atresia/ tracheoesophageal fistula | Chest and abdominal radiographs may show dilated proximal esophageal pouch and coiled proximal gastric tube. Abdominal gas is seen in atresia with tracheoesophageal fistula, while absence of abdominal gas indicates atresia without fistula. Esophagram with nonionic contrast media is the study of choice for looking for "H-type" fistula. It is associated with VACTERL (vertebral, anorectal, cardiac, tracheoesophageal, renal and limb anomalies). |
| Henoch-Schönlein purpura | Most common pediatric vasculitis. US is helpful to assess bowel involvement (bowel wall thickening), gall bladder hydrops, scrotal involvement, and complications like intussusception. MRI and CT can be used. |
| Hepatoblastoma | Most common pediatric hepatic malignancy. US shows heterogeneous mass in the liver with moderate vascularity and mass effect. CT scan reveals predominantly hypoattenuating mass, which can contain calcification. CT as well as MRI are accurate to assess the extent of liver involvement, portal vein invasion, and lymph nodal metastasis. |

| TABLE 29-1 | Gastrointestinal/Abdominopelvic Conditions: Recommended Imaging (*Continued*) |
|---|---|

| Condition | Imaging used |
|---|---|
| Hypertrophic pyloric stenosis | US is examination of choice, which shows the thickened and elongated pyloric muscle. Upper GI (UGI) examination can be used. |
| Inflammatory bowel disease | MR enterography is preferred over small bowel follow-through and useful to evaluate extent and degree of bowel inflammation and complications like abscess, fistula, and stricture. Diffusion-weighted MRI can distinguish acute vs. chronic inflammation.<br><br>CT enterography is equal as an alternative especially if sedation is needed for the MR. |
| Intestinal malrotation | Obstructive series is usually normal unless midgut volvulus is present; UGI study is recommended. Urgent imaging is a must. Ultrasound is useful in diagnosing volvulus. |
| Intussusception | Obstructive series may be useful in suggesting (mass effect) or excluding (air or stool in right colon and terminal ileum). US should establish the diagnosis. |
| Meckel diverticulum | Often difficult to diagnose. Nuclear medicine "Meckel scan" may demonstrate approximately 80-90% sensitivity and 90-95% specificity if there is gastric mucosa. CT with oral and IV contrast or MRI may demonstrate diverticulum. |
| Necrotizing enterocolitis | Serial abdominal radiographs every 4-6 hours may demonstrate pneumatosis, free peritoneal air, and portal vein gas. US is increasing being used. |
| Neuroblastoma | CT is recommended for initial staging and shows heterogeneous mass with enhancement and calcifications. The mass often crosses the midline and encases the vessels. CT is also helpful to assess osseous and liver metastases. MRI is comparable and can evaluate intraspinal extension of a mass. MIBG scan is helpful to detect metastatic disease. |
| Wilms tumor | Most common renal malignancy in young children. CT is done for initial staging. The mass enhances and tends to displace the adjacent vessels. Calcifications are rare, and tumor can extend into the renal veins and inferior vena cava. Lung metastases are common at presentation. MRI can be used to evaluate the tumor. |

| TABLE 29-2 | Selected Head and Neck Conditions: Recommended Imaging |
|---|---|

| Condition | Imaging used |
|---|---|
| Cervical spine trauma | Anteroposterior (AP) and lateral cervical spine radiographs (also odontoid view in children greater than age 6 years) are useful. Use CT if there is still question of fracture. If there is concern for ligamentous injury, flexion and extension lateral radiographs or MRI without contrast are necessary. |
| Cystic neck lesions | Thyroglossal duct cyst, dermoid, lymphatic malformation, and abscesses are the most common cystic lesions in the neck. US is preferred for initial evaluation of these cystic lesions. |
| Head trauma, epidural/ subdural hematoma | CT with and without IV contrast is used, with magnetic resonance imaging (MRI) if CT is inconclusive. |
| Orbital cellulitis | Orbital CT with IV contrast. |
| Retropharyngeal abscess | Soft tissue neck AP and lateral radiographs for initial evaluation. Typically, CT neck with IV contrast is used to further identify. |
| Stridor/croup, epiglottitis | Frontal and lateral soft tissue neck and chest radiographs show steeple sign of croup and the thumb sign of epiglottitis. |
| Stroke | CT without IV contrast is used to evaluate for bleeding and edema, MRI without contrast and magnetic resonance arteriogram for suspected hemorrhagic etiology, and for patient with sickle cell disease. |
| Ventriculoperitoneal shunt malfunction | Shunt series (radiographs of skull, chest, and abdomen) to access for discontinuity is useful, with MR or noncontrast head CT for ventricular sizes. |

- Water-soluble ionic contrast agents (e.g., Hypaque, Gastroview) are used when barium is contraindicated. Their advantage over barium is that they reabsorb from body cavities, but the disadvantage is that image quality is poorer.
  ○ They are hyperosmolar and may cause fluid shifts into the GI tract. This is usually well tolerated by the patient.
  ○ They should not be used when large volume aspiration is a possibility, as they may cause pulmonary edema.
- Water-soluble nonionic low-osmolar contrast agents (e.g., Omnipaque, Optiray) may be used orally in infants when the risk of aspiration is high or when GI leak is suspected. Nonionic contrast agents can be diluted to make them isotonic and still produce satisfactory image quality.

| TABLE 29-3 | Selected Other Conditions: Recommended Imaging |
|---|---|
| **Condition** | **Imaging used** |
| Child abuse | Complete skeletal survey may show multiple fractures in various stages of healing and metaphyseal corner, posterior rib, sternal, complex skull, and phalangeal fractures. All of these findings are highly suggestive of child abuse. CT or MRI of the head is useful to assess intracranial hemorrhage and skull fractures. |
| Pleural effusion | Frontal and lateral chest radiographs may be sufficient. Decubitus radiographs help demonstrate fluid mobility and amount. Use US if they are inconclusive or localization for drainage is required. Use CT with contrast if there is concern for empyema, loculated fluid, or necrotizing pneumonia. |
| Developmental dysplasia of the hip | Imaging is not preferable until patient is at least 2 weeks of age; earlier imaging is often inconclusive because of transient ligamentous laxity as a result of maternal hormones. US is the study of choice until age 6 months. AP radiograph of the pelvis after age 6 months. |
| Extremity deep vein thrombosis | Venous US with Doppler. |
| Langerhans cell histiocytosis (LCH) | Can affect single or multiple bones. Most common locations are skull, pelvis, femur, ribs, and humerus. Radiographs show lytic lesions with or without sclerotic rim. In the skull, lytic lesions have beveled edges. Floating teeth may be seen. Vertebra plana or vertebral body compression deformity in the spine. |
| Pulmonary embolism | CT with pulmonary embolism protocol is necessary, which requires excellent intravenous (IV) access for contrast. |
| Osteomyelitis | Radiographs are often negative in early acute osteomyelitis. MRI is preferred for diagnosis of acute osteomyelitis, which shows marrow edema, cortical breaks, subperiosteal, subcutaneous, and intramuscular tissue abscesses, fistulae, and sequestrum. |
| Scoliosis | Use scoliosis survey (AP total spine radiograph), adding lateral view if significant scoliosis, lordosis, or kyphosis. |
| Septic arthritis | Most common in hip, knee, and ankle joints. US is useful to diagnose the effusions. Effusions can be tapped under US or fluoroscopy guidance to obtain joint fluid for cytology and culture. MRI is useful. |

*(Continued)*

| TABLE 29-3 | Selected Other Conditions: Recommended Imaging (*Continued*) |
|---|---|
| Condition | Imaging used |
| Skeletal dysplasias | Skeletal survey will help establish the diagnosis. |
| Slipped capital femoral epiphysis | Adolescent boys and girls. AP and frog leg radiographs show extent and severity of slip, which is medial and posterior. MR in questionable cases. |
| Thoracic trauma | CT with IV contrast is the study of choice. In patients with minor trauma, chest radiographs may be sufficient. |
| Vascular and lymphatic malformations | US, CT, and MRI are useful to determine the type of vascular and lymphatic malformation, flow rates, extent of the lesion, and vascularity. |

## Intravenous Contrast Considerations

- The radiologist will help you determine appropriateness based on such factors as clinical indications and renal function.
- Contrast power injectors provide optimal imaging for all CTs, except for head CT, but these require a 22-gauge or larger needle, and preferably antecubital IV access. Hand IV lines and some central lines should be injected manually, which leads to suboptimal vessel opacification.
- Contrast is relatively contraindicated in patients with renal insufficiency (elevated creatinine and GFR), sickle cell crisis, or prior major anaphylactic allergic reaction to contrast.
- Patients with prior less severe contrast reactions may have IV contrast if premedicated.
  - According to the ACR Manual on Contrast Media recommendations, prednisone 0.5-0.7 mg/kg PO (maximum up to 50 mg) should be given 13 hours, 7 hours, and 1 hour prior to contrast injection. In addition, diphenhydramine 1.25 mg/kg PO (maximum up to 50 mg) may be given 1 hour prior to contrast injection.
  - Appropriate IV drug doses may be substituted for patients who cannot ingest PO medication.

## Magnetic Resonance Imaging Considerations

- Contraindications to MRI include presence of programmable implanted devices (e.g., pacemakers, cochlear implants), MRI-noncompatible aneurysm clips, and metallic fragments in the eye. Compatibility must also be considered for other implants, prostheses, metal objects, and some dark tattoos.
- Closed loop wires have a tendency to heat up during the examination. Skin staples are usually tolerated if they are taped securely.
- Some stents, filters, coils, and prosthetic valves require 6-8 weeks to allow tissue ingrowth before an MRI may be performed.
- IV gadolinium is relatively contraindicated in patients with renal insufficiency due to risk of nephrogenic systemic fibrosis (NSF).
- Patients usually must lie flat for 30-90 minutes or more and must be cooperative enough to lie still (or be sedated).

## CHEST RADIOGRAPHY

- Check for airspace opacities, thickened bronchial walls, pulmonary edema, increased or decreased pulmonary vascularity, pleural effusions, pneumothorax, heart size, midline trachea, side of aortic arch, rib fractures, and septal lines (Kerley B lines).
- Normal cardiothoracic ratio is 65% in infants and 55% in older children. A large thymic shadow is normal under the age of 2 years.
- Check aeration. Flattened or inverted diaphragm on lateral view suggests air trapping.
- Check for anomalies. Check on which side (left or right) the cardiac apex, aortic arch, stomach bubble, and liver shadow are located. Note any rib or vertebral anomalies.

### Evaluating for Airspace Opacities

- Check for subtle airspace opacities behind the diaphragm and heart on the frontal view. Normally, the borders of the heart and diaphragm are sharp, and the right and left heart shadows should be similar in density. Right middle lobe and lingular airspace opacities are adjacent to the heart and obscure the heart borders on frontal radiographs (silhouette sign).
- Airspace opacification is present if the lung projecting over the spine does not become increasingly darker inferiorly on lateral radiograph (spine sign).
- The normal thymus, which can be large and triangular in young children, is sometimes confused for upper lobe airspace opacity, especially on the right.
- Classic appearances of common entities
  - Viral pneumonia/bronchiolitis: hyperinflation, perihilar infiltrates, and thickened bronchial walls (Fig. 29-1).
  - Bacterial pneumonia: focal airspace opacity, lobar consolidation with air bronchograms (Fig. 29-2), and parapneumonic pleural fluid.

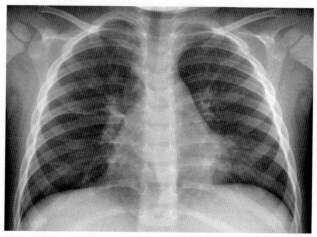

**Figure 29-1. Viral bronchiolitis.** Frontal view of the chest shows hyperinflation with perihilar infiltrates and peribronchial cuffing consistent with reactive airway disease. Notice associated subsegmental atelectasis in both lower lobes.

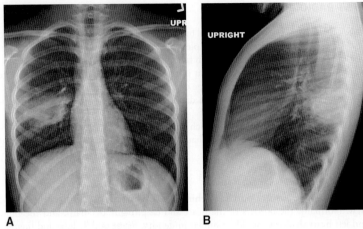

**A**    **B**

Figure 29-2. **Right lower lobe pneumonia.** Frontal (**A**) and lateral (**B**) radiographs of chest reveal airspace opacity with air bronchograms in superior segment of right lower lobe consistent with pneumonia.

- Atelectasis: linear opacities and volume loss.
- Round pneumonia: common in children below the age of 8 years due to incomplete development of collateral pathways. On radiographs, it appears as a circumscribed radiopacity with air bronchograms and tends to have slightly irregular margins. Superior segments of the lower lobes are the most common location.
- Acute chest syndrome (ACS): seen in sickle cell patients. Segmental, lobar, or multilobar consolidation with or without pleural effusion can be seen. The consolidation in ACS can progress rapidly, more so than in other bacterial pneumonias. Other radiographic signs of sickle cell disease are cardiomegaly and vertebral endplate infarcts (H vertebra), aseptic necrosis of humeral heads, and a small, calcified spleen.
- The appearance of viral or bacterial pneumonia and atelectasis can be similar, especially in infants.

### Evaluating Chest Radiographs from the Neonatal Intensive Care Unit

- Check every line and tube position.
- Check for pneumothorax.
- Check for classic appearances of common entities.
  - Transient tachypnea of the newborn: streaky densities extending from the hilar areas that tend to resolve in a few days and fluid in the minor fissure usually with normal lung volumes.
  - Hyaline membrane disease: diffuse ground glass or finely granular appearance, small lung volumes, air bronchograms, and no pleural fluid. With worsening opacification, consider patent ductus arteriosus or fluid overload.
  - Meconium aspiration pneumonia: usually in term or postterm newborns; hyperinflated lungs with patchy, coarse infiltrates. Postterm babies may have proximal humeral epiphyses present as a sign of maturity.
  - Neonatal pneumonia: variable appearance, including asymmetric airspace opacities, often with pleural effusions, and can simulate hyaline membrane disease. Group B streptococcus is a common pathogen.

## Checking for Free Air in the Chest

*Pneumothorax*

- Look for a thin sharp line representing the pleural surface, with air beyond the visceral pleura (air is darker, lucent, and without vessels) (Fig. 29-3).
- Other signs to look for are:
  - Deep sulcus sign: lateral costophrenic angle deepened with increased lucency (basilar pneumothorax).
  - Increased lucency over one lung (anterior pneumothorax).
  - Increased sharpness of cardiomediastinal border with lucency along the border (medial pneumothorax).
  - Mediastinal shift away from pneumothorax or hemidiaphragm depressed on side of the pneumothorax suggests tension. The amount of tension may vary depending on the size of the pneumothorax and the condition of the underlying lung. These radiographic findings of tension may not be present with positive end-expiratory pressure ventilation or very diseased noncompliant lungs.
- An upright or expiratory examination in cooperative patients and a lateral decubitus (opposite side down) view in uncooperative or intubated patients could be obtained to confirm pleural air.
- Pneumomediastinum: lucencies in the mediastinum with air outlining the heart borders, air on the undersurface of the thymus (Fig. 29-4), pulmonary artery (ring

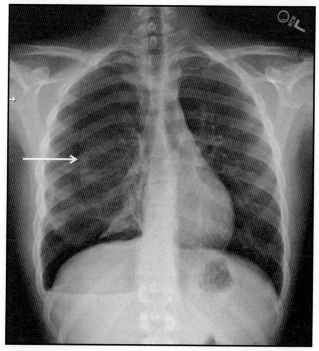

**Figure 29-3. Pneumothorax.** Frontal radiograph of the chest demonstrates a large right pneumothorax with collapse of right lung. Notice sharp pleural line (*arrow*) with absent pulmonary markings.

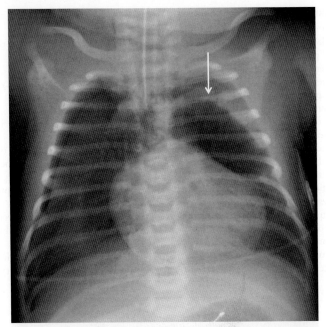

**Figure 29-4. Pneumomediastinum and pneumothorax.** Frontal radiograph of the chest shows lucency in mediastinum underlying thymus with elevation of thymus (*arrow*). Notice small right pneumothorax. Also, there is collapse of the left lower lobe in retrocardiac region.

around artery sign), aorta and diaphragm (continuous diaphragm sign), and air in the neck. On lateral decubitus radiographs, mediastinal free air does not move, unlike a pneumothorax.

- Pneumopericardium: air surrounding the heart with pericardium sharply outlined by air density on either side. The air parallels the heart including inferiorly. It does not extend above the level of ascending aorta.

### Checking for a Foreign Body

- Aspirated foreign bodies most often cause ipsilateral air trapping causing one lung to look more lucent. Occasionally lung or lobar collapse can occur. To evaluate for nonopaque/radiolucent foreign bodies, expiratory or both lateral decubitus chest radiographs are helpful. The latter are especially useful in infants and young children.
- An aspirated foreign body must always be suspected when one lung appears more lucent. Fluoroscopy or chest CT may be performed if radiographs are equivocal.

### CHEST COMPUTED TOMOGRAPHY AND MAGNETIC RESONANCE IMAGING

- Noncontrast CT is appropriate for evaluating pulmonary nodules, mild lung parenchymal disease, and airway disease.
- IV contrast optimizes evaluation of patients with more extensive pneumonias, pleural versus parenchymal disease, masses in the lungs or mediastinum, vascular anom-

alies, congenital heart disease (pre- and postoperative), chest trauma, pulmonary embolism, complex airspace disease, and bone tumors.

- High-resolution CT comprising of inspiratory and expiratory images can be performed to better characterize lung parenchymal disease especially interstitial lung diseases.
- MRI is used to evaluate the heart and great vessels and for pre-op pectus excavatum.

## ABDOMINAL RADIOGRAPHY

- Abdomen 1 view: Also known as the kidneys, ureters, and bladder (KUB) view, abdominal flat plate (AFP), or supine abdomen radiograph.
- Abdomen 2 view: Also known as an obstructive series (two views: supine and either upright or left lateral decubitus) and may include an upright chest view.
  - The supine radiograph is used to evaluate bowel gas pattern, masses, organ enlargement, colonic fecal matter, and abnormal calcifications (e.g., renal calculi, gallstones, and appendicoliths). The upright or left lateral decubitus views allow an evaluation for pneumoperitoneum and gas-fluid levels in the bowel.
  - Decubitus radiographs are usually taken in young children, whereas erect radiographs are usually taken in older children.

### Evaluating Bowel Gas Pattern

- Normal bowel gas pattern
  - Gas is seen in the stomach and nondilated small bowel and colon.
  - Crying infants often swallow air and have many loops of gas-filled nondilated proximal small bowel loops.
  - Small bowel folds completely encircle the bowel and colonic folds (haustra) only partially encircle the bowel.
  - The position of the bowel in the abdomen helps to separate large from small bowel in addition to small bowel valvulae conniventes and colonic haustral markings.
- Complete small bowel obstruction (Fig. 29-5)
  - The most important sign is dilated small bowel. The colon usually has little or no gas. Gas usually is not seen in the rectum. If gas is present in the rectum, it will not be distended.
  - The more loops of dilated small bowel, the more distal the obstruction.
- Partial or early small bowel obstruction
  - The small bowel is dilated but less than complete obstruction.
  - Some gas and stool are still seen in the colon and rectum.
- Ileus
  - The small and large bowels are dilated, with the large bowel dilated more prominently than the small bowel.
  - The patient may be postoperative.
- Intussusception: small bowel obstruction pattern, but may be a nonspecific bowel gas pattern
  - Classic findings are a soft tissue mass in the right upper quadrant just beyond the hepatic flexure with no recognizable right colonic gas or stool.
  - Gas- or stool-filled right colon is against the diagnosis.
  - Ultrasound confirms the diagnosis and is very accurate when done by an experienced examiner (see Fig. 29-6).

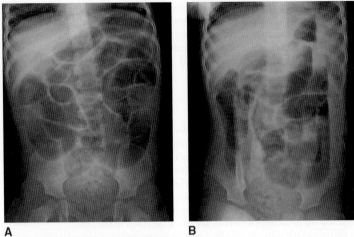

**A**          **B**

Figure 29-5. **Small bowel obstruction.** Frontal (**A**) and left lateral decubitus (**B**) views of the abdomen show multiple dilated bowel loops with a gasless rectosigmoid colon. The decubitus view shows scattered small bowel air-fluid levels in a pattern typical of distal small bowel obstruction.

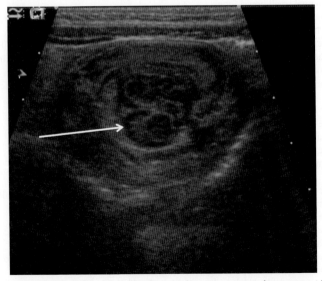

Figure 29-6. **Intussusception.** Grayscale ultrasound transverse image shows mass with target appearance with concentric hypo- and hyperechoic rims consistent with intussusception. Notice small lymph nodes in the intussusceptum (*arrow*).

- In patients without free air, peritonitis, or cardiovascular instability, an enema reduction is indicated, typically using air or water-soluble contrast agents. Reduction rates are around 90% in patients who are not obstructed.
- Necrotizing enterocolitis: look for pneumatosis in the bowel wall, typically in the colon (Fig. 29-7). Air in the bowel wall appears "bubbly" when it is subserosal and "linear" when it is submucosal in location. Also, look for portal venous gas and pneumoperitoneum (Fig. 29-8). The bowel may be dilated. Bowel loops may appear thickened and may not move on decubitus radiographs. Ultrasound is used to look for pneumatosis, thickened or thin bowel with diminished perfusion, complex peritoneal fluid suggesting perforation, and portal vein gas.
- Nonspecific bowel gas pattern: not normal but not clearly obstructed.
  - Usually a few loops of mildly dilated small bowel or a gasless abdomen.
  - This may be seen in many abdominal diseases such as gastroenteritis or pancreatitis.
- Remember, if dilated bowel loops are fluid filled, they may not be appreciated. Hence, a paucity of bowel gas may suggest a small bowel obstruction in the appropriate clinical setting.

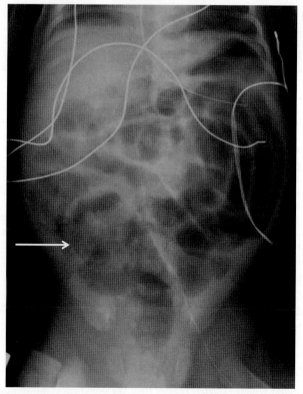

**Figure 29-7. Necrotizing enterocolitis.** Frontal radiograph of the abdomen shows lucencies predominantly in the right abdomen (*arrow*), compatible with pneumatosis intestinalis.

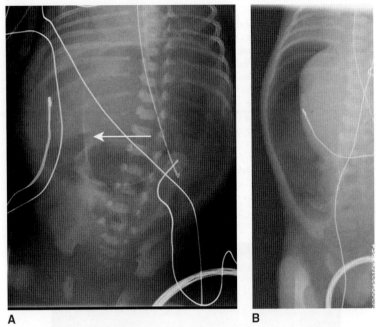

**A**　　　　　　　　　　　　　　　　　**B**

**Figure 29-8. Pneumoperitoneum.** Frontal view **(A)** of the abdomen shows a large lucency in abdomen. The falciform ligament (*arrow*) is visible since it is outlined by air. Left lateral decubitus (left side down) view **(B)** of the abdomen shows free peritoneal air lateral to the edge of the liver.

## Evaluating for Pneumoperitoneum

- Upright view: subdiaphragmatic gas. Adequate examination must include a portion of the chest and is more appropriate for older children.
- Left lateral decubitus view (Fig. 29-7): gas between liver and body wall. Adequate examinations must include the entire right abdomen.
- Supine view (Fig. 29-7): findings include sharp appearance of inferior liver edge; increased lucency, especially over the liver (football sign); falciform ligament outlined by air; visible inner and outer margins of bowel wall (Rigler sign); and air not conforming to typical bowel appearance such as in the subhepatic space.

## Evaluating Tubes and Lines

- Check all line positions.
  - Umbilical arterial catheter: courses caudally from umbilicus to internal iliac arteries and then cranially to aorta. There are two preferred positions:
    - Mid descending thoracic aorta (below ductus arteriosus) and above vertebral body T10 (usually T7-T9)
    - At the level of vertebral body L3 or L4 (below renal arteries and above aortic bifurcation)
  - Umbilical venous catheter: courses from the umbilicus cranially through the umbilical vein to ductus venosus to intrahepatic inferior vena cava. The preferred position is at the inferior vena cava/right atrial junction. Check for malpositioned catheters in the portal vein (left or right) and superior mesenteric vein.

- Endotracheal tube (ETT): The preferred position of the tip is below the thoracic inlet and above the carina. The ETT shifts with head position. As the head is flexed forward, the ETT passes lower in the trachea toward the carina, and as the head is extended posteriorly, the ETT will travel higher up in the trachea.
- ECMO arterial-venous (AV): The tip of the arterial catheter should be at or near the aortic arch (T4 level), and the tip of the venous catheter should be in the right atrium.
- ECMO venovenous (VV): The tip of the venous catheter should be in the right atrium.
- Nasogastric (NG) tube: Tip of the NG tube should be in the mid stomach with all side holes below the gastroesophageal junction.

## ABDOMINAL IMAGING

- Abdominal ultrasound
  - Assesses abdominal organs: liver, gallbladder, bile ducts, pancreas, spleen, kidneys, and bladder; sensitive for gallstones, renal stones, and fluid-filled bowel walls and their vascularity.
  - Can be performed at patient's bedside; keep patient NPO.
    - US is the first modality for evaluation of appendicitis (Fig. 29-9), intussusception, cholecystitis, liver lesions, renal pathologies, Henoch-Schönlein purpura, ovarian torsion, cysts, masses, and testicular pathologies.
- Abdominal/pelvic CT
  - Typically performed with IV contrast. Oral contrast useful for differentiation of small bowel from masses including abscesses. Keep patient NPO.
  - Evaluates abdominal solid organs (Fig. 29-10), intestines, mesentery, and retroperitoneum, and urinary tract very well; may be used in diagnosing bowel obstruction, abdominal trauma, masses (Fig. 29-11), inflammatory bowel disease, and pancreatitis.
  - Noncontrast CT for urinary tract stones.

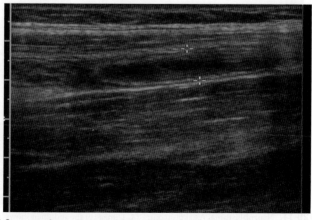

**Figure 29-9. Appendicitis.** Transverse **(A)** and longitudinal **(B)** ultrasound image of the right lower quadrant shows a noncompressible, tubular, blind-ending, hypoechoic structure, compatible with appendicitis. Normal appendix is compressible and measures <6 mm in diameter.

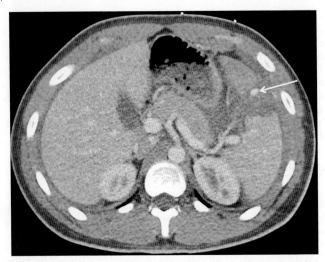

**Figure 29-10. Splenic trauma.** Axial CT image of the upper abdomen shows hypodensity involving spleen consistent with splenic laceration. Notice small enhancing focus (*arrow*) in the hypodensity suggestive of active extravasation.

- Ultrasound is preferable for characterizing adnexal and uterine pathology.
- Preferred for evaluating larger children and when ultrasound is equivocal including for appendicitis and to evaluate complications of appendicitis, such as abscess formation.

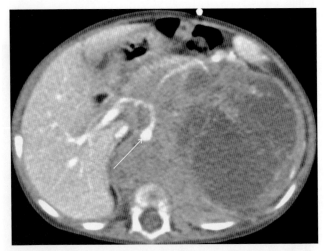

**Figure 29-11. Neuroblastoma.** Axial postcontrast CT image of the abdomen shows large heterogeneously enhancing mass in the retroperitoneum on left side crossing the midline and causing encasement and displacement of aorta and celiac axis (*arrow*) compatible with neuroblastoma.

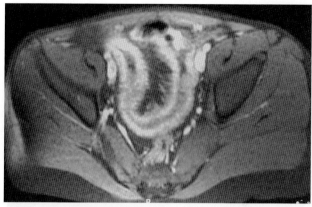

**Figure 29-12. Crohn disease.** Axial T1-weighted fat-suppressed MR enterography image through pelvis reveals circumferential bowel wall thickening involving distal ileum with enhancement. Notice engorged vessels in mesentery giving positive "comb sign."

- Abdominal/pelvic MRI
  - Use increasing. However, greater need for sedation than with CT.
  - MRCP is used to characterize pancreatic and biliary ductal anatomy.
  - MR enterography for evaluation of inflammatory bowel disease (Fig. 29-12).
  - MR imaging is useful for evaluation of a variety of abdominal abnormalities including appendicitis, solid organ masses, abscesses, and ovarian and uterine pathologies.

## GASTROINTESTINAL FLUOROSCOPIC EXAMINATIONS

- Fluoroscopic examinations can be performed with barium or water-soluble contrast.
- Examinations involve radiologist at patient's side performing the procedure.
- Patient should be NPO for 4 hours except in tiny premature infants.

### Speech Swallow Study

- Multiple food and liquid consistencies given with real-time fluoroscopic evaluation to assess which food types can be tolerated without aspiration
- Performed in conjunction with trained speech therapist

### Esophagram

Assesses the pharynx and esophagus for causes of dysphagia, strictures, foreign bodies, post-op tracheoesophageal fistula complications, vascular rings–double arch, right arch and aberrant left subclavian, and pulmonary artery sling. CT angiography is used to determine the exact abnormality.

### Upper Gastrointestinal Series

- Upper gastrointestinal (UGI) is the examination of choice for evaluating vomiting. Gastroesophageal reflux is the most common finding in vomiting children especially infants. UGI is used in the infant especially the newborn to exclude intestinal malrotation (Fig. 29-13) and midgut volvulus although ultrasound can be used for the

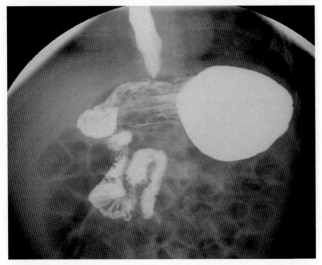

**Figure 29-13. Malrotation.** Upper GI examination with barium shows duodenojejunal junction near midline compatible with malrotation. Normally, D-J junction should cross midline and is located to the left of the left pedicle of L1 vertebra.

latter. Obstructions of the stomach, duodenum, and proximal jejunum can be diagnosed as well as ulcers, masses, duodenal webs, and SMA syndrome.
• When evaluating for hypertrophic pyloric stenosis (HPS), ultrasound is the first-line option (Fig. 29-14), but UGI can also be used.

### Small Bowel Follow-Through
• This procedure is used to evaluate the small intestine. It is usually performed in conjunction with an UGI examination.
    • Conditions assessed usually include inflammatory bowel disease, strictures, masses, and obstruction.
    • Small bowel obstruction can usually be diagnosed by plain radiographs of the abdomen, although small bowel studies and CT can be confirmatory.
• Contrast-enhanced abdominal and pelvic CT and MRI have markedly decreased the use of small bowel studies.

### Contrast Enema
• This fluoroscopic procedure is used to evaluate the colon for strictures, obstruction, masses, and constipation.
    • Evaluation of congenital obstruction such as Hirschsprung disease with sigmoid colon larger than rectum (Fig. 29-15), meconium ileus (Fig. 29-16), meconium plug syndrome (small left colon), distal bowel atresia, and post colostomy imperforate anus.
    • With intussusception, therapeutic reduction (with air or water-soluble contrast) is indicated. Since therapeutic reductions carry a risk of perforation, IV access and surgical consultation are needed.
• Active colitis is a relative contraindication to an enema.

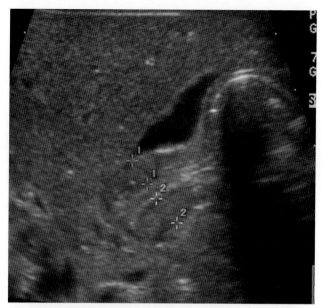

Figure 29-14. **Hypertrophic pyloric stenosis.** Ultrasound image of stomach reveals thickened pyloric wall and elongated pyloric channel consistent with HPS. Normal pyloric wall thickness measures <3 mm, and length measures <15 mm.

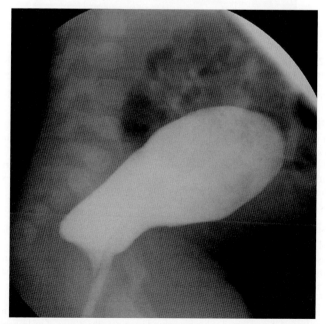

Figure 29-15. **Hirschsprung disease.** Hypaque enema shows small caliber rectum with dilated sigmoid colon with zone of transition at rectosigmoid junction consistent with Hirschsprung disease.

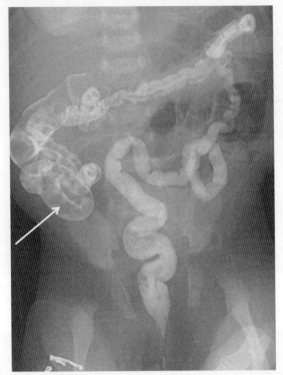

**Figure 29-16. Meconium ileus.** Hypaque enema shows filling defects (meconium) in distal ileal loops (*arrow*) with unused small caliber colon compatible with meconium ileus.

## GENITOURINARY IMAGING

### Voiding Cystourethrogram (VCUG)

- After the bladder is catheterized, fluoroscopy is performed during bladder filling and with spontaneous or voluntary voiding.
- A VCUG can identify and grade vesicoureteral reflux and diagnose obstruction including posterior urethral valves, bladder dyssynergia, or strictures. Urine should be clear of infection. The vesicoureteral reflux is graded I to V.
- Some centers use contrast ultrasound to diagnose reflux.

### Ultrasound

- Renal ultrasound
  - This examination is used to evaluate for age-appropriate kidney size, solid masses, cysts, hydronephrosis, scarring, stones, vascular occlusions, and diseases that alter renal echogenicity.
  - For the evaluation of prenatally detected hydronephrosis in neonates, US is performed at the age of 7-10 days unless the degree of prenatal hydronephrosis is moderate or large. US performed at birth may underestimate the degree of hydronephrosis.
  - CT is more sensitive for small solid masses and tiny calculi.

- Scrotal ultrasound
  - The examination of choice to assess for testicular or scrotal pathology, including testicular torsion, torsion of testicular appendage, trauma, masses, and infection.
  - Doppler evaluation is performed to assess blood flow.
- Pelvic ultrasound
  - The examination of choice for ovarian and uterine pathology.
  - Pediatric pelvic ultrasound is performed transabdominally. A full bladder is required.
    - Doppler evaluation is performed to assess blood flow.
    - Common indications include pelvic pain, ovarian torsion, tuboovarian abscess, pregnancy, ectopic pregnancy, adnexal masses, and uterine bleeding.

### Genitourinary Computed Tomography and Magnetic Resonance Imaging

- Stone protocol CTs are performed without oral or IV contrast to assess for renal and ureteral calculi and associated obstruction.
- Contrast CT is used to evaluate possible masses, pyelonephritis, obstruction, trauma, and anomalies of the genitourinary tract.
- MRI is increasingly used to diagnose tumors, pyelonephritis, masses, and function.

### SKELETAL IMAGING

- Bones are generally evaluated with plain radiographs.
- Radiographs of the skull, chest, abdomen, and extremities are performed for indications such as trauma, pain, tumors, osteomyelitis, slipped capital femoral epiphysis (SCFE) (Fig. 29-17), avascular necrosis, child abuse (Figs. 29-18 and 29-19), skeletal dysplasias (Fig. 29-20), and Langerhans cell histiocytosis.
- CT provides excellent bone detail and is better for complex fractures.

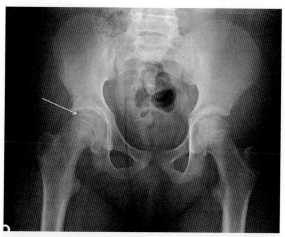

**Figure 29-17. Slipped capital femoral epiphysis.** Frontal radiograph of pelvis shows slipped capital femoral epiphysis on the right side (*arrow*). Notice that a line drawn along the lateral aspect of the right femoral neck does not intersect the lateral aspect of capital femoral epiphysis.

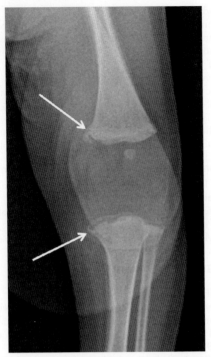

**Figure 29-18. Child abuse.** Frontal radiograph of knee reveals corner fractures (*arrows*) involving distal femoral and proximal femoral metaphyses, characteristic of child abuse.

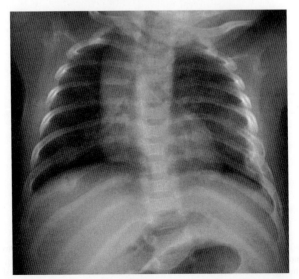

**Figure 29-19. Child abuse.** Frontal radiograph of chest reveals healing fractures involving right 7th and 8th ribs and left 6th, 7th, 8th, and 9th ribs suggestive of child abuse.

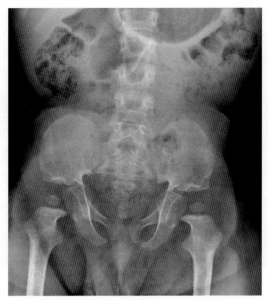

**Figure 29-20. Achondroplasia.** Frontal radiograph of the pelvis shows narrowing of the inter-pedicular distance inferiorly across lumbar spine, flattening and irregularity of the acetabular roofs, squaring of the iliac wings, and narrow sciatic notches compatible with achondroplasia. There is metaphyseal widening involving both femora.

- Ultrasound and MRI can be used for better soft tissue differentiation (Fig. 29-21).
- Hip ultrasound is added typically for two different indications:
  - To assess for dislocation (developmental dysplasia of the hip) in children <6 months of age.
  - To check for fluid in infants and children suspected of having a septic hip or other causes of hip effusion such as toxic/transient synovitis.
- Bone age can be normal, advanced, or delayed relative to chronologic age.
  - A single left hand radiograph is compared with an atlas of normal standard examples (Greulich and Pyle method).
  - Multiple radiographs of one side of the patient are taken to count ossification centers throughout the skeleton (Elgenmark method); this is more accurate in patients <2 years of age.

## NEUROIMAGING

- Neonatal head ultrasound is used to assess for intracranial hemorrhage (Fig. 29-22), hydrocephalus, periventricular leukomalacia, large arteriovenous shunts, developmental anomalies of the brain, extra-axial fluid collections, and gross brain maturity.
- Transcranial Doppler is helpful to evaluate the risk of stroke in children with sickle cell disease by assessing the blood flow velocities in the distal internal carotid or proximal middle cerebral artery.

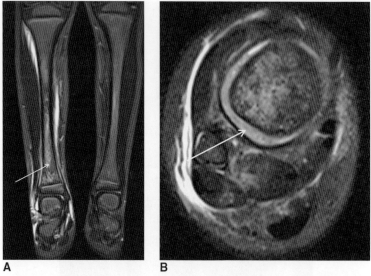

A        B

**Figure 29-21. Osteomyelitis.** Coronal T2-weighted fat-suppressed MR image **(A)** demonstrates bone marrow edema involving right femoral distal metadiaphysis (*arrow*) with associated soft tissue edema and effusion in right ankle joint. Axial T2-weighted MR image **(B)** shows subperiosteal collection surrounding distal femoral metaphysis compatible with subperiosteal abscess.

- Head CT
  - After the neonatal period, noncontrast head CT is the usual screening examination, including for hematomas (Fig. 29-23) and trauma (Fig. 29-24).
  - Contrast may be used to assess for tumors, but MRI is preferred for greater sensitivity.
  - MRI is used to evaluate seizures, tumors, congenital anomalies, strokes, and ventriculoperitoneal shunt dysfunction. Diffusion-weighted image (DWI) and apparent diffusion coefficient map (ADC) are more sensitive to acute ischemia.
- Spine CT is used for evaluating injury after plain radiographs as well as for assessing tumors, infections, and congenital vertebral deformities.
- Spine MRI is used for overall spine imaging, including spinal cord, intervertebral disks, and subarachnoid and epidural pathology. MRI is the examination of choice for tumors, tumor extension into spinal canal such as neuroblastoma, congenital anomalies, and epidural abscesses.
- Positron emission tomography is primarily used for tumor detection and surveillance and to locate seizure foci.

## NUCLEAR MEDICINE

- Nuclear medicine examinations can provide functional information that other imaging modalities cannot. However, anatomic detail is usually less than with other imaging modalities.
- Some nuclear medicine examinations can be performed portably.
- Bone scan
  - This scan is more sensitive than a radiograph but less specific for bone pathology. MRI is also excellent for bone pathology and is more specific.

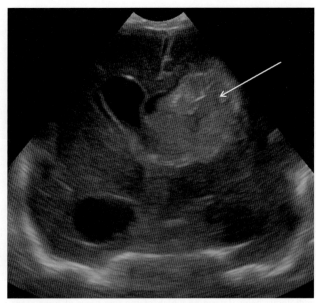

**Figure 29-22. Grade IV hemorrhage in preterm infant.** Coronal ultrasound image of the head reveals large hemorrhage in left caudothalamic groove with intraparenchymal extension in the left frontal lobe and basal ganglia (*arrow*) and ventricular dilatation consistent with grade IV hemorrhage.

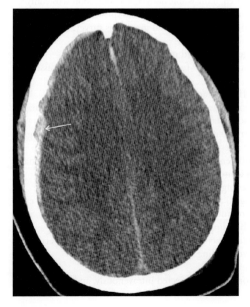

**Figure 29-23. Subdural hemorrhage.** Axial CT image of the head shows crescentic high attenuation blood along the frontoparietal region (*arrow*) with mild mass effect over anterior aspect of falx. Notice small subdural hemorrhage along the anterior interhemispheric fissure.

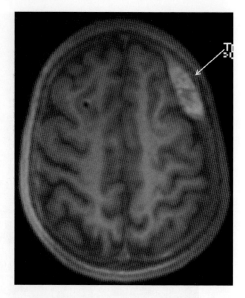

**Figure 29-24. Epidural hemorrhage.** T1-weighted axial image of the brain reveals hyperintense lenticular-shaped epidural hemorrhage in left frontal region (*arrow*).

- The radiologist helps determine which of the two types of bone scans is more appropriate.
  - Three-phase bone scan consists of blood flow, immediate uptake, and delay retention (about 2-4 hours after injection) imaging of a technetium-radiolabeled agent injected intravenously. The imaging of the first two phases is limited to the primary region of concern. Delayed imaging is often of the whole body. Usual indication is osteomyelitis (which can be multifocal in children via hematogenous spread) or occult fracture.
  - Delayed whole-body imaging is used for skeletal metastasis survey.
- Renal scan
  - A technetium-radiolabeled agent is injected intravenously.
  - Used to assess the relative contribution of function of each kidney and to assess for urinary obstruction.
- Hydroxy iminodiacetic acid (HIDA) scan
  - A technetium-radiolabeled agent is injected intravenously and the abdomen is imaged to evaluate for radiotracer hepatic uptake and excretion into the biliary system.
  - Some radiologists administer phenobarbital for a few days before imaging to improve sensitivity for biliary atresia. Patients should be kept NPO.
  - HIDA scans are useful for differentiating congenital biliary atresia from neonatal hepatitis and for diagnosis of acute or chronic cholecystitis.
- Tagged red cell scan for GI bleeding
  - Technetium-radiolabeled (tagged) red blood cells are injected intravenously to evaluate for bleeding over 60-90 minutes of imaging.
  - The patient must be actively bleeding to obtain a positive result.
  - Because GI bleeding is episodic, evacuation of bloody stools does not directly correlate with the timing of active bleeding.
- Meckel scan
  - A technetium-radiolabeled compound is injected intravenously, and the abdomen is imaged.

- This is a highly specific examination for Meckel diverticulum containing ectopic gastric mucosa.
- It does not require active bleeding.
- Lung scan
  - Usually a two-part examination.
    - Ventilation imaging with inhaled xenon gas or technetium-radiolabeled particles.
    - Perfusion imaging with technetium-labeled intravenously injected particles, which are trapped in small arterial branches.
- Used to evaluate for pulmonary embolism and lung transplantation surveillance.
- CT is the modality of choice for pulmonary embolism.

## INTERVENTION RADIOLOGY

- Venous access: ultrasound and fluoroscopy are used to insert peripherally inserted central catheter (PICC) and central venous lines.
- Gastrostomy or gastrojejunostomy catheters: can be placed or exchanged under fluoroscopic guidance in a minimally invasive manner under IV sedation or general anesthesia.
- Diagnostic angiography and angioembolization: digital subtraction angiography is useful for diagnosis and treatment of vascular malformations and preoperative embolization of vascular tumors.
- Needle biopsy: ultrasound and CT guidance used for renal, liver, thyroid, bone, lymph node, and lung biopsies.
- Abscess drainage: intra-abdominal abscesses can be drained in minimally invasive manner under ultrasound and CT guidance. Lung abscesses and abscesses in other sites such as extremities are also amenable to sampling and drainage under imaging guidance.
- Pleural fluid and ascites drainage: ultrasound guidance is used for sampling or drainage of pleural fluid and ascites.
- Percutaneous nephrostomies: obstructed renal pelvicalyceal system is drained by placement of pigtail drainage catheters inserted under fluoroscopic or ultrasound guidance.

## SUGGESTED READINGS

Coley BD, ed. Caffey's Pediatric Diagnostic Imaging. 13th Ed. Philadelphia, PA: Mosby Elsevier, 2019.

Donnelly LF, ed. Pediatric Imaging. 2nd Ed. Philadelphia, PA: Elsevier, 2017.

James CA, ed. Pediatric Radiology Casebase. New York, NY: Thieme, 2016.

Jatav A, et al. Intestinal obstruction in neonatal and pediatric age group (a clinico-pathological study). Int J Recent Sci Res 2015;6:5868–5874.

Kan JH, et al. Pediatric musculoskeletal imaging: beyond the basics. Ped Radiol 2013;43(supp):247–258.

Liszewski MC, Lee EY. Neonatal lung disorders: pattern recognition approach to diagnosis. Am J Roent 2018;210:964–975.

Maller V, et al. Neonatal head ultrasound a review and update—part 1. Ultrasound Q 2019;35:202–211.

Maller V, et al. Neonatal head ultrasound a review and update—part 2. Ultrasound Q 2019;35:212–223.

Swischuk LE, ed. Imaging of the Newborn, Infant, and Young Child. 5th Ed. Baltimore, MD: Lippincott Williams & Wilkins, 2003.

Viteri B, Calle-Toro JS, Furth S, et al. State-of-the-art renal imaging in children. Pediatrics 2020;145(2):e20190829. https://doi.org/10.1542/peds.2019-0829

# Rheumatologic Diseases

Tarin M. Bigley and Erica Schmitt

## INTRODUCTION

Pediatric rheumatology is a broad field that deals with disorders of the joints, connective tissues, muscles, and vasculature as well as autoimmune and autoinflammatory disorders.

## APPROACH TO THE CHILD WITH JOINT PAIN AND/OR SWELLING

• Joint pain is a common complaint in children.
• It is generally transient, secondary to trauma and/or increased activity.

### Etiology and Differential Diagnosis

• It is important to determine if the pain is secondary to joint, muscle, ligament, or bone or if it is referred pain.
• Joint pain (arthralgia) should be distinguished from arthritis, which has objective physical examination findings of limitation in the range of motion, effusion, warmth, and/or erythema.
• Joint pain may be due to various conditions depending on the number and kind of joints involved. Diagnostic considerations include:
  • Single joint (monoarticular):
    ○ Fracture
    ○ Hemarthrosis (primarily seen in sickle cell disease, trauma, bleeding diatheses such as hemophilia)
    ○ Infectious: septic joint, osteomyelitis, Lyme arthritis, or gonococcal infection
    ○ Inflammatory: juvenile idiopathic arthritis (JIA) or other inflammatory arthritis (e.g., sarcoidosis), chronic nonbacterial osteomyelitis
    ○ Malignancy: primary bone tumor or leukemia
  • Multiple joints (polyarticular)
    ○ Infectious: Lyme arthritis or *Neisseria gonorrhoeae*, viral infections (Parvovirus, Epstein-Barr virus, HIV, hepatitis B and C, arboviruses)
    ○ Inflammatory: JIA, immunoglobulin A vasculitis (IgAV, formerly Henoch-Schönlein purpura [HSP]), systemic lupus erythematosus (SLE), serum sickness–like reaction, sarcoidosis, inflammatory bowel disease (IBD)–associated arthritis, Kawasaki disease or other systemic vasculitis, autoinflammatory syndromes, chronic nonbacterial osteomyelitis
    ○ Malignancy: Leukemia
    ○ Polyarticular joint pain without significant swelling: hypermobility, pes planus, overuse injuries, osteochondroses, amplified musculoskeletal pain (AMP) syndrome, Celiac disease
    ○ Reactive arthritis: *Salmonella, Shigella, Yersinia, Campylobacter,* or *Chlamydia*
    ○ Rheumatic fever and poststreptococcal reactive arthritis (PSRA)
    ○ Rickets

- Hip involvement (rare as the sole presentation of an inflammatory arthritis in children)
  - Avascular necrosis: Legg-Calvé-Perthes disease, sickle cell disease, or chronic steroid use
  - Infectious: septic joint, Lyme arthritis, osteomyelitis
  - Inflammatory: IBD-associated arthritis, psoriatic arthritis, enthesitis-related arthritis
  - Slipped capital femoral epiphysis (SCFE)
  - Transient synovitis (formerly known as toxic synovitis)

## Laboratory Studies

*Initial Evaluation*

- Blood cultures: any time there is fever and new-onset joint pain
- Complete blood count (CBC):
  - Elevated white blood cells (WBCs): infection, inflammatory arthritis, malignancies
  - Cytopenias: SLE, malignancy
  - Microcytic anemia: IBD, systemic JIA
  - Thrombocytosis: systemic JIA
- Erythrocyte sedimentation rate (ESR) and C-reactive protein (CRP): elevated in infectious and inflammatory conditions; these are both nonspecific but can be useful for tracking established disease activity
- Renal function panel: SLE, vasculitis (e.g., IgAV, ANCA-associated vasculitis, Goodpasture syndrome)
- Antinuclear antibody (ANA): if there is clinical concern for SLE or with established diagnosis of JIA to stratify risk of uveitis (see JIA section)

## Joint Fluid Analysis (Table 30-1)

- For isolated effusions with fever, joint aspiration is necessary to exclude a septic joint and should be done quickly and before initiation of antibiotics if the patient is stable.

| TABLE 30-1 | Properties of Synovial Joint Fluid | | | |
|---|---|---|---|---|
| | **Normal** | **Noninflammatory** | **Inflammatory** | **Infectious** |
| Color | Colorless/ Straw | Straw/yellow | Yellow | Variable |
| Clarity | Clear | Clear | Clear to cloudy | Cloudy, turbid |
| White blood cell count (per µL) | <200 | <2000 | 2000-50,000 | >50,000 |
| % Neutrophils | <25% | <25% | >50% | >75% |
| Associated conditions | (normal) | Trauma, avascular necrosis | JIA, reactive arthritis, spondyloarthritis | Often bacterial, culture positive |

JIA, juvenile idiopathic arthritis.

- Do not consider a rheumatologic etiology or initiate steroids in a child with fever and joint effusion before conducting a thorough investigation for a septic joint or osteomyelitis.

## Imaging

- Plain film radiographs of involved joints may show evidence of trauma, arthritis, and bony abnormalities.
- Sonography is a sensitive technique that can identify joint effusion, synovitis, tenosynovitis, and enthesitis. It can be useful in acute settings to examine the hip joint and may be considered if multiple joints need to be imaged or if the child is unable to be sedated for an MRI.
- In cases where there is a history of trauma, concern for septic joint and/or osteomyelitis, or the diagnosis of arthritis is uncertain, a magnetic resonance imaging scan with and without contrast can be useful.

## Treatment

- A patient who presents with joint pain and fever should be presumed to have a septic joint or osteomyelitis until proven otherwise.
- A potentially septic joint or osteomyelitis is an emergency that requires prompt recognition, involvement of orthopedic surgery, radiologic imaging, and initiation of intravenous (IV) antibiotics once blood and synovial fluid (if appropriate) cultures are obtained.
- Drugs frequently used in rheumatology are described in Table 30-2.

## JUVENILE IDIOPATHIC ARTHRITIS

- JIA is a chronic inflammatory arthritis of unknown etiology.
- Several classification schemata exist. This disease may be classified into three main subsets: oligoarticular, polyarticular, and systemic (Table 30-3). Other types of JIA also include psoriatic arthritis, enthesitis-related arthritis (including juvenile spondyloarthritis), and undifferentiated arthritis. Other chronic conditions presenting with arthropathy include IBD and cystic fibrosis.

## Diagnosis

- JIA is a diagnosis of exclusion (see Table 30-3).
- Diagnosis requires arthritis in one or more joints for at least 6 weeks, age of onset <16 years, and exclusion of other causes of joint inflammation.
- Laboratory values are of little use in diagnosis but can help to exclude other diagnoses, and are for prognosis (e.g., increased risk of uveitis with a positive ANA), for further classification of established chronic arthritis (e.g., rheumatoid factor and HLA-B27), and for tracking disease activity (ESR, CRP, and CBC).

## Treatment

- Pharmacologic therapy
  - Anti-inflammatory agents
    - Nonsteroidal anti-inflammatory drugs (NSAIDs): Naproxen 20 mg/kg/day divided q12h *or* ibuprofen 40 mg/kg/day divided q6h. Patients should take this on a scheduled basis for initial therapy.

**TABLE 30-2  Common Drugs Used in Pediatric Rheumatology[a]**

| Drug | Mechanism/actions | Dosage | Major side effects |
|---|---|---|---|
| **NSAIDs** | | | |
| 1. Naproxen | Anti-inflammatory | 1. 20 mg/kg/day PO div. q12h (max 1 g/day) | Easy bleeding and bruising |
| 2. Ibuprofen | Cyclooxygenase enzyme inhibition | 2. 10 mg/kg/dose PO q6h (max 2.4 g/day) | Gastrointestinal: gastritis, bleeding |
| 3. Aspirin | | 3. 60-90 mg/kg/day PO div. q.i.d. (max 4 g/day) | Nephrotoxicity |
| | | | Pseudoporphyria (naproxen) |
| | | | Reye syndrome (aspirin) |
| **Corticosteroids** | | | |
| Triamcinolone acetonide (IA) | Anti-inflammatory | Varies, typically 10-40 mg per joint | Skin atrophy at site of injection; very rarely infection |
| Prednisone (PO) | Anti-inflammatory | Varies, 0.5-2 mg/kg/day PO | Cushing syndrome, growth delay, osteoporosis, avascular necrosis, cataracts and glaucoma |
| Methylprednisolone (IV) | Immunosuppressive (T cell) | Pulse dose: 30 mg/kg/day IV, maximum 1 g/day | |
| **Disease-Modifying Drugs** | | | |
| Methotrexate (PO, SC) | Inhibits purine synthesis | 10-15 mg/m² once weekly PO or SC (max 20-25 mg weekly) | Hepatotoxicity |
| | | | Cytopenias |
| Hydroxychloroquine (PO) | Unknown—interferes with neutrophil trafficking, lysosomal pH | 3-5 mg/kg/day (max 400 mg/day) | Retinal toxicity with long-term use |
| Colchicine (PO) | Interferes with microtubules | 0.3-1.8 mg/day (max 2.4 mg/day) | Abdominal pain, diarrhea |
| **Cytotoxic Agents** | | | |
| Cyclophosphamide (IV) | Alkylating agent | Varies, pulse therapy monthly is 500-1000 mg/m² IV | Cystitis, BM suppression |
| | Causes lymphopenia | | Increased risk of infection, Risk of infertility with high total dose |
| Cyclosporine (PO) | Thought to inhibit T-cell activation | Not standardized, dose based on goal trough levels | Nephrotoxicity, hypertension, hepatotoxicity |

*(Continued)*

**TABLE 30-2** Common Drugs Used in Pediatric Rheumatology[a] *(Continued)*

| Drug | Mechanism/actions | Dosage | Major side effects |
|------|-------------------|--------|--------------------|
| Mycophenolate mofetil (PO) | Inhibits de novo guanine nucleotide synthesis, reduces lymphocyte proliferation | 300–600 mg/m²/dose q12h (max 3 g/day) | GI toxicity, cytopenias, infection |
| **Biologic agents** | | | |
| Rituximab (IV) | Anti-CD20 mAb (anti-B cell) | Pediatric dosing not standardized, given as an IV infusion | Infusion reactions<br>Increased risk of infection including reactivation of JC virus |
| Intravenous immune globulin (IV) | Pooled human immunoglobulin | Up to 2 g/kg IV | Infusion reactions<br>Aseptic meningitis |
| Anakinra (SC, IV) | Soluble IL-1Ra (inhibits IL-1) | Varies; 1–2 mg/kg/day SC | Local injection site reactions |
| Canakinumab (SC) | Anti-IL-1β mAb | Varies; 2–4 mg/kg every 4–8 weeks SC | Local injection site reactions/ |
| Tocilizumab (SC, IV) | Anti-IL-6R mAb | Varies | Infusion or injection reaction, AST/ALT elevations, hyperlipidemia |
| **Anti-TNF-α agents** | | | **For all anti-TNF-α agents** |
| 1. (Enbrel) (SC) | Soluble TNF-α receptor | 1. 0.8 mg/kg SC weekly (max 50 mg weekly) | Infusion/injection site reactions |
| 2. Infliximab (Remicade) (IV) | Anti-TNF-α chimeric mAb | 2. 3–10 mg/kg IV q 4–8 weeks | Reactivation of tuberculosis |
| 3. Adalimumab (Humira) (SC) | Humanized anti-TNF-α mAb | 3. 10–40 mg SC every 2 weeks | Possible increased risk of malignancy |
| **Kinase inhibitors** | | | |
| Tofacitinib (PO) | Small molecule, predominantly inhibits JAK1 and JAK3 | 3.2–5 mg per dose, twice daily | Infection, lipid abnormalities |

[a]These medications are each used in a variety of rheumatologic diseases; many are investigational, and all should be given in consultation with a pediatric rheumatologist.

BM, bone marrow; IA, intra-articular; IV, intravenous; JAK, janus kinase; NSAID, nonsteroidal anti-inflammatory drug; PO, by mouth; SC, subcutaneous; TNF, tumor necrosis factor.

**TABLE 30-3** Classification of Juvenile Idiopathic Arthritis (JIA)

| | Oligoarticular | Polyarticular | Systemic |
|---|---|---|---|
| **Diagnostic criteria** | | | |
| Number of joints | ≤4 | ≥5 | Any number, usually >5 |
| Length of arthritis | 6 weeks | 6 weeks | 6 weeks |
| Others | | | Daily fever >39°C for at least 2 weeks |
| **Gender** | Female > male | Female > male | Male = female |
| **Peak age** | 1-3 years | 1-3 years and 9-14 years | 1-5 years, but may occur any time during childhood |
| **Extra-articular manifestations** | Systemic symptoms rare | Poor growth | Ill appearance |
| | Uveitis (15-30%) | Low-grade fever | Evanescent, erythematous macular rash |
| | | Fatigue | Serositis |
| | | Uveitis (2-20%) | Lymphadenopathy, hepatomegaly, and/or splenomegaly |
| | | | Pulmonary and cardiac disease |
| | | | Uveitis is rare |
| **Laboratory findings** | approximately 65% ANA+ | approximately 50% ANA+ | approximately 50% ANA+ |
| | Often normal, may have mildly ↑ ESR, CRP | ↑ ESR, CRP | ↑ WBC, platelets |
| | | ↑ WBC, platelets | ↓ hemoglobin |
| | | RF used to classify as RF+ or RF− disease | ↑ ESR, CRP |
| | | | Usually ANA and RF negative |
| **Prognosis** | Good, overall | Often chronic | Guarded initially |
| | ↑ uveitis with ANA+ | RF+ more severe | approximately 40% fully recover |

ANA, antinuclear antibody; CRP, C-reactive protein; ESR, erythrocyte sedimentation rate; RF, rheumatoid factor; WBC, white blood cell.
Adapted from Cassidy JT, et al. A study of classification criteria for a diagnosis of juvenile rheumatoid arthritis. Arthritis Rheum 1986;29(2):274–281; Petty RE, Laxer RM, Lindsley CB, et al. Textbook of Pediatric Rheumatology. 8th Ed. Philadelphia, PA: Elsevier Inc., 2021.

- ○ Intra-articular corticosteroids: First-line therapy for patients with oligoarticular arthritis in joints amenable to intra-articular injection. Many patients will experience 3+ months of remission following a joint injection with triamcinolone acetonide.
  - ○ Systemic corticosteroids: Used for flares unresponsive to other therapies or severe systemic manifestations; can be given orally or intravenously. Systemic corticosteroids are generally not used as a first-line therapy anymore due to the early use of biologic medications.
- Disease-modifying antirheumatic drugs (DMARDs)
  - ○ Methotrexate and leflunomide: need to monitor for liver injury and blood counts
  - ○ Antitumor necrosis factor-α agents (anti-TNF-α, biologic agents): etanercept, infliximab, adalimumab, and golimumab
  - ○ Other biologic medications: IL-1 inhibitors (anakinra, rilonacept, canakinumab), IL-6 receptor antibody (tocilizumab), CTLA4-Ig (abatacept), and Janus kinase (JAK)-inhibitors (tofacitinib)
- See Table 30-2 for dosages and further information for select medications.
- Special considerations for therapy of systemic JIA
  - Initial treatment is often instituted during hospitalization until systemic symptoms are under control.
  - NSAIDs may help to control pain and swelling but are not used alone.
  - Initial treatment often consists of steroids and methotrexate with a biologic medication.
  - Early use of biologic agents, especially inhibitors of the IL-1 or IL-6 pathways, may be beneficial in some patients.
- Other monitoring/therapies
  - Ophthalmology examinations for uveitis are necessary every 3-6 months for oligoarticular and polyarticular JIA, and yearly for systemic JIA. Children <6 years old with a positive ANA and oligoarticular disease are at highest risk for eye disease, which can be severe and may require escalation of therapy.
  - Physical therapy, occupational therapy, and psychological support can be important for long-term outcome. However, with improving therapies, fewer physical disabilities related to JIA now occur.

## Complications

- Most complications/emergencies are related to therapy for JIA, including infections associated with immunosuppressive therapy (corticosteroids and anti-TNF-α agents) or gastrointestinal bleeding related to NSAID use.
- Children with systemic JIA are often very ill and present with multiple extra-articular manifestations as described in Table 30-3.
- Macrophage activation syndrome is a rare life-threatening complication associated with systemic JIA and other autoimmune disorders. This syndrome is characterized by persistent fever, hepatosplenomegaly, lymphadenopathy, overwhelming systemic inflammation, disseminated intravascular coagulation, hepatic failure, and cytopenias; it can be fatal, and swift recognition and treatment in consultation with a pediatric rheumatologist and pediatric hematologist is necessary.
- Parenchymal lung disease is a more recently recognized complication of systemic JIA. Described entities include interstitial lung disease, pulmonary fibrosis, pulmonary arterial hypertension, and pulmonary alveolar proteinosis. Pulmonary involvement is associated with a poor prognosis.

## SYSTEMIC LUPUS ERYTHEMATOSUS

### Definition and Epidemiology

- SLE is an autoimmune inflammatory disorder characterized by dysregulation of innate and adaptive immunity with abnormalities noted in type-I interferon production, complement pathways, apoptosis, and immune complex deposition in multiple organs.
- It more commonly affects females after puberty.
- It can develop at any age, but very rarely occurs in children <5 years of age.

### Diagnosis and Laboratory Studies

- SLE is a clinical diagnosis. Classification criteria have been developed which require the presence of at least four or more clinical and/or laboratory criteria (Table 30-4; think **MD SOAP BRAIN**).

| TABLE 30-4 | Classification Criteria for Systemic Lupus Erythematous |
|---|---|

1. **M**alar rash: spares nasolabial folds and eyelids
2. **D**iscoid rash: usually on scalp or limbs
3. **S**erositis: pleuritis or pericarditis
4. **O**ral or nasal mucocutaneous ulcers: usually painless
5. **A**rthritis: two or more peripheral joints, nonerosive
6. **P**hotosensitivity: by history or examination
7. **B**lood: cytopenias (one of the following):
   - Hemolytic anemia
   - Leukopenia (<4000/μL) on two or more occasions
   - Lymphopenia (<1500/μL) on two or more occasions
   - Thrombocytopenia (<100,000/μL)
8. **R**enal disorder:
   - Proteinuria >0.5 g/day, **or**
   - Cellular casts
9. **A**NA: positive in the absence of medications known to cause drug-associated lupus
10. **I**mmunologic (one of the following):
    - Anti-dsDNA antibodies
    - Anti-Sm nuclear antigen
    - Antiphospholipid antibodies: anticardiolipin antibodies, lupus anticoagulant, or false-positive serologic test for syphilis for at least 6 months
11. **N**eurologic (one of the following):
    - Seizure
    - Psychosis

Adapted from Tan E, et al. The 1982 revised criteria for the classification of systemic lupus erythematosus. Arthritis Rheum 1982;25:1271–1277; Hochberg MC. Updating the American College of Rheumatology revised criteria for the classification of systemic lupus erythematosus. Arthritis Rheum 1997;40:1725.

- In addition to the laboratory criteria listed in Table 30-4 that are used for diagnosis and classification, the following can be used as markers to monitor disease activity and response to therapy in SLE.
  - C3 and C4. Low levels indicate increased disease activity.
  - CBC. Patients often have cytopenias.
  - dsDNA. Titers are often elevated and may be reflective of disease activity.
  - Kidney function. As many as 75% of children with SLE have lupus nephritis.
  - Antiphospholipid antibodies (may also be present in patients without SLE or other autoimmune disease). Patients are at increased risk for thrombotic events. Diagnosis of antiphospholipid syndrome is made based on a history of thrombosis or pregnancy loss or prematurity with persistent lupus anticoagulant, anticardiolipin (IgG or IgM) antibody, or β2-glycoprotein (IgG or IgM) antibody positivity 12 weeks apart.

## Treatment

- Goal: to control the immune response and treat organ-specific manifestations of the disease
- Pharmacologic therapies (for more information on specific agents, see Table 30-2)
  - Hydroxychloroquine: used in most patients, effective for musculoskeletal and mucocutaneous manifestations, reduces rate of disease flares and improve survival.
  - NSAIDs (use with caution if patients have renal disease)
  - Corticosteroids
    - Oral prednisone, 0.5-2 mg/kg/day taper until improvement of laboratory markers of disease control; may require long-term use
    - Pulse dosing of IV steroids are used for severe, acute organ involvement (i.e., brain, kidney, hematologic, and cardiopulmonary manifestations)
  - Immunosuppressive/cytotoxic agents: cyclophosphamide, mycophenolate, azathioprine, and cyclosporine
  - Biologic modifiers: rituximab (monoclonal anti-CD20 antibody), belimumab (monoclonal antibody against B-lymphocyte stimulating factor)
  - Anticoagulation: should be considered if patients have high titer antiphospholipid antibodies and a history of thrombosis. Warfarin is typically used for secondary thrombosis prevention

## Complications

- Patients with SLE can present with a variety of emergent conditions, including mesenteric vasculitis (presenting as acute abdominal pain); cardiac tamponade; Libman-Sacks endocarditis; pleural effusions; pulmonary hemorrhage; renal failure; and thrombosis with stroke or pulmonary embolism related to antiphospholipid syndrome.
- Immunosuppressive therapy makes these patients susceptible to infection.

## NEONATAL LUPUS

- This self-limited condition is seen in newborns as a result of transplacental passage of maternal autoantibodies (SSA and SSB; also known as Ro and La). This is a temporary acquired disease, and symptoms are generally limited to the skin and heart.
- The majority of mothers of these infants do not have SLE or a known connective tissue disorder but are more likely to develop these conditions in the future and should receive counseling.

- Clinical manifestations include an owl-eye rash, or ringworm-appearing rash (commonly on the face and scalp), congenital heart block, and less commonly liver disease or cytopenias (neutropenia most common).
- Treatment is generally supportive until maternal antibodies are gone (typically by 6-8 months of age). There is no consensus regarding prenatal and postnatal immunomodulatory management of cardiac manifestations, though treatment algorithms exist.
- If present, congenital heart block is usually permanent and may require a pacemaker.
- Infants do not appear to have an increased risk of developing SLE later in life but may be at increased risk for autoimmunity based on a genetic predisposition.

## JUVENILE DERMATOMYOSITIS

### Definition and Epidemiology

- Juvenile dermatomyositis is an autoimmune disorder characterized by inflammation of the muscle and skin resulting in proximal muscle weakness and characteristic skin lesions. The mechanism appears to be related to a vasculopathy (inflammation of the blood vessels).
- Before therapy with corticosteroids, one-third of patients died, but with therapy, current survival is >95%.
- The peak age of onset is approximately 7 years of age.
- The condition is seen more commonly in girls.

### Clinical Presentation

- Patients may present acutely with inability to walk because of muscle weakness; look for Gower sign on physical examination. Muscle involvement is typically symmetric and proximal (trunk, limb-girdle, anterior neck flexors).
- Characteristic rashes include a heliotrope rash with purplish discoloration of upper eyelids and periorbital edema, as well as Gottron's papules (shiny, scaly, erythematous dermatitis over the dorsum of the metacarpophalangeal, and proximal interphalangeal joints).
- Other findings may include fever, fatigue, and weight loss; dysphagia and dysphonia; arthralgias and arthritis; subcutaneous calcinosis, sometimes resulting in ulcerations; nail bed telangiectases, which are nearly pathognomonic; and vasculitis that affects visceral organs (GI bleeding) and skin. Interstitial lung disease can be seen in some types of JDM.
- Labs demonstrate elevated serum muscle enzymes. Myositis-specific antibodies may be present and can often predict clinical phenotypes and outcomes. Muscle biopsy may be needed at diagnosis, particularly if the presentation is atypical.
- Plain films may be used to characterize the extent of calcinosis, and MRI of the musculature (generally pelvis and thighs) has been used to aid in the diagnosis of JDM and to monitor disease activity.
- The disease course varies, with about one-third of patients following a monocyclic course, up to one-third follow a polycyclic course with multiple relapses and remissions, and the remainder have a chronic course with persistent disease activity despite treatment.

### Treatment

- Pharmacologic therapy. For more information on specific agents, see Table 30-2.
  - Corticosteroids: IV pulse or oral 1-2 mg/kg/day until symptoms improve (strength, muscle enzymes), then taper. However, these drugs may be required for years.

- Immunosuppressives/cytotoxic agents: methotrexate, hydroxychloroquine, cyclophosphamide, cyclosporine, and azathioprine have been used.
- Biologic modifiers: IVIG and rituximab (experimental) have been used with some success.

## Complications

- Prompt recognition of symptoms and treatment advances have significantly reduced the morbidity and mortality of this disease.
- However, patients are still at risk for cardiorespiratory failure because of muscle weakness, aspiration pneumonias, and organ damage such as gastrointestinal hemorrhage related to vasculitis. Other long-term complications include refractory calcinosis, lipodystrophy, osteoporosis, and interstitial lung disease.

## IMMUNOGLOBULIN A VASCULITIS (IGA VASCULITIS [IGAV], FORMERLY HENOCH-SCHÖNLEIN PURPURA)

### Definition and Epidemiology

- IgAV is characterized by a purpuric rash without evidence of coagulopathy, abdominal pain, arthritis or arthralgias, and renal involvement.
- It is a common vasculitis in children, usually occurring between the ages of 3 and 12 years.
- It is more frequent in winter months.
- It often follows a viral upper respiratory infection.

### Clinical Presentation and Diagnosis

- If other causes of purpura are excluded (e.g., infection, thrombocytopenia, DIC, and other vasculitides), IgAV can be diagnosed if palpable purpura is present (with lower limb predominance), plus at least one of the following (adapted from EULAR/PRINTO/PRES Criteria 2010):
  - Diffuse abdominal pain
  - Skin biopsy demonstrating leukocytoclastic vasculitis with IgA deposits or kidney biopsy demonstrating proliferative glomerulonephritis with IgA deposition
  - Arthritis or arthralgia
  - Renal involvement (hematuria, proteinuria)
- Other findings may include constitutional signs; intussusception and gastrointestinal bleeding; glomerulonephritis, which occurs in one-third of cases and usually resolves but can result in renal failure (kidney biopsy may be required); subcutaneous edema; and scrotal pain and swelling.

### Treatment

- Treatment is generally supportive and symptomatic.
- Corticosteroids may be effective, and short-term therapy may help with arthritis, orchitis, and gastrointestinal hemorrhage.
- Prophylactic corticosteroids do not appear to alter the long-term course of IgAV. However, treatment of gastrointestinal hemorrhage and renal complications is necessary.
- Children should be monitored for kidney involvement with a urinalysis and blood pressure every 1-2 weeks for the 1st month and then monthly for at least 6 months after diagnosis.

## RESULTS

- Most patients recover in 2-4 weeks, and the course of IgAV is usually benign. One-third of children experience recurrence with rash and abdominal pain, usually shortly after the initial episode.
- Less than 5% of patients with renal disease progress to renal failure and may require transplantation.

## ACUTE RHEUMATIC FEVER

### Etiology and Epidemiology

- This multisystem inflammatory process generally occurs 2-3 weeks after pharyngitis with group A β-hemolytic *Streptococcus* infection. It does not occur after cutaneous group A *Streptococcus* infections.
- Acute rheumatic fever (ARF) is thought to be caused by autoreactive antibodies directed against antigens from the *Streptococcus* bacteria that mimic host antigens.
- Peak age of incidence is 6-15 years.
- <2 cases per 100,000 school aged children in the United States (low-risk), higher in developing countries and low socioeconomic status.

### Laboratory Studies and Imaging

- Throat culture or rapid streptococcal test
- Streptococcal antibody titers (ASO and anti-DNAseB)
- Echocardiogram and EKG for patients with confirmed rheumatic fever and/or suspected cardiac disease

### Diagnostic Criteria

- Diagnosis of initial episode of ARF is based on the Jones criteria (Table 30-5). Evidence of prior streptococcal infection with two major criteria or one major and two minor criteria is necessary.
- The most recent modification to the Jones Criteria (2015) modifies several major and minor criteria for moderate- and high-risk populations and accounts for advances in echocardiography in the diagnosis of carditis.
- Patients with a history of ARF are at increased risk for recurrence of subsequent streptococcal infections and do not have to meet the Jones criteria for diagnosis of an acute exacerbation.

### Treatment

- Therapy consists of antibiotic therapy and treatment of carditis (if present) as well as prophylaxis against recurrent infection.
- Initial treatment is aimed at eliminating the streptococcal infection, even if cultures at the time of diagnosis are negative. **One** of the following is appropriate:
  - Benzathine penicillin G: 0.6 (<27 kg) or 1.2 (>27 kg) million international units IM once
  - Penicillin VK: 250 mg (<27 kg) or 500 mg (>27 kg) b.i.d.-t.i.d. for 10 days
  - Amoxicillin: 50 mg/kg once daily (maximum 1 g/day) for 10 days
  - Clindamycin 20 mg/kg/day PO divided t.i.d. (maximum 900 mg/day) for 10 days
  - Oral cephalosporin (first generation: cephalexin, cefadroxil) for 10 days

| TABLE 30-5 | The Jones Criteria for Rheumatic Fever—Criteria for Initial Diagnosis in Low-Risk Populations |
|---|---|

**Evidence of prior *Streptococcus* infection**

1. Positive throat culture or rapid streptococcal test

2. Elevated or rising streptococcal antibody titers (ASO and/or DNAse)

**Major criteria**

**J**oints: polyarthritis, generally migratory affecting knees, elbows, and wrists

♥ **C**arditis: valvular disease, pancarditis; can be clinical and/or subclinical

**N**odules-subcutaneous: painless, over extensor joint surfaces

**E**rythema marginatum: serpiginous erythematous rash with clear center

**S**ydenham chorea: sudden rapid movements of trunk and/or extremities

**Minor criteria**

1. Fever ($\geq$38.5°C)

2. Polyarthralgia

3. Prolonged PR interval

4. Elevated ESR $\geq$ 60 mm/hr and/or CRP $\geq$ 3.0 mg/dL

Adapted from Gewitz MH, Baltimore RS, et al.; American Heart Association Committee on Rheumatic Fever, Endocarditis, and Kawasaki Disease of the Council on Cardiovascular Disease in the Young. Revision of the Jones Criteria for the diagnosis of acute rheumatic fever in the era of Doppler echocardiography: a scientific statement from the American Heart Association. Circulation 2015;131(20):1806-1818. Erratum in: Circulation 2020;142(4):e65.

- Carditis. If there is evidence of carditis, initial treatment includes aspirin 80-100 mg/ kg/day div. q.i.d. and cardiology consultation.
  - Rheumatic heart disease can progress to acute congestive heart failure, and patients with carditis should be monitored closely for cardiovascular compromise.
  - Corticosteroids are sometimes used for severe carditis and congestive heart failure.
- Arthritis is usually self-limited and highly responsive to aspirin.
- Prophylaxis for rheumatic heart disease.
  - Prophylaxis is important for the prevention of recurrent infection and rheumatic heart disease and should be continued for a minimum of 5 years (American Heart Association [AHA] guidelines).
    - If heart disease does not develop, can consider discontinuation at age 21 or 5 years (whichever is longer). Consider longer treatment in high-risk populations (e.g., teachers, health care providers, military personnel).
    - If there is evidence of carditis with residual heart disease, patients may require prophylaxis for 10 years or until age 40 (whichever is longer), sometimes for life.
  - **One** of the following agents should be used:
    - Benzathine penicillin G: 0.6 (<27 kg) or 1.2 (>27 kg) IM every 3-4 weeks; this is the preferred therapy due to compliance.
    - Penicillin VK 250 mg PO b.i.d.
    - Erythromycin 250 mg PO b.i.d.
    - Sulfadiazine 0.5 g (<27 kg) or 1 g (>27 kg) PO daily.

## Poststreptococcal Reactive Arthritis

- Children who do not meet the criteria for ARF but have arthritis and a history of group A streptococcal pharyngitis may have PSRA.
- Unlike ARF, the arthritis in PSRA is nonmigratory, additive, and prolonged and does not respond to aspirin.
- Onset of arthritis with PSRA is typically within the first 2 weeks of streptococcal infection, in contrast to arthritis in ARF, which takes 2-3 weeks to develop.
- Treatment includes NSAIDs and sometimes corticosteroids for arthritis. Patients should receive treatment for their streptococcal infection.
- Consider prophylaxis for at least 1 year if there are no signs of carditis and repeating an echocardiogram 1 year after diagnosis to evaluate for carditis.

## KAWASAKI DISEASE

The cause of this acute vasculitis is unknown, but an infectious etiology is suspected.

### Clinical Presentation and Diagnosis

- Kawasaki is a clinical diagnosis. In the absence of another disease process, clinical features as described by the American Academy of Pediatrics (AAP) and the AHA include:
  - Fever (usually >39°C) for ≥5 days and at least four of the following:
    - Bilateral conjunctivitis (bulbar), nonexudative
    - Mucositis: erythema of the lips, cracked lips, strawberry tongue, or oropharyngeal erythema
    - Cervical lymphadenopathy, >1.5 cm; typically unilateral and solitary
    - Polymorphic erythematous rash
    - Changes in extremities: swelling, erythema, or periungual peeling
  - Exceptions
    - If there are coronary artery abnormalities, Kawasaki disease can be diagnosed with less than four of the above criteria.
    - Even with a positive viral PCR or culture, Kawasaki disease should still be considered if the patient is not improving.
  - Other associated symptoms
    - Central nervous system: irritability, lethargy, aseptic meningitis, and hearing loss
    - Cardiovascular: coronary artery abnormalities, aneurysms of other medium-sized vessels, pericarditis, congestive heart failure, and valvular abnormalities
    - Gastrointestinal: abdominal pain, diarrhea, vomiting, hepatic dysfunction, and gallbladder hydrops
    - Genitourinary: urethritis and perineal desquamating rash
    - Musculoskeletal: arthritis and arthralgias

### Atypical Kawasaki Disease

- Atypical (more properly called incomplete) KD should be considered in children with unexplained fever for >5 days who meet only 2 or 3 of the additional clinical criteria. Infants with Kawasaki disease typically have atypical disease and may manifest with only prolonged fever and additional vascular abnormalities.
- Guidelines suggested by the AAP and AHA include:
  - Treat and obtain an echocardiogram for patients with fever ≥5 days plus two to three clinical criteria, if CRP ≥ 3.0 mg/dL, or if ESR ≥ 40 mm/hr, **and** patients have three or more additional laboratory criteria:
    - Albumin ≤3.0 g/dL
    - Elevated alanine aminotransferase

- Anemia
- Thrombocytosis ≥450,000/μL
- WBC count ≥15,000 μL
- Sterile pyuria (≥10 WBC/HPF)
- If the patient does not have three additional laboratory criteria, obtain an echocardiogram if clinically indicated and treat if there are cardiac findings.
- Atypical Kawasaki disease is more common in infants, and echocardiography should be considered with fever for ≥7 days in infants ≤6 months of age regardless of lack of other clinical criteria.

## Laboratory Studies and Imaging

- No laboratory studies are diagnostic. Common abnormalities include an elevated ESR and CRP, sterile pyuria, hypoalbuminemia, anemia, thrombocytosis (usually after 7 days), and cerebrospinal fluid pleocytosis.
- It is essential to assess cardiac function and coronary arteries with an echocardiogram if Kawasaki disease is diagnosed or suspected. Repeat echocardiograms should be performed after treatment at routine intervals depending on the degree of initial cardiac involvement.

## Treatment

- Therapy should be initiated before day no. 10 of fever and preferably within the first 7 days, to reduce the risk of coronary artery disease from approximately 20% to 5%.
  - Standard therapy is aspirin and IVIG. Additional immune suppressants including corticosteroids should be considered for disease not responsive to two doses of IVIG, severe KD, or atypical KD.
- Pharmacologic therapy includes:
  - Aspirin:
    - Start with moderate- to high-dose aspirin 30-100 mg/kg/day divided four times daily (maximum 4 g/day).
    - Practice guidelines vary. It may be possible to switch to low-dose aspirin (3-5 mg/kg/day) 48 hours after resolution of fever.
    - Continue low-dose aspirin until markers of inflammation (i.e., ESR, CRP, thrombocytosis) have normalized or longer if there is cardiac involvement.
  - IVIG
    - Start with 2 g/kg in a single infusion.
    - Give a second dose if the fever continues ≥36 hours after treatment.
  - Corticosteroids and other immune suppressants
    - For patients with persistent fevers after IVIG and/or severe vasculitis, corticosteroids and other immune suppressants, including anti-TNF-α medications or cyclosporine, may be indicated.
  - Anticoagulation
    - This is necessary for patients with large coronary aneurysms or coronary artery thrombosis.
    - Aspirin, clopidogrel, dipyridamole, warfarin, and/or low-molecular-weight heparin can be used.

## Complications

- For patients without cardiac involvement, the outcome is excellent.
- For patients with cardiac involvement:
  - The highest risk for myocardial infarction is in the 1st year after diagnosis.
  - Approximately 50% of coronary lesions resolve after 1-2 years. Coronary or other medium-sized vessel aneurysms may rupture.

- Reactions to IVIG (e.g., anaphylaxis with IgA deficiency) may occur.
- Consultation with appropriate subspecialties (rheumatology, infectious diseases, and/or cardiology) may be important depending on the patient's clinical course.

## MULTISYSTEM INFLAMMATORY SYNDROME IN CHILDREN (MIS-C)

- Hyperinflammatory syndrome that occurs in children with a history of SARS-CoV-2 infection or exposure 2-6 weeks prior.
- Fever of ≥24 hours duration with involvement of two or more organ systems:
  - Cardiovascular (e.g., shock, myocarditis, coronary artery dilation, arrhythmia)
  - Respiratory (e.g., pneumonia, ARDS, pulmonary embolism)
  - Renal (e.g., AKI, renal failure)
  - Neurologic (e.g., headache, seizure, stroke, aseptic meningitis)
  - Hematologic (e.g., coagulopathy, cytopenias)
  - Gastrointestinal (e.g., abdominal pain, ascites, vomiting, diarrhea, hepatitis, ileus, gastrointestinal bleeding)
  - Dermatologic (e.g., erythroderma, mucositis, other rash)
- Common lab abnormalities: elevated inflammatory markers (ESR, CRP, and ferritin), cytopenias, elevated brain natriuretic peptide (BNP)
- Can present with or without Kawasaki-like features
  - Obtain an echocardiogram to evaluate for coronary artery dilation and cardiac dysfunction
- Treatment includes IVIG first line and corticosteroids first line or for continued fever >36 hours after IVIG. Addition of biologics such as anti-IL-1 or anti-IL-6 medications for refractory disease.

## AUTOINFLAMMATORY DISEASES/PERIODIC FEVER SYNDROMES

Autoinflammatory diseases (aka periodic fevers syndromes) are caused by abnormal innate immune signaling and characterized by recurrent episodes of fever without an infectious source (Table 30-6).

### Clinical Presentation and Diagnosis

- Patients present at a young age (generally <3 years) with well-characterized recurrent episodes of fever without infection.
- Associated symptoms may include abdominal pain, rash, joint pain, fatigue, sore throat, and/or lymphadenopathy.
- Periodic fever with aphthous stomatitis, pharyngitis, and adenitis (PFAPA) is a heterogeneous clinical syndrome of recurrent fevers associated with sore throat and cervical adenitis. Behçet disease also presents with aphthous stomatitis, but patients also typically have genital ulcers and are less likely to have fevers.
- Autosomal dominant and recessive genetic mutations have been discovered for some hereditary autoinflammatory diseases including tumor necrosis factor (TNF) receptor–associated periodic syndrome (TRAPS), familial Mediterranean fever (FMF), cryopyrin-associated periodic syndrome (CAPS), hyperimmunoglobulin D syndrome (HIDS), and deficiency of deaminase 2 (DADA2).

### Treatment

- Treatment varies based on the cause of the fever syndromes (Table 30-6).
- Corticosteroids often halt acute febrile episodes but are of limited use for long-term therapy.

| TABLE 30-6 | Genetic Cause and General Features of Autoinflammatory Diseases | | |
|---|---|---|---|
| Syndrome | Gene(s) involved | Clinical features | Treatment |
| PFAPA | No single gene | Periodic fevers, aphthous stomatitis, pharyngitis, adenitis. Often do not have all features. Symptoms improve with age. | Colchicine<br>Cimetidine<br>IL-1 inhibitors<br>Tonsillectomy |
| Behçet disease | No single gene | Oral and genital ulcers, pathergy, uveitis, arthralgias. Onset early in life—evaluate for *TNFAIP2* mutation. | Colchicine |
| TRAPS | *TNFRSF1A* (AD) | Migrating rash, conjunctivitis, abdominal pain, arthritis lasting for days-weeks | IL-1 inhibitors |
| FMF | *MEFV* (AR) | Recurrent episodes of fever, rash, arthritis/arthralgias, abdominal pain, pericarditis that last 12-72 hr with sporadic timing of flares. | Colchicine<br>IL-1 inhibitors |
| CAPS | *NLRP3* (AD) | FCAS: 2-3 days of fever, urticarial rash and arthralgia hours after cold exposure. Onset in late childhood. | IL-1 inhibitors |
| | | MWS: 2-3 days of fever, urticarial rash, arthritis/arthralgia, sensorineural hearing loss. Onset in infancy. | |
| | | NOMID: fever, arthritis and other skeletal abnormalities, HSM, developmental delay, constitutive urticarial-like rash. Neonatal onset. | |
| HIDS | *MVK* (AR) | Fevers, rash, cutaneous vasculitis, severe abdominal pain, vomiting, diarrhea, arthralgias, that last 3-7 days and occur every 2-12 weeks. Onset usually in infancy. | IL-1 inhibitors<br>IL-6 inhibitors<br>TNF-α inhibitors |
| DADA2 | *ADA2* (AR) | Recurrent fevers, livedo reticularis, HSM, vasculopathy, early-onset strokes. | TNF-α inhibitors<br>HSCT |

Abbreviations: TRAPS, TNF receptor–associated periodic syndrome; FMF, familial Mediterranean fever; CAPS, cryopyrin-associated periodic syndrome; HIDS, hyperimmunoglobulin D syndrome; DADA2, deficiency of deaminase 2; AD, autosomal dominant; AR, autosomal recessive; HSM, hepatosplenomegaly; HSCT, hematopoietic stem cell transplant.

## Complications

- CAPS can present with severe manifestations in infants including rash, arthropathy, encephalitis, and other neurologic symptoms.
- Amyloidosis can be a complication of long-term inflammation and has been associated with periodic fever syndromes.
- Treatment of FMF patients with colchicine has been shown to significantly reduce the risk of amyloidosis.

## CHRONIC PAIN SYNDROMES

- Encompasses a broad range of disorders in children including AMP, chronic abdominal pain, chronic fatigue syndrome, fibromyalgia, and other disorders of pain.
- Rheumatologists are often referred patients with AMP; however, the general treatment strategies are applicable to most chronic pain syndromes.

### Clinical Presentation and Diagnosis

- Risk factors for AMP include recent injury with immobility, female sex, psychological stress, and possibly genetics.
- Many patients are seen by multiple physicians prior to their diagnosis.
- Early recognition and diagnosis of chronic pain syndromes is important to avoid unnecessary diagnostic testing and stress.

### Treatment

- The goal of treatment is to both improve pain and activities of daily living.
- The mainstay of treatment in children includes:
  - Increased physical activity including exercise and often physical and occupational therapy (PT and OT). Patients should be counseled that increased activity may initially worsen their symptoms, but regular exercise is critical for improvement.
  - Establish a regular routine including school attendance and participation in activities.
  - Sleep hygiene with avoidance of electronics in bed and a regular sleep/wake schedule.
  - Patients may benefit from psychological counseling for coping strategies and cognitive behavioral therapy.
  - In general, analgesics are not useful for many chronic pain disorders.
  - Some patients require more intensive therapy in the inpatient or outpatient setting with daily PT and OT.

## SUGGESTED READINGS

Gerber MA, Baltimore RS, Eaton CB, et al. Prevention of rheumatic fever and diagnosis and treatment of acute Streptococcal pharyngitis: a scientific statement from the American Heart Association Rheumatic Fever, Endocarditis, and Kawasaki Disease Committee of the Council on Cardiovascular Disease in the Young, the Interdisciplinary Council on Functional Genomics and Translational Biology, and the Interdisciplinary Council on Quality of Care and Outcomes Research: endorsed by the American Academy of Pediatrics. Circulation 2009;119(11):1541–1551.

Gewitz MH, Baltimore RS, et al.; American Heart Association Committee on Rheumatic Fever, Endocarditis, and Kawasaki Disease of the Council on Cardiovascular Disease in the Young.

Revision of the Jones Criteria for the diagnosis of acute rheumatic fever in the era of Doppler echocardiography: a scientific statement from the American Heart Association. Circulation 2015;131(20):1806–1818. Erratum in: Circulation 2020;142(4):e65.

Heiligenhaus A, Minden K, Tappeiner C, et al. Update of the evidence based, interdisciplinary guideline for anti-inflammatory treatment of uveitis associated with juvenile idiopathic arthritis. Semin Arthritis Rheum 2019;49(1):43–55.

Kaushik A, Gupta S, Sood M, et al. Systematic review of multisystem inflammatory syndrome in children associated with SARS-CoV-2 infection. Pediatr Infect Dis J 2020;39(11):e340.

McCrindle BW, Rowley AH, Newburger JW, et al. Diagnosis, treatment, and long-term management of Kawasaki disease: a scientific statement for health professionals from the American Heart Association. Circulation 2017;135(17):e927–e999.

Ozen S, Pistoria O, Iusan SM, et al. EULAR/PRINTO/PRES criteria for Henoch-Schonlein purpura, childhood polyarteritis nodosa, childhood Wegener granulomatosis, and childhood Takayasu arteritis: ankara 2008. Part II: final classification criteria. Ann Rheum Dis 2010;69:798–806.

Petty RE, Laxer RM, Lindsley CB, et al. Textbook of Pediatric Rheumatology. 8th Ed. Philadelphia, PA: Elsevier Inc., 2021.

Tan EM, Cohen AS, Fries JF, et al. The 1982 revised criteria for the classification of systemic lupus erythematosus. Arthritis Rheum 1982;25:1271–1277.

Wu JQ, Lu MP, Reed AM. Juvenile dermatomyositis: advances in clinical presentation, myositis-specific antibodies and treatment. World J Pediatr 2020;16(1):31–43.

## RHEUMATOLOGY WEB SITES

The American College of Rheumatology, http://www.rheumatology.org/
The Arthritis Foundation, http://www.arthritis.org/
Autoinflammatory Alliance, http://autoinflammatory.org/
Pediatric Rheumatology European Section, http://www.pres.org.uk/

# Sedation

Mythili Srinivasan and Robert M. Kennedy

## INTRODUCTION

- Goals of sedation include alleviation of procedure-related pain and anxiety, reduction of psychological trauma and its sequelae, immobility when necessary to complete the procedure, and maintenance of patient safety with limitation of sedation-related complications.
- There is an increased need for procedural sedation in pediatrics.
  - Many procedures and imaging studies require patient cooperation with little to no movement, while others require pain control and the need for reduced anxiety and relaxation.
  - Because of developmental status and age-related behaviors in children, completing these procedures often requires moderate, deep, or dissociated sedation. This chapter will be focused on these levels of sedation.
- Sedative medications should never be prescribed and administered at home, either before or after the procedure. This is associated with increased risks of respiratory depression and death. It is strongly discouraged by the American Academy of Pediatrics (AAP).
- Although many institutions have sedation protocols in place, the safest practice for administering procedural sedation is a designated pediatric sedation service or unit run by experienced sedation providers trained in airway management and sedation techniques.
  - Sedations in the emergency department setting are considered "urgent" and children frequently are not fully fasted. Ketamine is a good option for these sedations since it provides excellent analgesia, relative preservation of protective airway reflexes, and cardiopulmonary function, but providers must be prepared to manage emesis, laryngospasm, and other adverse events.
  - Sedation providers should have immediate access to extra personnel in case of life-threatening adverse events and availability of providers experienced in advanced airway skills if needed.
  - Pediatric-sized airway equipment should be readily available, as well as an oxygen source and emergency medications.
- During procedural sedation—from the time a sedative drug is administered until the child awakens—continuous monitoring of cardiopulmonary function by both electronic monitors and medical providers trained in sedation and pediatric advanced life support is necessary.
- PS provider should not be performing any significant role in the procedure, so as not be distracted from the airway and observation of the patient.
- However, for brief easily interruptible procedures being performed under **moderate sedation**, the sedation provider may assist with the procedure, while a sedation trained RN or EMP-T monitors the patient's vital functions and is ready to initiate supportive care, as needed. This should be done in accordance with the local hospital procedural sedation guideline.

- Sufficient qualified personnel (in addition to the practitioner(s) performing the procedure) must be present to:
  - provide the moderate, deep, or dissociative sedation
  - monitor the patient
  - manage sedation-related complications, if any
  - recover and discharge the patient
- When patients who are considered at high risk for sedation complications are encountered, involvement of an anesthesiologist is recommended.
- This chapter is meant to serve as a reference for physicians trained in sedation. It should not be considered all-inclusive of the subject or a substitute for formal sedation training before participating in sedation-related patient care.

## DEFINITIONS

- The following are definitions from American Society of Anesthesiologists (ASA), AAP, American College of Emergency Physicians (ACEP), and Joint Commission guidelines. In general, the deeper the level of sedation, the greater the risk of cardiopulmonary depression and adverse events.
  - Minimal sedation: a drug-induced state during which patients respond normally to verbal commands. Although cognitive function and coordination may be impaired, ventilatory and cardiovascular functions are unaffected.
  - Moderate sedation/analgesia: a drug-induced depression of consciousness during which patients respond purposefully to verbal commands, either alone or accompanied by light-to-moderate tactile stimulation. No interventions are required to maintain a patent airway, and spontaneous ventilation is adequate. Cardiovascular function is usually maintained.
  - Deep sedation/analgesia: a drug-induced depression of consciousness during which patients cannot be easily aroused or respond purposefully following repeated or painful stimulation. The ability to maintain ventilatory function independently may be impaired. Patients may require assistance in maintaining a patent airway, and spontaneous ventilation may be inadequate. Cardiovascular function is usually maintained.
  - **Dissociative sedation:** ketamine-induced depression of consciousness in which the central nervous system is isolated from outside stimuli (e.g., pain, sight, sound). The resulting trance-like cataleptic state is characterized by potent analgesia, sedation, and amnesia while maintaining cardiovascular stability and relative preservation of spontaneous respirations and protective airway reflexes.

## STAGES OF SEDATION AND RECOVERY

- **Presedation:** physical examination, evaluation of medical history and past sedation/anesthesia experiences, sedation plan, and informed consent; gathering of equipment, medications, and obtaining intravenous (IV) access.
- **Sedation**
  - Induction: administration of sedation/analgesia (higher risk of apnea or laryngospasm at this phase). The sedation provider should not leave the patient's bedside from this point on.
  - Maintenance: maintaining effective depth of sedation
    - This may require additional doses or titration of medications, keeping in mind the length of the procedure (avoid prolonging sedation) and the type of agent needed (analgesic vs. anxiolytic/hypnotic).

- Continuous cardiorespiratory monitoring and recording of vital signs every 5 minutes is necessary during moderate, deep, and dissociated sedation.
  - Continuous monitoring with end-tidal capnography is encouraged for all deep and dissociated sedations and highly recommended if supplemental oxygen is to be administered.
  - Level of consciousness and responsiveness to painful procedures should also be continually monitored.
  - A sedation score should be recorded every 15 minutes until the patient is ready for discharge or transfer. A common score used is the University of Michigan Sedation Scale (see reference by Malviya et al. in Suggested Readings):
    – 0 = awake and alert
    – 1 = minimally sedated: tired/sleepy, appropriate response to verbal conversation and/or sound
    – 2 = moderately sedated: somnolent/sleeping, easily aroused with light tactile stimulation or a simple verbal command
    – 3 = deeply sedated: deep sleep, arousable with purposeful response to significant physical stimulation
    – 4 = unarousable or nonpurposeful response to significant physical stimulation
- Emergence: recovering from effects of sedation. The patient should be fully monitored with the provider or sedation credentialed nurse at bedside (higher risk of laryngospasm at this phase).
- **Recovery**
  - Phase I (deep sedation with recovery score ≥3; see Table 31-1 for Aldrete recovery scoring system). Continuous monitoring and recording of vital signs every 5 minutes is necessary.
    - Sedation, pain, and recovery scores are documented every 15 minutes.
    - The transition to phase II recovery begins when the level of consciousness is consistent with moderate sedation (sedation score of 2); the patient is clinically stable and vital signs are at baseline (+/− 20%); supplemental $O_2$, airway, ventilation, and cardiovascular support are not required; and the Aldrete recovery score is 8 with pain score of 6 or less.
  - Phase II (minimal to moderate sedation with sedation score ≤2): recovery provider must be immediately available.
    - Vital signs and sedation/recovery score are recorded every 15 minutes until conclusion of phase II recovery.
    - Pain and recovery scores are documented at end of phase II recovery.
    - Noninvasive blood pressure monitoring and electrocardiogram may be waived if they are disruptive to patient and recovery care, provided the vital signs are stable.
    - Phase II recovery concludes with discharge once standard discharge criteria are met by the patient. Care can be transferred to responsible parent/legal guardian/inpatient care team.

## Discharge/Transfer Criteria

- It is suggested that the following criteria be met before discharge from sedation:
  - Vital signs at baseline +/− 20%
  - No respiratory distress
  - $Spo_2$ at baseline (+/−3%) or ≥95% on room air
  - Motor function baseline or sits/stands with minimal assistance
  - Fluids/hydration normal and no emesis/nausea

| TABLE 31-1 | Aldrete Scoring System for Recovery from Sedation[a] | |
|---|---|---|
| **Condition** | | **Score** |
| **Activity** | | |
| Able to move four extremities voluntarily or on command | | 2 |
| Able to move two extremities voluntarily or on command | | 1 |
| Able to move zero extremities voluntarily or on command | | 0 |
| **Respirations** | | |
| Able to deep breathe and cough freely | | 2 |
| Dyspnea or limited breathing | | 1 |
| Apneic | | 0 |
| **Circulation** | | |
| Blood pressure +/− 20% of presedation level | | 2 |
| Blood pressure +/− 20-50% of presedation level | | 1 |
| Blood pressure +/− 50% or more of presedation level | | 0 |
| **Consciousness** | | |
| Fully awake | | 2 |
| Arousable with verbal stimulation | | 1 |
| Not responding | | 0 |
| **Color** | | |
| Pink | | 2 |
| Pale, dusky, blotchy, jaundiced | | 1 |
| Cyanotic | | 0 |

[a]Need score of 9 for discharge or 8 for admission.
From Aldrete JA, Kroulik D. A postanesthetic recovery score. Anesth Analg 1970;49:924–934.

- Aldrete recovery score ≥9 for discharge, ≥8 for admission to a hospital floor, where monitoring is not one-to-one (see Table 31-1)
- Pain score ≤4/10 for discharge or ≤6/10 for admission (or pain score reduced 50% postprocedure)
- Sedation score ≤1 for discharge or ≤2 for admission; with no naloxone or reversal agents given for 2 hours
- It is important to stress to parents that after sedation, children should not climb, bathe, or swim alone; be left alone in a car seat; or participate in activities requiring physical coordination for 24 hours.

## PRESEDATION EVALUATION

Goals are to identify the difficult airway, that is, any anatomic characteristics that would make it difficult to provide positive pressure ventilation or intubation, if necessary; assess any cardiac, respiratory, or neurologic risk factors for adverse responses to sedation medications; and prevent sedation complications.

## History

- The history and physical examination should determine any risks versus benefits of sedation. Problems to be discussed with an attending physician experienced in sedation or anesthesia include concerns regarding the history and physical examination; any patients ASA class III, IV, or V (see later discussion for ASA classification system); or any patients with cardiopulmonary instability that may worsen with sedation.
- Past medical history should focus on systemic conditions affecting sedation outcome as well as identify contraindications to certain medications:
  - Cardiac history: congenital heart disease, history of arrhythmias, past radiologic or surgical interventions, current cardiac medications, and blood pressure issues.
  - Respiratory issues: current or recent upper or lower respiratory infection, history of wheezing, recurrent pneumonia, any respiratory medications/inhalers, history of croup, prematurity or prolonged intubation, chronically enlarged tonsils, snoring, obstructive sleep apnea, pneumothorax, or any potential airway masses/tumors/hemangiomas.
  - Gastrointestinal issues: history of gastroesophageal reflux disease, frequent vomiting, motion sickness or prolonged vomiting after prior sedation or anesthesia, history of delayed gastric emptying, bowel obstruction, gastroparesis, melena, or known gastrointestinal blood loss.
  - Neurologic disorders: epilepsy—last seizure, seizure frequency and characteristics, typical epileptic rescue treatment, and current anticonvulsant therapy. VP shunt (malfunction prevents use of ketamine).
  - Neuromuscular disease: degree of respiratory musculature compromise, muscular myopathy or dystrophy, any cardiac involvement, potential $K^+$ imbalance, history of respiratory disease/infections.
  - Renal disease: potential electrolyte disturbances, decreased renal function significant enough to require changes in medication dosage or dosing intervals, hypoalbuminemia secondary to renal losses, hypertension, dehydration, history of oliguria or anuria, and need for intermittent bladder catheterization with associated latex sensitivity.
  - Liver disease: hepatic dysfunction that may impact drug metabolism, hepatomegaly that may impact lung tidal volumes, history of esophageal varices, or ascites.
  - Hematology/oncology disease
    - Most recent complete blood count/electrolytes, last chemotherapy regimen, and any in-situ central lines. History of vitamin B12 deficiency and family history of methylene tetrahydrofolate deficiency which can be potential contraindications for nitrous oxide sedation.
    - Porphyria: if present, avoid barbiturates.
  - Endocrine disease
    - Diabetes—current blood glucose level, diabetic medications and last dose, recent electrolytes if hyperglycemic
    - Thyroid disease—recent TSH and T4, assessment of patient symptoms of hyper/hypothyroidism
    - Adrenal disease—current medication management and stress dosing requirements
  - Genetic disease: Many syndromes are associated with cardiac, renal, and metabolic derangements as well as craniofacial/airway abnormalities. Medical conditions of specific syndrome should be reviewed prior to proceeding with sedation.

- Psychiatric disease: Patients with a history of schizophrenia or other psychoses may have an exacerbation of the psychosis with use of ketamine.
- Recent surgeries: Examples include recent tympanoplasty or retinal eye surgery, which are contraindications for nitrous oxide sedation.
- Current medications
  ○ It is important to be aware of the drug metabolism so that adverse events due to drug-drug interactions can be avoided.
  ○ Oxycodone, midazolam, and ketamine, and fentanyl are few examples of sedation medications that undergo phase I metabolism via cytochrome P-450 enzymes.
  ○ Drugs that are substrates, inhibitors, or inducers of these enzymes can alter the metabolism of oxycodone, midazolam, ketamine, and fentanyl.
  ○ For example, protease inhibitors are potent inhibitors of cytochrome P-450 enzymes CYP3A4. Midazolam is extensively metabolized by CYP3A4, and coadministration with protease inhibitors results in a fourfold increase in midazolam bioavailability and may result in prolonged sedation.
- Importance of past sedation/anesthesia records
- **Sedation/anesthesia records should be reviewed** as available to assess size of endotracheal tubes (ETTs) and laryngoscope blades needed, any difficulty with mask ventilation or intubation, and any adverse medication reactions or unexpected outcomes caused by sedation or anesthesia.
- History of postsedation or postoperative nausea or vomiting.
- Sedative agents used in past (if known) and any complications/parental concerns.
- Family history of adverse reactions or events during sedation or anesthesia particularly addressing malignant hyperthermia (**relevant if using succinylcholine**).

## Classification Systems
### Mallampati Classification System
- During presedation evaluation, each patient should be assigned a Mallampati score, with the understanding that each classification is associated with anticipation of increasingly difficult airway management. There are four classes (Fig. 31-1). Class 4 is considered the most difficult.
- Mallampati scoring should be done during the physical examination in conjunction with determination of neck mobility, ability to open mouth without temporomandibular joint or jaw pathology, dentition status, mouth and tongue size, and cricoidmandible distance. This is done by asking the child to open the mouth and stick out the tongue as far as possible without use of tongue blades or assistance. Many young children are unable to perform this task.
- This helps give the sedation provider an idea of degree of difficulty in managing the airway if mask ventilation or intubation should become necessary.

### ASA Physical Status Classification
- During presedation evaluation, each patient may be assigned an ASA score to determine the physiologic status of the patient before sedation; increasing score correlates with increasing risk of adverse events during anesthesia; for nonscheduled sedations, an "E" is added to indicate the sedation was for an emergent/urgent condition:
  - Class I: normal healthy patient with no chronic medical conditions

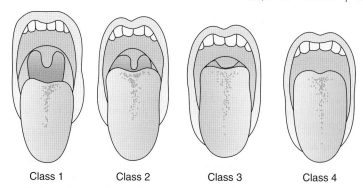

| Class 1 | Class 2 | Class 3 | Class 4 |

**Figure 31-1. Mallampati classification system for use during presedation evaluation.** (From Mallampati S, Gatt S, Gugino L, et al. A clinical sign to predict difficult tracheal intubation: a prospective study. Can Anaesth Soc J 1985;32(4):429–434.)

- Class II: patient with a mild to moderate but well-controlled medical condition, such as asthma or diabetes under good control
- Class III: patient with severe systemic disease such as cardiac disease with border-line blood pressure control or on inotropes, seizure disorder with frequent seizures
- Class IV: patient with severe systemic disease that is life threatening
- Class V: moribund patient with little chance of survival; surgery is a last effort to save life
- Patients with class I, II, or III status require specialty trained and experienced sedation physicians: patients with class III, IV or V status warrant consultation with anesthesiology colleagues.

## High-Risk Problems
- Medical conditions
  - ASA classes III, IV, or V
  - Potential airway obstruction: enlarged tonsils/adenoids, history of loud snoring, obstructive sleep apnea, foreign body aspiration or ingestion, airway abscess, oral or pharyngeal trauma, known or suspected airway masses, suspected epiglottitis
  - Poorly controlled asthma
  - Morbid obesity (>2 times ideal body weight)
  - Cardiovascular conditions (shock, cyanosis, congestive heart failure, history of congenital heart disease)
  - History of prematurity with residual pulmonary, cardiovascular, gastrointestinal, or neurologic problems
  - Neurologic conditions such as poorly controlled seizures, global hypotonia, history of ventilatory assistance +/− tracheostomy, inability to control secretions or history of aspiration, hypertonia with inability to lie supine to access airway, and central apnea
  - Gastrointestinal conditions: uncontrolled gastroesophageal reflux, poor gastrointestinal motility, and surgical abdomen
  - Age <3 months
  - Pregnancy or suspected pregnancy

- Current URI, especially febrile, purulent rhinorrhea, or wheezing that does not clear with one albuterol treatment
- Neuromuscular disease
- Procedures requiring deep sedation in patients with a full stomach
- Conditions that put patients at risk for failed sedation
  - Severe developmental delay
  - Behavioral issues or severe psychologic/psychiatric disease
  - History of failed sedation, oversedation, or paradoxical response to sedatives (hyperactive)

## Screening for Acute Illness

- Patients should be screened for acute illnesses that may increase their risk for sedation-related adverse events.
- When acute illness is detected, the sedation provider must weigh the increased risks of sedation against the need for the diagnostic or therapeutic procedure.
- If the procedure is considered elective, the following guidelines are suggested:
- **Indications for cancellation or delay of elective sedations include the following:**
  - Illness with fever >100.4°F (38°C) within 24 hours
  - Active infection with cardiopulmonary compromise
  - Active vomiting within 12 hours of sedation
  - Any respiratory infection with persistent wheezing **not** cleared by one albuterol treatment
- Rescheduling recommendations for delay include the following:
  - Asthma without underlying infection: 7 days.
  - Asthma with infectious component: 3 weeks.
  - URI with cough/congestion: 3 weeks.
    - URI symptoms may increase the risk of laryngospasm, bronchospasm, and hypoxia during sedation.
    - Mild URI symptoms alone (nonpurulent rhinitis, afebrile status, cough that clears) may not be an indication to cancel or delay a procedure; sedation management should reflect anticipation of above potential complications.
    - Severe URI (febrile, purulent discharge, wet cough) should prompt consideration of cancellation; discussion with advanced sedation provider to review the risks versus the urgency of the procedure is advised. Elective procedures should be cancelled.
  - Fever: back to baseline >24 hours and acting well.
  - Emesis: resolved for 24 hours and tolerating clear liquids, normal urine production, and adequate signs of euvolemia.
  - Croup: 3 weeks, with presedation visit to primary care physician.
  - Pneumonia: 4 weeks after resolution of symptoms.
  - Influenza: 3 weeks after resolution of symptoms.
  - Bronchiolitis: 6 weeks after resolution with presedation visit to primary care physician.
  - Children with known infection (e.g., otitis/tonsillitis): >24 hours without fever and on pharmacotherapy, if warranted.
  - These recommendations are subject to modification by the sedation provider based on urgency of the elective procedure, individual patient history, and local hospital guidelines.

## PEDIATRIC AIRWAY AND POSITIONING

### Anatomy
- The larynx is at the level of C3-C6 and serves as the area of phonation. It also protects the lower airways from contents of the oropharynx.
- The larynx is made of distinct cartilages: thyroid, cricoid, arytenoids, corniculates, and epiglottis.
- The vocal cords lie beneath the overhang of the epiglottis, at the level of the thyroid cartilage.
- The opening between the true vocal cords is the glottic opening, where intubation tubes are passed. This is the narrowest part of the airway in children >10 years of age. In children <10 years of age, the airway is narrowest at the level of the cricoid ring, just below the vocal cords.
- Receptors sensitive to mechanical and chemical stimuli lie in the trachea and are involved in regulating rate and depth of breathing, as well as causing cough and bronchoconstriction reflexive actions.
- Positioning of the pediatric airway is complicated in infants by a large occiput size in relation to body size, a large tongue in relation to mouth size, and vocal cords, which are angled anteriorly in comparison to adults. The larynx is more cephalad than in adults, with narrowing below the vocal cords.

### Positioning Techniques
- Avoid head flexion or extreme head extension.
- Place towel roll underneath shoulders (if infant or toddler) to align airway, to achieve "sniffing" position.
- Adult-sized patients may require roll underneath head instead of shoulders to align airway. Obese children may require additional padding beneath the head.

### Identifying the Potentially Difficult Airway
- Head: prominent occiput or misshapen skull
- Back: moderate to severe scoliosis or kyphosis
- Neck: short neck, fat neck, poor cervical mobility, neck masses, and cervical collar or traction in place
- Face: craniofacial abnormalities such as small mouth opening, short mandible, large tongue, narrow palate (associated with difficult airways), cleft palate, or conditions that reduce the space in which to displace the tongue to visualize the glottis
- Airway: history of snoring, stridor, hoarseness, drooling, enlarged tonsils, or leaning forward to open airway
- Past medical history: history of prolonged intubation, airway tumors/hemangiomas/inflammation, obesity, craniofacial syndromes, or hypothyroidism
- Syndromes: craniofacial syndromes such as Crouzon, Apert, Goldenhar, or Pierre Robin syndromes; Down, Turner, or Hurler/Hunter syndromes

## AIRWAY EQUIPMENT, MEDICATIONS, AND PERSONNEL

### Equipment
*It is recommended to have books (code books) or tables with precalculated weight-based estimates of airway equipment and medication doses immediately available.*

*At Bedside or Immediately Available*
- ETTs: three (estimated size for weight, plus one size above and below).
  - Size in Code Book or calculate size by:
  - Uncuffed ETT : (16 + age)/4. Cuffed ETT is ½ size smaller.
- Laryngeal mask airway (LMA).
- Oral and nasopharyngeal airways.
- Laryngoscope plus curved and straight blades, check to confirm fully operational.
- Rolled towel for positioning if needed.
- Stylets.
- Clean syringes and needles for additional medications.

*In Room*
- Suction unit, turned on
- Anesthesia bag (continuous positive airway pressure [CPAP] bag) with appropriate mask size assembled and attached to 10 L oxygen
- Nasal cannula +/− ETCO$_2$ with **full** oxygen tank to accompany patient during transport
- Continuous cardiorespiratory monitoring (transport monitor if needed)
- IV setup or IO readily available in case of loss of IV access or if vascular access is emergently needed when sedation medications are administered orally or by inhalation

## Medications (Immediately Available)
- Emergency medications
  - Succinylcholine (20 mg/mL)
  - Atropine (0.4 mg/mL)
  - Epinephrine 0.1 mg/mL for small children or 1 mg/mL for adult size patient
  - Naloxone (0.4 mg/mL)
  - Flumazenil (0.1 mg/mL)
- Sedation medications (see Tables 31-2 and 31-3 for sedation medications and dosing). Sedation physician should:
  - be ready with extra medication doses as anticipated
  - have normal saline, with 10-mL syringes, available for flushing medications
  - review medication doses for reversal, if applicable (i.e., flumazenil or naloxone) (Table 31-4)
  - review succinylcholine dose for severe laryngospasm

## Personnel Required
- The AAP recommends that one nurse, one sedationist/anesthesiologist, and one proceduralist (if one is warranted) should be present.
- Observing the patient and monitoring vital signs should be the sole job of the sedationist during procedural sedation.
- Emergency department sedation is unique due to several factors: (1) procedures are urgent/emergent, (2) often only a single physician may be present to provide sedation and perform the procedure, and (3) there is immediate availability of trained personnel in the ED to assist in case of complications. Due to these factors, exceptions are often made to personnel requirements for procedural sedation in the ED by the local governing bodies in charge of procedural sedation.
- Following sedation, the patient should be monitored, with vital signs recorded every 5 minutes until awake, then every 15 minutes until the patient has reached baseline mental status. A designated recovery area should be staffed and equipped appropriately in case of airway compromise during recovery.

**TABLE 31-2** Common Sedation and Analgesic Medications

| Drug | Onset | Route | Dosing | Contraindications | Duration of action | Comments |
|------|-------|-------|--------|-------------------|--------------------|----------|
| **Sedative/Hypnotics** | | | | | | |
| Propofol | 15-30 sec | IV | For use only by propofol credentialed/anesthesia-approved attending physicians | Egg allergy (relative). History of difficult airway; if cardiac, renal, metabolic, mitochondrial, or pulmonary disease, discuss with anesthesia. | 3-5 min if no infusion | Can cause profound respiratory depression, apnea, and hypotension |
| Midazolam | 2-3 min | IV | 6 months to 6 years: 0.05 mg/kg (anxiolysis) and 0.1 mg/kg (sedation); may titrate doses at 0.05 mg/kg to maximum of 0.6 mg/kg; **consider maximum of 2 mg unless anesthesiologist involved.**<br><br>6-12 years: 0.025-0.05 mg/kg initially (anxiolysis) and 0.05-0.1 mg/kg (sedation); maximum single dose of 2.5 mg, to a maximum of 0.4 mg/kg; **consider max dose of 4 mg total unless anesthesiologist involved.** | History of paradoxical reaction | 45-60 min IV<br>60-90 min PO | Can cause respiratory depression, bradycardia, and hypotension.<br><br>Serum levels increased with cimetidine, protease inhibitors, erythromycin, clarithromycin, and antifungals. |

(Continued)

TABLE 31-2  Common Sedation and Analgesic Medications (Continued)

| Drug | Onset | Route | Dosing | Contraindications | Duration of action | Comments |
|------|-------|-------|--------|-------------------|--------------------|----------|
| | 20-30 min | PO | 0.25-0.5 mg/kg once only (max dose of 10 mg) | | | Anxiolytic doses should not exceed 2-4 mg total; sedation doses should not exceed 10 mg total. |
| Pentobarbital | 3-5 min | IV | 1st dose 2.5 mg/kg; may repeat 1.25 mg/kg three times to max of 7.5 mg/kg OR 200 mg total | History of paradoxical reaction; porphyria. Apnea when used with other agents. | 15-45 min IV 60-240 min PO | May cause arrhythmias or respiratory depression |
| | 15-60 min | PO/PR | (<4 year) 3-6 mg/kg to max 100 mg total. (>4 year) 1.5-3 mg/kg to max 100 mg total | Not recommended in congestive heart failure, hypotension, or liver failure | | |
| **Analgesics** | | | | | | |
| Fentanyl | 2-3 min | IV | 0.5-1 µg/kg. Administer over 30-60 sec; may repeat q2-3 min to desired effect, with a maximum dose of 100 µg in 30-min span. Consult experienced sedation attending if larger dose is required in larger patients. | Apnea when used with other agents, especially benzodiazepines (midazolam). Adjust dose in renal failure. Consultation with anesthesia advised with bradycardia, hypotension, or respiratory depression as effects of fentanyl may be deleterious. | 30-60 min | Rapid infusion may cause chest wall rigidity and/or respiratory depression. |

| Drug | Onset | Route | Dose | Cautions/Contraindications | Duration | Notes |
|---|---|---|---|---|---|---|
| Ketamine | 1 min | IV | 0.5-1.0 mg/kg to repeat as needed every 5-10 min | Contraindicated in patients with increased intracranial pressure, recent craniotomy, hypertension, aneurysm, thyrotoxicosis, or schizophrenia. Can cause hypertension, tachycardia, nystagmus, nausea/vomiting, salivation, and emergence reaction. | Dissociation: 15-30 min. Recovery: 90-150 min. | Use with caution in patients with seizure disorder. |
| Nitrous oxide | 2-5 min | mask | Most sedations are performed using 70% $N_2O$; often patients are premedicated with 0.1-0.2 mg/kg oxycodone (max dose 10 mg) to augment depth of sedation. | Laryngospasm can occur. Contraindicated in patients with pneumothorax, intestinal obstruction, recent ear/eye/sinus/cranial surgery, increased intracranial pressure, craniofacial or sinus injury, pregnancy, vitamin B12 deficiency, methylene tetrahydrofolate deficiency. | <5 min | Adverse effects include nausea and vomiting, diaphoresis, and hallucinations. Long-term use is associated with megaloblastic anemia, myeloneuropathy, and impaired fetal development. |

*(Continued)*

**TABLE 31-2** Common Sedation and Analgesic Medications (*Continued*)

| Drug | Onset | Route | Dosing | Contraindications | Duration of action | Comments |
|------|-------|-------|--------|-------------------|--------------------|----------|
| Morphine | 5-10 min | IV | 0.05-0.15 mg/kg q 10-20 min, max dose 4-6 mg. Use lower doses in opioid naive patients. Peak effect at 20 min.<br><br>May be used to provide analgesia, not a preferred agent for sedation. | Use with caution in patients with known or suspected obstructive sleep apnea, hypotension, cardiac disease, and respiratory depression. Can cause histamine release with itching, bronchospasm. | 180-300 min | Adverse effects include nausea and vomiting, itching, central nervous system or respiratory depression, miosis, biliary spasm, increased intracranial pressure, and hypotension/bradycardia. Use naloxone for reversal. |
| Oxycodone | 30-60 min | PO | 0.1-0.2 mg/kg for hospital dosing; prescription dosing is limited to 0.05-0.1 mg/kg/dose—max dose 10 mg. Consult pain specialist if patient opioid tolerant. | Use with caution in patients with renal disease, hypotension, cardiac disease, and respiratory disease. | 120-180 min | |

| TABLE 31-3 | Antinausea Agents[a] | | |
|---|---|---|---|
| **Antinausea medications** | **Class** | **Route** | **Dose** |
| Ondansetron (Zofran) | Antiserotonin | IV/PO | 0.15 mg/kg q8h |
| Diphenhydramine (Benadryl) | Antihistamine | PO/IV | 0.5-1 mg/kg q6h (max 50 mg) |

[a]Some sedation procedures may be complicated by postprocedure nausea and vomiting. Medications can be given to help counteract these side effects and decrease complications. Be aware that antihistamines may worsen postsedation drowsiness.

| TABLE 31-4 | Emergency Drugs[a] |
|---|---|
| **Drug** | **Dose** |
| Atropine | 0.02 mg/kg/dose IV q 3-5 min (0.1 mg minimum dose, maximum 0.5 mg). |
| Epinephrine | 0.01 mg/kg/dose (or 0.1 mL/kg of 1:10,000) IV/IO q 3-5 min. |
| Flumazenil | 0.01 mg/kg IV (max dose 0.2 mg) over 15 sec; may repeat this dose 4 times to a maximum of 3 mg. |
| | Monitor for resedation; use with caution in patients on benzodiazepine therapy for seizures because flumazenil may induce seizure. |
| Naloxone | 0.01-0.02 mg/kg IV, may repeat every 2-3 min as needed. Maximum dose 2 mg: partial reversal to reestablish ventilation but maintain analgesia. |
| | Full reversal: <20 Kg: 0.1/mg/kg/dose, ≥20 Kg or >5 years: 2 mg/dose, adults: 0.4 mg-2 mg/dose. Full reversal may result in severe pain, hypertension, tachycardia, etc. |
| | Monitor for resedation. |
| Rocuronium | 1 mg/kg, maximum dose of 100 mg. |
| Succinylcholine | 1-2 mg/kg/dose IV/IO (maximum 150 mg) for paralysis for intubation; 0.1-0.5 mg/kg/dose for laryngospasm. |
| | Contraindicated in children with burns >48 hours old, neuromuscular disease, hyperkalemia, muscular dystrophy, suspected increased intracranial pressure, or prolonged immobilization; these patients should be discussed with anesthesia before any sedation and may require anesthesia level care. |

[a]Drug math:
1:100,000 = 10 μg/mL = 0.01 mg/mL
1:10,000 = 100 μg/mL = 0.1 mg/mL
1:1000 = 1000 μg/mL = 1 mg/mL

## RECOGNIZING INEFFECTIVE VENTILATION

- Administration of supplemental oxygen during sedation reduces the risk of hypoxic injury by delaying onset of hypoxemia if respiratory depression or apnea should occur. However, supplemental oxygen use often delays recognition of ineffective breathing since oxygen saturations do not drop for several minutes, even during apnea. It is thus recommended that $ETCO_2$ be monitored when supplemental oxygen is used. $ETCO_2$ monitoring detects respiratory depression/apnea more rapidly than does pulse oximetry or direct observation. When the patient is breathing room air, oxygen saturation by pulse oximetry can be used as a proxy for ventilation if $ETCO_2$ is unavailable.
- The mouth, nose and chest wall should be visible during sedation. This allows for rapid visualization of emesis and apnea.
- Signs of ineffective ventilation include the following:
  - Color changes: perioral and facial paleness. Cyanosis is not noted until oxygen saturations drop to 85% or lower.
  - Chest wall movement: decrease seen with respiratory depression or apnea, increase seen with laryngospasm or upper airway obstruction. Abdominal breathing: "See-saw" retractions are a sign of upper airway obstruction.
  - Snoring/upper airway sounds: These are signs of upper airway obstruction and require airway repositioning, jaw thrust, placement of oral or nasal airway, or possibly placement of a more definitive airway (i.e., LMA or ETT).
  - Pulse oximetry tone, decreasing pitch indicates dropping oxygen saturations. Use of the tone allows observation of the patient instead of the monitor.
  - End-tidal capnography: $ETCO_2$ should read 30-50 mm Hg unless metabolic derangement is present. Loss of $ETCO_2$ waveform is the earliest warning sign of apnea/obstruction.
    - Decreased $ETCO_2$ may indicate poor ventilation and obstruction versus apnea.
    - Increased $ETCO_2$ may indicate poor ventilation and inadequate respiratory rate.
    - Loss of wave form associated with chest wall movement indicates upper airway obstruction such as laryngospasm.

## SEDATION CHECKLIST

- Time out: Verify patient information, medical record, and procedure to be performed with the family/guardian/patient and the medical team.
- Complete sedation record to document
  - History of the present illness: diagnosis, reason for sedation
  - Past medical history (relevant to sedation)
  - Past sedation/anesthesia history/records
  - Drug allergies/sensitivities
  - Current medications
  - Review of systems
  - Laboratory tests
  - Baseline vital signs
  - Physical examination
  - NPO status (Table 31-5)
  - ASA classification
  - Mallampati classification
  - Informed consent

| **TABLE 31-5** Nothing-by-Mouth (NPO) Guidelines for Elective Sedation[a] | |
|---|---|
| | Time |
| Clear liquids | 2 hr |
| Breast milk | 4 hr |
| Fortified breast milk/formula/solids | 6 hr |

[a]These guidelines are strictly adhered to for all elective sedations, and any NPO violations are rescheduled or delayed until criteria are met.
Clear liquids: water, sugar water, Kool-aid, Pedialyte, soda, apple or grape juice without pulp, Gatorade.
Solids: all food, cow milk, unstrained fruit juices, tube feedings, candy, and gum.
*Source:* Courtesy of St. Louis Children's Hospital.

- Develop and document assessment and plan for performing sedation. Inform parents and team members of plan.
- Perform checklist before performing sedation. (Think **SOAP ME.**)
  **S**uction: Yankauer catheter with power "on" and tested.
  **O**xygen: nasal cannula, CPAP bag available with oxygen source.
  **A**irway: size-appropriate nasopharyngeal and oropharyngeal airways, ETTs, and LMA. Functional laryngoscope blades and stylets are available.
  **P**harmacy: intubation medications, emergency medications including succinylcholine with known doses/concentrations. Have normal saline flush available.
  **M**onitors: pulse oximetry, noninvasive blood pressure, $ETCO_2$ as appropriate, and ECG monitoring on patient. Have stethoscope available.
  **E**quipment: any anticipated special equipment. Have code cart/airway cart available and nearby.
- Have anesthesia and code team contact numbers ready and available should assistance be needed.
- Ensure appropriately staffed and equipped recovery area for postsedation monitoring.
- Have responsible attending physician and proceduralist in room or immediately available and aware that sedation is about to begin.
- Have IV line in place for intravenous sedation techniques, check flow before administering medications.
- Preoxygenate as appropriate (if $ETCO_2$ monitor will be used).
- If all checklist items have been completed, the patient is ready for sedation. **Before starting sedation, be sure to double-check the sedative agent dose for age and weight as well as for maximum doses.** Be sure to note times of medications and any premedications given. Vital signs are recorded every 5 minutes in sedation record.
- Document any sedation-related complications: any airway repositioning or nasopharyngeal/oral airways, need for larger than usual drug dosing to achieve sedation, any signs of airway obstruction (snoring, desaturation, poor chest rise), or difficult mask ventilation or intubations. This is valuable information for the next sedationist/anesthesiologist.

## ADVERSE EVENTS DURING SEDATION

### Upper Airway Obstruction/Laryngospasm

- Stridor indicates partial obstruction; complete obstruction will be silent.

- Reposition using chin lift or jaw thrust.
- Consider oral airway placement.
- Apply CPAP bag and mask. Hold continuous pressure at 15-20 mm Hg. By distending the pharynx, this may partially open the larynx and allow air exchange. This is successful treatment for most brief laryngospasm associated with sedation.
- ***Call for help.***
- If no response, give succinylcholine 0.25-0.5 mg/kg. Note, succinylcholine typically is not kept in Code Carts as it is refrigerated when rarely used.
- Positive pressure ventilation with bag-mask may be needed only briefly as the patient recovers from stage II anesthesia or is sedated more deeply with additional medication, for example, propofol. Both strategies reduce the likelihood of laryngospasm.
- If the child cannot be oxygenated, proceed to intubation. Once the airway is secured, consider nasogastric tube placement for gastric decompression.

## Apnea with or without Hypoxia

- Reposition using chin lift or jaw thrust.
- Administer 100% oxygen.
- Decrease or discontinue infusion rate of sedative, if applicable.
- Give a painful sternal rub to stimulate.
- If no spontaneous breathing, ventilate with CPAP or ambu-type bag-mask.
- ***Call for help.***
- Consider flumazenil or naloxone as appropriate
  - Flumazenil: 0.01 mg/kg IV (maximum dose 0.2 mg) over 15 seconds; may repeat this dose 4 times to a maximum of 3 mg. Caution, may precipitate a seizure in patients on benzodiazepines for seizure or anxiety.
  - Naloxone: 0.01-0.02 mg/kg IV, may repeat every 2-3 minutes as needed. The goal is to titrate with naloxone until the patient begins to breathe; full reversal may cause hypertension and severe pain.
    - **If unable to ventilate**, for example, rigid chest, give naloxone 0.1 mg/kg IV or succinylcholine 1-2 mg/kg IV, or 4 mg/kg IM if no vascular access.
  - Perform intubation if necessary.

## Hypotension (a decrease in systolic blood pressure by >20%)

- To increase blood pressure, consider etiologies.
  - Sedation medication adverse effect
  - Allergic reaction: see protocol
  - Cardiac rhythm disturbance
  - Shock or poor perfusion

### *Hypovolemia*

- Rapidly infuse 20 mL/kg normal saline or lactated Ringer's solution if no contraindications (cardiac, renal, or pulmonary disease); reassess BP, HR, capillary refill; repeat as needed.
- Change blood pressure cuff cycling rate to every 1-3 minutes until blood pressure is stabilized.
- Consider decreasing infusion rate of sedation agent (as applicable).
- If no response, turn off sedation drug infusion and allow recovery.
- Consider inotrope or vasopressor infusion and transfer to ICU if hypotension unresponsive to interventions.

## Allergic Reaction (Anaphylaxis)

- Place patient in Trendelenburg position; administer 100% oxygen.
- *Call for help.*
- Give epinephrine 1 mg/mL IM—anterior lateral thigh.
  - <10 kg = 0.01 mg/kg.
  - 10-25 kg = 0.15 mg.
  - 25 kg = 0.3 mg.
  - IM is preferred over IV.
  - If anaphylactic symptoms persist, may repeat epinephrine dose every 5-15 minutes as needed.
  - Consider IV epinephrine continuous infusion after third IM dose.
- Give 20-mL/kg IV bolus of normal saline; repeat as necessary.
- If respiratory state compromised, it may be necessary to give nebulized albuterol (2.5 or 5 mg in 3 mL normal saline) or intubate if severe respiratory involvement.
- As soon as possible, administer the following:
  - H-1 receptor antagonist (cetirizine PO: 6 months to <2 years, 2.5 mg; 2-5 years, 5 mg; >5 years, 10 mg)
  - If unable to take PO cetirizine, diphenhydramine 1 mg/kg IV [maximum dose 50 mg]
  - H-2 receptor antagonist (e.g., famotidine: 1 mg/kg PO [max 40 mg] or IV [max 20 mg])
  - Corticosteroids (methylprednisolone 1 mg/kg IV [max 80 mg] q12h or prednisone 2 mg/kg PO q24h)
- Observe for 6-24 hours to watch for late-phase rebound symptoms.

## Aspiration

Significant aspiration is likely to occur quietly. An actively vomiting patient probably has protective airway reflexes. Passive regurgitation of gastric contents due to esophageal relaxation is more likely associated with clinically significant aspiration. This may occur during very deep sedation with opioids and propofol and during paralysis for intubation and may not be appreciated until gastric contents are seen within the mouth.

- Turn head/body to side and suction immediately; interrupt procedure as needed.
- Turn off infusion medication (if applicable) and allow for recovery.
- Administer oxygen as needed, watching for signs of laryngospasm; if persistent desaturation, may need definitive airway (ETT) to facilitate PEEP administration.
- Obtain chest radiograph to evaluate for signs of aspiration if clinically indicated (new cough, tachypnea, new oxygen requirement, lung auscultation findings).
- Admit for overnight hospitalization for observation if any new oxygen requirement present.

## SUGGESTED PROTOCOLS FOR PROCEDURAL SEDATION

**For intensely painful procedures**: (fracture reduction, burn debridement, abscess incision and drainage, peripherally inserted central catheter placement, etc.)

- Ketamine provides dissociative sedation, analgesia, and amnesia for the procedure and is an ideal agent for painful procedures.

- *Ketamine IV* more effectively reduces patient distress during intensely painful procedures and causes less respiratory depression than fentanyl- or propofol-based techniques.
- Intravenous administration is preferred when multiple or prolonged attempts likely will be needed to complete the procedure, thus increasing potential need for additional doses of ketamine.
- Time of recovery is reduced by administering a smaller initial dose (1 mg/kg) followed by a half doses as needed.
- An *initial ketamine dose 1 mg/kg (maximum dose 50 mg) administered over 5 seconds* results in dissociated sedation for 3-5 minutes with recovery sufficient for discharge in many patients by 20-25 minutes.
- Additional half doses can be administered as needed.
- Emergence dysphoria occurs in 5-10% of children.
- Routine coadministration of benzodiazepine or antisialagogue is no longer recommended.

**For minimal to moderately painful procedures** (burn dressing change, abscess I&D, urinary catheter placement, IV start, fracture reduction with hematoma block):

- **Nitrous oxide**, inhaled, provides analgesia, amnesia, and sedation.
- Local anesthesia is often necessary and provides additional analgesia.
- Moderate sedation can be achieved using 50-70% nitrous oxide as a single agent.
- Deeper sedation may be achieved by premedication with 0.2 mg/kg oxycodone PO, maximum dose 10 mg or intranasal fentanyl 1-2 μg/kg, maximum dose 100 μg. Note, coadministration of an opioid increases likelihood of emesis; ondansetron does not blunt this effect.
- It is best to wait 45-60 minutes after oral oxycodone or 15 minutes after IN fentanyl administration to start nitrous sedation so that peak effect of the opioid is achieved at start of nitrous oxide administration.
- It takes 1-2 minutes to reach the peak effect of nitrous oxide.
- To reduce environmental exposure, maintain a tight seal of the mask on the child' face.
- In addition, provide 100% oxygen at end of nitrous sedation for at least 2-3 minutes to scavenge the exhaled nitrous oxide and residual nitrous oxide in the system.

**For nonpainful procedures requiring patient immobility** (MRI, bone scan, etc):

- *Propofol and dexmedetomidine* provide sedation. However, propofol does not provide any analgesia, and dexmedetomidine provides minimal analgesia. These agents are used for nonpainful procedures requiring immobility.
- In most hospitals, these agents are only used by anesthesiologists, critical care physicians, or emergency medicine physicians.
- Protocols for the use of these agents are beyond the scope of this chapter.

## SUGGESTED READINGS

Al-alami AA, Zestos MM, Baraka AS. Pediatric laryngospasm: prevention and treatment. Curr Opin Anaesthesiol 2009;22(3):388–395.

American Society of Anesthesiologists. Continuum of depth of sedation: definition of general anesthesia and levels of sedation/analgesia. Available at http://www.asahq.org/standards/20. htm. Accessed February 13, 2001.

Bhatt M, Johnson DW, Chan J, et al. Risk factors for adverse events in emergency department procedural sedation for children. JAMA Pediatr 2017;171(10):957–964.

Chinta SS, Schrock CR, McAllister JD, et al. Rapid administration technique of ketamine for pediatric forearm fracture reduction: a dose-finding study. Ann Emerg Med 2015;65(6):640.

Clark M, Brunick A. Handbook of Nitrous Oxide and Oxygen Sedation. 5th Ed. St. Louis, MO: Elsevier Inc., 2020. ISBN: 9780323567428.

Coté CJ, Wilson S; American Academy of Pediatrics, American Academy of Pediatric Dentistry. Guidelines for monitoring and management of pediatric patients before, during, and after sedation for diagnostic and therapeutic procedures. Pediatrics 2019;143(6):e20191000.

Gooden CK, Lowrie LH, Jackson BF, eds. The Pediatric Procedural Sedation Handbook. New York: Oxford University Press, 2018.

Green SM, Leroy PL, Roback MG, et al.; International Committee for the Advancement of Procedural Sedation. Guidelines: an international multidisciplinary consensus statement on fasting before procedural sedation in adults and children. Anaesthesia 2020;75:374–385. doi:10.1111/anae.14892

Green SM, Roback MG, Kennedy RM, et al. Clinical practice guideline for emergency department ketamine dissociative sedation: 2011 update. Ann Emerg Med 2011;57(5):449–461.

Green SM, Roback MG, Krauss B, et al. Predictors of airway and respiratory adverse events with ketamine sedation in the emergency department: an individual-patient data meta-analysis of 8,282 children. Ann Med 2009;54(2):158–168; e151–e154.

Hampson-Evans D, Morgan P, Farrar M. Pediatric laryngospasm. Paediatr Anaesth 2008;18(4):303–307.

Joint Commission on Accreditation of Healthcare Organizations. Standards and intents for sedation and anesthesia care. In: Revisions to Anesthesia Care Standards, Comprehensive Accreditation Manual for Hospitals. Oakbrook Terrace, IL: Joint Commission on Accreditation of Healthcare Organizations, 2001. Available at http://www.jcaho.org/standard/aneshap.html. Accessed February 13, 2001.

Luhmann J, Schootman M, Luhmann S, et al. A randomized comparison of nitrous oxide plus hematoma block versus ketamine plus midazolam for emergency department forearm fracture reduction in children. Pediatrics 2006;118(4):e1078—e1086.

Malviya S, Voepel-Lewis T, Tait AR, et al. Depth of sedation in children undergoing computed tomography: validity and reliability of the University of Michigan Sedation Scale (UMSS). Br J Anaesth 2002;88:241–245.

Mason KP, ed. Pediatric Sedation Outside of the Operating Room: A Multispecialty International Collaboration. 3rd Ed. New York: Springer Science+Business Media LLC, 2021. ISBN 978-3-030-58405-4.

Tobias JD. Applications of nitrous oxide for procedural sedation in the pediatric population. Pediatr Emerg Care 2013;29:245–265.

# Appendix A
## Immunization Guidelines, 2022

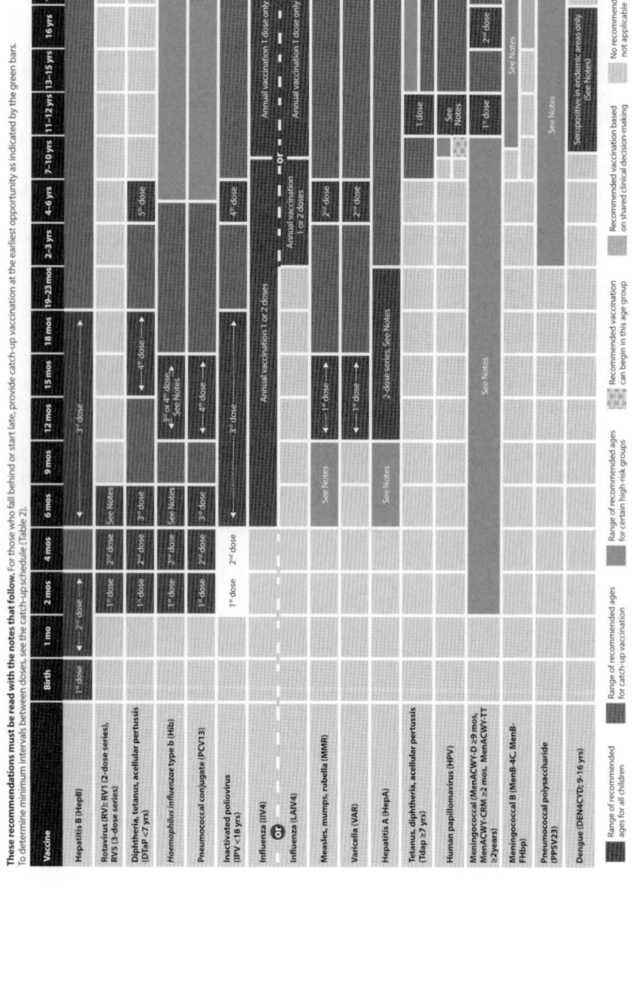


**Figure A-1 Recommended immunization schedule for persons aged 0-18 years.** (Reprinted from Centers for Disease Control and Prevention. Recommended Child and Adolescent Immunization Schedule for ages 18 years or younger, 2022. Available at https://www.cdc.gov/vaccines/schedules/downloads/child/0-18yrs-combined-schedule-bw.pdf.)

Recommended Catch-up Immunization Schedule for Children and Adolescents Who Start Late or Who Are More than 1 Month Behind, United States, 2022

The table below provides catch-up schedules and minimum intervals between doses for children whose vaccinations have been delayed. A vaccine series does not need to be restarted, regardless of the time that has elapsed between doses. Use the section appropriate for the child's age. **Always use this table in conjunction with Table 1 and the Notes that follow.**

| Vaccine | Minimum Age for Dose 1 | Dose 1 to Dose 2 | Dose 2 to Dose 3 | Dose 3 to Dose 4 | Dose 4 to Dose 5 |
|---|---|---|---|---|---|
| | | | **Children age 4 months through 6 years** | | |
| | | | Minimum Interval Between Doses | | |
| Hepatitis B | Birth | 4 weeks | 8 weeks and at least 16 weeks after first dose minimum age for the final dose is 24 weeks | | |
| Rotavirus | 6 weeks Maximum age for first dose is 14 weeks, 6 days | 4 weeks | 4 weeks maximum age for final dose is 8 months, 0 days | | |
| Diphtheria, tetanus, and acellular pertussis | 6 weeks | 4 weeks | 4 weeks | 6 months | 6 months |
| Haemophilus influenzae type b | 6 weeks | **No further doses needed** if previous dose was administered at age 15 months or older **4 weeks** if first dose was administered before the 1st birthday **8 weeks (as final dose)** if first dose was administered at age 12 months through 14 months. | **No further doses needed** if previous dose was administered at age 15 months or older **4 weeks** if current age is younger than 12 months and first dose was administered at younger than age 7 months and at least 1 previous dose was PRP-T (ActHIB®, Pentacel®, Hiberix®), Vaxelis® or unknown **8 weeks and age 12 through 59 months (as final dose)** if current age is younger than 12 months and first dose was administered at age 7 through 11 months; OR if current age is 12 through 59 months and first dose was administered before the 1st birthday and second dose was administered at younger than 15 months; OR if both doses were PedvaxHIB® and were administered before the 1st birthday | **8 weeks (as final dose)** This dose only necessary for children age 12 through 59 months who received 3 doses before the 1st birthday. | |
| Pneumococcal conjugate | 6 weeks | **No further doses needed for healthy children** if previous dose was administered at age 24 months or older **4 weeks** if first dose was administered before the 1st birthday **8 weeks (as final dose for healthy children)** if first dose was administered at the 1st birthday or after | **No further doses needed** for healthy children if previous dose was administered at age 24 months or older **4 weeks** if current age is younger than 12 months and previous dose was administered at <7 months old **8 weeks (as final dose for healthy children)** if previous dose was administered between 7–11 months (wait until at least 12 months old); OR if current age is 12 months or older and at least 1 dose was administered before age 12 months | **8 weeks (as final dose)** This dose only necessary for children age 12 through 59 months who received 3 doses before age 12 months or for children at high risk who received 3 doses at any age. | |
| Inactivated poliovirus | 6 weeks | 4 weeks | **4 weeks** if current age is <4 years **6 months (as final dose)** if current age is 4 years or older | **6 months (minimum age 4 years for final dose)** | |
| Measles, mumps, rubella | 12 months | 4 weeks | | | |
| Varicella | 12 months | 3 months | | | |
| Hepatitis A | 12 months | 6 months | | | |
| Meningococcal ACWY | 2 months MenACWY-CRM 2 months MenACWY-D 2 years MenACWY-TT | 8 weeks | See Notes | See Notes | |
| | | | **Children and adolescent age 7 through 18 years** | | |
| Meningococcal ACWY | Not applicable (N/A) | 8 weeks | | | |
| Tetanus, diphtheria, and acellular pertussis | 7 years | 4 weeks | **4 weeks** if first dose of DTaP/DT was administered before the 1st birthday **6 months (as final dose)** if first dose of DTaP/DT or Tdap/Td was administered at or after the 1st birthday | **6 months** if first dose of DTaP/DT was administered before the 1st birthday | |
| Human papillomavirus | 9 years | Routine dosing intervals are recommended. | | | |
| Hepatitis A | N/A | 6 months | | | |
| Hepatitis B | N/A | 4 weeks | **8 weeks and at least 16 weeks after first dose** | | |
| Inactivated poliovirus | N/A | 4 weeks | **6 months** A fourth dose is not necessary if the third dose was administered at age 4 years or older and at least 6 months after the previous dose. | A fourth dose of IPV is indicated if all previous doses were administered at <4 years or if the third dose was administered <6 months after the second dose. | |
| Measles, mumps, rubella | N/A | 4 weeks | | | |
| Varicella | N/A | 3 months if younger than age 13 years. 4 weeks if age 13 years or older | | | |
| Dengue | 9 years | 6 months | | | |

**Figure A-2 Catch-up immunization schedule for persons aged 4 months to 18 years who start late or who are >1 month behind.** (Reprinted from Centers for Disease Control and Prevention. Recommended Child and Adolescent Immunization Schedule for ages 18 years or younger, 2022. Available at https://www.cdc.gov/vaccines/schedules/downloads/child/0-18yrs-combined-schedule-bw.pdf.)

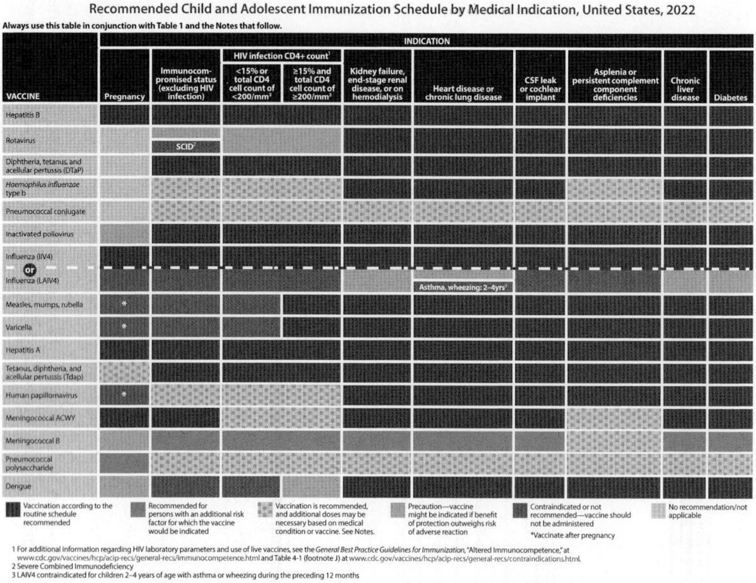

Recommended Child and Adolescent Immunization Schedule by Medical Indication, United States, 2022

Always use this table in conjunction with Table 1 and the Notes that follow.

**Figure A-3** **Recommended child and adolescent immunization schedule by medical indication.** (Reprinted from Centers for Disease Control and Prevention. Recommended Child and Adolescent Immunization Schedule for ages 18 years or younger, 2022. Available at https://www. cdc.gov/vaccines/schedules/downloads/child/0-18yrs-combined-schedule-bw.pdf.)

- 9vHPV, 4vHPV, or 2vHPV for routine vaccination of females 11 or 12 years[1] of age and females through 26 years of age who have not been vaccinated previously or who have not completed the 3-dose series.
- 9vHPV or 4vHPV for routine vaccination of males 11 or 12 years[1] of age and males through 21 years of age who have not been vaccinated previously or who have not completed the 3-dose series.
- 9vHPV or 4vHPV vaccination for men who have sex with men and immunocompromised men (including those with HIV infection) through age 26 years if not vaccinated previously.

---

[1]Can be given starting at 9 years of age.

# Appendix B
**Developmental Milestones**

| Month | Social/Emotional | Language/Communication | Cognitive | Movement/Physical |
|---|---|---|---|---|
| 2 | • Calms down when spoken to or picked up<br>• Looks at your face<br>• Seems happy to see you when you walk up to her<br>• Smiles when you talk to or smile at her | • Makes sounds other than crying<br>• Reacts to loud sounds | • Watches you as you move<br>• Looks at a toy for several seconds | • Holds head up when on tummy<br>• Moves both arms and legs<br>• Opens hands briefly |
| 4 | • Smiles on his own to get your attention<br>• Chuckles (not yet a full laugh) when you try to make her laugh<br>• Looks at you, moves, or makes sounds to get or keep your attention | • Makes sounds like "oooo," "aahh" (cooing)<br>• Makes sounds back when you talk to him<br>• Turns head towards the sound of your voice | • If hungry, opens mouth when she sees breast or bottle<br>• Looks at hands with interest | • Holds head steady without support when you are holding her<br>• Holds a toy when you put it in his hand<br>• Uses her arm to swing at toys<br>• Brings hands to mouth<br>• Pushes up onto elbows/forearms when on tummy |
| 6 | • Knows familiar people<br>• Likes to look at self in mirror<br>• Laughs | • Takes turns making sounds with you<br>• Blows "raspberries" (sticks tongue out and blows)<br>• Makes squealing noises | • Puts things in her mouth to explore them<br>• Reaches to grab a toy he wants<br>• Closes lips to show she doesn't want more food | • Rolls from tummy to back<br>• Pushes up with straight arms when on tummy<br>• Leans on hands to support himself when sitting |

9

- Is shy, clingy, or fearful around strangers
- Shows several facial expressions, like happy, sad, angry, and surprised
- Looks when you call her name
- Reacts when you leave (looks, reaches for you, or cries)
- Smiles or laughs when you play peek-a-boo

- Makes a lot of different sounds like "mamamama" and "bababababa"
- Lifts arms up to be picked up

- Looks for objects when dropped our of sight (like his spoon or toy)
- Bangs two things together

- Gets to a sitting position by herself
- Moves things from one hand to her other hand
- Uses fingers to "rake" food towards himself
- Sits without support

12

- Plays games with you, like pat-a-cake

- Waves "bye-bye"
- Calls a parent "mama" or "dada" or another special name
- Understands "no" (pauses briefly or stops when you say it)

- Puts something in a container, like a block in a cup
- Looks for things he sees you hide, like a toy under a blanket

- Pulls up to a stand
- Walks, holding onto furniture
- Drinks from a cup without a lid, as you hold it
- Picks things up between thumb and pointer finger, like small bits of food

(Continued)

| Month | Social/Emotional | Language/Communication | Cognitive | Movement/Physical |
|---|---|---|---|---|
| 15 | • Copies other children while playing, like taking toys out of a container when another child does<br><br>• Shows you an object she likes<br><br>• Claps when excited<br><br>• Hugs stuffed doll or other toy<br><br>• Shows you affection (hugs, cuddles, or kisses you) | • Tries to say one or two words besides "mama" or "dada", like "ba" for ball or "da" for dog<br><br>• Looks at a familiar object when you name it<br><br>• Follows directions given with both a gesture and words. For example, he gives you a toy when you hold out your ahnd aand say, "Give me the toy."<br><br>• Points to ask for something or to get help | • Tries to use things the right way, like a phone, cup, or book<br><br>• Stacks at least two small onjects, like blocks | • Takes a few steps on his own<br><br>• Uses fingers to feed herself some food |
| 18 | • Moves away from you, but looks to make sure you are close by<br><br>• Points to show you something interesting<br><br>• Puts hands out for you to wash them<br><br>• Looks at a few pages in a book with you<br><br>• Helps you dress him by pushing arm through sleeve or lifting up foot | • Tries to say three or more words besides "mama" or "dada"<br><br>• Follows one-step directions without any gestures, like giving you the toy when youo say, "Give it to me." | • Copies you doing chores, like sweeping with a broom<br><br>• Plays with toys in a simple way, like pushing a toy car | • Walks without holding on to anyone or anything<br><br>• Scribbles<br><br>• Drinks from a cup without a lid and may spill sometimes<br><br>• Feeds herself with her fingers<br><br>• Tries to use a spoon<br><br>• Climbs on and off a couch or chair without help |

**24 (2 years)**

- Notices when others are hurt or upset, like pausing or looking sad when someone is crying
- Looks at your face to see how to react in a new situation

- Points to things in a book when you ask, "Where is the bear?"
- Says at least two words together, like "More milk."
- Points to at least two boyd parts when you ask him to show you
- Uses more gestures than just waving and pointing, like blowing a kiss or nodding yes

- Holds something in one hand while using the other hand; for example, holding a container and taking the lid off
- Tries to use switches, knobs, or buttons on a toy
- Plays with more than one toy at the same time, like putting toy food on a toy plate

- Kicks a ball
- Runs
- Walks (not climbs) up a few stairs with or without help
- Eats with a spoon

**30 (2.5 years)**

- Plays next to other children and sometimes plays with them
- Shows you what she can do by saying, "Look at me!"
- Follows simple routines when told, like helping to pick up toys when you say, "It's clean-up time."

- Says about 50 words
- Says two or more words, with one action word, like "Doggie run"
- Names things in a book when you point and ask, "What is this?"
- Says words like "I", "me", or "we"

- Uses things to pretend, like feeding a block to a doll as if it were food
- Shows simple problem-solving skills, like standing on a small stool to reach something
- Follows two-step instructions like "Put the toy down and close the door."
- Show he knows at least one color, like pointing to a red crayon when you ask, "Which one is red?"

- Uses hands to twist things, like turning doorknobs or unscrewing lids
- Takes some clothes off by himself, like loose pants or an open jacket
- Jumps off the ground with both feet
- Turns book pages, one at a time, when you read to her

*(Continued)*

| Month | Social/Emotional | Language/Communication | Cognitive | Movement/Physical |
|---|---|---|---|---|
| 36 (3 years) | • Calms down within 10 minutes after you leave her, like at a childcare drop off<br><br>• Notices other children and joins them to play | • Talks with you in conversation using at least two back-and-forth exchanges<br><br>• Asks "who", "what", "where", or "why" questions, like "Where is mommy/daddy?"<br><br>• Says what action is happening in a picture or book when asked, like "running", "eating", or "playing"<br><br>• Says first name, when asked<br><br>• Talks well enough for others to understand, most of the time | • Draws a circle, when you show him how<br><br>• Avoids touching hot objects, like a stove, when you warn her | • Strings items together, like large beads or macaroni<br><br>• Puts on some clothes by himself, like loose pants or a jacket<br><br>• Uses a fork |

| 48 (4 years) | • Pretends to be something else during play (teacher, superhero, dog)<br>• Asks to go play with children if none are around, like "Can I play with Alex?"<br>• Comforts others who are hurt or sad, like hugging a crying friend<br>• Avoids danger, like not jumping from tall heights at the playground<br>• Likes to be a "helper"<br>• Changes behavior based on where she is (place of worship, library, playground) | • Says sentences with four or more words<br>• Says some words from a song, story, or nursery rhyme<br>• Talks about at least one things that happened during his day, like "I played soccer."<br>• Answers simple questions like "What is a coat for?" or "What is a crayon for?" | • Names a few colors of items<br>• Tells what comes next in a well-known story<br>• Draws a person with three or more body parts | • Catches a large ball most of the time<br>• Serves himself food or pours water, with adult supervision<br>• Unbuttons some buttons<br>• Holds crayon or pencil between fingers and thumb (not a fist) |

(Continued)

| Month | Social/Emotional | Language/Communication | Cognitive | Movement/Physical |
|---|---|---|---|---|
| 60 (5 years) | • Follows rules or takes turns when playing games with other children<br><br>• Sings, dances, or acts for you<br><br>• Does simple chores at home, like matching socks or clearing the table after eating | • Tells a story she heard or made up with at least two events. For example, a cat was stuck in a tree and a firefighter saved it<br><br>• Answers simple questions about a book or story after you read or tell it to him<br><br>• Keep s aconversation going with more than three back-and-forth exchanges<br><br>• Uses or recognizes simple rhymes (bat-cat, ball-tall) | • Counts to 10<br><br>• Names some numbers between 1 and 5 when you point to them<br><br>• Uses words about time, like "yesterday", "tomorrow", "morning", or "night"<br><br>• Pays attention for 5 to 10 minutes during activities. For example, during story time or making arts and crafts (screen time does not count)<br><br>• Writes some letters in her name<br><br>• Names some letters when you point to them | • Buttons some buttons<br><br>• Hops on one foot |

Adapted from Zubler JM, Wiggins LD, Macias MM, et al. Evidence-Informed Milestones for Developmental Surveillance Tools. *Pediatrics.* 2022;149(3):e2021052138.

# Appendix C
## Growth Charts

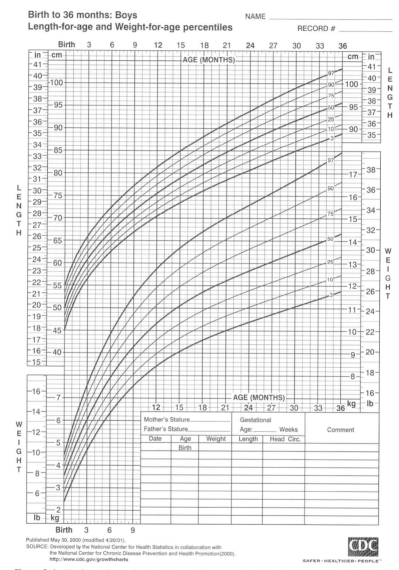

**Birth to 36 months: Boys**
**Length-for-age and Weight-for-age percentiles**

NAME _____

RECORD # _____

Published May 30, 2000 (modified 4/20/01).
SOURCE: Developed by the National Center for Health Statistics in collaboration with
the National Center for Chronic Disease Prevention and Health Promotion(2000).
http://www.cdc.gov/growthcharts

**Figure C-1.  Birth to 36 months: boys' length-for-age and weight-for-age percentiles.** (*Source*: National Center for Health Statistics in collaboration with the National Center for Chronic Disease Prevention and Health Promotion, May 30, 2000. Modified April 20, 2001.)

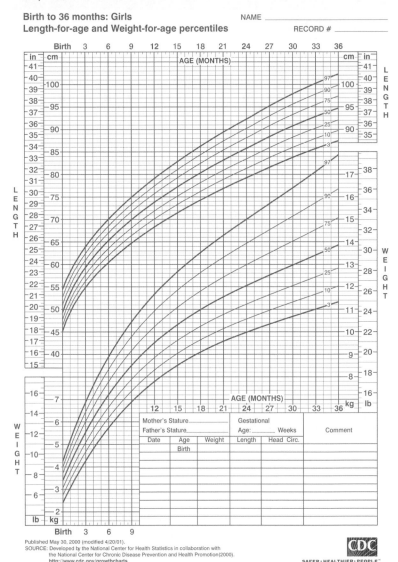

**Figure C-2. Birth to 36 months: girls' length-for-age and weight-for-age percentiles.** (*Source*: National Center for Health Statistics in collaboration with the National Center for Chronic Disease Prevention and Health Promotion, May 30, 2000. Modified April 20, 2001.)

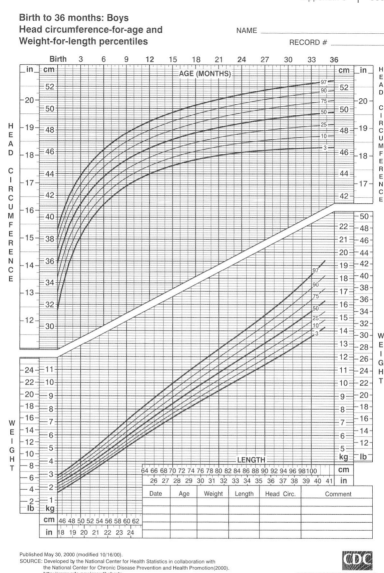

**Birth to 36 months: Boys**
**Head circumference-for-age and**
**Weight-for-length percentiles**

NAME _____

RECORD # _____

Published May 30, 2000 (modified 10/16/00).
SOURCE: Developed by the National Center for Health Statistics in collaboration with
   the National Center for Chronic Disease Prevention and Health Promotion(2000).
   http://www.cdc.gov/growthcharts

**Figure C-3. Birth to 36 months: boys' head circumference-for-age and weight-for-length percentiles.** (*Source*: National Center for Health Statistics in collaboration with the National Center for Chronic Disease Prevention and Health Promotion, May 30, 2000. Modified April 20, 2001.)

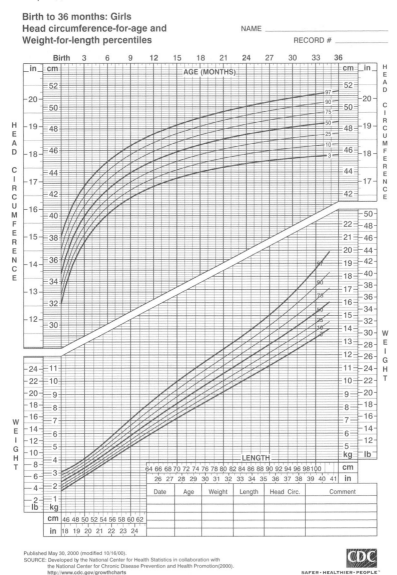

**Birth to 36 months: Girls**
**Head circumference-for-age and**
**Weight-for-length percentiles**

NAME _____

RECORD # _____

**Figure C-4. Birth to 36 months: girls' head circumference-for-age and weight-for-length percentiles.** (*Source*: National Center for Health Statistics in collaboration with the National Center for Chronic Disease Prevention and Health Promotion, May 30, 2000. Modified April 20, 2001.)

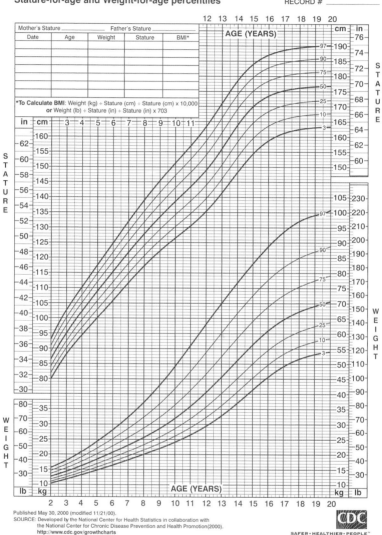

**Figure C-5. Two to twenty years: boys' stature-for-age and weight-for-age percentiles.** (*Source*: National Center for Health Statistics in collaboration with the National Center for Chronic Disease Prevention and Health Promotion, May 30, 2000. Modified April 20, 2001.)

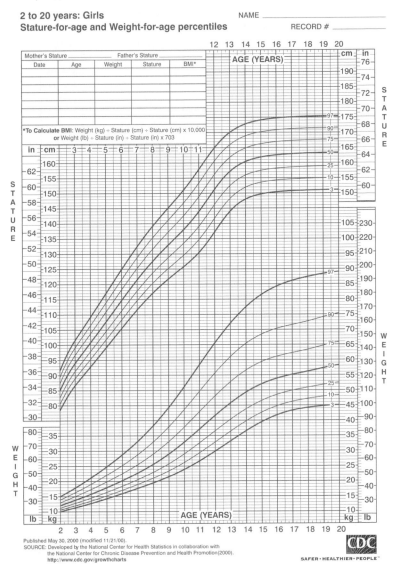

**Figure C-6. Two to twenty years: girls' stature-for-age and weight-for-age percentiles.**
(*Source*: National Center for Health Statistics in collaboration with the National Center for Chronic Disease Prevention and Health Promotion, May 30, 2000. Modified April 20, 2001.)

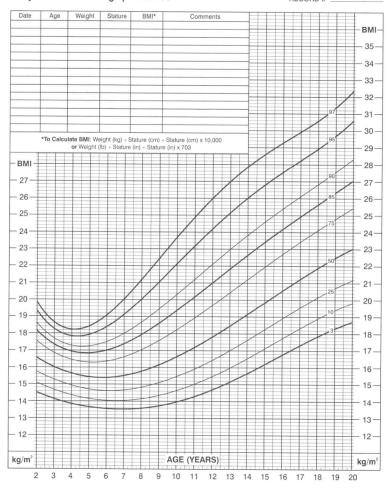

## 2 to 20 years: Boys
## Body mass index-for-age percentiles

NAME _____

RECORD # _____

*To Calculate BMI: Weight (kg) ÷ Stature (cm) ÷ Stature (cm) x 10,000
or Weight (lb) ÷ Stature (in) ÷ Stature (in) x 703

Published May 30, 2000 (modified 10/16/00).
SOURCE: Developed by the National Center for Health Statistics in collaboration with
the National Center for Chronic Disease Prevention and Health Promotion(2000).
http://www.cdc.gov/growthcharts

SAFER·HEALTHIER·PEOPLE™

**Figure C-7. Two to twenty years: boys' body mass index (BMI)-for-age percentiles.** (*Source*: National Center for Health Statistics in collaboration with the National Center for Chronic Disease Prevention and Health Promotion, May 30, 2000. Modified April 20, 2001.)

**2 to 20 years: Girls**
**Body mass index-for-age percentiles**

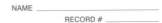
NAME _____
RECORD # _____

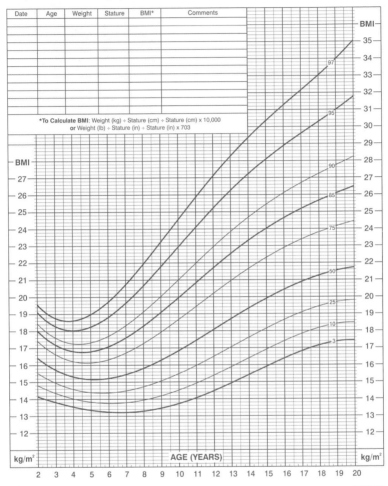

*To Calculate BMI: Weight (kg) ÷ Stature (cm) ÷ Stature (cm) x 10,000
or Weight (lb) ÷ Stature (in) ÷ Stature (in) x 703

Published May 30, 2000 (modified 10/16/00).
SOURCE: Developed by the National Center for Health Statistics in collaboration with
the National Center for Chronic Disease Prevention and Health Promotion(2000).
http://www.cdc.gov/growthcharts

SAFER · HEALTHIER · PEOPLE™

**Figure C-8. Two to twenty years: girls' body mass index (BMI)-for-age percentiles.** (*Source*: National Center for Health Statistics in collaboration with the National Center for Chronic Disease Prevention and Health Promotion, May 30, 2000. Modified April 20, 2001.)

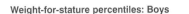

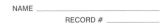

## Weight-for-stature percentiles: Boys

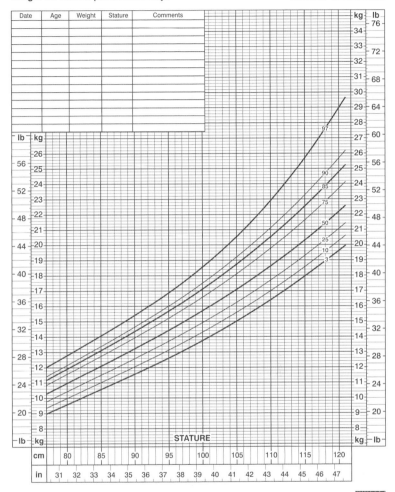

Published May 30, 2000 (modified 10/16/00).
SOURCE: Developed by the National Center for Health Statistics in collaboration with
the National Center for Chronic Disease Prevention and Health Promotion(2000).
http://www.cdc.gov/growthcharts

**Figure C-9. Boys' weight-for-stature percentiles.** (*Source*: National Center for Health Statistics in collaboration with the National Center for Chronic Disease Prevention and Health Promotion, May 30, 2000. Modified April 20, 2001.)

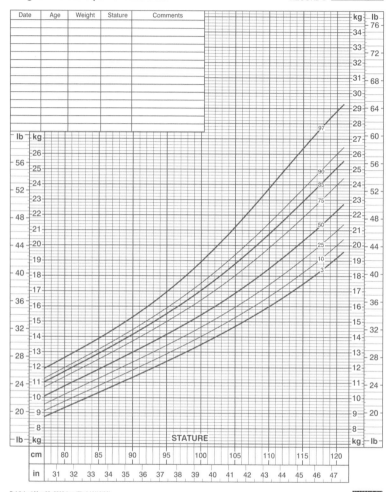

**Weight-for-stature percentiles: Girls**

NAME _____

RECORD # _____

Published May 30, 2000 (modified 10/16/00).
SOURCE: Developed by the National Center for Health Statistics in collaboration with
the National Center for Chronic Disease Prevention and Health Promotion (2000).
http://www.cdc.gov/growthcharts

**Figure C-10. Girls' weight-for-stature percentiles.** (*Source*: National Center for Health Statistics in collaboration with the National Center for Chronic Disease Prevention and Health Promotion, May 30, 2000. Modified April 20, 2001.)

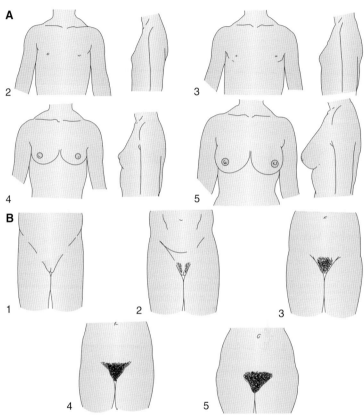

**Figure D-1. Female tanner stages. A.** Female breast development. Sex maturity rating *1* (not shown): prepubertal; elevation of papilla only. Sex maturity rating *2*: breast buds appear; areola is slightly widened and projects as small mound. Sex maturity rating *3*: enlargement of the entire breast with no protrusion of the papilla or the nipple. Sex maturity rating *4*: enlargement of the breast and projection of areola and papilla as a secondary mound. Sex maturity rating *5*: adult configuration of the breast with protrusion of the nipple; areola no longer projects separately from the remainder of the breast. **B.** Female pubic hair development. Sex maturity rating *1*: prepubertal; no pubic hair. Sex maturity rating *2*: straight hair extends along the labia and, between rating *2* and *3*, begins on the pubis. Sex maturity rating *3*: pubic hair increased in quantity, darker, and present in the typical female triangle but in smaller quantity. Sex maturity rating *4*: pubic hair more dense, curled, and adult in distribution but less abundant. Sex maturity rating *5*: abundant, adult-type pattern; hair may extend onto the medial part of the thighs. (Adapted from Tanner JM. Growth at Adolescence. 2nd Ed. Oxford: Blackwell, 1962; reprinted from Silbert-Flagg J, Pillitteri A. Maternal and Child Nursing, 8th Ed. Philadelphia: Wolters Kluwer, 2017.)

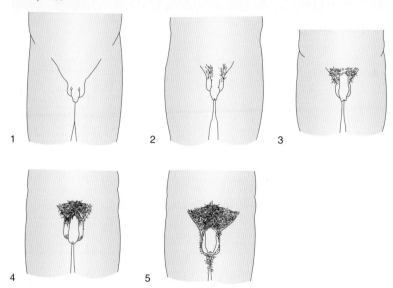

**Figure D-2. Male tanner stages.** Male genital and pubic hair development. Ratings for pubic hair and for genital development can differ in a typical boy at any given time because pubic hair and genitalia do not necessarily develop at the same rate. Sex maturity rating *1*: prepubertal; no pubic hair; genitalia unchanged from early childhood. Sex maturity rating *2*: light, downy hair develops laterally and later becomes dark; penis and testes may be slightly larger; scrotum becoming more textured. Sex maturity rating *3*: pubic hair has extended across the pubis; testes and scrotum are further enlarged; penis is larger, especially in length. Sex maturity rating *4*: more abundant pubic hair with curling; genitalia resemble those of an adult; glans has become larger and broader; scrotum is darker. Sex maturity rating *5*: adult quantity and pattern of pubic hair, with hair present along inner borders of thighs; testes and scrotum are adult in size. (Adapted from Tanner JM. Growth at Adolescence. 2nd Ed. Oxford: Blackwell, 1962; reprinted from Silbert-Flagg J, Pillitteri A. Maternal and Child Nursing, 8th Ed. Philadelphia: Wolters Kluwer, 2017.)

# Appendix E
## Phototherapy/Exchange Transfusion Guidelines

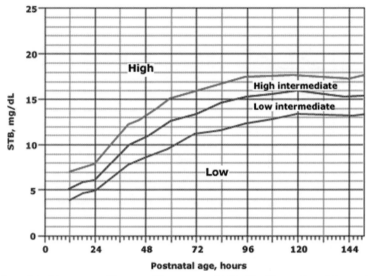

**Figure E-1. Nomogram of hour-specific serum total bilirubin.** (*Source*: From Subcommittee on Hyperbilirubinemia. Management of hyperbilirubinemia in the newborn infant 35 or more weeks of gestation. Pediatrics 2004;114:297. ©2004 The American Academy of Pediatrics.)

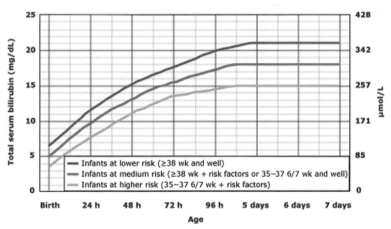

**Figure E-2. Total serum bilirubin guideline for phototherapy.** (*Source*: From Subcommittee on Hyperbilirubinemia. Management of hyperbilirubinemia in the newborn infant 35 or more weeks of gestation. Pediatrics 2004;114:297. ©2004 The American Academy of Pediatrics.)

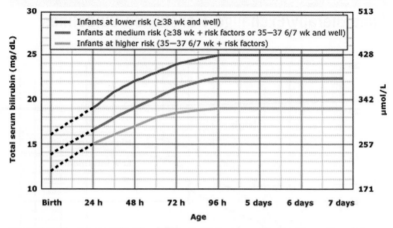

Figure E-3. **Total serum bilirubin guideline for exchange transfusion.** (*Source*: From Subcommittee on Hyperbilirubinemia. Management of hyperbilirubinemia in the newborn infant 35 or more weeks of gestation. Pediatrics 2004;114:297. ©2004 The American Academy of Pediatrics.)

# Appendix F
**Hypertension in Children and Adolescents**

**TABLE F-1  BP Levels for Boys by Age and Height Percentile**

| Age (y) | BP percentile | SBP (mm Hg) Height percentile or measured height | | | | | | | DBP (mm Hg) Height percentile or measured height | | | | | | |
|---|---|---|---|---|---|---|---|---|---|---|---|---|---|---|---|
| | | 5% | 10% | 25% | 50% | 75% | 90% | 95% | 5% | 10% | 25% | 50% | 75% | 90% | 95% |
| 1 | Height (in) | 30.4 | 30.8 | 31.6 | 32.4 | 33.3 | 34.1 | 34.6 | 30.4 | 30.8 | 31.6 | 32.4 | 33.3 | 34.1 | 34.6 |
| | Height (cm) | 77.2 | 78.3 | 80.2 | 82.4 | 84.6 | 86.7 | 87.9 | 77.2 | 78.3 | 80.2 | 82.4 | 84.6 | 86.7 | 87.9 |
| | 50th | 85 | 85 | 86 | 86 | 87 | 88 | 88 | 40 | 40 | 40 | 41 | 41 | 42 | 42 |
| | 90th | 98 | 99 | 99 | 100 | 100 | 101 | 101 | 52 | 52 | 53 | 53 | 54 | 54 | 54 |
| | 95th | 102 | 102 | 103 | 103 | 104 | 105 | 105 | 54 | 54 | 55 | 55 | 56 | 57 | 57 |
| | 95th + 12 mm Hg | 114 | 114 | 115 | 115 | 116 | 117 | 117 | 66 | 66 | 67 | 67 | 68 | 69 | 69 |
| 2 | Height (in) | 33.9 | 34.4 | 35.3 | 36.3 | 37.3 | 38.2 | 38.8 | 33.9 | 34.4 | 35.3 | 36.3 | 37.3 | 38.2 | 38.8 |
| | Height (cm) | 86.1 | 87.4 | 89.6 | 92.1 | 94.7 | 97.1 | 98.5 | 86.1 | 87.4 | 89.6 | 92.1 | 94.7 | 97.1 | 98.5 |
| | 50th | 87 | 87 | 88 | 89 | 89 | 90 | 91 | 43 | 43 | 44 | 44 | 45 | 46 | 46 |
| | 90th | 100 | 100 | 101 | 102 | 103 | 103 | 104 | 55 | 55 | 56 | 56 | 57 | 58 | 58 |
| | 95th | 104 | 105 | 105 | 106 | 107 | 107 | 108 | 57 | 58 | 58 | 59 | 60 | 61 | 61 |
| | 95th + 12 mm Hg | 116 | 117 | 117 | 118 | 119 | 119 | 120 | 69 | 70 | 70 | 71 | 72 | 73 | 73 |
| 3 | Height (in) | 36.4 | 37 | 37.9 | 39 | 40.1 | 41.1 | 41.7 | 36.4 | 37 | 37.9 | 39 | 40.1 | 41.1 | 41.7 |
| | Height (cm) | 92.5 | 93.9 | 96.3 | 99 | 101.8 | 104.3 | 105.8 | 92.5 | 93.9 | 96.3 | 99 | 101.8 | 104.3 | 105.8 |
| | 50th | 88 | 89 | 89 | 90 | 91 | 92 | 92 | 45 | 46 | 46 | 47 | 48 | 49 | 49 |
| | 90th | 101 | 102 | 102 | 103 | 104 | 105 | 105 | 58 | 58 | 59 | 59 | 60 | 61 | 61 |
| | 95th | 106 | 106 | 107 | 107 | 108 | 109 | 109 | 60 | 61 | 61 | 62 | 63 | 64 | 64 |
| | 95th + 12 mm Hg | 118 | 118 | 119 | 119 | 120 | 121 | 121 | 72 | 73 | 73 | 74 | 75 | 76 | 76 |

**Age 4**

Systolic BP (mm Hg):

| | 38.8 | 39.4 | 40.5 | 41.7 | 42.9 | 43.9 | 44.5 |
|---|---|---|---|---|---|---|---|
| Height (in) | 38.8 | 39.4 | 40.5 | 41.7 | 42.9 | 43.9 | 44.5 |
| Height (cm) | 98.5 | 100.2 | 102.9 | 105.9 | 108.9 | 111.5 | 113.2 |
| 50th | 90 | 90 | 91 | 92 | 93 | 94 | 94 |
| 90th | 102 | 103 | 104 | 105 | 105 | 106 | 107 |
| 95th | 107 | 107 | 108 | 108 | 109 | 110 | 110 |
| 95th + 12 mm Hg | 119 | 119 | 120 | 120 | 121 | 122 | 122 |

Diastolic BP (mm Hg):

| | 38.8 | 39.4 | 40.5 | 41.7 | 42.9 | 43.9 | 44.5 |
|---|---|---|---|---|---|---|---|
| Height (in) | 38.8 | 39.4 | 40.5 | 41.7 | 42.9 | 43.9 | 44.5 |
| Height (cm) | 98.5 | 100.2 | 102.9 | 105.9 | 108.9 | 111.5 | 113.2 |
| 50th | 48 | 49 | 49 | 50 | 51 | 52 | 52 |
| 90th | 60 | 61 | 62 | 62 | 63 | 64 | 64 |
| 95th | 63 | 64 | 65 | 66 | 67 | 67 | 68 |
| 95th + 12 mm Hg | 75 | 76 | 77 | 78 | 79 | 79 | 80 |

**Age 5**

Systolic BP (mm Hg):

| | 41.1 | 41.8 | 43.0 | 44.3 | 45.5 | 46.7 | 47.4 |
|---|---|---|---|---|---|---|---|
| Height (in) | 41.1 | 41.8 | 43.0 | 44.3 | 45.5 | 46.7 | 47.4 |
| Height (cm) | 104.4 | 106.2 | 109.1 | 112.4 | 115.7 | 118.6 | 120.3 |
| 50th | 91 | 92 | 93 | 94 | 95 | 96 | 96 |
| 90th | 103 | 104 | 105 | 106 | 107 | 108 | 108 |
| 95th | 107 | 108 | 109 | 109 | 110 | 111 | 112 |
| 95th + 12 mm Hg | 119 | 120 | 121 | 121 | 122 | 123 | 124 |

Diastolic BP (mm Hg):

| | 41.1 | 41.8 | 43.0 | 44.3 | 45.5 | 46.7 | 47.4 |
|---|---|---|---|---|---|---|---|
| Height (in) | 41.1 | 41.8 | 43.0 | 44.3 | 45.5 | 46.7 | 47.4 |
| Height (cm) | 104.4 | 106.2 | 109.1 | 112.4 | 115.7 | 118.6 | 120.3 |
| 50th | 51 | 51 | 52 | 53 | 54 | 55 | 55 |
| 90th | 63 | 64 | 65 | 65 | 66 | 67 | 67 |
| 95th | 66 | 67 | 68 | 69 | 70 | 70 | 71 |
| 95th + 12 mm Hg | 78 | 79 | 80 | 81 | 82 | 82 | 83 |

**Age 6**

Systolic BP (mm Hg):

| | 43.4 | 44.2 | 45.4 | 46.8 | 48.2 | 49.4 | 50.2 |
|---|---|---|---|---|---|---|---|
| Height (in) | 43.4 | 44.2 | 45.4 | 46.8 | 48.2 | 49.4 | 50.2 |
| Height (cm) | 110.3 | 112.2 | 115.3 | 118.9 | 122.4 | 125.6 | 127.5 |
| 50th | 93 | 93 | 94 | 95 | 96 | 97 | 98 |
| 90th | 105 | 105 | 106 | 107 | 109 | 110 | 110 |
| 95th | 108 | 109 | 110 | 111 | 112 | 113 | 114 |
| 95th + 12 mm Hg | 120 | 121 | 122 | 123 | 124 | 125 | 126 |

Diastolic BP (mm Hg):

| | 43.4 | 44.2 | 45.4 | 46.8 | 48.2 | 49.4 | 50.2 |
|---|---|---|---|---|---|---|---|
| Height (in) | 43.4 | 44.2 | 45.4 | 46.8 | 48.2 | 49.4 | 50.2 |
| Height (cm) | 110.3 | 112.2 | 115.3 | 118.9 | 122.4 | 125.6 | 127.5 |
| 50th | 54 | 54 | 55 | 56 | 57 | 57 | 58 |
| 90th | 66 | 66 | 67 | 68 | 68 | 69 | 69 |
| 95th | 69 | 70 | 70 | 71 | 72 | 72 | 73 |
| 95th + 12 mm Hg | 81 | 82 | 82 | 83 | 84 | 84 | 85 |

**Age 7**

Systolic BP (mm Hg):

| | 45.7 | 46.5 | 47.8 | 49.3 | 50.8 | 52.1 | 52.9 |
|---|---|---|---|---|---|---|---|
| Height (in) | 45.7 | 46.5 | 47.8 | 49.3 | 50.8 | 52.1 | 52.9 |
| Height (cm) | 116.1 | 118 | 121.4 | 125.1 | 128.9 | 132.4 | 134.5 |
| 50th | 94 | 94 | 95 | 97 | 98 | 98 | 99 |
| 90th | 106 | 107 | 108 | 109 | 110 | 111 | 111 |
| 95th | 110 | 110 | 110 | 111 | 112 | 115 | 116 |
| 95th + 12 mm Hg | 122 | 122 | 123 | 124 | 126 | 127 | 128 |

Diastolic BP (mm Hg):

| | 45.7 | 46.5 | 47.8 | 49.3 | 50.8 | 52.1 | 52.9 |
|---|---|---|---|---|---|---|---|
| Height (in) | 45.7 | 46.5 | 47.8 | 49.3 | 50.8 | 52.1 | 52.9 |
| Height (cm) | 116.1 | 118 | 121.4 | 125.1 | 128.9 | 132.4 | 134.5 |
| 50th | 56 | 56 | 57 | 58 | 58 | 59 | 59 |
| 90th | 68 | 68 | 69 | 70 | 70 | 71 | 71 |
| 95th | 71 | 71 | 72 | 73 | 73 | 74 | 74 |
| 95th + 12 mm Hg | 83 | 83 | 84 | 85 | 85 | 86 | 86 |

(Continued)

**TABLE F-1** BP Levels for Boys by Age and Height Percentile *(Continued)*

| Age (y) | BP percentile | SBP (mm Hg) | | | | | | | DBP (mm Hg) | | | | | | |
|---|---|---|---|---|---|---|---|---|---|---|---|---|---|---|---|
| | | Height percentile or measured height | | | | | | | Height percentile or measured height | | | | | | |
| | | 5% | 10% | 25% | 50% | 75% | 90% | 95% | 5% | 10% | 25% | 50% | 75% | 90% | 95% |
| 8 | Height (in) | 47.8 | 48.6 | 50 | 51.6 | 53.2 | 54.6 | 55.5 | 47.8 | 48.6 | 50 | 51.6 | 53.2 | 54.6 | 55.5 |
| | Height (cm) | 121.4 | 123.5 | 127 | 131 | 135.1 | 138.8 | 141 | 121.4 | 123.5 | 127 | 131 | 135.1 | 138.8 | 141 |
| | 50th | 95 | 96 | 97 | 98 | 99 | 99 | 100 | 57 | 57 | 58 | 59 | 59 | 60 | 60 |
| | 90th | 107 | 108 | 109 | 110 | 111 | 112 | 112 | 69 | 70 | 70 | 71 | 72 | 72 | 73 |
| | 95th | 111 | 112 | 112 | 114 | 115 | 116 | 117 | 72 | 72 | 73 | 74 | 75 | 75 | 75 |
| | 95th + 12 mm Hg | 123 | 124 | 124 | 126 | 127 | 128 | 129 | 84 | 85 | 85 | 86 | 87 | 87 | 87 |
| 9 | Height (in) | 49.6 | 50.5 | 52 | 53.7 | 55.4 | 56.9 | 57.9 | 49.6 | 50.5 | 52 | 53.7 | 55.4 | 56.9 | 57.9 |
| | Height (cm) | 126 | 128.3 | 132.1 | 136.3 | 140.7 | 144.7 | 147.1 | 126 | 128.3 | 132.1 | 136.3 | 140.7 | 144.7 | 147.1 |
| | 50th | 96 | 97 | 98 | 99 | 100 | 101 | 101 | 57 | 58 | 59 | 60 | 61 | 62 | 62 |
| | 90th | 107 | 108 | 109 | 110 | 112 | 113 | 114 | 70 | 71 | 72 | 73 | 74 | 74 | 74 |
| | 95th | 112 | 112 | 113 | 115 | 116 | 118 | 119 | 74 | 74 | 75 | 76 | 76 | 77 | 77 |
| | 95th + 12 mm Hg | 124 | 124 | 125 | 127 | 128 | 130 | 131 | 86 | 86 | 87 | 88 | 88 | 89 | 89 |
| 10 | Height (in) | 51.3 | 52.2 | 53.8 | 55.6 | 57.4 | 59.1 | 60.1 | 51.3 | 52.2 | 53.8 | 55.6 | 57.4 | 59.1 | 60.1 |
| | Height (cm) | 130.2 | 132.7 | 136.7 | 141.3 | 145.9 | 150.1 | 152.7 | 130.2 | 132.7 | 136.7 | 141.3 | 145.9 | 150.1 | 152.7 |
| | 50th | 97 | 98 | 99 | 100 | 101 | 102 | 103 | 59 | 60 | 61 | 62 | 63 | 63 | 64 |
| | 90th | 108 | 109 | 111 | 112 | 113 | 115 | 116 | 72 | 73 | 74 | 74 | 75 | 75 | 76 |
| | 95th | 112 | 113 | 114 | 116 | 118 | 120 | 121 | 76 | 76 | 77 | 77 | 78 | 78 | 78 |
| | 95th + 12 mm Hg | 124 | 125 | 126 | 128 | 130 | 132 | 133 | 88 | 88 | 89 | 89 | 90 | 90 | 90 |

| Age | | Systolic BP (mm Hg) — Percentile of Height | | | | | | | Diastolic BP (mm Hg) — Percentile of Height | | | | | | |
|---|---|---|---|---|---|---|---|---|---|---|---|---|---|---|---|
| 11 | Height (in) | 53 | 54 | 55.7 | 57.6 | 59.6 | 61.3 | 62.4 | 53 | 54 | 55.7 | 57.6 | 59.6 | 61.3 | 62.4 |
| | Height (cm) | 134.7 | 137.3 | 141.5 | 146.4 | 151.3 | 155.8 | 158.6 | 134.7 | 137.3 | 141.5 | 146.4 | 151.3 | 155.8 | 158.6 |
| | 50th | 99 | 99 | 101 | 102 | 103 | 104 | 106 | 61 | 61 | 62 | 63 | 63 | 63 | 63 |
| | 90th | 110 | 111 | 112 | 114 | 116 | 117 | 118 | 74 | 74 | 75 | 75 | 75 | 76 | 76 |
| | 95th | 114 | 114 | 116 | 118 | 120 | 123 | 124 | 77 | 78 | 78 | 78 | 78 | 78 | 78 |
| | 95th + 12 mm Hg | 126 | 126 | 128 | 130 | 132 | 135 | 136 | 89 | 90 | 90 | 90 | 90 | 90 | 90 |
| 12 | Height (in) | 55.2 | 56.3 | 58.1 | 60.1 | 62.2 | 64 | 65.2 | 55.2 | 56.3 | 58.1 | 60.1 | 62.2 | 64 | 65.2 |
| | Height (cm) | 140.3 | 143 | 147.5 | 152.7 | 157.9 | 162.6 | 165.5 | 140.3 | 143 | 147.5 | 152.7 | 157.9 | 162.6 | 165.5 |
| | 50th | 101 | 101 | 102 | 104 | 106 | 108 | 109 | 61 | 62 | 62 | 62 | 62 | 63 | 63 |
| | 90th | 113 | 114 | 115 | 117 | 119 | 121 | 122 | 75 | 75 | 75 | 75 | 75 | 76 | 76 |
| | 95th | 116 | 117 | 118 | 121 | 124 | 126 | 128 | 78 | 78 | 78 | 78 | 78 | 79 | 79 |
| | 95th + 12 mm Hg | 128 | 129 | 130 | 133 | 136 | 138 | 140 | 90 | 90 | 90 | 90 | 90 | 91 | 91 |
| 13 | Height (in) | 57.9 | 59.1 | 61 | 63.1 | 65.2 | 67.1 | 68.3 | 57.9 | 59.1 | 61 | 63.1 | 65.2 | 67.1 | 68.3 |
| | Height (cm) | 147 | 150 | 154.9 | 160.3 | 165.7 | 170.5 | 173.4 | 147 | 150 | 154.9 | 160.3 | 165.7 | 170.5 | 173.4 |
| | 50th | 103 | 104 | 105 | 108 | 110 | 111 | 112 | 61 | 60 | 61 | 62 | 63 | 64 | 65 |
| | 90th | 115 | 116 | 118 | 121 | 124 | 126 | 126 | 74 | 74 | 74 | 75 | 76 | 77 | 77 |
| | 95th | 119 | 120 | 122 | 125 | 128 | 130 | 131 | 78 | 78 | 78 | 78 | 80 | 81 | 81 |
| | 95th + 12 mm Hg | 131 | 132 | 134 | 137 | 140 | 142 | 143 | 90 | 90 | 90 | 90 | 92 | 93 | 93 |
| 14 | Height (in) | 60.6 | 61.8 | 63.8 | 65.9 | 68.0 | 69.8 | 70.9 | 60.6 | 61.8 | 63.8 | 65.9 | 68.0 | 69.8 | 70.9 |
| | Height (cm) | 153.8 | 156.9 | 162 | 167.5 | 172.7 | 177.4 | 180.1 | 153.8 | 156.9 | 162 | 167.5 | 172.7 | 177.4 | 180.1 |
| | 50th | 105 | 106 | 109 | 111 | 112 | 113 | 113 | 60 | 60 | 62 | 64 | 65 | 66 | 67 |
| | 90th | 119 | 120 | 123 | 126 | 127 | 128 | 129 | 74 | 74 | 75 | 77 | 78 | 79 | 80 |
| | 95th | 123 | 125 | 127 | 130 | 132 | 133 | 134 | 77 | 78 | 79 | 81 | 82 | 83 | 84 |
| | 95th and 12 mm Hg | 135 | 137 | 139 | 142 | 144 | 145 | 146 | 89 | 90 | 91 | 93 | 94 | 95 | 96 |

*(Continued)*

**TABLE F-1  BP Levels for Boys by Age and Height Percentile (Continued)**

| Age (y) | BP percentile | SBP (mm Hg) Height percentile or measured height | | | | | | | DBP (mm Hg) Height percentile or measured height | | | | | | |
|---|---|---|---|---|---|---|---|---|---|---|---|---|---|---|---|
| | | 5% | 10% | 25% | 50% | 75% | 90% | 95% | 5% | 10% | 25% | 50% | 75% | 90% | 95% |
| 15 | Height (in) | 62.6 | 63.8 | 65.7 | 67.8 | 69.8 | 71.5 | 72.5 | 62.6 | 63.8 | 65.7 | 67.8 | 69.8 | 71.5 | 72.5 |
| | Height (cm) | 159 | 162 | 166.9 | 172.2 | 177.2 | 181.6 | 184.2 | 159 | 162 | 166.9 | 172.2 | 177.2 | 181.6 | 184.2 |
| | 50th | 108 | 110 | 112 | 113 | 114 | 114 | 114 | 61 | 62 | 64 | 65 | 66 | 67 | 68 |
| | 90th | 123 | 124 | 126 | 128 | 129 | 130 | 130 | 75 | 76 | 78 | 79 | 80 | 81 | 81 |
| | 95th | 127 | 129 | 131 | 132 | 134 | 135 | 135 | 78 | 79 | 81 | 83 | 84 | 85 | 85 |
| | 95th and 12 mm Hg | 139 | 141 | 143 | 144 | 146 | 147 | 147 | 90 | 91 | 93 | 95 | 96 | 97 | 97 |
| 16 | Height (in) | 63.8 | 64.9 | 66.8 | 68.8 | 70.7 | 72.4 | 73.4 | 63.8 | 64.9 | 66.8 | 68.8 | 70.7 | 72.4 | 73.4 |
| | Height (cm) | 162.1 | 165 | 169.6 | 174.6 | 179.5 | 183.8 | 186.4 | 162.1 | 165 | 169.6 | 174.6 | 179.5 | 183.8 | 186.4 |
| | 50th | 111 | 112 | 114 | 115 | 115 | 116 | 116 | 63 | 64 | 66 | 67 | 68 | 69 | 69 |
| | 90th | 126 | 127 | 128 | 129 | 131 | 131 | 132 | 77 | 78 | 79 | 80 | 81 | 82 | 82 |
| | 95th | 130 | 131 | 133 | 134 | 135 | 136 | 137 | 80 | 81 | 83 | 84 | 85 | 86 | 86 |
| | 95th and 12 mm Hg | 142 | 143 | 145 | 146 | 147 | 148 | 149 | 92 | 93 | 95 | 96 | 97 | 98 | 98 |
| 17 | Height (in) | 64.5 | 65.5 | 67.3 | 69.2 | 71.1 | 72.8 | 73.8 | 64.5 | 65.5 | 67.3 | 69.2 | 71.1 | 72.8 | 73.8 |
| | Height (cm) | 163.8 | 166.5 | 170.9 | 175.8 | 180.7 | 184.9 | 187.5 | 163.8 | 166.5 | 170.9 | 175.8 | 180.7 | 184.9 | 187.5 |
| | 50th | 114 | 115 | 116 | 117 | 117 | 118 | 118 | 65 | 66 | 67 | 68 | 69 | 70 | 70 |
| | 90th | 128 | 129 | 130 | 131 | 132 | 133 | 134 | 78 | 79 | 80 | 81 | 82 | 82 | 83 |
| | 95th | 132 | 133 | 134 | 135 | 137 | 138 | 138 | 81 | 82 | 84 | 85 | 86 | 86 | 87 |
| | 95th and 12 mm Hg | 144 | 145 | 146 | 147 | 149 | 150 | 150 | 93 | 94 | 95 | 97 | 98 | 98 | 99 |

Use percentile values to stage BP readings according to the scheme (elevated BP: ≥90th percentile; stage 1 HTN: ≥95th percentile; and stage 2 HTN: ≥95th percentile + 12 mm Hg). The 50th, 90th, and 95th percentiles were derived by using quantile regression on the basis of normal-weight children (BMI < 85th percentile).

**TABLE F-2** BP Levels for Girls by Age and Height Percentile

| Age (y) | BP percentile | SBP (mm Hg) Height percentile or measured height | | | | | | | DBP (mm Hg) Height percentile or measured height | | | | | | |
|---|---|---|---|---|---|---|---|---|---|---|---|---|---|---|---|
| | | 5% | 10% | 25% | 50% | 75% | 90% | 95% | 5% | 10% | 25% | 50% | 75% | 90% | 95% |
| 1 | Height (in) | 29.7 | 30.2 | 30.9 | 31.8 | 32.7 | 33.4 | 33.9 | 29.7 | 30.2 | 30.9 | 31.8 | 32.7 | 33.4 | 33.9 |
| | Height (cm) | 75.4 | 76.6 | 78.6 | 80.8 | 83 | 84.9 | 86.1 | 75.4 | 76.6 | 78.6 | 80.8 | 83 | 84.9 | 86.1 |
| | 50th | 84 | 85 | 86 | 86 | 87 | 88 | 88 | 41 | 42 | 42 | 43 | 44 | 45 | 46 |
| | 90th | 98 | 99 | 99 | 100 | 101 | 102 | 102 | 54 | 55 | 56 | 56 | 57 | 58 | 58 |
| | 95th | 101 | 102 | 102 | 103 | 104 | 105 | 105 | 59 | 59 | 60 | 60 | 61 | 62 | 62 |
| | 95th + 12 mm Hg | 113 | 114 | 114 | 115 | 116 | 117 | 117 | 71 | 71 | 72 | 72 | 73 | 74 | 74 |
| 2 | Height (in) | 33.4 | 34 | 34.9 | 35.9 | 36.9 | 37.8 | 38.4 | 33.4 | 34 | 34.9 | 35.9 | 36.9 | 37.8 | 38.4 |
| | Height (cm) | 84.9 | 86.3 | 88.6 | 91.1 | 93.7 | 96 | 97.4 | 84.9 | 86.3 | 88.6 | 91.1 | 93.7 | 96 | 97.4 |
| | 50th | 87 | 87 | 88 | 89 | 90 | 91 | 91 | 45 | 46 | 47 | 48 | 49 | 50 | 51 |
| | 90th | 101 | 101 | 102 | 103 | 104 | 105 | 106 | 58 | 58 | 59 | 60 | 61 | 62 | 62 |
| | 95th | 104 | 105 | 106 | 106 | 107 | 108 | 109 | 62 | 63 | 63 | 64 | 65 | 66 | 66 |
| | 95th + 12 mm Hg | 116 | 117 | 118 | 118 | 119 | 120 | 121 | 74 | 75 | 75 | 76 | 77 | 78 | 78 |
| 3 | Height (in) | 35.8 | 36.4 | 37.3 | 38.4 | 39.6 | 40.6 | 41.2 | 35.8 | 36.4 | 37.3 | 38.4 | 39.6 | 40.6 | 41.2 |
| | Height (cm) | 91 | 92.4 | 94.9 | 97.6 | 100.5 | 103.1 | 104.6 | 91 | 92.4 | 94.9 | 97.6 | 100.5 | 103.1 | 104.6 |
| | 50th | 88 | 89 | 89 | 90 | 91 | 92 | 93 | 48 | 48 | 49 | 50 | 51 | 53 | 53 |
| | 90th | 102 | 103 | 104 | 104 | 105 | 106 | 107 | 60 | 61 | 61 | 62 | 63 | 64 | 65 |
| | 95th | 106 | 106 | 107 | 108 | 109 | 110 | 110 | 64 | 65 | 65 | 66 | 67 | 68 | 69 |
| | 95th + 12 mm Hg | 118 | 118 | 119 | 120 | 121 | 122 | 122 | 76 | 77 | 77 | 78 | 79 | 80 | 81 |

(Continued)

**TABLE F-2** BP Levels for Girls by Age and Height Percentile *(Continued)*

| Age (y) | BP percentile | SBP (mm Hg) Height percentile or measured height | | | | | | | DBP (mm Hg) Height percentile or measured height | | | | | | |
|---|---|---|---|---|---|---|---|---|---|---|---|---|---|---|---|
| | | 5% | 10% | 25% | 50% | 75% | 90% | 95% | 5% | 10% | 25% | 50% | 75% | 90% | 95% |
| 4 | Height (in) | 38.3 | 38.9 | 39.9 | 41.1 | 42.4 | 43.5 | 44.2 | 38.3 | 38.9 | 39.9 | 41.1 | 42.4 | 43.5 | 44.2 |
| | Height (cm) | 97.2 | 98.8 | 101.4 | 104.5 | 107.6 | 110.5 | 112.2 | 97.2 | 98.8 | 101.4 | 104.5 | 107.6 | 110.5 | 112.2 |
| | 50th | 89 | 90 | 91 | 92 | 93 | 94 | 94 | 50 | 51 | 51 | 53 | 54 | 55 | 55 |
| | 90th | 103 | 104 | 105 | 106 | 107 | 108 | 108 | 62 | 63 | 64 | 65 | 66 | 67 | 67 |
| | 95th | 107 | 108 | 109 | 109 | 110 | 111 | 112 | 66 | 67 | 68 | 69 | 70 | 70 | 71 |
| | 95th + 12 mm Hg | 119 | 120 | 121 | 121 | 122 | 123 | 124 | 78 | 79 | 80 | 81 | 82 | 82 | 83 |
| 5 | Height (in) | 40.8 | 41.5 | 42.6 | 43.9 | 45.2 | 46.5 | 47.3 | 40.8 | 41.5 | 42.6 | 43.9 | 45.2 | 46.5 | 47.3 |
| | Height (cm) | 103.6 | 105.3 | 108.2 | 111.5 | 114.9 | 118.1 | 120 | 103.6 | 105.3 | 108.2 | 111.5 | 114.9 | 118.1 | 120 |
| | 50th | 90 | 91 | 92 | 93 | 94 | 95 | 96 | 52 | 52 | 53 | 55 | 56 | 57 | 57 |
| | 90th | 104 | 105 | 106 | 107 | 108 | 109 | 110 | 64 | 65 | 66 | 67 | 68 | 69 | 70 |
| | 95th | 108 | 109 | 109 | 110 | 111 | 112 | 113 | 68 | 69 | 70 | 71 | 72 | 73 | 73 |
| | 95th + 12 mm Hg | 120 | 121 | 121 | 122 | 123 | 124 | 125 | 80 | 81 | 82 | 83 | 84 | 85 | 85 |
| 6 | Height (in) | 43.3 | 44 | 45.2 | 46.6 | 48.1 | 49.4 | 50.3 | 43.3 | 44 | 45.2 | 46.6 | 48.1 | 49.4 | 50.3 |
| | Height (cm) | 110 | 111.8 | 114.9 | 118.4 | 122.1 | 125.6 | 127.7 | 110 | 111.8 | 114.9 | 118.4 | 122.1 | 125.6 | 127.7 |
| | 50th | 92 | 92 | 93 | 94 | 96 | 97 | 97 | 54 | 54 | 55 | 56 | 57 | 58 | 59 |
| | 90th | 105 | 106 | 107 | 108 | 109 | 110 | 111 | 67 | 67 | 68 | 69 | 70 | 71 | 71 |
| | 95th | 109 | 109 | 110 | 111 | 112 | 113 | 114 | 70 | 71 | 72 | 72 | 73 | 74 | 74 |
| | 95th + 12 mm Hg | 121 | 121 | 122 | 123 | 124 | 125 | 126 | 82 | 83 | 84 | 84 | 85 | 86 | 86 |

**Age 7**

| BP Percentile | SBP (mm Hg) by Height Percentile | | | | | | | DBP (mm Hg) by Height Percentile | | | | | | |
|---|---|---|---|---|---|---|---|---|---|---|---|---|---|---|
| Height (in) | 45.6 | 46.4 | 47.7 | 49.2 | 50.7 | 52.1 | 53 | 45.6 | 46.4 | 47.7 | 49.2 | 50.7 | 52.1 | 53 |
| Height (cm) | 115.9 | 117.8 | 121.1 | 124.9 | 128.8 | 132.5 | 134.7 | 115.9 | 117.8 | 121.1 | 124.9 | 128.8 | 132.5 | 134.7 |
| 50th | 92 | 93 | 94 | 95 | 97 | 98 | 99 | 55 | 55 | 56 | 57 | 58 | 59 | 60 |
| 90th | 106 | 106 | 107 | 109 | 110 | 111 | 112 | 68 | 68 | 69 | 70 | 71 | 72 | 72 |
| 95th | 109 | 110 | 111 | 112 | 113 | 114 | 115 | 72 | 72 | 73 | 73 | 74 | 74 | 75 |
| 95th + 12 mm Hg | 121 | 122 | 123 | 124 | 125 | 126 | 127 | 84 | 84 | 85 | 85 | 86 | 86 | 87 |

**Age 8**

| BP Percentile | SBP (mm Hg) by Height Percentile | | | | | | | DBP (mm Hg) by Height Percentile | | | | | | |
|---|---|---|---|---|---|---|---|---|---|---|---|---|---|---|
| Height (in) | 47.6 | 48.4 | 49.8 | 51.4 | 53 | 54.5 | 55.5 | 47.6 | 48.4 | 49.8 | 51.4 | 53 | 54.5 | 55.5 |
| Height (cm) | 121 | 123 | 126.5 | 130.6 | 134.7 | 138.5 | 140.9 | 121 | 123 | 126.5 | 130.6 | 134.7 | 138.5 | 140.9 |
| 50th | 93 | 94 | 95 | 97 | 98 | 99 | 100 | 56 | 56 | 57 | 59 | 60 | 61 | 61 |
| 90th | 107 | 107 | 108 | 110 | 111 | 112 | 113 | 69 | 70 | 71 | 72 | 72 | 73 | 73 |
| 95th | 110 | 111 | 112 | 113 | 115 | 116 | 117 | 72 | 73 | 74 | 74 | 75 | 75 | 75 |
| 95th + 12 mm Hg | 122 | 123 | 124 | 125 | 127 | 128 | 129 | 84 | 85 | 86 | 86 | 87 | 87 | 87 |

**Age 9**

| BP Percentile | SBP (mm Hg) by Height Percentile | | | | | | | DBP (mm Hg) by Height Percentile | | | | | | |
|---|---|---|---|---|---|---|---|---|---|---|---|---|---|---|
| Height (in) | 49.3 | 50.2 | 51.7 | 53.4 | 55.1 | 56.7 | 57.7 | 49.3 | 50.2 | 51.7 | 53.4 | 55.1 | 56.7 | 57.7 |
| Height (cm) | 125.3 | 127.6 | 131.3 | 135.6 | 140.1 | 144.1 | 146.6 | 125.3 | 127.6 | 131.3 | 135.6 | 140.1 | 144.1 | 146.6 |
| 50th | 95 | 95 | 97 | 98 | 99 | 100 | 101 | 57 | 58 | 59 | 60 | 60 | 61 | 61 |
| 90th | 108 | 108 | 109 | 111 | 112 | 113 | 114 | 71 | 71 | 72 | 73 | 73 | 73 | 73 |
| 95th | 112 | 112 | 113 | 114 | 116 | 117 | 118 | 74 | 74 | 75 | 75 | 75 | 75 | 75 |
| 95th + 12 mm Hg | 124 | 124 | 125 | 126 | 128 | 129 | 130 | 86 | 86 | 87 | 87 | 87 | 87 | 87 |

**Age 10**

| BP Percentile | SBP (mm Hg) by Height Percentile | | | | | | | DBP (mm Hg) by Height Percentile | | | | | | |
|---|---|---|---|---|---|---|---|---|---|---|---|---|---|---|
| Height (in) | 51.1 | 52 | 53.7 | 55.5 | 57.4 | 59.1 | 60.2 | 51.1 | 52 | 53.7 | 55.5 | 57.4 | 59.1 | 60.2 |
| Height (cm) | 129.7 | 132.2 | 136.3 | 141 | 145.8 | 150.2 | 152.8 | 129.7 | 132.2 | 136.3 | 141 | 145.8 | 150.2 | 152.8 |
| 50th | 96 | 97 | 98 | 99 | 101 | 102 | 103 | 58 | 59 | 59 | 60 | 61 | 61 | 62 |
| 90th | 109 | 110 | 111 | 112 | 113 | 115 | 116 | 72 | 73 | 73 | 73 | 73 | 73 | 73 |
| 95th | 113 | 114 | 114 | 116 | 117 | 119 | 120 | 75 | 75 | 76 | 76 | 76 | 76 | 76 |
| 95th + 12 mm Hg | 125 | 126 | 126 | 128 | 129 | 131 | 132 | 87 | 87 | 88 | 88 | 88 | 88 | 88 |

*(Continued)*

**TABLE F-2  BP Levels for Girls by Age and Height Percentile (Continued)**

| Age (y) | BP percentile | SBP (mm Hg) Height percentile or measured height | | | | | | | DBP (mm Hg) Height percentile or measured height | | | | | | |
|---|---|---|---|---|---|---|---|---|---|---|---|---|---|---|---|
| | | 5% | 10% | 25% | 50% | 75% | 90% | 95% | 5% | 10% | 25% | 50% | 75% | 90% | 95% |
| 11 | Height (in) | 53.4 | 54.5 | 56.2 | 58.2 | 60.2 | 61.9 | 63 | 53.4 | 54.5 | 56.2 | 58.2 | 60.2 | 61.9 | 63 |
| | Height (cm) | 135.6 | 138.3 | 142.8 | 147.8 | 152.8 | 157.3 | 160 | 135.6 | 138.3 | 142.8 | 147.8 | 152.8 | 157.3 | 160 |
| | 50th | 98 | 99 | 101 | 102 | 104 | 105 | 106 | 60 | 60 | 60 | 61 | 62 | 63 | 64 |
| | 90th | 111 | 112 | 113 | 114 | 116 | 118 | 120 | 74 | 74 | 74 | 74 | 74 | 75 | 75 |
| | 95th | 115 | 116 | 117 | 118 | 120 | 123 | 124 | 76 | 77 | 77 | 77 | 77 | 77 | 77 |
| | 95th + 12 mm Hg | 127 | 128 | 129 | 130 | 132 | 135 | 136 | 88 | 89 | 89 | 89 | 89 | 89 | 89 |
| 12 | Height (in) | 56.2 | 57.3 | 59 | 60.9 | 62.8 | 64.5 | 65.5 | 56.2 | 57.3 | 59 | 60.9 | 62.8 | 64.5 | 65.5 |
| | Height (cm) | 142.8 | 145.5 | 149.9 | 154.8 | 159.6 | 163.8 | 166.4 | 142.8 | 145.5 | 149.9 | 154.8 | 159.6 | 163.8 | 166.4 |
| | 50th | 102 | 102 | 104 | 105 | 107 | 108 | 108 | 61 | 61 | 61 | 62 | 64 | 65 | 65 |
| | 90th | 114 | 115 | 116 | 118 | 120 | 122 | 122 | 75 | 75 | 75 | 75 | 76 | 76 | 76 |
| | 95th | 118 | 119 | 120 | 122 | 124 | 125 | 126 | 78 | 78 | 78 | 78 | 79 | 79 | 79 |
| | 95th and 12 mm Hg | 130 | 131 | 132 | 134 | 136 | 137 | 138 | 90 | 90 | 90 | 90 | 91 | 91 | 91 |
| 13 | Height (in) | 58.3 | 59.3 | 60.9 | 62.7 | 64.5 | 66.1 | 67 | 58.3 | 59.3 | 60.9 | 62.7 | 64.5 | 66.1 | 67 |
| | Height (cm) | 148.1 | 150.6 | 154.7 | 159.2 | 163.7 | 167.8 | 170.2 | 148.1 | 150.6 | 154.7 | 159.2 | 163.7 | 167.8 | 170.2 |
| | 50th | 104 | 105 | 106 | 107 | 108 | 108 | 109 | 62 | 62 | 63 | 64 | 65 | 65 | 66 |
| | 90th | 116 | 117 | 119 | 121 | 122 | 123 | 123 | 75 | 75 | 75 | 76 | 76 | 76 | 76 |
| | 95th | 121 | 122 | 123 | 124 | 126 | 126 | 127 | 79 | 79 | 79 | 79 | 80 | 80 | 81 |
| | 95th + 12 mm Hg | 133 | 134 | 135 | 136 | 138 | 138 | 139 | 91 | 91 | 91 | 91 | 92 | 92 | 93 |
| 14 | Height (in) | 59.3 | 60.2 | 61.8 | 63.5 | 65.2 | 66.8 | 67.7 | 59.3 | 60.2 | 61.8 | 63.5 | 65.2 | 66.8 | 67.7 |
| | Height (cm) | 150.6 | 153 | 156.9 | 161.3 | 165.7 | 169.7 | 172.1 | 150.6 | 153 | 156.9 | 161.3 | 165.7 | 169.7 | 172.1 |

Blood Pressure Levels for Boys by Age and Height Percentile — Ages 15–17

| Age | BP Percentile / Height | | | | | | | |
|---|---|---|---|---|---|---|---|---|
| **15** | 50th | 105 | 106 | 107 | 108 | 109 | 109 | 109 |
| | 90th | 118 | 118 | 120 | 122 | 123 | 123 | 123 |
| | 95th | 123 | 123 | 124 | 125 | 126 | 127 | 127 |
| | 95th + 12 mm Hg | 135 | 135 | 136 | 137 | 138 | 139 | 139 |
| | Height (in) | 59.7 | 60.6 | 62.2 | 63.9 | 65.6 | 67.2 | 68.1 |
| | Height (cm) | 151.7 | 154 | 157.9 | 162.3 | 166.7 | 170.6 | 173 |
| | 50th | 63 | 63 | 64 | 65 | 66 | 66 | 66 |
| | 90th | 76 | 76 | 76 | 76 | 77 | 77 | 77 |
| | 95th | 80 | 80 | 80 | 80 | 81 | 81 | 82 |
| | 95th + 12 mm Hg | 92 | 92 | 92 | 92 | 93 | 93 | 94 |
| **16** | Height (in) | 59.9 | 60.8 | 62.4 | 64.1 | 65.8 | 67.3 | 68.3 |
| | Height (cm) | 152.1 | 154.5 | 158.4 | 162.8 | 167.1 | 171.1 | 173.4 |
| | 50th | 106 | 107 | 108 | 109 | 110 | 110 | 110 |
| | 90th | 119 | 120 | 122 | 123 | 124 | 124 | 124 |
| | 95th | 124 | 125 | 125 | 127 | 128 | 128 | 128 |
| | 95th + 12 mm Hg | 136 | 137 | 137 | 139 | 140 | 140 | 140 |
| | 50th | 64 | 64 | 65 | 66 | 66 | 67 | 67 |
| | 90th | 76 | 76 | 76 | 77 | 78 | 78 | 78 |
| | 95th | 80 | 80 | 80 | 81 | 82 | 82 | 82 |
| | 95th + 12 mm Hg | 92 | 92 | 92 | 93 | 94 | 94 | 94 |
| **17** | Height (in) | 60.0 | 60.9 | 62.5 | 64.2 | 65.9 | 67.4 | 68.4 |
| | Height (cm) | 152.4 | 154.7 | 158.7 | 163.0 | 167.4 | 171.3 | 173.7 |
| | 50th | 107 | 108 | 109 | 110 | 110 | 110 | 111 |
| | 90th | 120 | 121 | 123 | 124 | 124 | 125 | 125 |
| | 95th | 125 | 125 | 126 | 127 | 128 | 128 | 128 |
| | 95th + 12 mm Hg | 137 | 137 | 138 | 139 | 140 | 140 | 140 |
| | 50th | 64 | 65 | 65 | 66 | 66 | 67 | 67 |
| | 90th | 76 | 77 | 77 | 78 | 78 | 78 | 78 |
| | 95th | 80 | 80 | 81 | 81 | 82 | 82 | 82 |
| | 95th + 12 mm Hg | 92 | 92 | 93 | 93 | 94 | 94 | 94 |

Use percentile values to stage BP readings according to the scheme (elevated BP: ≥90th percentile; stage 1 HTN: ≥95th percentile; and stage 2 HTN: ≥95th percentile + 12 mm Hg). The 50th, 90th, and 95th percentiles were derived by using quantile regression on the basis of normal-weight children (BMI < 85th percentile).

## TABLE F-3 Updated Definitions of Blood Pressure Categories and Stages

**For children aged 1 to <13 years**

Normal BP: <90th percentile

Elevated BP: ≥90th percentile to <95th percentile or 120/80 mm Hg to <95th percentile (whichever is lower)

Stage 1 HTN: ≥95th percentile to <95th percentile + 12 mm Hg, or 130/80 to 139/89 mm Hg (whichever is lower)

Stage 2 HTN: ≥95th percentile + 12 mm Hg, or ≥140/90 mm Hg (whichever is lower)

**For children aged ≥13 years**

Normal BP: <120/<80 mm Hg

Elevated BP: 120/<80 to 129/<80 mm Hg

Stage 1 HTN: 130/80 to 139/89 mm Hg

Stage 2 HTN: ≥140/90 mm Hg

Reproduced with permission from Pediatrics, 140(3): e20171904, Copyright © 2017 by the AAP. [published correction appears in Pediatrics, 2017;140(6):e20173035].

# Appendix G
## Common Procedures
Akshaya J. Vachharajani

- Make yourself comfortable. This is the most important aspect of beginning a procedure.
- If *you* are uncomfortable, the procedure will take longer and is more likely to be unsuccessful.
- For all the procedures described below
  - Perform a time-out.
  - Wear a mask.
  - Wear a sterile gown and sterile gloves after scrubbing.
  - Prepare and drape the skin with povidone-iodine under aseptic precautions.

### UMBILICAL ARTERY CATHETERIZATION

#### Indications
- Monitoring of arterial blood gases and blood pressure
- Administering total parenteral nutrition (TPN) or hypertonic solutions

#### Complications
- Hemorrhage (from line displacement)
- Thrombosis
- Infection
- Ischemia/infarction of lower extremities, bowel, or kidney
- Arrhythmia
- Hypertension

#### Line Placement and Catheter Length
- With a high line, place the tip of the catheter above the diaphragm, between T6 and T9 (above the renal and mesenteric arteries). This approach is less prone to complications.
- Use the formula to determine catheter length (high line):

$$\text{Catheter length (cm)} = (3 \times \text{birth weight (kg)} + 9)$$

#### Procedure
- Determine the catheter length.
- Restrain infant. Using sterile technique, "prep" and drape umbilical cord and adjacent skin.
- Flush catheter with sterile saline (after attaching a three-way stopcock) before insertion to avoid air embolism.
- Place sterile umbilical tape around the base of the cord. Cut through cord horizontally about 1.5-2.0 cm above the skin. Tighten umbilical tape to stop bleeding.
- Identify the one large, thin-walled vein and the two smaller, thicker-walled arteries. Use curved-tip forceps to gently open and dilate one of the arteries.

- Grasp catheter approximately 1 cm from the tip with toothless forceps and insert catheter into artery to the desired length. Feed catheter into artery using gentle pressure.
  - Do not force the catheter.
  - Forcing the catheter may create a false luminal tract.
- Secure catheter with a suture through the cord and around the catheter.
- Confirm catheter position with a radiograph. The catheter may be pulled back but not advanced once the sterile field is broken.

## UMBILICAL VEIN CATHETERIZATION

### Indications
- Administering crystalloids or colloids in the labor and delivery room to resuscitate neonates in shock
- Rapidly administering medications
- Administering hypertonic fluids or TPN

### Complications
- Hemorrhage from line displacement or vessel perforation
- Infection
- Air embolism
- Arrhythmia
- Portal vein thrombosis and portal hypertension (delayed complication)
- Pleural and pericardial effusion and pericardial tamponade

### Line Placement and Catheter Length
- Place the catheter in the inferior vena cava above the level of the ductus venosus and the hepatic veins and below the level of the left atrium. Practically, this means at the level of the right dome of the diaphragm.
- Use the formula to determine catheter length:

  Catheter length (cm) $= [0.5 \times$ length of the umbilical artery catheter (cm)$] + 1$

### Procedure
- Follow procedure steps for umbilical artery catheter placement up to identifying the artery. In this case, identify the thin-walled vein and insert the catheter.
  - Gently advance catheter to desired distance.
  - Do not force the catheter because this may cause a false luminal tract.
- Secure catheter as in umbilical artery catheter placement.
- Confirm catheter placement with a radiograph.
- In the delivery room, where speed of placing the umbilical line is essential, insert the catheter to 5 cm in a term infant (or until you can first draw back blood easily); this is sufficient.

## LUMBAR PUNCTURE

### Indications
- Diagnosing meningitis (suspected sepsis in neonates, apnea and bradycardia, evaluation of neonates or children with positive blood cultures)
- Relieving increased intracranial pressure (ICP) in neonates with hydrocephalus (serial lumbar punctures)

## Contraindications

- Increased ICP
  - If signs or symptoms of increased ICP are present (papilledema, retinal hemorrhage, trauma with associated head injury), perform computed tomography (CT) before lumbar puncture. In neonates, increased ICP is not a major contraindication as the fontanelle is open and the risk of cerebellar herniation is low. CT scan is rarely performed in neonates.
  - Lumbar puncture should not be performed in very sick neonates who do not tolerate the required positioning.
- Bleeding diathesis
  - Platelet count >50,000/µL is preferable.
  - Correction of clotting factor deficiencies before lumbar puncture prevents spinal cord hemorrhage and potential paralysis.
- Overlying skin infections, which may inoculate the cerebrospinal fluid (CSF)

## Complications

- Dry tap or traumatic tap (most common complication).
- Headache.
- Acquired epidermal spinal cord tumor caused by implantation of epidermal material into spinal canal if no stylet used on skin entry.
- Local back pain.
- Infection.
- Bleeding.
- Herniations associated with increased ICP. Cerebellar tonsillar herniation is not a dreaded complication in neonates who have an open anterior fontanelle.

## Procedure

- Position the child either in the sitting position or in the lateral recumbent position with the hips, knees, and neck flexed. Monitor cardiorespiratory status for compromise.
- Locate either the L3-L4 or L4-L5 interspace by drawing an imaginary line between the two iliac crests.
- Clean the skin with povidone-iodine, and drape the child in sterile fashion.
- Use a 20- to 22-gauge spinal needle of desired length.
- Anesthetize the overlying skin and subcutaneous tissue with 1% buffered lidocaine.
- Puncture midline just caudal to palpated spinous process, angling the needle slightly cephalad and toward the umbilicus. Advance the needle slowly; withdraw the stylet every few millimeters to check for CSF flow.
- If resistance is met (i.e., you hit bone), withdraw the needle to the skin and redirect the angle of the needle.
- Send CSF for appropriate studies (tube 1 for culture and Gram stain, tube 2 for glucose and protein, tube 3 for cell count and differential, and tube 4 for saved CSF or any additional specialized studies). The tube with the clearest CSF should be sent for cell count regardless of its number.
- To measure CSF pressure, patient must be lying straight (not curled up) on his or her side. Once free flow of CSF is established, attach the manometer and measure CSF pressure.

## CHEST TUBE PLACEMENT AND THORACENTESIS

### Indications
Tension pneumothorax and pleural effusion

### Complications
- Pneumothorax or hemothorax
- Bleeding or infection
- Pulmonary contusion or laceration
- Puncture of the diaphragm, liver, or spleen

### Procedure
*Needle Decompression*
- For tension pneumothorax, decompress by inserting a 23-gauge butterfly or 22-gauge angiocatheter at the second intercostal space in the midclavicular line, taking aseptic precautions.
- Insert the needle or the angiocatheter attached to a three-way stopcock open to the syringe, and aspirate as the needle is advanced. Stop advancing the needle as soon as air is aspirated in the syringe. Stop aspirating after the syringe is full of air, and turn the stopcock off and empty the syringe.
- Turn the stopcock in line with the syringe and start aspirating again. Repeat until no air is aspirated.

*Chest Tube Placement*
- Position child supine or with affected side up.
- Identify the entry point, which is the third to fifth intercostal space in the mid to anterior axillary line, usually at the level of the nipple. (Be careful to avoid breast tissue.)
- Locally anesthetize skin, subcutaneous tissue, chest wall muscles, and parietal pleura with lidocaine.
- Make an incision at the desired insertion point, and bluntly dissect through tissue layers until the superior portion of the rib is reached. (This avoids the neurovascular bundle on the inferior portion of each rib.)
- Push a hemostat over the top of the rib, through the pleura, and into the pleural space. Enter the pleural space cautiously. Spread hemostat to open, place chest tube in clamp, and guide into entry point.
- Insert the tube.
  - For a pneumothorax, insert the tube anteriorly toward the apex of the opposite lung.
  - For a pleural effusion, direct the tube inferiorly and posteriorly.
- Secure the tube with purse-string sutures.
- Attach the tube to the drainage system with −20 to −30 cm of water pressure.
- Apply a sterile occlusive dressing.
- Confirm position with a chest radiograph. A lateral chest radiograph is needed to confirm that the tip of the chest tube is in the anterior mediastinum especially if evacuating a pneumothorax.

*Thoracentesis*
- Confirm fluid in pleural space with clinical examination, chest radiography, or sonography. Confirm that the volume of the fluid is large enough to be drained.
- Place child in sitting position leaning over a table if possible. Otherwise, place child supine.
- Identify the point of entry in the seventh intercostal space and posterior axillary line.
- "Prep" and drape area under aseptic precautions.
- Anesthetize skin, subcutaneous tissue, chest wall muscles, and pleura with lidocaine.
- Advance an 18- to 22-gauge intravenous catheter or large-bore needle attached to a syringe and a stopcock and then "walk" the needle over the top of the rib into the pleural space while providing steady negative pressure.
- Aspirate fluid.
- After removing the needle or catheter, place an occlusive dressing and obtain a chest radiograph to rule out iatrogenic pneumothorax.

## SUTURING

### General Information
- Lacerations to be sutured should be <6 hours old (12 hours on the face).
- Usually, bite wounds should not be sutured.
- The longer sutures are left in place, the greater the potential for scarring and infection.
- Plastic surgery should be considered with any laceration involving the face, lips, hands, genitalia, mouth, or orbital area, including deep lacerations with nerve damage; stellate lacerations; flap lacerations; lacerations involving the vermilion border; lacerations with questionable tissue viability; and large, complex lacerations.

### Procedure
- Remove foreign bodies.
- Examine area for exposed nerves, tendons, and bone.
- Perform a neurovascular examination.
- Remember to ask about tetanus status and immunize if needed.
- Irrigate wound with copious amounts of sterile saline to clean area. (This is the most important step to prevent infection.)
- Apply anesthetic.
  - Injectable
    - No end-artery supply: 1% lidocaine with 1% epinephrine; maximum dose is 7 mg/kg.
    - End-artery supply: 1% lidocaine without epinephrine; maximum dose is 3-5 mg/kg.
  - Topical: lidocaine, epinephrine, tetracaine (LET), lidocaine (ELA-Max)
- Débride any necessary areas.
- Begin suturing (Table G-1).
- Apply antibiotic ointment and sterile dressing.

| TABLE G-1 | Suture Requirements for Lacerations by Location | |
|---|---|---|
| Location | Suture (monofilament) | Removal (days) |
| Face | 6-0 | 3-5 |
| Scalp | 4-0 or 5-0, consider staples | 5-7 |
| Eyelid | 6-0 or 7-0 | 3-5 |
| Eyebrow | 5-0 or 6-0 | 3-5 |
| Trunk | 4-0 or 5-0 | 5-7 |
| Extremities | 4-0 or 5-0 | 7 |
| Joint surface | 4-0 | 10-14 |
| Hand | 5-0 | 7 |
| Sole of foot | 3-0 or 4-0 | 7-10 |

## APPLICATION OF SKIN ADHESIVES

- Appropriate uses: low-tension areas
- Inappropriate uses: high-tension areas, contaminated wounds, wounds across mucocutaneous junctions, animal or human bites, or wounds with evidence of infection

### Procedure
- Clean and dry area.
- Achieve hemostasis.
- Approximate wound edges.
- Squeeze adhesive onto wound edges and then apply in a circular motion around wound.
- Apply at least three layers, allowing each layer to dry between applications.

### Postapplication
- Do not apply dressing. None is needed, and adhesive falls off in 5-10 days.
- Avoid topical ointments.
- Do not scrub or submerse area.

## SUGGESTED READINGS

Dieckman R, Fisher D, Selbst S. Pediatric Emergency and Critical Care Procedures. St. Louis, MO: Mosby-Year Book, 1997.
The Cochrane Database of Systematic Reviews. 2005: Issue 4. http://www.cochrane.org/reviews

# Index

*Note*: Page numbers followed by *f* refer to figures; page numbers followed by *t* refer to tables.